Mary York

Nursing: From Concept to Practice

JANET-BETH McCANN FLYNN, R.N., M.S.N.
Doctoral Student, School of Education
The Catholic University of America
Lecturer, George Mason University
Formerly:
Assistant Professor of Nursing, George Mason University

PHYLLIS BURROUGHS HEFFRON, R.N., M.S.N.
Professional Nurse/Education Specialist
Office of Academic Affairs
Veteran's Administration
Washington, D.C.
Formerly:
Assistant Professor, The Catholic University School of Nursing
Lecturer, The University of Maryland School of Nursing

Brady Communications Company, Inc. • Bowie Maryland 20715
A Prentice-Hall Publishing Company

Nursing: From Concept to Practice

Publishing Director: David A. Culverwell
Acquisitions Editor: Richard A. Weimer
Production Editor/Text Design: Lisa G. Kolman
Manufacturing Director: John A. Komsa
Art Director/Cover Design: Don Sellers, AMI
Assistant Art Director: Bernard Vervin
Photography: George Dodson

Copy Editor: Elyse Finger
Indexer: William O. Lively
Typesetter: Carver Photocomposition, Arlington, VA
Printer: R. R. Donnelley & Sons, Harrisonburg, VA
Typefaces: Aster Roman (text) & Memphis Bold (display)

Library of Congress Cataloging in Publication Data

Flynn, Janet-Beth, 1944–
    Nursing, from concept to practice.

    Bibliography: p.
    Includes index.
    1. Nursing. I. Heffron, Phyllis, 1941–
II. Title. [DNLM: 1. Nursing Process. WY 100 F648n]
RT41.F55 1983   610.73   83-15918
ISBN 0-89303-719-2

ISBN 0-89303-719-2

Prentice-Hall International, Inc., London
Prentice-Hall Canada, Inc., Scarborough, Ontario
Prentice-Hall of Australia, Pty., Ltd., Sydney
Prentice-Hall of India Private Limited, New Delhi
Prentice-Hall of Japan, Inc., Tokyo
Prentice-Hall of Southeast Asia Pte. Ltd., Singapore
Whitehall Books, Limited, Petone, New Zealand
Editora Prentice-Hall Do Brasil LTDA., Rio de Janeiro

Printed in the United States of America

84 85 86 87 88 89 90 91 92 93 94   10 9 8 7 6 5 4 3 2

CONTENTS

PREFACE

This book is designed as an introduction to selected concepts that have built the foundation for professional nursing. This foundation encompasses various philosophies, theories, concepts, and frameworks that give nurses the ability to provide quality nursing care. Once acquired and understood, this type of knowledge enables nurses to analyze situations, draw conclusions, make decisions, and solve problems.

The concepts chosen for this text represent those topics that are fundamental to professional nursing practice. The principal goal in planning for and writing this book has been to consolidate these concepts in one text, and present them theoretically using a systems theory and adaptation approach as they relate to the nursing process.

The book is divided into four major sections as follows:

Part I   Professional Aspects of Nursing & Health Care
Part II   Concepts of Communication
Part III Concepts Related to the Care of Individuals
Part IV Social Systems, The Environment, and Nursing

Part One has been designed to give the reader a thorough understanding of the nursing profession today as it relates to theory, the health care system, and current professional issues. The Nursing Process is presented as the basic working framework within which nursing knowledge is applied. Part Two begins to narrow the focus slightly and presents subjects fundamentally important to establishing the nurse/patient relationship and accomplishing nursing goals and objectives. Part Three focuses on the care of individuals and includes concepts that can be used in a large variety of clinical settings. Topics for this section were chosen primarily on the basis of their applicability across a wide range of patient situations, conditions, and age. Concepts related to specific pathologies or specialized levels of care are not included. Suicide is presented (within the Crisis chapter) because of its significance as a national problem and for its potential development in adolescents, the elderly, and in adverse health conditions. The last section contains four global concepts; family, groups, community, and the environment. These concepts are presented as integral components of holistic nursing and health care.

Distributive and episodic health care are discussed in Chapter 3 within the traditional model, i.e., outpatient setting versus inpatient setting. However, an effort has been made to present each concept in such a way that it can be applied in either setting. Throughout the book, the authors have sought to reflect nursing's present day professional achievements and accompanying changes in roles and responsibilities.

The terms client and patient are used interchangeably throughout the text. The frequent use of the feminine pronoun when referring to the nurse and masculine pronoun when referring to the client is not intended to imply sex role stereotypes; rather it is meant to enhance clarity of reading. All of the chapters contain behavioral objectives, content outlines, glossaries, study questions, and annotated bibliographies. Additionally some chapters contain assessment tools to enhance clinical practice. Most of the chapters in parts 2, 3, and 4 are further divided into two sections: a comprehensive, definitive overview of the concept, and a nursing process approach for applying the concept to practice. The traditional four step nursing process structure (assessment, planning, implementation, and evaluation) is used consistently and examples of nursing diagnoses are presented where appropriate.

While not identified in a step-by-step procedural format, technical skills are identified throughout the chapters within the framework of the nursing process sections. Likewise, growth and development is not addressed as a separate entity but discussed as a part of selected chapters.

We gratefully acknowledge the help of those who have encouraged and supported us: our nursing colleagues and former teachers; our contributing authors for their excellent work and continued faith in us; and our families, in particular, who have given us strength and perseverance through their love and confidence in us. We also would like to acknowledge the staff at Robert J. Brady Company, particularly Lisa Kolman, Edie Plunkett, and Rick Weimer. Their willingness to involve us in all aspects of the publishing process has been gratifying and we value the knowledge we have gained from it.

We appreciate and acknowledge Patricia Grim and Vickie Reed for their conscientious efforts in typing much of the manuscript.

Writing this book has given us a greater appreciation for the contributions of nursing leaders and renewed our spirits for the future of nursing.

CONTRIBUTING AUTHORS

Rose K. Cringle R.N., Ph.D.
Research Associate
Maryland Psychiatric Research Center
Catonsville, Maryland

Sister Rosemary Donley, Ph.D., R.N., F.A.A.N.
Dean of Nursing
The Catholic University of America
Washington, D.C.

Joann M. Eland, M.A., Ph.D., R.N.
Assistant Professor
The University of Iowa College of Nursing
Iowa City, Iowa

Janet-Beth McCann Flynn, R.N., M.S.N.
Doctoral Student, School of Education
The Catholic University of America
Lecturer, George Mason University
    Formerly:
    Assistant Professor of Nursing, Catholic
    University of America

Helen V. Foerst, R.N., B.S., M.A.
Deputy Chief Nurse
Office of the Assistant Secretary for Health
United States Public Health Service

Edna M. Fordyce, R.N., M.N., Ed.D.
Associate Professor
Department of Nursing
Towson State University
Towson, Maryland

Phyllis Burroughs Heffron, R.N., M.S.N.
Professional Nurse/Education Specialist
Office of Academic Affairs
Veteran's Administration
Washington, D.C.

Formerly:
Assistant Professor, The Catholic University School of Nursing
Lecturer, The University of Maryland School of Nursing

Marion R. Johnson, R.N., M.S.N.
Assistant Professor
College of Nursing
University of Iowa
Iowa City, Iowa

Carol N. Knowlton, R.N., M.S.N.
Assistant Dean
School of Nursing
The Catholic University of America
Washington, D.C.

Sally Laliberté, R.N., M.S.N., C.N.M.
Private Practice In Midwifery
Greenbelt, Maryland

Elizabeth A. McFarlane, R.N., D.N.Sc.
Assistant Professor
The Catholic University of America
Washington, D.C.

Nancy S. McKelvey, R.N., M.S.N.
Director of Educational Programs
American Society for Psychoprophylaxis
    in Obstetrics/Lamaze
Arlington, Virginia

Cynthia E. Northrop, R.N., M.S., J.D.
Attorney at Law
Laurel, Maryland

Nancie H. Pardue, R.N., M.S.N., C.C.R.N.
Doctoral Candidate, Nursing

The Catholic University of America
Washington, D.C.

Marie Lawrence Rawlings, R.N., M.S.N.
Certified Clinical Specialist in Psychiatric/
  Mental Health Nursing
Washington Veterans Administration Medical Center
Washington, D.C.

Joan M. Roche, M.S.N., Ph.D.
Associate Professor of Nursing
Marymount College of Virginia
Arlington, Virginia

M. Gaie Rubenfeld, R.N., M.S.
Assistant Professor
School of Nursing
The Catholic University of America
Washington, D.C.

Mary Ann Schroeder, R.N., D.N.Sc.
Assistant Professor
Community Health Nursing
The Catholic University of America
Washington, D.C.

Linda Manglass Shapiro, R.N., M.S.N., C.S.
Nurse Therapist
Crisis Center, Psychiatric Institute
Washington, D.C.
Assistant Clinical Professor
Georgetown University
Washington, D.C.

Mary B. Walsh, R.N., M.S.N.
Associate Professor
The Catholic University of America
School of Nursing
Washington, D.C.

Eliza M. Wolff, R.N., Dr. P.H.
Office of Geriatrics and Extended Care
Veterans Administration
810 Vermont Avenue, N.W.
Washington, D.C.

Helen Yura, R.N., Ph.D., F.A.A.N.
Professor and Graduate Program Director
Department of Nursing
Old Dominion University
Norfolk, Virginia

Section 1

Professional Aspects of Nursing & Health Care

The practice of nursing has evolved through the ages along with cultures, societies, and countries. American nursing has undergone profound changes during this process, particularly in recent times, as influences such as science and technology have advanced our way of life and given rise to changing health care needs and delivery.

This section focuses on the state of the art in professional nursing today. It provides a historical perspective of early American nursing leaders and significant events that have been instrumental in the long process of attaining professional status. Nursing education is addressed from a historical perspective as well, and describes present day educational programs and their diversities. Nursing roles, set-tings for practice, legal aspects, and accountability are all addressed in terms of their evolution towards a professional status in today's society.

The importance of theory building in nursing and the need for nurses to understand current theories and concepts is addressed in Chapter One. Systems theory and the concepts of adaptation provide examples of theories applicable to nursing as well as give a comprehensive knowledge base of these theories. Specific nursing theories are presented in Chapter Nine and the significance of theory building in nursing is re-emphasized.

Professional nursing is currently practiced within a logical step-by-step framework called the Nursing Process. Within this framework the nurse applies her knowledge about theories and concepts and, in combination with her knowledge about the patient, uses learned skills to help individuals with nursing and health care needs. The expert presentation of the Nursing Process in this section is highlighted by the introduction of human needs theory and provides a clear illustration of the relationship of theory to nursing practice. Health assessment and the health care system are addressed separately and serve to complete the picture of the nurse and the professional nursing system as it exists today.

1

Theory, Concept, and Process

Janet-Beth McCann Flynn
Phyllis B. Heffron

CHAPTER OUTLINE

OBJECTIVES

At the completion of this chapter the reader will be able to:

- Define the terms theory, concept, and process.
- Compare and contrast the terms theory, concept, and process.

GLOSSARY

Concept—General, intangible, and symbolic ways of referring to reality.

Philosophy—A set of beliefs that are acquired and interpreted throughout a lifetime of experiences with reality.

Process—The act of continuously moving along in order to meet a predetermined goal or set of goals.

Theory—Systematically related set of statements or concepts that describe, explain, and predict the real world.

INTRODUCTION

Man's quest for knowledge is a never ending process, but the acquisition of facts alone is not enough to facilitate adaptation. Facts need a unifying theme to pull them together into a larger system of viewing life and giving them meaning. This is why we have large bodies of knowledge such as philosophies, theories, and concepts.

Philosophies, theories, and concepts organize facts into a structured framework for viewing reality. Once these have been organized and defined, a mechanism must be defined to put the organized frameworks into action. This action phase is called **process.**

Nurses need to understand philosophies, theories, concepts, and processes because nursing is a discipline based on using and integrating bodies of knowledge in order to assess what is needed or, to deliver health care.

This chapter describes the terms philosophy, theory, concept, and process.

PHILOSOPHY

A philosopher is one who loves wisdom. **Philosophy** is the study of wisdom, of fundamental knowledge, and of the process by which we construct our outlook on life. It is also the study of how people acquire beliefs.[1] The basic beliefs and values that give meaning to our experiences come from a lifetime of learning through interpersonal contact, religion, education, and the environment.

As nurse authors Yura and Walsh observe, these beliefs and values determine the manner by which persons relate to each other, the way they work with each other and—to bring the point home—the way nurses care for clients.[2] A person's philosophy, whether or not that person is able to recognize and articulate it as such, is a

set of beliefs and values that direct behavior and attitude. It can be thought of as a multifaceted lens through which we observe, comprehend, and evaluate the seemingly random events that go on around us—a lens through which we see things as good, evil, healthful, sick, socially or professionally appropriate, irresponsible, and so forth.

Individuals use their philosophy of life to orient themselves to the world around them. Nurses, as they work with clients, families, and groups, come into contact with some of the most profound issues that affect human life—suicide, child abuse, abortion, and euthanasia, to name a few. Studying philosophy helps individuals to reflect on personal belief systems and provides a framework for examining one's own value system. "An awareness and understanding of one's own philosophy and values and a deliberate expression of one's own beliefs about man are fundamental to the performance of quality nursing."[3]

THEORY

Riehl and Roy define a theory as a "scientifically acceptable general principle which governs practice or is proposed to explain observed facts."[4] Yura and Walsh write that a "theory is a systematically related set of statements that describes, explains, and predicts parts of the empirical or real world."[5]

From a philosophical viewpoint, a theory is a proposed structuring of reality, not reality itself, and is used to guide, explain, and predict reality.[6,7] Theories can be verbalized and communicated to others. They are structures for passing on knowledge. Examples of well-known theories include Albert Einstein's Theory of Relativity, Issac Newton's Theory of Gravitation, and Sigmund Freud's Psychoanalytic Theory.

Generally speaking, a theory is a "set of beliefs for which there is some, but not completely supporting, evidence."[8] It is a set of untested ideas that results from speculations about reality.[9] Theories are testable and therefore refutable and alterable.[10] Theory guides research through the generation of expected or predicted outcomes (hypothesis) of interventions. A theory is therefore supported or not supported by the empirical data that is obtained through the research it generates. When theories are proved, they become laws. Physical scientific theories are easier to prove than human based theories. Disciplines, such as chemistry and physics, have more laws than social sciences, such as sociology, psychology, and nursing.

Theories have many purposes. They provide a systematic way of viewing reality. They guide research and provide a framework for evaluation. In addition to guiding practice and identifying research problems, theory provides a basis for evaluating and selecting proposed innovative methods or practices.[11]

The nursing profession needs theories to organize and integrate what is known about man, health, illness, and nursing. These theories can provide a structured systematic way of examining and directing nursing practice. Theories are the primary force in elevating nursing from a skill oriented job into a bona fide profession. Over the past 20 years, many nursing theorists (see Chapter 9) have struggled to define the nature of nursing and identify its professional purpose through the development of theoretical frameworks.

According to Ellis, the purposes of developing theories of nursing are to facilitate the differentiation between fact and pseudofact and to structure the conveying of facts from other professions.[12] Nursing theory provides the framework to integrate knowledge from the biological and psychological aspects of man.

Ellis provides another reason for nurses to be concerned with theory and theory development. She writes that theory di-

rects practice, and through practice, observations can be made that provide the opportunity for theory evaluation.[13]

Theories generally are arrived at by two major processes.* One process is that of **deductive reasoning.** Deductive reasoning is the method of looking initially at the general or universal idea, and then moving to the specific or particular. In **inductive reasoning,** the other major process, the direction is reversed. First, the specific or particular action is identified, and then conclusions are drawn about general or universal ideas.

For example, it is observed that people who smoke cigarettes have a higher incidence of lung cancer than those who do not smoke. Is this deductive or inductive reasoning? In what direction does the flow of information take place? Does the process move from the general to the specific or vice versa? In the case of smoking, the process is from the particular (people who smoke) to the general (lung cancer). Therefore, this example demonstrates the inductive method. An example of the deductive method would be to consider that resistance to infection is best in healthy people. Therefore, it can be deduced that people who are chronically ill with a kidney disease probably would be more likely to catch colds than people who are generally healthy.

Some nursing theorists use the deductive method and others use the inductive method. According to Dickoff and James, the determination of what kind of nursing theory is needed for professional practice is dependent upon professional purpose.[14] They write that a professional person, as opposed to a technician, is one who shapes reality rather than one who experiences reality. Nursing theory must therefore be

---

*Major portion of discussion on reasoning from unpublished manuscript by Dr. MaryAnn Schroeder.

based upon an action orientation and have a purpose.[15]

Dickoff and James suggest that theories evolve through a series of stages or levels, and during development, each higher level presupposes the existence of theories at a lower level.[16] The first level of theory development is the factor isolating stage, in which relevant facets or concepts of the theories are identified and named. The second level of theory development is observing and noting the relationship between the concepts that were named in stage one. In the third level, concepts are related to each other in such a way that predictions about outcomes can be made. Finally, after the predictive theory is defined, the highest level of theory development is reached. This is called the situation producing theory, and its purpose is to produce situations in which predicted outcomes are obtained.

According to Riehl and Roy, nursing has not "yet reached the point of clear development on all four levels of theory," but nurses are able to use the elements of situation producing theory to provide the elements for nursing practice.[17]

Theories rarely occur in isolation, but rather, usually reflect the time and culture in which they are conceived. In other words, theories are the products of the milieu in which they happen. Two concepts that express these environmental or evolutional aspects of the climate in which theories arise are the German words **Zeitgeist** and **Weltanschauung**.* Zeitgeist means the general moral and intellectual state of a culture. It denotes the trends of taste characteristic of a given era. Zeitgeist is the spirit of the times—the fashion. Weltanschauung is the prevailing philosophy of life, a type of world view or manner of looking at the universe. For example, theories generated in an era of unrest and upheaval, such as in wartime, might reflect

concepts regarding anxiety and attempts by individuals to make themselves more comfortable. Theories may support the philosophy of the time or refute it. But it is the rare theory that appears indifferent to the intellectual or philosophical climate of the era.

CONCEPTS

Concepts are the building blocks of theories. They are general thoughts or ideas that are intangible and can be thought of as a symbolic or abstract way of referring to reality.[18,19] Concepts are words that describe objects, properties, events, and relationships among them.[20]

Concepts indicate the subject matter of theory and are defined by the specific theory.[21] Conceptual meanings are understood only within the framework of the theory of which they are a part.[22] Examples of concepts from nursing theories include self care, adaptation, interaction, and interdependence. Each theory must define its own concepts, as these vary from theory to theory.

Concepts develop as a part of a theory and are refined as the knowledge base of the theory expands. Refinement of concepts is an ongoing process that, according to Hardy, involves not only sharpening of theoretical and operational definitions, but also modifying existing theory. Concepts are refined by relating the theoretical world to the real world, by organizing many concrete items into a smaller number of classes, and by relating diverse concepts within a more general system of concepts.[23]

Concepts are necessary in nursing in order to relate theory to practice. Horgan, in 1967, researched selected nursing periodicals from 1950–1965 and found that, between 1960–1965, 18 concepts appeared.[24] Horgan defined a concept of nursing as an expression of ideas that summarize the theorists view of elements and

---

*This discussion from unpublished manuscript by Dr. MaryAnn Schroeder.

components of nursing and the nursing process. As time passes and nurses become more sophisticated, more concepts will be defined. Since this particular study was completed, the literature has been rich with concepts and theories. Many of the major nursing theories have been formalized during this time as well. If nursing is to continue to develop as a health care profession, identification of concepts and research to support them is essential.

PROCESS

Process is the action phase of a conceptual framework or theory. It is the act of moving forward to meet a goal. The very term "process" indicates continuous movement through a succession of stages until the goal or the outcome has been accomplished. According to Bevis, process is also a change that uses feedback as one proceeds toward the objective.[25] The feedback into the process is due to the data being collected from the environment. How this data analysis is carried out relates to the theoretical or conceptual framework and its definition.

Yura and Walsh write that the perception of a process as an action suggests a power behind the action or someone who strives to complete the action.[26] Therefore there is control over the action and a systematic movement toward completion. Conscious attention and effort must be exerted in order to complete the process and meet the predetermined goal. The action of moving, or the process, must be based on a needs assessment. Without a goal to direct the process, it would become disorganized and perhaps useless.[27]

Since nursing is action directed and goal oriented, it has a process, a systematic way of providing assistance to patients. It is based upon assessment of patients' needs, making plans with the patients to meet these needs, carrying out the plan, and evaluating its success. Without this systematic process, nursing would lack clarity and be potentially ineffective.

SUMMARY

Man needs a structure to be able to organize the hundreds of thousands of facts accumulated during life. Philosophies, theories, and concepts serve this purpose. They are frameworks for viewing and making sense of reality.

Nurses need philosophies, theories, and concepts because nursing is a field of diverse facts that need to be related to specific nursing actions. Through theory development, nursing is advancing professionally. Through application, theory becomes reality.

Process is the action phase of a conceptual framework or theory. The nursing process is the action phase in applying nursing concepts in practice. It is an organized framework for systematic problem solving and is goal directed. Without a systematic and comprehensive theory, process cannot be effective.

STUDY QUESTIONS

1. What is a theory?

2. How do concepts relate to theory?

3. What is process?

4. Why do nurses need theories and concepts?

REFERENCES

1. Van Cleve Morris and Young Pai, **Philosophy and the American School.** 2nd Ed. (Boston: Houghton Mifflin Company, 1976) p. 4.

2. Helen Yura and Mary Walsh, **The Nursing Process.** 3rd Ed. (New York: Appleton-Century-Crofts, 1978) p. 16.

3. **Ibid.**

4. Joan P. Riehl and Sr. Callista Roy, **Conceptual Models for Nursing Practice.** (New York: Appleton-Century-Crofts, 1974) p. 3.

5. Yura and Walsh, **Nursing Process.** p. 16.

6. J. Dickoff and P. James, "A Theory of Theories: A Postition Paper." **Nursing Research**, 17 (1968) pp. 197–203.

7. Riehl and Roy, **Conceptual Models.** 1974. p. 3.

8. Morris and Pai, **Philosophy.** p. 4.

9. Dorothea E. Orem (Ed.), **Concept Formulation in Nursing: Process and Product.** (Boston: Little, Brown, and Co., 1979) p. 55.

10. Margaret Newman, **Theory Development in Nursing.** (Philadelphia: F.A. Davis Co., 1979) p. 6.

11. C.H. Patterson, **Foundations for a Theory of Induction and Educational Psychology** (New York: Harper & Row, Publishers, 1977) p. 4.

12. R. Ellis, "Characteristics of Significant Theorists," **Nursing Research**, 17, (1968) pp. 217–222.

13. **Ibid.**

14. J. Dickoff and P. James, "A Theory of Theories: A Position Paper," **Nursing Research**, 17 (1968) pp. 197–203.

15. **Ibid.**

16. **Ibid.**

17. Riehl and Roy, **Conceptual Models.** 1974. p. 5.

18. Yura and Walsh, **Nursing Process.** p. 18.

19. A. Jacox, "Theory Construction in Nursing: An Overview," **Nursing Rsearch**, 23 (1974) pp. 4–13.

20. **Ibid.** p. 5.

21. **Ibid.** p. 5.

22. M. E. Hardy, "Theories: Components, Development, Evaluation," **Nursing Research**, 23 (1974) pp. 100–106.

23. **Ibid.** p. 101.

24. M.V. Horgan, "Concepts about Nursing in Selected Nursing Literature from 1950–1965." Unpublished Masters Thesis, The Catholic University of America, School of Nursing, Washington, D.C. 1967.

25. E.O. Bevis, **Curriculum Building in Nursing—A Process.** (St. Louis: The C.V. Mosby Co., 1973) p. 9.

26. Yura and Walsh, **Nursing Process.** p. 19.

27. Ibid.

ANNOTATED BIBLIOGRAPHY

Ellis R: **Characteristics of Significant Theories.** Nurs Res 17:3:217–222; May–June 1968. This classic article reviews the key components of theories.

Hardy ME: **Theories: Components, Development, Evaluation.** Nurs Res 23:2: 100–197; March–April 1974. This article discusses basic terms, selection, and evaluation of nursing theories.

Jacox A: **Theory Construction in Nursing: An Overview.** Nurs Res 23:1:4–13; January–February 1974. This article reviews how scientific knowledge is developed and organized into theories.

Jones PS: **An Adaptation Model for Nursing Practice.** Am J Nurs 78:11:1900–1905; November 1978. This article discusses the conceptual framework of adaptation. It provides an excellent and brief review of the relevant literature and suggests a tool for assessment.

Newman MA: **Theory Development in Nursing.** Philadelphia, F. A. Davis Co., 1979. This brief and excellent book discusses how theories are developed.

Riehl JP, Roy C: **Conceptual Models for Nursing Practice,** New York, Appleton-Century-Crofts, 1974. This text is a collection of contributed chapters that discuss several of the major nursing theories.

2

General Systems Theory and Adaptation

Phyllis B. Heffron

CHAPTER OUTLINE

OBJECTIVES

At the completion of this chapter the reader will be able to:

- Define each term in the glossary.
- Discuss, using examples, the meaning of the phrase "a whole is greater than the sum of its parts."
- Describe the relationships between feedback, steady state, and equifinality.
- Distinguish between homogeneity and ordered differentiation in systems in terms of entropy and negentropy.
- Explain the concept of adaptation as it relates to general systems theory.
- Identify six system processes that contribute to the adaptation of open systems.
- Identify four ways that psychosocial adaptation can be measured.
- Explain the importance of social and anthropological adaptation, and provide examples of each.
- Discuss a general concept of man, using general systems terminology and the principles of adaptation.
- Explain how a general systems approach can be applied to the concept of health care.
- Describe three ways in which the theories of systems and adaptation have had an influence on nursing education.

GLOSSARY

Adaptation—a dynamic, ongoing, and life sustaining process whereby living things continually adjust to environmental changes.

Adaptation Theory—the body of knowledge that describes and predicts concepts and principles about adaptation, its process, relationships, and consequences.

Anthropological adaptation—the cultural adaptation of particular groups of people to environmental forces over time and space.

Biological adaptation—the adaptation of living things to their environment for the ultimate purpose of reproduction and survival.

Boundary—a real or imaginary line of demarcation that separates one system from another and from its environment.

Closed system—a system that does not change or allow any input or output exchanges with the environment; also used to describe relatively closed groups.

Dynamic equilibrium—a state of balance in living systems that is ever-changing due to continual environmental movements and subsequent cyclical processes of input, throughput, and output.

Ecological adaptation—the adaptation of living things that emphasizes man as a part of nature, constantly influencing and being influenced by his internal and external environment. Through it, man is allowed to live in harmony with nature.

Energy—the capacity for doing work; the product of a force (e.g., thermal, electrical, chemical), that acts on a body.

Entropy—a systems energy state that measures the system's tendency toward disorder.

Equifinality—a systems principle stating that the system tends toward equilibrium and can arrive at a final goal through various methods and from different initial states.

Evolution—the historic and ongoing process of how living things have changed or adapted over the ages, since life began.

Feedback—a systems process, circular in nature, whereby system outputs are monitored and regulate subsequent input decisions.

General Adaptation Syndrome (GAS)—a predictable and specific set of reactions that occur generally when the body is confronted by a stressor.

General systems theory—a universal theory of wholeness that explains the relationships between wholes and parts and describes the characteristics and processes of systems and their functions.

Holism—pertaining to the idea of wholeness and interrelatedness of component parts in a whole system.

Holistic Health Care—health care that takes into consideration the bio/psycho/social and spiritual needs of the client and provides for all dimensions of health—preventive, rehabilitative, and primary care.

Homeodynamics—the continuous ex-

GLOSSARY Continued

change of energy between man and his environment. Used synonymously with steady state.

Humanism—pertaining to the idea of universally applicable human characteristics; of needs, feelings, and responses that signify the total experience of being a person.

Input—any form of information, matter, or energy that enters into the system through its boundary, from the environment.

Negentropy—a systems energy state that measures the system's tendency toward order.

Open system—a system with an open or semipermeable boundary that allows a free exchange of input and output between the system and its environment.

Physiological adaptation—the ongoing process by which internal bodily functions are regulated and ad-

justed to maintain homeostasis.

Psychological adaptation—the ongoing process by which man sustains a balance in his mental and emotional states of being.

Social adaptation—the continual adjustment and adaptation of man to other people and community groups in the social environment.

Steady state—a state of balance or internal constancy that signifies that a system is in harmony with its environment.

Stress—an ever present and dynamic state of reaction that results from systems' interactions with their environments; a non-specific response of the body to any demand made on it.

Stressor—any factor or agent that is responsible for or intensifies a stress state.

INTRODUCTION

The nursing profession has experienced many changes over the past two decades. One of the most exciting and fundamental changes has been in the area of theory building and conceptualization in nursing.

The purpose of this chapter is to introduce the student to two general and universally applicable theories that have been widely studied and used by nurses in the past few years—general systems theory and adaptation theory. These two theories were chosen for use in this textbook to orient the student to the definition and function of theories in general. General systems theory and adaptation theory are both concrete examples that can accomplish this orientation, and they can be explained, illustrated, and understood within the context of many concepts.

The second reason these two theories were chosen is that they are basic to a wide variety of nursing concepts, and they are a part of or form the structural framework of much of the thinking and writing going on in nursing today. They have a great deal to offer, and practicing professionals, as well as nursing students will benefit from a basic understanding and appreciation of their ideas and principles. Systems theory, in particular, is widely used in textbooks, in professional literature, and in educational programs.

GENERAL SYSTEMS THEORY

Overview and Significance

Our modern world is so complex that we

cannot comprehend it as a single phenomenon or entity. As a result, we tend to fragment it into understandable, manageable pieces. This fragmentation can be seen in science, which is broken down into elements such as chemistry, physics, microbiology, and sociology. In governments we have the division of states, regions, counties, and townships. In the human body there are organ systems, organs, tissues, cells, and genes.

General systems theory explains the breaking of whole things into parts and gaining knowledge about how the parts work together in "systems." It explains the relationships between wholes and parts, describes pertinent concepts about them, and makes predictions about how these "parts of wholes" will function, behave, and react. The terms **general systems theory** and **systems theory** will be used interchangeably in this text.

The basic concepts and ideas of general systems theory were explicitly proposed in the 1950s by scientists from a wide variety of disciplines. Ludwig von Bertalanffy emerged as one of the primary theorists, and went on to develop and introduce systems theory as a universal theory, applicable to many fields of study. The theoretical framework gives us generalizations about systems from which concepts, principles, and models can be transformed to work for a particular discipline. Psychology, biology, education, and computer science are all examples of fields that use systems theory and its applications.

Definition of a System

Bertalanffy defines a system as a set of interacting elements.[1] These interacting elements, or components, may or may not serve a different function, but ultimately they all serve a common purpose—to contribute to the overall goal of the system. In general systems theory, this is one of the most fundamental properties of a system.

Families provide us with an excellent example of how this works. Given that the typical components of a family are the mother, father, and children, we can say this family system is a set of interacting components. Each member has a unique role and function that contributes to the overall functioning of the system (e.g., keeping members safe, fed, clothed, loved, socialized).

Likewise, a mechanical system, such as a bicycle, also has related components that interact. The wheels, pedals, bearings, and brakes all function separately, but ultimately serve to provide a vehicular system.

From these examples we also can understand another part of the definition of a system. In systems the whole is always greater than the sum of its parts. In other words, each part standing by itself has a certain meaning or value that is enhanced or altered, i.e., it becomes "greater," when it is in interaction with the other system elements. In systems, elements work together in such a way that a change in one element may affect the meaning or use of other elements, as well as of the total system. For example*, consider a man with one leg: the only way he can propel himself is by hopping on that one leg. Next, consider a man with two legs: if the two legs are seen simply as a collection of single legs, then the best we can expect that man to do is to hop twice as fast as the man with one leg. But if he uses his two legs together as a system, he can run—an activity unique to the system, not simply the sum of individual characteristics. The earlier example of the bicycle as a mechanical system also illustrates this point.

The Hierarchy of Systems

Systems are hierarchical in nature and

---

*Example from unpublished Masters Thesis, Michael H. Heffron.

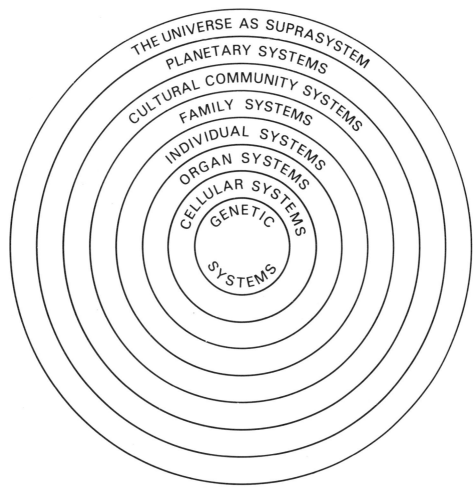

Figure 2-1.   A common systems hierarchy.

are composed of interrelated subsystems. Each subsystem is made up of lower subsystems, until some lowest-level subsystem is reached, or at the other end, some highest-level suprasystem. In most living systems, the bottom line for the elementary, or the top line for the suprasystem is somewhat arbitrarily drawn. Atoms, for example, are elementary subsystems in many systems, but to the nuclear physicist, they are complex systems. Figure 2-1 illustrates a broad and common systems hierarchy.

The assignment of systems, therefore, as subsystems or suprasystems, is relative to the focus of study. For example, nursing might be considered a *subsystem*, within the realm of a health care system, but a *system* in the realm of a hospital setting.

Boundaries

In systems theory, **boundaries** are real or imaginary lines of demarcation that separate one system from another or a system from its environment. These boundaries help provide a sense of order to the overall concept of a system. Examples of boundaries are skin around a body system, or a brick wall around a prison system. Boundaries serve as a point of exchange between what goes into and what goes out of the system.

Input, Output, and Throughput

Input and **output** are processes by which a system is able to communicate and react with its environment (i.e., with what is outside but interactive with a system). Input can be defined as any form of information, energy, or material that enters into the system through its boundary. Output is any energy, information, or matter that is transferred to the environment.

Throughput is a process that occurs at some point between the input and output processes. It enables the input to be transformed in such a way that it can be used readily by the system. When food is put into the human system by way of the mouth, for example, it immediately is subjected to a transformation process as the teeth mechanically grind it and the enzyme ptyalin chemically alters it. Without this and the subsequent processes of throughput, such as internal digestion and metabolism, the initial input could not be made into useful forms of energy for system survival. The throughput process is often referred to as transformation and occurs in manners and degrees of complexity that are highly specific to each organism or system.

Open and Closed Systems

One of the most important concepts advanced in general systems theory is the distinction between open and closed systems. An open system is one in which there is freedom and space for the movement of energy, matter, and information into and out of the system—through the system boundary. The boundaries in open systems often are described as *semipermeable*, because they are necessarily equipped to be selective about the movement of input and output. This crucial process of selectivity is discussed further in the sections of this chapter on feedback and equilibrium.

The input and output process in open systems might involve nutrients and wastes, in an animal or plant system, or pieces of information, in a library system. A business system may be described as an open system with the exchange of goods and services the input and output. Likewise, the exchange of feelings, verbally or through body language, in a group system would help classify it as an open system.

All living systems are by nature open systems; their very survival depends on a continuous exchange of energy, and they are constantly in a state of change. Open systems may vary in their degree of openness, both from system to system and within the same system. Hibernating bears, for example, breathe in oxygen and give off carbon dioxide, but there is little other interaction with the environment until spring. Amoebas and other one-celled animals are highly open systems at all times.

Closed systems are theoretically just the opposite of open systems. A closed system would experience no input from the environment nor give any output. It would not change under any circumstances. If openness and closeness were on a continuum, such as in Figure 2-2, all systems would be somewhere in between. In reality, no totally closed system has ever been known to exist. The terminology "closed system" is used in scientific literature, however, and it is important to keep in mind that it may or may not be in accordance with the definition found in general systems theory. The social sciences, in particular, often make reference to families, particular groups, or societies, as being closed systems. What they mean is that the system in question is *relatively* closed to outside influence or exchange. This might be said about a club or religious group, for example; that only admits members who meet some narrow criteria or that isolates itself from general society.

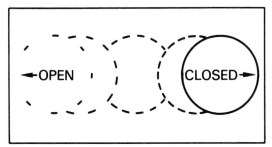

Figure 2-2. An illustrated continuum of open and closed systems.

Steady State, Dynamic Equilibrium

Open systems have to maintain a special balance within themselves in order to survive. This special balance is referred to as the system's **steady state** or **dynamic equilibrium.** In the human body system, for example, we can find many instances of this. Maintenance of body temperature, the normal salinity and pH of body fluids, or the proper amount of sugar in the blood and urine are all examples of how the healthy body is in a physiological balance. Psychologically, man also must adapt and maintain a steadiness and balance in his emotional life. Too much expression of anger, for example, may lead to violent, survival threatening behavior and alienation by others, whereas too little expression of anger may lead to gastric ulcers, headaches, or other somatic problems.

The concept of steady state does not imply elementary steadiness as one might think of an unmoving hand or an unchanging course at sea. On the contrary, the steady state in systems theory is always associated with the continual input/throughput/output cycle and, while balanced, it is never static. **Homeostasis** is another term that is often used syn-onymously with steady state, and it too may be misleading in this regard. Stasis clearly implies a stationary or stagnant state, contradictory to the dynamic nature of the steady state in open systems. Used specifically within the physiological context from which it originates, homeostasis is a time honored and acceptable term. It seems to lose some of its appropriateness, however, as it is adapted for use in describing the whole of man's interactions with his environment in a broad and extended way. **Homeodynamics** is yet another term used in describing man's dynamic state of balance. Homeodynamics is defined as the continuous exchange of energy between man and his environment that characterizes life itself—its growing, changing, and learning.[2] Whichever terminology is used, and you will see all of these terms used in this text as well as in the general literature, the principle is the same: In open systems there is a life sustaining balance at all levels that is maintained through the continual input and output exchange process within the environment.

Feedback

The maintenance of the steady state is highly dependent on a mechanism called **feedback.** Feedback is a system's self regulatory process, circular in nature, whereby system outputs are monitored, and the result is used to control subsequent input. It is not unlike the feedback mechanism that occurs in the communication process where there is interaction between the sender and the receiver; or in perception theory, whereby input messages are encoded, processed, and decoded with the help of feedback to promote adaptation and a system steady state.[3]

Examples of the feedback mechanism can be found within individual, community, family, and group systems. Persons interacting with their various community systems receive feedback via rules, regulations, and laws. For example, a driver in a great hurry may drive through a stoplight, be stopped by a policeman, and be given a traffic ticket. The act of getting the ticket is the feedback, which probably causes the driver to modify input behavior when re-entering the transportation system.

Children within a family system receive feedback from parents regarding their behavior. The harmony and steady state of the family depends greatly on how this feedback is used.

The feedback mechanism is always at work in maintaining the homeodynamic balance of physiological systems and subsystems. The presence or absence of hormones, for example, acts as feedback information for the maintenance of the menstrual cycle, the growth process, the regulation of certain blood chemistry, and so forth. The autonomic nervous system, one of the body's most crucial internal homeodynamic mechanisms, uses a feedback mechanism to balance the effects of its sympathetic and parasympathetic centers, the consequences of which regulate, for example, heart and respiratory rates, secretion of digestive juices, and constriction or dilation of the pupils.

Equifinality

Open systems tend toward a dynamic equilibrium that allows them to maintain their functions and survive. An important principle of systems theory, which is also a characteristic of the steady state, is the principle of equifinality.

Equifinality is a goal seeking process in which the system strives to reach a particular final state or goal, regardless of the means. A classic example is in the growth and morphogenesis of organisms, particularly the case of identical mammalian twins occurring from one ovum. The goal is the fully formed organism, which can be reached in either of two ways—from a single egg or from half of a divided egg.[4]

The chapters on Family Concepts and Group Concepts provide illustrations of equifinality and how groups of people tend to be goal seeking, reach their goals in different ways, and have the potential for changing from their original states. In addition, individual behavior also reflects an equifinality. Coping mechanisms, for example, that help us to adapt and reduce stress, are highly varied and used by individuals in differing combinations and degrees. One person may seek out the company of a listening friend to reduce stress or anxiety (maintain a steady state), while another person may have a glass of wine, meditate, or take a walk. A third person may do a combination of these. The process is goal seeking, and the same goal can be reached through different methods.

Energy, Entropy, and Negentropy

Energy, as a concept in general systems theory, may be looked at from several viewpoints. A basic dictionary definition of **energy** is the capacity to do work. Traditionally, energy is further defined in terms of its source, e.g., the sun or the wind. It also can be talked about in terms of its method of action, what it looks like, what kind of qualitative effect it has, and how much is needed by whom or what. In systems theory, we look additionally and very specifically at the maintenance of adequate amounts of energy and its distribution and movement.

We have noted that open systems are constantly in a dynamic state as the processes of input, throughput, and output are recurring. As these processes continue, the differentiated features of individual components in the systems may tend to lose their distinctiveness, their individuality, and to blend together with the other system components into a homogeneous entity. Contrary to what may be our first intuitive feeling about this process, this tendency toward homogeneity is a tendency toward disorder—that is, a breakdown of organized distinctions. This tendency is called **entropy.** It can be defined as a measure of the tendency toward disorder in a system. Conversely, negative entropy or **negentropy**, occurs when the system is tending toward order and increasing organization. Negentropy is defined as a measure of a system's tendency toward order.

In order to understand these concepts more clearly, it is important to recognize what order and disorder really mean in terms of living systems, and how systems are affected by entropy and negentropy. Increasing organization, as defined within the context of a system, is an ordered differentiation of system elements, as opposed to homogeneity. Thus, entropy may be understood as dissipation of energy or a diversion of that energy required to maintain the differentiation of system components. If allowed to predominate, it will cause a system to run down and fail to accomplish meaningful goals. Negentropy, on the other hand, allows the system to differentiate or distinguish its energy flow and provide for order and purpose. Input energy is transformed uniquely and carefully, according to a more specific plan, and there is differentiation or increased organization as system goals are attained.

Yura and Walsh provide an illustration of what these concepts mean as they discuss the use of entropy as measurement of an individual's health state. Health state is equated with the steady state or systems goal, i.e., the goal of a healthy living system is to maintain a steady state as negentropy is maximized and the human organism tends toward order.[5] The human organism, in order to seek and maintain health, must expend energy to understand and define what "good" health is in its particular situation, identify a plan for working toward this goal, mobilize the means for reaching it, and then carry it out. All of these steps take organization as the person (system) interacts with the environment and adapts to the goal of steady state or "good" health. Negentropy is maximized when this is the case.

ADAPTATION THEORY

Definition of Adaptation

The concept of adaptation has been around for many years, as we have studied and observed ourselves in relation to the world around us. A basic encyclopedic definition of **adaptation** in a general biological context is the adjustment of living matter to environmental conditions and to other living things. There are many recorded descriptions and references to adaptation, and in almost all contexts it is characterized as a dynamic process that effects change and involves interaction and response. Human adaptation is much more complex than that of other animals, and occurs on three levels—internally (the self), socially (with others), and physically (biochemically by nature).[6] Adaptation is thought by many scientists to be perhaps the one attribute that most clearly distinguishes the concept of life from the concept of inanimate matter.[7]

Within a general systems framework, adaptation is a process that must be ongoing to ensure the survival of living, open systems; it is the process that fosters regulatory mechanisms in systems and works toward a homeodynamic goal or steady state. The processes of input, throughput, and output, as well as feedback, negentropy, and equifinality, are the major system processes that are associated with and contribute to the adaptation of open systems.

Because it is used in so many disciplines and is present in all forms and aspects of life, adaptation means many things to many people.[8] Biologists, sociologists, psychologists, and physicians are among the numerous professionals who use adapta-

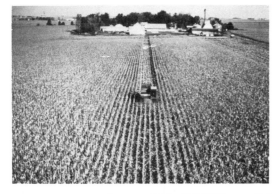

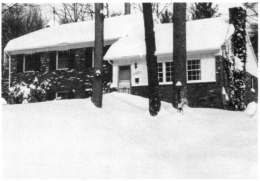

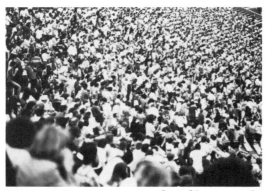

Figure 2-3.   Some examples of human adaptation.

tion and apply its principles. This interest and recognition are invaluable to the study of man and to such fields as nursing because they allow adaptation to be looked at holistically, as a process that affects the whole person, and not just selected parts.

To understand adaptation theory in its broadest sense, it is important to understand more about how the various disci-plines view it and make its application meaningful. For the purpose of this discussion, we will look briefly at adaptation theory as developed in biology, physiology, and selected areas of nursing, psychology, and the social sciences.

BIOLOGICAL ADAPTATION

Biology, the study of life, gives us one of the broadest ranges of information and understanding about adaptation theory. Charles Darwin studied the adaptation of many life forms as he was formulating his famous theory of evolution. He observed that most organisms produce far more offspring than can possibly survive. Those that survive do so because they are best adapted to cope with their environment. Among these survivors, some are better adapted than others, and these would leave the greater number of offspring; the principle of natural selection.[9] Natural selection, according to Darwin, is the process that supports **evolution.** Evolution is the historic and ongoing process of change and adaptation of living things since life began. The well-adapted survivors have passed on accumulated changes to their offspring, and for three billion years, living things have been adapting through succeeding generations to their environment and each other.[10]

Biology is ultimately concerned about the survival of living things. Various animals and plants are adapted for securing their food and for surviving extremes of temperature and water supplies. The cactus, for example, is adapted for survival in hot, dry climates. Animals like fish and birds each show anatomical adaptations that suit them for life in the water or in the air. Camels are not only built to withstand heat and scarcity of water, but they also have a second row of thick eyelashes that gives them protection against sandstorms.

Ecology, which is the study of plants and animals in relation to their total environment, is concerned with both anatomical and physiological adaptation. Human ecology, which is most relevant to nursing, provides us with additional information on physical, cultural, technological, social, and behavioral adaptation.[11] Within human ecology, people are viewed as open systems in constant interaction with their environments. Their responses to various environmental conditions—weather, temperature, air quality, water purity, noise, toxic substances—are all concerns of adaptation that have become profound and threatening issues in present day society. Such manmade environmental hazards as high-speed automobiles, chemicals, drugs, and nuclear devices unfortunately are teaching us much about maladaptation as well as adaptation.

Physiological Adaptation

Physiology, a branch of biology, involves the functions, maintenance, and reproduction of living organisms. It is concerned basically with cellular function and the internal environment of the body. Adaptation at this level is looked at within the context of maintaining intracellular homeostasis (i.e., preserving the correct fluid composition and temperature in order for the cells to carry on their functions). As these cellular systems are grouped together into tissue systems, organs, and so forth, the homeodynamic processes are different; as systems' goals change, environmental exchanges become more complex, and there is a need for more intricate mechanisms of adaptation.

Earlier in this chapter, several of the common homeostatic mechanisms present in human physiology were identified as helping to maintain the body's steady state. One of these is kidney filtration, which provides an excellent example of the complexities of physiological adaptation. Brunner brings out this complexity by describing quantitatively the filtering and excretion processes that go in a typically healthy person at rest. Within a 24-hour period, as a result of the recirculation of about 3 liters of plasma per minute through the kidney, 170 liters of water, 170 grams of glucose, and 560 grams of sodium, and other substances are filtered. Of these amounts, virtually the same exact percentages are either excreted or reabsorbed, according to cellular or other systems requirements for homeostasis.[12] This is not to mention the myriad of other possible inputs to this system such as drugs or excess water, to which healthy kidneys can adapt.

Thus far, adaptation has been defined as a homeodynamic process in which various body systems adjust to their exchanges and interactions with other internal systems and external environmental exchanges.

Stress and Adaptation

Within living systems, stress can be defined in numerous ways. It is a difficult term to describe, as a single phenomenon or typologically, such as psychological, physiological, or sociological stress. Furthermore, stress can be viewed as both a cause and an effect.[13] We often say that illness imposes a stressful condition on our bodies and, at the same time, we refer to stress as the cause of the illness. Dr. Hans Selye, a physiologist who studied stress extensively, offers a definition of stress as both an effect and, through his term **stressor,** as a cause. Selye defines stress as the nonspecific response of the body to any demand made on it, and a stressor as any factor or agent that is responsible for or intensifies a stress state.[14] Because stress causes the body to change in some way, the need for adaptation is created. The responses or adaptations that take place can be chemical, structural, or both. The chapter on Anxiety, Fear, and Stress elaborates on stress and adaptation and specifies adaptive and maladaptive mechanisms that may take place.

Psychosocial Adaptation

Psychosocial adaptation involves the way a person adjusts mentally and emotionally as a self-system, as a person relating to others, and to society in general. These relationships include thinking, acting, and feeling, and can be measured, to a very large degree, by the state of a person's identity, personal esteem, and level of fulfillment. All of these psychological "states" can be quite complex and never can be totally separated from other kinds of adaptation, such as physiological and biochemical. Also, not as much research has been done in the area of social and psychological adaptation as in **physiological** homeostasis and there are not as many guidelines as to which variables are important.[15]

Presently, more is being studied and written about the application of adaptation principles to psychosocial issues. Selye's General Adaptation Syndrome theory, for example, has been applied by a number of nurse-authors to the area of psychosocial assessment.[16–18]

In addition, the application of general adaptation concepts is being used to describe and present issues in the study of nursing.[19–22] Social adaptation has been addressed from the viewpoint of medical sociology, as has anthropological and family adaptation.[23–25] The following discussion will outline briefly some of the recent ideas regarding the psychosocial adaptation of man.

Sister Callista Roy, a nurse theorist, developed a systems adaptation model for the practice of nursing. The Roy model views man as a bio/psycho/social being and describes his adaptation as occurring in four modes. Three of these, the self-concept mode, the interdependence mode, and the role mode, are concerned with the ways

man adapts psychosocially. The self-concept mode addresses such areas as esteem, self-concept, and ego integrity. The interdependence mode deals with how man adapts to others. Changes in relationships, such as death or separation, can disrupt the giving and receiving of affection, social resources, and other need fulfilling activities. The role mode addresses how man adapts to the various and changing roles he must perform to maintain a homeodynamic balance within himself, his family, and society. Any change in role, such as a new job or new baby, requires adaptation to bring the system back into balance. Adaptation processes will be geared to changing any lost or maladaptive behaviors related to these changes.[26,27]

Psychological adaptation is defined by Murray and Zentner in terms of behavioral adequacy and the attainment of appropriate human relationships. Adaptation is achieved through the processing of the conscious self (ego), the unconscious self (id), and the inner self (superego). These are primarily defense mechanisms that allow the person to adjust to and cope with stressful situations. Adaptation, according to these authors, can be evaluated using Selye's General Adaptation Syndrome. (Refer to Chapter 21 for a definition of the GAS or General Adaptation Syndrome.) During the Alarm Phase, for example, there may be heightened awareness mixed with mild anxiety. The manifestation of anxiety during this stage may increase to varying levels, including agitation and hallucinations. The introduction of defense mechanisms, such as rationalization or denial, signals adaptation and the beginning of the Resistance Phase. If the person is unable to use any coping mechanisms, some type of mental illness is likely to ensue, and the Exhaustion Phase sets in. As in the physiological GAS, the person may go back and forth between the three phases, but repeated experiences in the Exhaustion Phase eventually can lead to death.[28]

Lancaster talks about the full range of adaptation behavior within the context of an ecological framework. She defines adaptation as a dynamic, active process by which the individual living system meets its basic needs within a constantly changing environment. In order to understand and promote adaptation of mental health needs, Lancaster identifies specific psychological, sociocultural, and technological adaptive mechanisms, in addition to the basic physiological mechanisms. Examples of psychological adaptive mechanisms are such things as traditional psychoanalytic defense mechanisms, e.g. denial, repression, learning, and problem solving. Sociocultural adaptive mechanisms reflect the person's need for belonging and socializing in groups, and include social norms, role identification, and ethical values. Technological adaptive mechanisms might include mood altering drugs, hearing aids, and biofeedback devices.[29]

David Mechanic, a prominent medical sociologist, defines social adaptation as a process that requires a person's psychological capacities, skills, and qualities to meet and adjust to the demands of his physical and social environments.[30] This kind of adaptation is a highly complex process within human systems. Not only does man vary in his own individual qualities, skills, and abilities, but the demands of his social environment (other people, groups, community organizations, and institutions) are all highly variable, and often inconsistent and unpredictable. Take, for example, the social adaptation of people who are hospitalized. The social demands of hospitalization include such things as the relinquishment of privacy, adherence to predetermined eating, bathing, and sleeping schedules, the separation from familiar people, and tolerance of often uncomfortable examinations and treatments. These demands seem relatively beyond the tolerance limits of people accustomed to leading an independent life over which they

exert control. For these people, adaptation may be difficult in the hospital setting and may depend on complex coping mechanisms. Yet there are some people who, because of previous stressful events or other factors may adapt quickly and gratefully to the role of being a dependent patient in a hospital. Other factors that affect this kind of social adaptation are the prior experiences the individual has had in adapting to similar situations, how family and friends have adapted, and what one's values are in regard to such issues as privacy and authority. This list of variables appears endless when considering adaptation within this kind of sociocultural framework.

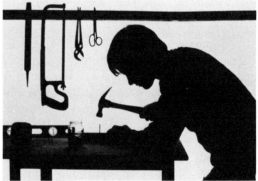

Figure 2-4.   Tools are important components in sociocultural adaption.

Anthropology offers us yet another broad and comprehensive view of adaptation theory. Similar to biological adaptation, anthropological adaptation refers to the capacity of a particular group to tolerate selective forces in its environment and to master environmental problems by developing effective structures, behaviors, and forms of social organization. Man, in contrast to other living systems, relies more heavily on "learned" ways of adapting rather than on instinctive or inherited methods. Human populations can make complex and extensive changes in a relatively short period of time. As new tools, ideas, and ways of living emerge, cultural adaptation takes place.[31] Culture can be viewed as a determinant of adaptation.[32]

Anthropology looks at man and adaptation longitudinally as well as comprehensively. Through a time and space perspective, man's adaptation is seen in relation to the past, present, and future. As this knowledge is gained and combined with geographical, physical, and sociocultural aspects, a unique and comparative view of man and adaptation emerges.[33]

NURSING IMPLICATIONS

The ideas and principles within systems theory and adaptation have had considerable influence on nursing and the health professions. In nursing these theories have provided useful frameworks for the definition of major concepts and sound theoretical foundations for education and practice.

The remaining portion of this chapter will focus on how systems and adaptation theory have been applied in the areas of health care, clinical practice, and nursing education.

Man's Adaptive Nature

Systems and adaptation theory allow man to be viewed within a dynamic, humanistic, and holistic framework. **Holism** and **holistic** are terms that reflect the idea of wholeness and the interrelatedness of component parts in a whole system. **Humanistic** refers nonjudgmentally to the qualities and essences of being human and to universal human characteristics, such as beliefs, values, and feelings.

Human beings are complex organisms made up of distinct groups and subgroups of related components. The interplay between these human components (i.e., behaviors, feelings, and thoughts), as well as structural and physiological human aspects, involve many unique and complementary relationships that are at the very

core of human adaptation. Together, these systems and adaptation provide for a viable and comprehensive view of man.

In the nursing profession, man is frequently viewed from a holistic and dynamic perspective. In this way, man can be looked at within the context of his own individual system, as well as other systems and subsystems in the environment. From this broad and ecological viewpoint, nurses can better understand some of the complexities of human behavior and better meet patients' needs. Patients undergoing planned admissions to the hospital, for example, show highly diverse reactions to seemingly simple procedures such as filling out forms, securing valuables, and going for x-rays. A second look at these reactions, from a systems viewpoint, can provide insight into some of the reasons for them. Attitudes and fears from childhood (psychological subsystem), present economic situations (economic social system or self-social subsystem), and previous community experiences (community systems) are some examples of systems interactions that might influence a person's reactions.

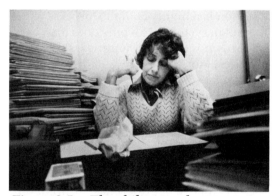

Figure 2-5.   The ability to adapt to stressful situations is dependent on interactions from all of man's subsystems.

Living systems are goal seeking. They have the potential for growth and development and are allowed flexibility and variance as they pursue their goals. Goals are reached through careful organization and channeling of energy for effective interaction (adaptation) between all the parts. Nursing practice is benefited and enhanced in many settings by looking at man in this way. The community health nurse, for example, looks at goal seeking and growth within the context of a wide variety of man's subsystems. Here, clients may be individuals, family groups, or the community at large. All three of these entities are systems within themselves and subsystems of one another that are constantly striving to reach certain goals—all within the context of how they should relate with, depend on, and help each other. Consider an elderly crippled widow who wishes to remain at home, despite her inability to care completely for herself and follow a medication regime. The community health nurse is able to help this client reach her goal of partial self-care by contacting two family members and another community agency for help. Through mutual planning and health teaching by the nurse, the client feels supported and is able to remain semi-independent during her convalescence.

In another instance, the surgical intensive care nurse must look critically at man's physiological goals. In this case, the physiological system will dictate certain priorities of care as homeostasis returns and tissues are repaired, but a look at the psychosocial subsystems will be equally important in promoting the overall return to health. By assessing such things as the will to live, the degree and source of any psychic stress, and family attitudes toward the patient's illness, the nurse is acknowledging that mind and body are not separate, but function and respond as a whole unit.

Nursing theorists have given additional evidence of the usefulness of systems and adaptation theory as a way of looking at man. Orem, for example, views man as a system with an internal physical, psycho-

logical, and social nature, that all react to the external elements—the environment.[34] Sister Callista Roy, whose systems adaptation model was mentioned earlier, sees man holistically as a bio/psycho/social being who adapts according to various modes or components. These modes of adaptation correlate with the characteristics of each component subsystem of man.

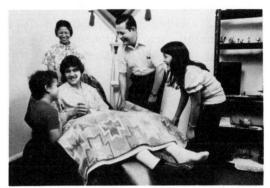

Figure 2-6.   Man is a bio/psycho/social and spiritual being.

Nursing as an Adaptive System

A systems adaptation framework also can help to define and clarify the scope of professional nursing.

The practice of nursing takes place in a variety of settings and in a number of ways. A necessary and major facet of this practice is the **nursing process.** Inspired by several theories, one of which is general systems theory, the nursing process is an organized problem solving approach by which nurses interact with their clients to promote adaptation. Found in virtually every contemporary nursing book, it is a step-by-step goal seeking process that is hierarchical in nature and uses a feedback mechanism. The four phases or steps of the nursing process are fully described in The Nursing Process chapter. The advancement of this process has benefited nursing in unparalleled ways. It is described as the essence and core of nursing and provides the profession with a positive self concept;

one that functions in an organized and adaptable fashion, from a scientific base.[35]

Health Care and Holism

Professional nurses carry out the nursing process interactively and interdependently within a larger system called the health care system. In American society, the term health care system identifies a confusing and highly complex network of health and medical components that vary greatly in their goals, meanings, and actual functions. The chapter on Health Care System elaborates on this and provides insights into its subsystems and the relationships among them. In the past few years, the ideas and principles of general systems theory have helped numerous groups of people think about the plan for a more comprehensive kind of health care system.

Holistic health and **holistic health care** are terms that became very popular during the 1960s, when many people began to voice dissatisfaction with the existing structures of health care and other American institutions. Holistic health care involves the whole person within their environment and reflects the systems concept that the whole is greater than the sum of its parts. It is mandated to consider all the components of health as an open system—health promotion, health education and prevention, health maintenance, and restorative/rehabilitative care. Nurses and other advocates of the holistic approach feel that all of these components are equally important in the process of identifying health needs, planning for care and intervention, and in evaluating the results.

Selye's research and findings on stress and adaptation helped to further thinking on the merits of holistic health care. His book, **The Stress of Life**, increased the interest in stress and stress related illnesses. Both health professionals and health consumers became more concerned about the

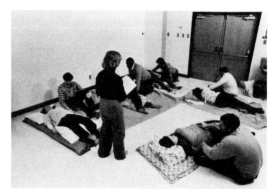

Figure 2-7. Health teaching is a part of holistic health care.

totality of stress; of its being the consequence of many interactions with the environment (e.g., chemical, biological, psychological, physical, sociocultural), with potentially damaging effects on the body. This interest and concern has helped cause the evolution of a holistic orientation in nursing, as well as foster a more holistic approach in medicine and other health professions.

Nursing Education

In nursing education, models such as systems theory and adaptation have proven to be very important and useful as teaching frameworks within which man, nursing, and health care can be explained.

An early example of this can be seen in the writings of Florence Nightingale. Although Nightingale's methods of nursing are not explicitly identified as theoretical and are less well known than her other contributions in nursing education, she used a framework of thought similar to that of adaptation theory. Her philosophy included frequent references to the effects of the environment on the patient and how these effects could hamper or help the healing process. In her nurse's training program, she stressed the importance of fresh air, sunshine, pure water, and a clean, quiet environment. In essence, she said

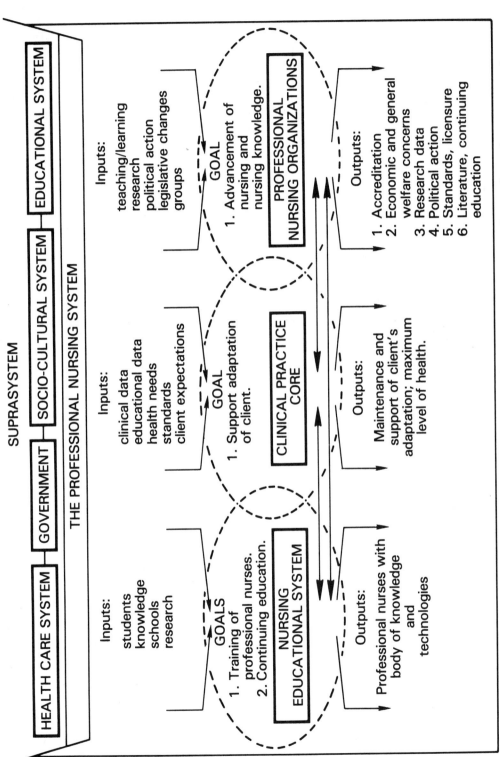

Figure 2-8. Systems Adaptation Model of the *Professional Nursing System* as used in a baccalaureate nursing program. Adapted from *The CUA Systems Adaptation Model,* 1978.

that if these elements are poorly attended to, patients will have to expend too much of their available energy to adapt to the environment rather than to get well.[36,37]

Although a number of early nursing leaders, such as Nutting and Robb, wrote about nursing as a more humanistic and integral science, the medical model remained the dominant theoretical framework for nursing until fairly recently. In the 1950s and 1960s, conceptual frameworks of intrapersonal theory and human needs theory were advanced. Both of these conceptual frameworks were holistic in nature and embraced basic adaptation principles, although neither general systems theory or adaptation theory were specifically credited.

In the 1970s, nursing leaders and educators began to develop and publish more information on theory development and evaluation. Nursing theories were identified as foundations for nursing education, and some baccalaureate nursing programs adopted a specific theory on which to base their curriculum.

One example of such curriculum is the Catholic University of America's School of Nursing's **Systems Adaptation Model.** The undergraduate faculty developed a conceptual framework for the curriculum based on Roy's adaptation model. Man and nursing were identified holistically as open, living systems that act on and influence each other, and adaptation was considered as the theoretical basis for this relationship. The curriculum model was developed using Roy's adaptive modes, and definitive descriptions of the self, family, professional nursing, health care, community, and group systems were stated. Individual, family, and community assessment tools were developed, and students were taught to use the nursing process within a systems adaptation framework.[38]

The principles of systems theory also has had some influence on the arrangement, organization, and placement of courses within nursing curriculums. For many years, nursing courses have been arranged exclusively in a categorical manner, such as medical nursing, surgical nursing, psychiatric nursing, and so forth. This type of categorization tends not to reflect the holistic nature of man and nursing, even though these courses might contain more integration than their titles suggest. Another approach, the integrated curriculum, is now used by many schools. Within this type of program, for example, the beginning psychiatric concepts of communication and self-esteem might be integrated along with general principles of health assessment in a first year clinical nursing course. Family health care might be in the focus of another beginning course, which would allow the integration of these concepts plus additional maternal and child health concepts. Within this type of curriculum, students might do home visits on patients they cared for in the hospital setting, rather than restricting this activity to a community health course.

Most curriculums in nursing education contain a mixture of some of these approaches and some of the more traditional ones. It does seem clear, however, that both general systems theory and adaptation theory have had an influence on schools of nursing and, in some cases, are being used as theoretical frameworks for curriculum guidance.

As was mentioned at the beginning of the section on general systems theory, the basic systems conceptual framework allows for a universality and common basis of understanding between different fields of study. This attribute has tremendous benefits for nursing as well as other service oriented subsystems of the health care system. Professionals from many disciplines must develop shared meanings and understandings in order to function in an interdependent teamwork fashion and achieve mutual goals of health care.[39] Additionally, nurses, psychologists, physicians, and social workers, for example, can benefit from a shared and interdisciplinary language to span conceptual gaps in knowledge and relate to one another's research more effectively.

Adaptation theory, as the basis for systems integrity and survival, also perpetuates a common basis of understanding across disciplinary boundaries. Together, these theoretical frameworks have been applied and have influenced the nursing profession in numerous ways.

SUMMARY

A system is made up of a set of interdependent and mutually interacting components that have a common goal. The end product or whole system is always greater than the sum of its parts.

Systems are arranged hierarchically in terms of other systems and may be classified as subsystems, systems, or suprasystems. Boundaries are lines of demarcation, visible or invisible, that enclose a system's parts and differentiate it from the environment and other systems.

Systems can be open or closed. Open systems are those that relate freely with the environment and allow for the continual exchange of matter, energy, and information across their boundaries. This input material undergoes varying degrees of transformation inside the system, called throughput, which converts it to usable forms of energy. Any material that leaves the system and is returned to the environment is called output. All living systems are open systems in nature, although the term closed system is sometimes used in the social sciences to refer to isolated or relatively closed groups of people.

Living systems show a remarkable capacity to maintain a constant balance or dynamic equilibrium within themselves. This balanced condition may be referred to as the system's steady state or homeostasis

and is necessary for survival of the system. A newer term, homeodynamics, emphasizes the nature of this balance in terms of continual change (i.e., the system is constantly exchanging input, and output remains stable).

Feedback is a self-regulatory process in which a system obtains information from or about its output which is then used to monitor its input. It is a circular mechanism and is largely responsible for the maintenance of the steady state.

Living systems exhibit a goal-seeking behavior known as the principle of equifinality. As a result of this property, systems tend toward equilibrium and can arrive at a final state via different routes and from different initial conditions. Equifinality also contributes toward the maintenance of the steady state and is necessary for the growth and integrity of the system.

Energy is a major concept in general systems theory and is described in terms of its type and state of distribution and movement. Entropy is a systems energy state which measures the tendency toward disorder in a system, and if allowed to predominate, will cause the system to degenerate and die. Negentropy is a systems energy state which measures its tendency toward order and increasing organization; negentropy allows a system to differentiate its energy in a purposeful way and progress toward a goal.

Adaptation is the process in which living matter adjusts and makes changes in response to interactions with the environment. It is a dynamic and creative process in man, described theoretically by a number of disciplines.

In general systems theory adaptation is an umbrella-term encompassing system processes that lead to the steady state. All open living systems require adaptation for continued functioning and systems survival.

Likewise in the fields of biology and ecology, adaptation connotes the adjustment and survival of living things, to each other and to environmental conditions. Ecology views adaptation holistically, to include all aspects of living organisms.

Psychosocial adaptation refers to that part of human adaptation that involves man's emotional stability and the quality of his interactions with other people and society in general. Adaptive processes within this realm are highly complex because of the great number of variables that are available; the uniqueness of psychological variables within each individual, in combination with all respective characteristics of society, gives rise to this sometimes unpredictable and inconsistent state of affairs.

Anthropological adaptation provides a broad view of human adaptation. The reactions of selected groups of people to all aspects of their environment are studied and looked at in a sociocultural framework over time. Adaptive mechanisms are described comparatively and according to various cultural characteristics.

Many of the basic concepts of professional nursing can be explained and understood within the frameworks of general systems theory and adaptation. Man can be seen as an open living system made up of interrelated parts that are in constant interaction with the environment. Additionally, man is a goal seeking organism that uses many feedback mechanisms for self-regulation and maintenance of a homeodynamic steady state.

Adaptation is necessary for man's survival and can be used as a measurement tool in the assessment of health status and planning for nursing care. Health care is described as holistic when it takes into consideration the bio/psycho/social and spiritual needs of man and provides for, or makes referrals for care in all these areas.

In nursing education, systems and adaptation frameworks are used in the teaching/learning process. There is also a trend toward holistic types of course integration in professional curriculums. This philosophy reinforces the concepts of man as an open system and of nursing as a process that promotes adaptation within a holistically structured health care system.

Finally, the universality of both of these theories has been a major factor in their capacity to influence nursing. By perpetuating a common basis of understanding across disciplinary boundaries, general systems theory in particular has helped to increase the knowledge base of nursing and foster a holistic approach in the pursuit of professionalism.

STUDY QUESTIONS

1. Describe a family you know in terms of components, boundaries, input, output, feedback, and steady state.

2. Develop a chart showing the hierarchy of systems and subsystems within your school of nursing.

3. List as many examples as you can of behaviors, mechanisms, or factors that have contributed to an increase in your personal negentropy status in the past 48 hours.

4. Describe two homeostatic mechanisms within the human body and list adaptive behaviors and mechanisms for each.

5. Write a short critique of your own health care needs in the past year. From a systems perspective, were they met in a holistic fashion? Why or why not?

6. Interview two classmates regarding their experience of coming to college for the first time. Compare their various reactions to the processes of social adaptation and methods that helped them cope and adapt.

REFERENCE LIST

1. Ludwig von Bertalanffy, **General Systems Theory** (New York, New York: Braziller 1968) p.55.
2. Arlyne B. Saperstein and Margaret A. Frazier, **Introduction to Nursing Practice** (Philadelphia, Pennsylvania: F.A. Davis Co., 1980) p.88.
3. Helen Yura and Mary B. Walsh, **The Nursing Process** (New York, New York: Appleton-Century-Crofts, 1973) p.65.
4. Bertalanffy, **General Systems**, p.40.
5. Yura and Walsh, **Nursing Process.**
6. Philip K. Bock, **Modern Cultural Anthropology** (New York: Alfred A. Knopf, Inc., 1969) p.209.
7. René Dubos, **Man Adapting** (New Haven, Connecticut: Yale University Press, 1965) p.256.
8. Dubos, **Man Adapting,** p.257.
9. Theodore W. Torrey, **Morphogenesis of the Vertebrates** (New York, New York: John Wiley and Sons, Inc., 1971) p.5.
10. Malcolm E. Weiss, **Clues to the Riddle of Life** (New York: Hawthorn Books, Inc., 1968), pp. 25, 29.
11. Jeanette Lancaster, **Community Mental Health Nursing, An Ecological Perspective** (St. Louis: The C.V. Mosby Co., 1980)
12. Lillian Brunner and Doris Suddarth, **Textbook of Medical-Surgical Nursing** (Philadelphia, Pennsylvania: J.B. Lippincott Co., 1980) pp.106–107.
13. Marjorie L. Byrne and Lida F. Thompson, **Key Concepts for the Study and Practice of Nursing** (St. Louis, Missouri: The C.V. Mosby Co., 1972) p.42.
14. Hans Selye, **The Stress of Life,** revised edition (New York, New York: McGraw-Hill Book Co., 1976).
15. Lancaster, **Community Mental Health Nursing.**
16. Ellen M. Feeley, Moira S. Shine, and Sharon B. Sloboda, **Fundamentals of Nursing Care** (New York: D. Van Norstrand Co., 1980) pp.179–180.
17. Ruth B. Murray and Judith P. Zenter. **Nursing Concepts for Health Promotion.** 2nd ed. Englewood Cliffs, N.J.: Prentice-Hall, Inc. 1979. pp.44–45,48.
18. Byrne and Thompson, **Key Concepts,** pp.44,45, 48.
19. Jeanine R. Auger, **Behavioral Systems and Nursing** (Englewood Cliffs, N.J.: Prentice-Hall Inc., 1976) pp.51, 162, 168.
20. Lancaster, **Community Mental Health,** pp.52–54.
21. Clark, **Mental Health Aspects,** pp.4–6, 69.
22. Joan P. Riehl, Sister Callista Roy, **Conceptual Models for Nursing Practice** (New York, New York: Appleton-Century-Crofts, 1974) pp.135–151.
23. Madeleine M. Leininger, **Nursing and Anthropology: Two Worlds to Blend** (New York, New York: John Wiley and Sons, 1970) p.5.
24. Murray and Zentner, **Nursing Concepts,** pp.179–180.
25. David Mechanic, **Medical Sociology** (New York, New York: The Free Press, 1968) pp.2, 57, 68, 179.
26. Riehl and Roy, **Conceptual Models,** pp.135–138.
27. Baccalaureate Curriculum Subcommittee, The Catholic University of America School of Nursing, **CUA Systems Adaptation Model** (The Catholic University of America, 1978) pp. 16, 19, 22.
28. Murray and Zentner, **Nursing Concepts,** pp.170–174.
29. Lancaster, **Community Mental Health,** pp.52–54.
30. Mechanic, **Medical Sociology,** p.57.
31. Bock, **Modern Cultural Anthropology,** pp.208,209.
32. Murray and Zentner, **Nursing Concepts,** p.175.
33. Leininger, **Nursing and Anthropology,** pp.208,209.
34. Julia B. George, Chairperson, The Nursing Theories Conference Group, **Nursing Theories** (Englewood Cliffs, N.J.: Prentice-Hall, Inc., 1980) p.66.
35. Yura and Walsh, **The Nursing Process,** p.1.
36. George, **Nursing Theories,** pp.33.
37. Frances T. Smith, "Florence Nightingale: Early Feminist," **American Journal of Nursing,** (May 1981) pp.1023–24.
38. **CUA Systems Adaptation Model,** 1978.
39. Lillian DeYoung, **Dynamics of Nursing** (St. Louis, Missouri: The C.V. Mosby Co., 1981) p.68.

ANNOTATED BIBLIOGRAPHY

Auger JR: **Behavioral Systems and Nursing,** Englewood Cliffs, Prentice-Hall, Inc., 1976. This text presents a behavioral systems approach to nursing practice. General systems theory is discussed as is the structure and function of behavior. An assessment tool and case examples are included.

Byrne ML, Thompson LF: **Key Concepts for the Study and Practice of Nursing,** St. Louis, The C.V. Mosby Co., 1972. This text uses a systems approach to identify concepts that can provide a frame of reference for nursing practice. There are good explanations of both systems and adaptation terminology. The authors use many examples to clarify the relationship between systems, adaptation, behavior, and nursing.

Hall JE, Weaver BR: **Distributive Nursing Practice: A Systems Approach to Community Health,** Philadelphia, J.B. Lippincott Co., 1977. This entire text uses a general systems theory approach to community health nursing. Chapters 3 and 4 give clear explanations of general systems concepts and provide examples of how they can be applied to components of nursing practice.

King I: **A Theory For Nursing Systems, Concepts, Process,** New York, John Wiley and Sons, 1981. A conceptual framework is presented by linking nursing concepts essential to understanding nursing as a system with health care systems. There are sections on social systems, personal systems, interpersonal systems, and goal attainment. A good reference for understanding how to use a systems framework in nursing.

3

Nursing: Past and Present

Janet-Beth Flynn
Helen Foerst
Phyllis B. Heffron

CHAPTER OUTLINE

OBJECTIVES

At the completion of this chapter, the reader will be able to:

- Define the terms in the glossary.
- Discuss the historic development of nursing.
- Describe Florence Nightingale's impact on modern nursing.
- Discuss the roles played by early leaders in nursing in the United States.
- Discuss how nursing was advanced by wars.
- Compare and contrast the Landmark studies.
- Identify and describe the different types of nursing education programs.
- Compare and contrast episodic nursing roles with distributive nursing roles.
- Discuss the meaning of the expanded role in nursing.
- Discuss international nursing roles.
- Discuss solutions for the problem of reality shock.
- Identify relevant issues on the question of nurse shortages.
- Identify the stages of burnout.
- Identify four ways in which computers can assist nursing practice.

GLOSSARY

Burnout—a stress-induced syndrome affecting experienced nurses characterized by general job frustration, fatigue, depression, irritability, and other physical symptoms.

Dependent Nursing Actions—actions that nurses carry out as a result of written or verbal orders of others on the health care team.

Distributive Care—care directed towards health maintenance and illness prevention; usually takes place in an outpatient facility, the home, or community setting.

Episodic Care—care directed toward a cure and that usually takes place in a hospital or other inpatient setting.

Health—a dynamic state of being that moves back and forth on a continuum.

Health-Illness Continuum—a hypothetical, graduated scale intended to measure an individual's total health status, as he perceives it.

Illness—a state of being in which an optimal health state, for a variety of reasons, is not being maintained.

Independent Nursing Actions—those actions performed by nurses based primarily on professional knowledge and judgments.

Interdependent Nursing Actions—those that nurses perform in collaboration with others on the health care team.

Medical Model—a framework of health care based on pathophysiological states, disease classification, and physical diagnosis.

Nursing Information System—a collection of computerized programs that contain nursing and selected patient and medical data. The system may or may not be a part of a larger medical information system used to record, review, monitor, and analyze these data.

Primary Care—health care that takes place at the time of the client's initial contact with the health care system or health provider. It usually takes place in an office or clinic setting, but may take place on admission to a hospital.

Reality Shock—the experiences and feelings a newly graduated nurse or a nurse returning to the workforce after an extended leave often faces due to differences between expectations of the employer and preparedness of the nurse. Reality shock is partially a result of the quick transition from classroom to workplace.

Wellness—ever-changing growth toward fulfilling an individual's potential, considering individual needs, abilities, and disabilities.

INTRODUCTION

The concept of nursing combines a richness of ideas, theories, and methodologies. Nursing is a complex system with various meanings that operate from numerous levels and facets. On one level, nursing is a professional occupation that provides a unique and vital service to society. It is a scientific discipline that studies and produces information about man and his environment, human health and adaptation, and the nature of nursing. On another level, nursing is a process of practical skills that require intelligence, dexterity, logic, and creativity. Additionally, those who practice nursing, and many who receive its services, describe nursing on a spiritual level; a level that embodies warmth and caring, empathy, personal ethics, and the give and take of human sharing.

It is a combination of all these things, along with history, educational processes, and professional roles that provide nurses with perspectives from which to view and understand the concept of nursing.

This chapter provides an overview of the history of nursing and nursing education. The basic concepts of health and illness are addressed, as are emerging patterns in the definition of nursing and the scope of nursing practice. Several pertinent dilemmas and contemporary issues also will be discussed.

Health and Illness

In order to think about the concept of nursing and what it means to deliver nursing and health care, the basic terms of health and illness, and more recently wellness, need to be understood. These terms describe subjectively a person's general state of being and are all relative according to a wide range of variables. Health and illness mean different things to different people and, consequently, it becomes important for nurses to deliberately formulate their own definitions.

Health traditionally has been viewed in terms of disease, pain, illness, or injury. This framework of thought, commonly referred to as the medical model, is based on an organized and precise classification of signs, symptoms, syndromes, and specifically named diseases that represent some type of physiological or psychological pathology. This model has dominated western medical and nursing schools for many years. Hospitals commonly use a medical classification system for assigning patients to rooms. Courses are taught on immunol-

ogy, cardiology, and ophthalmology. Many health insurance companies require patients to be assigned an official medical code before they can be reimbursed for health care.

In 1971, the World Health Organization (WHO) adopted a new definition of health in its official constitution. The WHO definition was comprehensive, and specifically stated that "health is a state of complete physical, mental, and social well being and not merely the absence of disease or infirmity."[1] During this time period, American consumers were becoming more interested in having a voice in their health care, and there was an increasing awareness regarding the effects of social and psychological stress on the body. The holistic health movement, which started in the 1960s, coined the term "high level wellness"—a concept that expanded and offered a whole new way of approaching health and health care.[2]

According to the holistic health model, **health** is seen as a dynamic state of being that, for each individual, moves back and forth on a continuum. Figure 3-1 illustrates this hypothetical and graduated scale, commonly called the **health-illness continuum.** This scale is intended to measure the total health picture as the individual perceives it—not as a judgment by the health care provider. **Wellness** is defined as ever changing growth toward fulfilling an individual's potential, considering individual needs, abilities, and disabilities.[3] A key assumption in holistic health is that the perception of health is an individual decision, promoting self-responsibility and self-control. Health and illness are not mutually exclusive, as defined within this model. A person with a disease process, such as cancer, may place himself at different places along the wellness continuum at different times—including optimal health if he feels he is functioning to his highest potential relative to his condition.

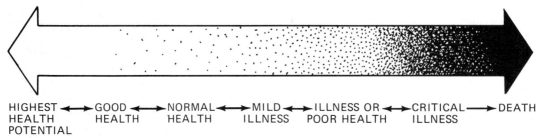

HIGHEST ⟷ GOOD ⟷ NORMAL ⟷ MILD ⟷ ILLNESS OR ⟷ CRITICAL ⟶ DEATH
HEALTH   HEALTH   HEALTH   ILLNESS   POOR HEALTH   ILLNESS
POTENTIAL

Figure 3-1.   The Health-Illness Continuum.

The holistic view of health has gained a great deal of popularity among health care professionals, particularly nurses. In addition to the symptoms and signs of illness, people who assess wellness look at a wide variety of health behaviors. Health behaviors are things a person does to understand his health state, maintain an optimal state of health, prevent illness and injury, and reach his maximum physical and mental potential. Behaviors such as eating habits, exercise, attention to signs of illness, following treatment advice, and avoiding known health hazards such as smoking are all examples. The ability to relax, emotional maturity, productivity, and self-expression are other examples that reflect one's total health picture.

A number of significant influences impact the health status and behavior of individuals, families, and groups of people. Among these are environmental influences, such as air and water pollution, educational level, occupation, income level, cultural influences including religion and family practices, and individual characteristics, such as age, physical and mental maturity, genetic factors, and personality. The geographic area in which one resides may affect health and behavior, e.g., affinity for natural disasters, such as floods and earthquakes, and dry climates versus tropical climates; each having characteristically high incidences of certain health problems. Additional societal factors (substance abuse), mass communica-

tion influences (TV advertising of health care products), and periods of political unrest (wars) may have a tremendous impact on health. The list of health behavior variables is almost inexhaustible when one considers the impact of the total environment as well as the inner workings of each individual. If nurses understand as much as possible about these influences and the resulting effects on their clients, they will be better able to communicate and carry out appropriate nursing actions.

Nurses give health care in a variety of settings; some emphasize a medical orientation to health, such as acute care facilities, and others emphasize a more holistic approach, such as primary care clinics, preventive health centers, and specialized agencies like birthing centers and hospices. Many health care institutions and agencies are a combination of both models of care, and it is often the individual practitioner who sets the tone and assists the client in gaining a realistic understanding of what "health" means in his circumstance.

Given nursing's long history of involvement in general health care and the close personal nature of the nursing role, holistic health and wellness represent new variations on an old theme. A main difference is increased vocal support by the public and other health care groups, and the continued demand for more personalized, total health care. The nursing profession is meeting this challenge.

A Definition of Nursing

Nursing has been defined in many ways and by many people since its earliest days. There are as many definitions of nursing as there are nursing leaders and state legislatures that license nurses.[4] Others that define nursing include schools of nursing, health care institutions, and professional organizations.

There was a time when nurses functioned primarily as physician's helpers. At the present time, independent and theory based practice are emergent characteristics of nursing. Figure 3-2 presents a number of selected definitions of nursing that reflect some of these changes and provide insight into how people define nursing.

Narrow and Buschle state that the content of a definition of nursing should meet the following criteria:

- description of its uniqueness
- consistency with current practices and laws
- reflection of a philosophy or set of beliefs.[5]

Throughout this textbook, the reader will learn about nursing relative to many specific concepts. Each concept contributes ideas that help to define nursing as it is viewed today and will shed light on one or more of the above criteria.

In 1980 the American Nurses' Association issued a public statement on the nursing profession that affirmed nursing's social responsibility and delineated the nature and scope of nursing practice. The following definition of nursing was asserted: *Nursing is the diagnosis and treatment of human responses to actual or potential health problems.*[6] This definition is one that maintains the orientation of nurses to the provision of care that promotes well-being in the people served and, at the same time, reflects the influence of nursing theory.

As with the concepts of health, wellness, and illness, each nurse eventually develops her own definition of nursing. An understanding of these concepts, and how each of the remaining concepts in the text interrelates with nursing will provide beginning nurses a basis from which to formulate their own definitions of nursing.

HISTORY OF NURSING

Early History

The history of caring for the sick is as old as mankind. Skeletons dating from the Neolithic period show evidence of amputations, tooth extraction, and opening of the skull surgically. Nursing originally developed to fulfill the needs of society, and to care for the sick and weak members of the group. Caring methods were based on what the people believed caused disease and injury and on what they believed about life. Over the years, technology changed what man believed and practiced, and as these changes occurred, changes occurred in care of the sick.

In the earliest records found, there is little evidence that nursing existed as a separate occupation, but it often was integrated as part of the practice of medicine men, priests, and priestesses, midwives, and wise women.[7,8] Care of the sick in the home was primarily delegated to the women in the family, but it was probably the duty of all the adults in the household to offer advice about care and treatment.

About 3500 B.C. an ancient Indian book used to record health and medical knowledge identified nurses as a special group of agents in the curing process. The nurses were rarely women, but their qualifications were similar to that of nurses today: knowledge, intelligence, responsibility, and high ethical standards.

SELECTED DEFINITIONS OF NURSING

Source	Definition
Florence Nightingale 1860	Nursing is a noncurative practice in which the patient is put in the best condition possible for nature to act.
Isabel Hampton Robb 1893	The hands of the nurse are the physician's hands lengthened out to minister to the sick. Her watchful presence at the bedside is a trained vigilance supplementing and perfecting his watchful care; her knowledge of his patient's condition an essential element in the diagnosis of disease; her management of the patient, the practical side of medical science. If she fails to appreciate her duties, the physician fails in the same degree to bring aid to his patient.
Education Committee for Curriculum Guide 1917	"Health" nursing is just as fundamental as "sick" nursing and the prevention of disease at least as important a function of the nurse as the care and treatment of the sick. . . . The nurse is essentially a teacher and an agent of health.
Committee on Curriculum of the National League of Nursing Education 1937	The word "nursing" can also be interpreted broadly to mean health conservation in its widest senses, including the care of normal children and adults; the nursing or nurture of the mind and spirit as well as the body; health education as ministration to the sick; the care of the patient's environment, social as well as physical; and health service to families and communities as well as to individuals.
Sister Olivia M. Gowan 1944	Nursing in its broadest sense may be defined as an art and a science which involves the whole patient—body, mind, and spirit; promotes his spiritual, mental, and physical health by teaching and by example; stresses health education and health preservation as well as ministration to the sick; involves the care of the patient's environment—social and spiritual as well as physical; and gives health service to the family and community as well as to the individual.
Frances Reiter 1961	. . . the nature of nursing . . . a disciplined art, an eclectic science and a personal service to patients that has long-term human value and social worth.
Virginia Henderson 1966	The unique function of the nurse is to assist the individual, sick or well, in the performance of those activities contributing to health or its recovery (or to peaceful death) that he would perform unaided if he had the necessary strength, will, or knowledge, and to do this in such a way as to help him gain independence as rapidly as possible.

Source	Definition
American Nurses' Association Committee for the Study of Credentialing in Nursing 1979	Nursing is defined as a health nurturing discipline: a field of study which encompasses the total occupation of nurturing the health of human beings, sick or well, through assistance with the activities that the human being cannot do or does not have the knowledge to do for himself, or to a peaceful death.
Dorothea Orem 1980	Nursing has as its special concern the individual's need for self-care action and the provision and management of it on a continuous basis in order to sustain life and health, recover from disease or injury, and cope with their effects.

Figure 3-2. Selected Definitions of Nursing.

References

Gertrude Torres, "Florence Nightingale" in *Nursing Theories,* (Englewood Cliffs: Prentice Hall, Inc., 180) p. 29.

Isabel A. Hampton, et al., "Educational Standards for Nurses" in *Nursing of the Sick, 1893.* Lucille Petry, consulting editor (New York: McGraw-Hill Book Co., 1949) pp. 2,3

The Education Committee of the National League of Nursing Education, *Standard Curriculum for Nursing Schools* (New York: The League, 1919).

Committee on Curriculum of the National League of Nursing Education, *A Curriculum Guide for Schools of Nursing* (New York: The League, 1937).

Sister Olivia M. Gowan, The Catholic University of America, School of Nursing, unpublished papers: 1944.

Frances Reiter, *Improvement of Nursing Practice* (New York: American Nurses Association, 1961).

Virginia Henderson, *The Nature of Nursing* (New York: The McMillan Co., 1966).

Committee for the Study of Credentialing in Nursing: A New Approach, Staff Working Papers Vol. II (Kansas City, Mo.: The American Nurses Association, 1979).

Dorothea E. Orem, *Nursing: Concepts of Practice,* 2nd ed. (New York: McGraw-Hill Book Company, 1980).

Medicine and caring for the sick were advanced by the ancient Egyptians chiefly by Imhotep, physician to the Pharaoh of the Third Dynasty. When Egypt came under Greek influence, the Greek and Egyptian philosophies of care for the sick were blended, and medicine advanced. Aesculapius, the greatest physician in Greek history, was made a god, and remains shrouded in mythology. The first person recorded to have contributed to medicine was Hippocrates (460–370 B.C.). His chief contribution to medicine was to change the concept of magic in medicine into a more concrete science. He taught physicians to use assessment skills to gather data about their patients rather than using the old practices based on myth and superstition.

Women began to care for the sick during the Greek era. Hygeia was the daughter of Aesculapius and later, goddess of health. She is said to have been the first to have provided health care for the sick in temples, where they came for her help. There is no written reference, however, to any organized nursing group at this time.

Judaism and Christianity considered the care of the sick and dependent a priority. Lay deaconesses, appointed by bishops of the early Christian church, visited the sick, much like today's visiting nurse. These appointments were highly esteemed and given to women of high social standing who provided nursing care as part of their humanitarian responsibilities. No formal education was expected or provided for these early nurses. It was assumed that the women used the skills they had acquired as wives and mothers. Gradually, the care of the sick and poor was assumed by a variety of religious orders.

During the Middle Ages (500–1500 A.D.), medicine in Europe was divided into two areas: lay medicine and ecclesiastical medicine; the latter centered around monasteries. As the Middle Ages advanced, the concept of nursing was identified and became an organized service. Three groups provided nursing services: military orders, regular orders, and secular orders. All of these groups worked under the auspices of the Roman Catholic church, which profoundly influenced all of their activities, since most of these religious nursing orders were founded for ministering purposes. It was during the Middle Ages that the first hospitals were built for the care of the sick.

The Military Orders. Certain military orders were founded to travel with and assist the crusaders, and the nursing knights were as skilled in the use of bandages as swords.[9] These knights were men from the Knights of St. John, the Teutonic Knights, and the Knights of St. Lazarus. There were three corresponding orders for women that tended female patients. The female nurses did not travel with the crusaders, but began hospitals in Europe.

The Regular Orders. Men and women of God established monasteries in which they organized hospices to care for orphans, the poor, and the sick. The uncertainty and insecurity of the Middle Ages caused people to seek protection behind moats and walls. Thus, nurses of this period cared for the institutionalized sick and did little to

bring nursing to the homebound.

The crusaders gained knowledge about illness from the Arabs, and the sick were separated and cared for, and the modern hospital had its origin. A small group of volunteer sisters in 650 A.D. began the Hotel Dieu (hospital) in Paris. This nursing order, the Augustinian Sisters, received no formal training (except for their apprenticeship), worked long hours, and were permitted no recreational activities. They provided basic care for their patients.

The Secular Orders. Secular orders were developed for the primary purpose of delivering nursing services to the ill and indigent. Individuals who entered these orders did not have to give up social standing, ties, relationships, or take vows of chastity. They primarily devoted their lives to a religious order in their home town without giving up rights as a citizen. One of the duties of these men and women was to provide nursing services in hospitals and homes. Many of the nurses were from wealthy or noble families and were highly educated in scriptures, philosophy, and language. In lay orders, no permanent vows were made, but nurses accepted year-long "contracts" instead. At the end of the designated time, they could rededicate, resign to marry, or take up another occupation.

The Reformation. Nursing continued much in the same manner up to the Protestant Reformation (beginning around 1500 A.D.). During this time, medicine underwent a renaissance. Leonardo da Vinci began a study of human anatomy. Many of his discoveries dispelled myths about illness, and care of the sick took a new direction. During this time, nursing reached a high level of organization in the religious, lay, and military orders. Unfortunately, these orders did not last, because during the Reformation, most religious orders were disbanded by the state, and the churches, monasteries, and hospitals were closed. In England alone, over 100 hospitals were closed, and no provision was made for care of the poor and the sick.[10]

When the demand for care of the sick became too great, hospitals were reopened under the direction of lay persons. However there was no honor in caring for the sick and gentlemen and gentlewomen no longer joined. Many of the new nurses were criminals, debtors, or other social outcasts. These "nurses," who were predominately women, worked off debts or jail sentences through nursing duties. They had no preparation or education in the care of the sick, and nursing entered its darkest days. There was little opportunity for advancement; work hours were long (sometimes extending to 48 hours at a time), the work hard, and the wages low. Nurses had no commitment to their patients, not to mention commitment to advancing the profession.

One final factor in the decline of the nursing profession during the age of Reformation was the social structure and the status of women within that structure. Under the auspices of the church, women had been given freedom to move about in society and were permitted to create careers for themselves. Nursing was seen as a noble occupation through which to contribute to society.

With the Reformation came a different view. A woman's place was seen as in the home, and nothing was felt to be more fulfilling than being a wife and a mother. Any designated women's work, such as care of the sick, would have been unthinkable to most women because of the social status of nursing. Another factor keeping women at home was the great amount of work required to obtain food and clothing and maintain a home. This left little free time for education or work outside of the home. Those women who were forced to work outside of the home usually entered domestic services. By leaving nursing to those who

could not receive employment elsewhere, nursing remained very much in the dark, not emerging again until the 18th century.

The Eighteenth Century. Social changes in the 18th century, caused primarily by the industrial revolution, brought about many needed changes in nursing. New lands were being settled during this time, and people began to immigrate to the European colonies in the new world.

Cities were built around manufacturing centers, and large numbers of workers were needed to build houses and factories and to work in the factories. As a result, large hospitals were required to accommodate the increased number of injuries and illnesses.

Prior to this period, society was more or less divided into the extremes of an upper and a lower class, with few individuals in between. As industrialization continued, a large middle class developed. With the rise of this middle class came a new social consciousness directed toward helping poor and lower class individuals who had great needs and few resources. As a result, the upper and middle classes began to engage in charitable acts, such as caring for the sick. The emancipation of women emerged along with general trends for personal freedom during the industrial revolution and this movement greatly assisted the evolution of nursing professionally.

The emancipation of women had four main facets: judicial, political, educational, and occupational. First, in order to be emancipated, women had to be equal with men in the eyes of the law. Second, women needed to be able to vote. Third, they needed to be able to be admitted to and educated in professional schools in order to enter the work force. Lastly, women needed access to the work force. These four facets could not have been carried out prior to the industrial revolution, which gave individuals more free time for pursuits beyond food gathering and basic family maintenance. Nursing might well have remained a task oriented craft without the strength and opportunity for advancement this movement provided.

The Nineteenth Century. During the 19th century, as a result of advances in medicine, social outcry regarding nursing, and the emancipation of women, nursing began to advance. The era of modern nursing began. In the British Isles, Ireland can be credited with the first systematic nursing institutions. These were the Irish Sisters of Charity started by Mary Aikenhead, and the Sisters of Mercy founded by Catherine M. Auley.

The need for better nurses was also identified in Germany around the same time. Theodor Fliedner, a minister, recognized the need for systematic training of nurses to care for the sick and, in 1836, bought a large house and converted it into a hospital. By 1842 the hospital had expanded to 200 beds with 120 nurses.

To be admitted to the Fliedner program, the prospective student had to be 18, in good health, and of high moral character. The course of study took three years to complete, and this program is considered to be the first of the systematically organized nursing schools.

The school and hospital flourished, and in 1846 Fliedner established nursing schools in London and, in 1850, Pittsburgh, Pennsylvania, and Milwaukee, Wisconsin. These schools were instrumental in advancing the idea of organized nursing education, and their excellent training programs did much to raise the level of nursing care and contribute to the respectability of nursing as a profession. Consequently, the profession of nursing was able to begin recruiting capable students from the middle and upper classes.

Florence Nightingale

Florence Nightingale is often referred to as the mother of modern nursing. Her contribution to nursing was profound, especially considering the status of nursing during her lifetime and the hardships of the time. She promoted health and hygiene, made reforms in military and civilian hospitals, and developed a philosophy of nursing based on wellness and health promotion.[11]

Born in Florence, Italy, in 1820, of wealthy parents, Florence Nightingale grew up in England. She was a gifted, precocious, and strong minded individual with a strong religious and social conscience.[12] Biographies differ as to when Miss Nightingale decided to enter nursing, but all agree on the factors that appear to have had the most influence upon her. First, "she became conscious of the harder side of life—of suffering, pain, and deprivation."[13] By 1843, she was caring for the sick and poor near one of her family's homes, much to the distress of her family. Her mother's reaction was, "Are you sure you would not like to be a kitchen maid?"[14] and her sister "declared that she was dying . . . and Florence's behavior was killing her."[15] The second influence on Nightingale was her Oxford prepared father who encouraged her and educated her as equally as the highly educated men of her day. Under his guidance, by the time she was 17 she had received an education in the classics, ancient and modern languages, literature, natural and social sciences, politics, economics, mathematics, and statistics. This home education was actually much like the curriculum in many colleges today and was a good basis for her later nursing practice. It also set her apart from the wealthy ladies of her era and as a consequence, she was bored with them and the passive role of women in Victorian England. In a monograph entitled *Cassandra*, Miss Nightingale described women as "sitting around a table in a drawing room, looking at paintings, doing worsted work and reading little books, or taking a little drive." When night comes Cassandra states "women suffer—

even physically . . . from the accumulation of nervous energy, which having had nothing to do during the day, makes them feel . . . as if they were going mad."[16]

The third influence was the visits she made with her mother to the sick. According to Woodham-Smith, a Nightingale biographer, "these sojourns initiated an unsatiable yearning in Nightingale to pursue this work in depth."[17] Stewart writes that, "even though she went into society and was wooed by highly eligible suitors, she never swerved from her early determination to study nursing. Partly to distract her from this idea, she was sent to the continent and there met a number of interesting and distinguished people who stimulated and broadened her interest in social reform. Wherever she went she studied social conditions, found how people lived, and noted what was being done to help them. She also visited . . . hospitals and nursing systems in many countries. . . ."[18]

In 1846, Nightingale learned of the Kaiserworth Deaconesses, a widely regarded health care institution in Germany, and she decided to devote herself to nursing. Aware that she lacked clinical education, she searched for an English agency that would be accepted by her family. Finally, in 1851 at age 31, parental consent was granted for a period of three months study at the Kaiserworth Deaconess in Germany under the excellent supervision of Pastor Fliedner and his wife. She was impressed with the organization and the purpose of this agency, but felt that her three-month education was not enough. In 1853 she enrolled with the Sisters of Charity in Paris, but became ill and had to leave. After this brief stay with the Sisters, she finally overruled her family and accepted the charge position in a private nursing home for sick governesses.

Her genius for nursing, politics, and organization became evident at once; she reorganized the nursing home. As soon as she had it running smoothly, Nightingale again visited hospitals, and at this point became interested in reforming nursing. She realized that before nursing reform could begin, some type of school for educating reliable and qualified nurses was needed. At the same time, she was being consulted by social reformers and physicians who were also beginning to see the need for qualified nurses. Plans for improving nursing education had to be put aside, however, because in 1854 a cholera epidemic broke out in England, and Florence Nightingale volunteered to care for the sick and dying. It was during this epidemic that she learned a great deal about epidemiology.

In 1854, war in the Crimea broke out. The British, French, and Turks were fighting against the Russians over possession of the Crimean Peninsula and access to the Black Sea. As the war progressed, it became apparent that the British military had organizational difficulties and was deficient in providing for the wounded.

Nightingale wrote to the Minister of War, Sidney Herbert, and volunteered her services. In October 1854, Florence Nightingale was appointed Superintendent of the Female Nursing Establishment of the English General Hospitals in Turkey.[19] She had 40 nurses in her charge when they landed at Scutari (New Istanbul) in November 1854. The hospital was overcrowded with wounded soldiers lying on the floor, still in their bloody uniforms. Supplies were virtually nonexistent, food was scarce, and plumbing and sewage were inadequate.

The nurses initially were refused admission to the wards by the physicians, but as the number of wounded and dying increased, the doctors turned to Nightingale and her nurses for assistance. Nursing and sanitary reforms initiated by Nightingale brought the death rate down from 42 to 2 percent within six months.[20]

She set up diet kitchens, established a laundry and a laboratory, and procured medical supplies and beds. She further reorganized the army service by starting a post office, so that soldiers and their families could communicate. She also began a savings fund for the men. She provided for rest and recreation, instituted care for the soldiers' families who had followed them to the war, and established convalescent camps. Once these units were thriving, Nightingale went to the front lines where she contracted Crimean fever (probably typhus or typhoid), and almost died. During her slow recovery, she consistently refused to leave the Crimea and left only when the last contingent of nurses left Scutari.

One of the important outcomes of the Crimean war was the conviction that nurses needed organized education. Nightingale's work was respected widely, and in 1855, the Duke of Cambridge set up the Nightingale Fund for the purpose of educating nurses. Due to another illness, it was several years before she actually established this first school of nursing. She never did fully recover from this undisclosed illness and apparently spent the rest of her life in self imposed isolation but worked unceasingly on nursing reform. In 1859 she published *Notes on Nursing*, to orient thinking on the meaning of nursing.[21] Finally, in 1860, a Nightingale School of Nursing was opened in conjunction with St. Thomas' Hospital in London. It was financed by the Nightingale Fund. Students were to be women of good character. The objective of the school was to educate nurses for hospital nursing, home visiting, and to produce nurses who were able to educate other nurses.

The entire program of education lasted one year and included medical and nursing lectures and supervised practice. Some of the concepts taught were revolutionary to the time and included mental health, family and community health, nutrition, hygiene, and general health promotion. Nightingale recognized pain and suffering as harmful to health, made observations about the value of sleep, and encouraged the use of color and flowers in hospitals.

Finally, Nightingale influenced modern nursing by developing her own philosophy of nursing, that nursing is an art that requires an organized, practical, and scientific basis for practice. She also felt that nurses are the "skilled servant in medicine, surgery, and hygiene, *not* the skilled servant of physicians. . . ."[22]

Through a life dedicated to nursing, Florence Nightingale set the stage for the evolution of modern nursing. Much of her basic philosophy has been incorporated into modern practice, and many of her principles are today's nursing goals: maintain health, maintain nutrition, observe accurately, provide a healthful environment, consider each person as an individual, and practice nursing as an art not, as a servant to others on the health care team.

NURSING IN AMERICA

While nursing was evolving in Europe, it was evolving in America as well. In colonial America there were no real hospitals. Most of the nursing care delivered to the sick was carried on in the home by the women of the household. Some areas of the colonies had more organized nursing services, some religiously influenced, but the details of their role is unclear. In New York City, "nurses" sought out the sick and provided comfort measures.[23] These so-called nurses had no formal education, primarily because no formal nursing schools existed in the American colonies.

During the 17th and 18th centuries, colonial hospitals began to open, as either almshouses or pesthouses, hospitals for contagious diseases.[24] These pesthouses were built in most of the major cities of the country to reduce the spread of disease.

As a rule, most physicians received their training as apprentices of practicing physicians, not in colleges or hospitals. At the end of the period of apprenticeship, the person was able to open his own practice. A few physicians, however, were educated in Europe, and by the close of the colonial days, two medical schools had been established in the colonies: The Medical College of Philadelphia in 1765, and the medical department of King's College in 1767.[25]

In later years, wars helped to advance the credibility of nursing services and the role of nursing, but at the time of the Revolutionary War, there was not even an identifiable group of nurses. Usually, women followed the men into battle and performed services, such as cooking, binding wounds, and helping with the ill. Chaplains were charged with the task of recommending cleanliness as a virtue conducive to health.[26] The idea of women as nurses, providing skilled nursing care on the battlefield, did not arise until the Crimean War, when Florence Nightingale took to the field with her group of nurses.

In 1751 the first real hospital was founded in Philadelphia, and other general hospitals soon followed. By 1850, many hospitals had been established but were thought of as agencies solely for the care of the sick and the poor. They were viewed as places for delivering care, not cures; infections and cross contamination were common occurrences. Nurses in these early hospitals were usually lower class women who regarded nursing the sick as drudgery rather than as a professional calling.[27]

In this period before the Civil War, medical standards declined as a result of a fast growing population, urbanization, poor sanitation, and few adequately educated physicians. By the time of the Civil War, Americans began to hear about Florence Nightingale and her work in the Crimean War. Within three weeks of the outbreak of the Civil War on April 14, 1861, 100 women had been selected to take a short nursing course to be able to assist the wounded.

Dorothea Lynde Dix (1803–1887), already well-known for her work on behalf of the mentally ill, was appointed as superintendent of the nurses. Although not a nurse herself, she earned this position for her unceasing humanitarianism. She established the first Nurse Corps of the United States Army. An allowance of $12 per month was paid to these nurses, who came mostly from either Protestant or Catholic orders.[28] Eventually 10,000 nurses participated in the Civil War, but not all of them were employed by the U.S. Army. Only about 3,000 of them served in this official capacity. Several hundred from religious orders served. A third group consisted of women hired to do menial hospital chores. A fourth group consisted of those wives, mothers, and sisters who initially became involved because they wished to take an active part in the conflict. This latter group served throughout the War and were unpaid. Other groups consisted of black nurses employed by the U.S. Government for $10 a month and women employed by various relief agencies.

In the South, there was no organized effort to obtain nurses, therefore the bulk of nursing duties was filled by infantrymen, who were detailed against their wishes to this type of duty.[29]

In the North, the nursing system had its defects, and physicians did not approve of women in hospitals or on the battlefield, but it was clear that the soldier patients were grateful for the nurses. The Civil War clearly established the need for nurses in the health care system and the need for organized nursing schools in the United States.

After the Civil War, nurses led a movement to establish nursing schools in the United States. During the postwar years, hospital schools of nursing began to develop. The instructors were generally physicians in these early schools, and instruction generally took place at the bedside. Based on the guidelines of the Nightingale Schools, the first American school for nurses' training was established in September 1872 at the New England Hospital for Women and Children in Boston, Massachusetts. The students worked from 5:30 am until 9:00 pm, and their rooms were located near the wards, so they could be called at night if they were needed.[30] In October 1873, the first diploma of nursing in the United States was awarded.

During the 1870s, other schools of nursing opened in New York, New Haven, and Boston. It was during this time that nurses adopted a standard nursing uniform consisting of a long dress of a somber color, white collar, cuffs, apron, and cap. This practice was begun partially for economical reasons and partially for neatness. By 1890 uniforms were an established custom, and each training school had a distinctive uniform, cap, and pin. Nurses continued to wear their uniform, cap, and pin after graduation. Patients and physicians began to recognize these and to equate them with the various schools. The distinctive cap and pin became a symbol of pride for nurses for the high standards of nursing education in their schools.[31,32] Today not all nurses wear caps, but many proudly wear their nursing school pin.

In 1893, the superintendent of nursing at the Farrand Training School at Harper Hospital in Detroit felt that nurses needed something beyond a uniform to direct their pride to nursing.[33] She led the committee that composed "The Florence Nightingale Pledge" (See Figure 3-3.) It was first used in 1893 by the graduating class. This pledge remains a part of nursing today, and many nurses recite it at a capping ceremony, dedication to nursing ceremony, or graduation. Although written nearly 100 years ago, it still clarifies many of the ideals of nursing today.

The Spanish-American War began in April 1898 and ended in August of the same year. The United States was unprepared for this war with Spain and had an army of only 28,000. The President sought congressional authorization to increase the Army's numbers to over 200,000. The Army, unable to supply trained hospital corpsmen so

I solemnly pledge myself before God, and the presence of this assembly: to pass my life in purity and to practice my profession faithfully. I will abstain from whatever is deleterious and mischievous, and will not take or knowingly administer any harmful drug. I will do all in my power to maintain and elevate the standard of my profession and will hold in confidence all personal matters committed to my keeping and all family affairs coming to my knowledge in the practice of my calling. With loyalty will I endeavor to aid the physician in his work and devote myself to the welfare of those committed to my care.[34]

Figure 3-3.   The Nightingale Pledge

quickly for such a large number, was forced to look elsewhere. At the time, a plan to organize a nurse corps was established. Thousands of applications were received from young and old, trained and untrained. Each application was processed and filed. Only those educated in a school of nursing were formally sought to fill positions as Army nurses. More than 1,500 were accepted and were paid $30 a month plus a ration allowance.

The Spanish naval squadron was defeated and the short war formally ended on August 12, 1898. The majority of soldiers were discharged, and the Army nurses were no longer needed. By 1900, only 202 nurses remained, but through the actions of influential women and prominent nurses, legislation was passed to establish the Army Nurse Corps permanently.[35] In 1908, the Navy established a Nurses Corps in much the same way.

During the early 20th century, millions of immigrants, mostly from Europe, flooded America. Many settled in the cities and took low-paying industrial jobs. This led to many public health problems. The already poor health care system was taxed beyond belief, as were sanitary and other municipal services. Crowded areas of cities degenerated into slums. Epidemics of typhus, scarlet fever, smallpox, and typhoid fever were rampant, and many died as a result of these and other communicable diseases.

Health conditions and historic happenings of this period gave rise to many new roles for nurses, and many nurses who would later become famous contributed during this time to nursing's struggle toward professionalism.

Early Leaders in American Nursing

During the late 19th and early 20th century, nursing began to emerge as a profession. Attention was paid to social welfare, and traditional roles of women were changing. Industry was growing, and cities were expanding. America was now ripe for the development of nursing education and nursing service.

A number of foresighted early nursing leaders struggled to make nursing a recognized and honored profession. These courageous women selflessly dedicated their lives and their careers to advancing nursing.

Isabel Adams Hampton Robb (1860–1910) was born in Ontario, Canada, where she attended public school. Later she began her career as a teacher, at the time, the only career acceptable for women.

This career did not satisfy her, however. She was restless and ambitious. At one point she told her sister that if she were a man, she would be Premier of Canada.[36]

She went to nursing school at Bellevue Hospital Training School in New York City in 1881, and was more interested in the academics related to nursing than the clinical application. Upon graduation, she worked for a short time as a supervisor of nursing and then spent about 1½ years as a staff nurse in Rome, caring for English and American travelers.

It was during this time that Hampton became convinced that nurses needed a firm foundation on which to build a clinical practice. After her return to the United States, she set as her goal the raising of standards of nursing education. She accepted a position as superintendent of the Illinois Training School for Nurses, where she introduced two important reforms. First, she planned the curriculum in graduated steps so that nursing students began with simple concepts and practices and advanced to complex. Second, she arranged for the students to affiliate with other hospitals to gain more experience.

When the Johns Hopkins Training School of Nurses was founded in Baltimore, Maryland, in 1889, she was appointed as its principal. There, she organized the work so that the students' day was limited to 12 hours, including two hours for recreation.[37]

In 1893, her reputation earned her the chairmanship of the nursing section of the Congress of Hospitals and Dispensaries. Within this organizational body, nursing leaders worked toward the formation of nursing associations. At the close of the Congress, she invited the superintendents of the training schools to join her in the formation of a nursing organization. This group called itself the American Society of Superintendents of Training Schools for nurses and was chaired by Miss Hampton, who subsequently served on the executive board.[38]

In July of 1894, Isabel Hampton married Dr. Hunter Robb.[39] Although her colleagues thought her marriage would interfere with her contribution to nursing, she continued in active pursuit of her hopes for the future of nursing.

Robb believed that staff nurses needed their own organization, and since the goals of the Superintendents were quite different, she organized a new group. In 1896, she became the first president of the new nursing organization, the Nurses Associated Alumnae of the United States and

Canada. After the birth of her son, she helped establish university affiliation for nursing education.

At the turn of the century, Robb made another valuable contribution to nursing when she became one of the founders of the *American Journal of Nursing*. In 1910, Isabel Hampton Robb died at age 50 in a street accident. She had been active in nursing for almost 30 years and made a great contribution in assisting nursing to emerge into a profession.

Mary Adelaide Nutting (1858–1948) was a graduate of the first class of the Johns Hopkins Training School for nurses. Later as superintendent of this school, she carried out many of the reforms begun by her predecessor. In 1896, she established the three-year curriculum, the eight-hour day for student nurses, and abolished the monthly allowance they received.[40]

Miss Nutting firmly believed that nursing education needed two major reforms: provision of financial support for schools of nursing, and separation of the nursing schools from the hospital nursing service department. Both of these are beliefs held by nurses at present.

Mary Adelaide Nutting's contributions to nursing were diversified. She is remembered in particular for her collection of historical works of nursing; *The History of Nursing*, a four-volume work coauthored with Lavinia Dock; the creation of the Department of Nursing and Health at Teachers College, Columbia University, the first professional school of nursing in the world; her interest in nursing organizations throughout the world; and the development of the International Council of Nurses.

Lillian Wald (1867–1940) was a pioneer in the field of public health nursing. She was born in Ohio, and received a good education, according to the standards of the day. In 1889, she entered the New York Hospital School of Nursing and graduated two years later. She worked in nursing for a short time and then entered medical school which she later dropped out of to help the destitute sick. She related the following story:

> "A little girl led me . . . between . . . reeking houses . . . past odorous fishstands for the streets were a market place . . . unclean, . . . past evil smelling, uncovered garbage cans, . . . where so many little children played. The child led me through a tenement hallway . . . and . . . into the sickroom. All the maladjustments of our [society] . . . seemed epitomized in this . . . journey and what was found at the end of it. Although the sick woman lay on a wretched, unclean bed, soiled with a hemorrhage two days old, they were not deranged human beings. . . . That morning's experience was a baptism of fire. Deserted were the laboratory and the academic work of the calling. I never returned to them . . . conditions such as these were allowed because people did not know, and for me there was a challenge to know and tell . . . such horrors would cease to exist."[41]

In 1893 Lillian Wald, along with her classmate Mary Brewster, founded the Henry Street Settlement in the tenement district of New York. The purpose of the Settlement was to improve the lives of the poor using a variety of methods. The nurses who worked out of the house on Henry Street, visited the sick, concerned themselves with living conditions, and sought to keep school children healthy.

Lillian Wald was also a public crusader and an avid fundraiser. She was an accomplished speaker and was interested in the election of political officials who would assist the poor with legislation geared toward correcting those problems she, as a nurse, perceived. Her interest and influence led to the development of courses in public health at Columbia University.

Wald had many ideas about how nurses could help people stay well, and the development of the nursing service of the Metropolitan Life Insurance Company and the Town and Country Nursing Service of the American Red Cross are both credited to her.[42] She also introduced the concept of school nursing.

In 1912, Wald founded the National Organization of Public Health Nursing and was its first president. She encouraged the federal government to promote child health. Wald was truly a farsighted individual who did much to improve the health of the people and promote the concept of public health nursing.

Lavinia Lloyd Dock (1858–1956), another important nurse leader, was born in 1858 in Pennsylvania. Both of her parents were well educated, and they educated all of their children equally. When she chose to enter nursing, the community in which she lived was shocked. One person exclaimed "but I always thought the Dock girls were ladies."[43]

In 1886, after graduation from the Bellevue Training School for Nurses in New York City, she became the night supervisor there. She observed the difficulties that student nurses had with drugs and solutions and wrote one of the first pharmacology texts for nurses, *Materia Medica for Nurses*.[44] The book was extremely successful, selling over 100,000 copies.[45]

Lavinia Dock met Isabel Hampton during her years at Bellevue, and when Hampton became superintendent at Johns Hopkins, she asked Dock to be her assistant. Later she joined Lillian Wald in the Henry Street Settlement. She was highly committed to social reform and had a strong feeling for the poor in the New York slums. Miss Dock confronted legislators but became disillusioned when she found that women had little power and, consequently, little influence. She concluded that only the vote would bring power to women, and she devoted more than 20 years to this cause.

Miss Dock was a pacifist. She was the editor of the *American Journal of Nursing's* Foreign Department during World War I and never mentioned the war, to demonstrate her protest.

As she grew older she retired from nursing but always remained alert. She fell and fractured her hip in March 1956, when she was 98, and died one month later. She campaigned during her life for the benefit of nurses, women, and mankind. She was one of the great women leaders in the early part of this century.

Annie W. Goodrich (1876–1955) graduated in 1892 from the New York Hospital Training School for Nurses, and became an outstanding educator, taking many important teaching and superintendent positions in New York City. In 1910 she became a state inspector of nurse training schools in New York City, and in 1914, an assistant professor at Teachers College, Columbia University.

During those years she worked with other nursing leaders in national and international nursing organizations to develop nursing into a profession. Internationally recognized for her excellence in nursing, she served as president of the International Council of Nurses (ICN) from 1912–1915.

In 1916 she became the director of the Visiting Nurse service of the Henry Street Settlement. During these years she worked closely with both Adelaide Nutting and Lillian Wald. The three women were known as "The Great Trio," because of their deep involvement with the movement of nursing toward professionalism.

In 1918, Goodrich was granted a leave of absence from Henry Street to make a survey of U.S. Army military hospitals with nursing departments. Later that year, when the U.S. Army organized a nursing school, she was appointed its first dean. She was also one of the founders of the Vassar Training Program during World War I.

The need for nurses was great during World War I and an appeal was sent out to college women to assist in the war effort; Vassar College offered its facilities. The two-year program with a 12-week preclinical summer session influenced by Adelaide

Nutting. After this course, students were assigned to general hospitals as regular students. The response was overwhelming. Four hundred and thirty women from 115 colleges in 41 states answered the call. Their enthusiasm made the program extremely successful and created an interest in nursing in colleges and universities throughout the country.[46]

After World War I, Annie Goodrich returned to Henry Street and to nursing education. She was selected as dean at the Yale University School of Nursing and remained there until her retirement in 1934. In that year she was also elected president of the newly formed Association of Collegiate Schools of Nursing.

Isabel Maitlana Stewart (1878–1963) was born in Canada and educated in the public schools. She taught in local schools before entering nursing at the Winnipeg General Hospital Training School. She graduated in 1903 and practiced as a private duty nurse, district nurse, and nursing supervisor.

She was attracted to the United States by an article in the *American Journal of Nursing* written by Adelaide Nutting. She entered a curriculum in hospital economics at Teachers Hospital, Columbia University, in 1908, and in 1913, she was the first nurse to receive a master's degree from that institution. She remained at Columbia throughout her career, finally succeeding Adelaide Nutting as the Helen Hartley Foundation Professor of Nursing Education, and as director of the department in 1925. She retained this position for 22 years.

She was interested in new developments in nursing and nursing education, and her greatest contribution to nursing was as an educator. She felt that students should receive some formal nursing education before entering the clinical area.

Isabel Stewart was a member and officer of many professional organizations. The idea of the Association of Collegiate

Schools of Nursing (ACSN) is credited to her. She was active in the National League for Nursing Education (NLNE) and the International Council of Nurses.

Isabel Stewart was interested in developing a standard curriculum for nursing and did much of the NLNE work that produced the Curriculum Guide in 1917 (later revised in 1927 and 1937). This guide was used during World War I to develop the Army Training School for Nurses. She served as chairperson of the Vassar Training Camp Program throughout World War I.

During World War II, she chaired several important committees of the National Nursing Council for War Service and was quite forceful in bringing about the Cadet Nursing Corps.

During these years she authored several books and pamphlets and, in 1916, became the first editor of the Department of Nursing Education of the *American Journal of Nursing*.

In 1963, Isabel Maitland Stewart died following a heart attack at her home. She was 85. This leader in the field of nursing worked long and hard to improve the level of nursing education in the United States and the world. In her honor, the Department of Nursing Education at Teachers' College, Columbia University, established the Isabel Stewart Professional Chair in Nursing Research.

Julie Catherine Stimson (1881–1948) was born in New England and received an education in the public schools in St. Louis, Missouri. She received a B.A. from Vassar in 1902 and then continued her studies in biology at California University. She met Annie Goodrich, was impressed with her, and as a consequence, she entered the New York Hospital Training School in 1908. In 1917, Stimson received an M.A. in sociology, biology, and education at Washington University in St. Louis, Missouri, making her extremely well-educated as a nurse.

Stimson's first nursing job was as the Superintendent of Nurses at Harlem Hospital. There she became aware of the health needs of the poor, and developed a social service department at that hospital.

She went on to become the Superintendent of Nurses at Barnes and Children's Hospital from 1913 to 1917 where she also established social services departments.

In 1917, Julia Stimson became an Army nurse and was sent to France to work with the English forces where she became the Chief Red Cross nurse in France. After World War I ended, Annie Goodrich, Dean of the Army Training School asked Stimson to take over that position. She did and held the position until 1933 when the school closed. In addition to this role, she became the Superintendent of the Army Nurse Corps.

With the help of legal advisors, military advisors, the public, and the Votes for Women Amendment to the Constitution (1920), the Army nurses appealed to Congress for a change in status. They were victorious and were accorded officer rank, Miss Stimson receiving the rank of Major. It was not until World War II, however, that nurses received full rank privileges and salaries on the same basis as the men.

Major Stimson did much to raise the public image of the nurse and played an important role in recruiting college-educated women for the Army Nurse Corps.

After retiring from the Army she was active in both the National League for Nursing and the American Nurses' Association. With the outbreak of World War II she returned to serve as a recruiter for the Army Nurse Corps and received the rank of Colonel, the first woman to achieve this rank.

Mary May Roberts (1877–1959) was born in Michigan, grew up in a small town, and received a public school education. She graduated first in her class from high school and desired a college education, but the family could not afford it. Although her father did not really want her to be a nurse, she entered the Jewish Hospital Training School for Nursing in Cincinnati, Ohio and graduated in 1899.

Her early career was spent in a variety of positions: clinic nurse, assistant superintendent, and private duty nursing. During World War I she joined the American Red Cross and recruited nurses, and later served as chief nurse at the Army School of Nursing at Camp Sherman, Ohio.

She returned to school, fulfilling an earlier dream, and obtained a B.S. degree from Teachers College at Columbia University. Upon graduation in 1921 she was appointed as coeditor of the *American Journal of Nursing*. In 1923, she was named editor, a position she retained until retirement in 1949. Under her watchful eye the *Journal* weathered the storms of the depression and World War II, increasing its circulation from 20,000 to 100,000.

Her goal was to produce a quality, literary journal directed to nurses at the bedside. She wanted nurses kept abreast with the latest developments in science and in the profession, and learned of her readers' needs by questioning them directly or by letter and telegram. She used the *Journal* to publish and support the Goldmark Report of 1923. (See Landmark studies.) After her retirement she wrote a book on the history of American nursing.

Stella Goostray (1886–1969) was born in the United States and educated in the public school system in Boston. She entered the work force as an assistant editor for an Episcopal magazine. When the United States entered World War I she entered nursing school hoping to be assigned to Europe. She began her studies in Boston, but contracted typhoid fever and had to drop out; she was strong enough to reenter in 1917 and graduated in 1920.

Miss Goostray entered Teachers College when Adelaide Nutting was teaching nursing administration there. She and Mary Roberts were classmates. In 1926 she earned a B.S. degree. During the years that she was completing her degree requirements at Teachers College, she took a position as an instructor at the Philadelphia General Hospital (PGH) School of Nursing.

She returned to Boston in 1926 and assumed the position of Superintendent of both the Children's Hospital School of Nursing and the Nursing Service of the hospital, where she remained until 1946.

Her contributions to nursing included improving the quality of nursing education and nursing service by hiring more qualified nurses and introducing auxiliary workers into the health care system.

Nationally, Stella Goostray was on the NLNE's education committee, was on the Board of directors of ANA, and was a member of the board of directors of *American Journal of Nursing*. She also served as chair for the Subcommittee on Nursing at the White House Conference on Child Health and Protection (1930).[48]

She was interested in the accreditation of schools of nursing and served on the Committee on the Grading of Nursing Schools. In 1933 her masters thesis dealt with the significance of accreditation. From 1942 until 1946 she chaired the National Council for War Services which planned nursing services during World War II.

In addition to all of her other roles she contributed to nursing literature by writing at least seven books with content ranging from mathematics, pharmacology, and chemistry to histories of nursing.

Helen Lathrop Bundge (1906–1969) was born and educated in Wisconsin. Miss Bundge went on to study at the University of Wisconsin from which she received a B.A. in sociology in 1928. In 1930 she received a Graduate Nurse Certificate from the same institution.

Upon graduation she became head nurse at Wisconsin General Hospital and later taught at the School of Nursing at the University of Wisconsin where she became assistant director.

She was awarded a M.A. in 1936 and earned an Ed.D. in 1949 from Teachers College. While at Teachers College she was a student of Isabel Stewart and was noticed by Adelaide Nutting.

The major thrust of Helen Bundge's contribution to nursing was in the area of nursing research. In 1952 the Rockefeller Foundation established the Institute of Research and Service in Nursing Education and she was appointed as its director. She believed that it was every nurse's role to contribute to nursing's body of knowledge through research.[49]

It was through her interest in informing nurses about nursing research that the prestigious journal, *Nursing Research*, came into being in 1952. She became its first editor and chairman of the 23 member editorial board. This journal continues to remain a well-respected publication in today's nursing literature.

Lydia Williams Hall (1906–1969) was born in New York and grew up in Pennsylvania. She graduated in the 1920s from the York (Pennsylvania) School of Nursing, and later earned a B.S. in public health nursing and an M.A. in natural science from Teachers College, Columbia University.

She later held a position as instructor at the York School of Nursing and as a pediatric supervisor. After moving to New York she worked as a staff nurse, head nurse, and supervisor at both St. Mark's Hospital and the Visiting Nurse Service of New York.[50]

Lydia Williams married Reginald Hall, and continued to be active in nursing, developing an interest in chronicity and rehabilitation. Although an administrator and an educator she was most noted for her interest in nursing theory. She began her theory development in the 1950s when there were no known or published nursing theorists. One of her colleagues at Columbia, Hildegard Peplau, published her own first writings in 1952. Dorothy Johnson's writings appeared in 1959 and Ida Orlando and Martha Rogers' in 1961.[51]

Mrs. Hall believed that nursing practice should be based on a theoretical framework. She also believed that nurses should develop their own theories and not have another discipline define a framework for them. Both of these ideas are widely accepted and supported by nurses today.

She developed her theory and implemented it at the Loeb Center for Nursing and Rehabilitation of Montefore Hospital and Medical Center in New York in 1963. One of the major forces of her framework in nursing autonomy.

These nursing leaders are but a few of the women who dedicated their lives to bringing nurses and nursing into the arena of professionalism. Others have worked within their various places of employment, within the professional organizations, and through the political process to strengthen and advance the state of nursing. Every hospital and every school of nursing has had behind it a nurse who strove to upgrade the professional status of nursing and bring it into the 20th century as a viable and autonomous profession.

It is also important to mention that great numbers of women who chose to work as staff nurses made their professional contributions within hospitals and the community. Throughout the first half of the century these nurses often worked under difficult employment conditions and societal prejudices, yet continued to carry on a hopeful and growth inspiring spirit regarding their profession.

HISTORIC LANDMARK STUDIES IN NURSING

Evaluation is an important aspect of the activities of any professional group or occupation. Around the turn of the century, there began what was to become a series of landmark evaluation studies in nursing and nursing education. With the coming of industrialization, the demand for adequate health care increased rapidly, as social, political, and economic changes affected people's values and lifestyles in the 20th century. The early work of Florence Nightingale and her philosophy of patient care had enlightened people to the realities and possibilities of better health care, particularly within the hospital setting. Nurses, as a group, were becoming more visible, and they began to distinguish themselves as an essential part of the health care system.

There have been numerous efforts to examine the practice of nursing and to evaluate the methods of nursing education. Unfortunately, relatively few studies have come to the attention of the nation or had a significant impact on the development of the profession. Those that have generally are referred to as landmark nursing studies.

The Goldmark Report

Prior to World War I nursing had been severely criticized by medical groups, which either believed nurses were undertrained or overtrained, and all believing that the profession was failing to produce nurses prepared to provide quality patient care.[52] Nursing leaders, however, identified the need for broader educational programs to prepare nurses for roles in the expanding health care system, but their requests went unheeded. In 1911, several nurses appealed to the Carnegie Foundation to conduct an impartial, scientific study of the system of nursing education similar to the Carnegie Foundation's study of medical education (The Flexner Report) completed the year before.[53] In 1912, Adelaide Nutting reported poor education practices and substandard living and working conditions in nursing schools throughout the country.[54] Her report had little impact at the time, but it brought attention to the plight of nursing education.

In 1918, Nutting brought her concerns about nursing and nursing education to the Rockefeller Foundation, highlighting the lack of nurses to provide adequate public health nursing. This meeting brought about the establishment of the Committee for the Study of Nursing Education. This group, made up of doctors, nurses, and individuals interested in public health was chaired by C.E.A. Winslow of Yale University, but most of the work was done by his secretary, a social researcher, Ruth Goldmark. The final report of this committee, known as the Goldmark Report, became the first landmark study of nursing. Originally, the committee had been established to study the educational requirements of public health nursing, but because of the complexity of nursing, it was expanded in 1920 to include all of nursing. The Committee was given the charge to "survey the entire field occupied by the nurse and other workers of related type; to form a conception of the tasks to be performed and the qualifications necessary for their execution and on the basis of such a study . . . to establish sound minimum educational standards for each type of nursing service for which there appears to be a vital social need.[55]

Due to the constraints of time and money, only 23 representative hospital schools of nursing and 49 public health agencies were analyzed. The results of this study were published in 1923, and many conclusions were drawn from the findings:

1. Public health was a neglected subject.
2. Public health was an attractive field and efforts should be made to attract young women of high credentials.
3. Attempts to lower educational standards would bring danger to the public.
4. Steps should be taken for the definition and licensure of a subsidiary level of nursing service, possibly to assist under the direction of the trained nurse.
5. Hospital training schools were not organized on a basis conforming to the standards accepted in other fields and nursing education was frequently sacrificed for hospital services.
6. It was possible to reduce the period of hospital training to 28 months if students had to meet the criteria of a high school diploma for admission into nursing school, therefore attracting students of high quality.
7. Leaders in nursing should receive additional training beyond basic nursing courses.
8. Strengthening university schools of nursing for training leaders was important to further nursing education.
9. When licensure of a subsidiary grade of nursing was provided, schools for training should be established.
10. Development of adequate nursing service was dependent on securing funds for the development of nursing education.

These conclusions encompassed all of nursing practice, and although the suggestions were constructive, the report criticized all phases of nursing. The Committee's findings were not widely published, so the public remained uninformed as to the conditions in nursing and the need for change.

Although the Report failed to initiate changes in nursing, it led to endowment of the Yale University School of Nursing by the Rockefeller Foundation.

The Grading Committee Report

The Committee in the Grading of Nursing Schools was established in 1926 in conjunction with the National League of Nursing Education, the American Nurses Association, the National Organization for Public Health Nursing, American Medical Association, American College of Surgeons, American Hospital Association, and American Public Health Association. May Burgess was appointed as its director. She was regarded highly by nurses and other health care providers.

The stated purpose of the Committee was to "study the ways and means for ensuring an ample supply of nursing services, of whatever type and quality needed for an adequate care of the patient, at a price within his reach."[57] This included grading schools, studying the work of nurses, defining the duties falling within the realm of nursing practice, identifying supply and demand for nursing service, and the problems of public health nursing.

The original purpose of the Committee, the grading of nursing schools, "meant that certain minimum standards agreed to by the Committee had to be met by the school if they were to be considered qualified to prepare graduates for the nursing profession. It was impossible to decide minimum standards until it was known what abilities graduate nurses should possess, and those abilities could not be determined until it was understood what the graduate would be called on to do in practice."[58] Therefore, grading had to be based on a careful study of nursing education and nursing practice.

Based on the above decision, the Committee planned to divide its goals into three projects: a study of supply and demand for graduate nurses, an analysis of what nurses did and how they should be prepared, and the grading of schools of nursing. The Committee planned to carry each goal to completion and publish the findings in separate reports. The Committee worked for seven years and produced three reports: *Nurses, Patients, and Pocketbooks*, in 1928, *An Activity Analysis of Nursing*, in 1934, and *Nursing Schools Today and Tomorrow*, also in 1934.

The first report, *Nurses, Patients, and Pocketbooks*, was 600 pages long and identified the problems of supply and demand of nursing service and made recommendations to improve the economic problems of the emerging nursing profession.

In the process of gathering data on the nursing schools, the Committee found that requirements for entry into nursing school were minimal, many not even requiring a high school diploma; the dropout rate was quite high; many schools were small and associated with hospitals that were too small to provide an adequate clinical experience; the student workday was long and the work week longer than in other professions; and the number of qualified instructors was extremely low. These findings demonstrated that nursing schools existed in order to staff hospitals and not to educate nurses.[59] Furthermore, the study found a tremendous number of undereducated nurses, leading to chronic unemployment in the field. Salaries were low, hours long, and working conditions poor. Complaints of a nursing shortage were based on maldistribution of nurses, and nurses not qualified to meet the identified health care needs.[60]

Recommendations of the Committee included:

- Reduce and improve the number of nurses.

- Replace students with graduate nurses in the hospitals.

- Help hospitals meet the costs of employing graduate nurses.

- Get public support for the above.

The results of this report were well received by nursing, medicine, and the public, because of the variety of groups represented on the Committee and the large number and distribution of nursing schools that were surveyed.

The second report, *An Activity Analysis of Nursing* (1934), found that job analysis was essential before nursing schools could be graded. The Committee wanted to learn what nurses actually did and the knowledge base necessary for performance in order to improve and standardize the educational programs in schools across the nation.

In 1934, the final report, *Nursing Schools Today and Tomorrow*, was published. This work, the grading of schools, was based on the information gathered in the two preceding reports. Once the essentials that constituted a good school of nursing were selected, schools were contacted for information concerning their curricula. Then they were ranked, based on their response to a self-report questionnaire. This enabled the Committee to be objective, because the score was based on statistical data. The final grade received by each school was based on each school's comparative standing on each item studied, indicating where it stood in relation to the top school. [61] Three separate gradings were done on nursing schools nationwide, but school participation was strictly voluntary. A school was only graded by its own request. The Committee did not so much desire the assigning of a rank to the school, but to stimulate a desire in the school to seek improvements where they were needed.[62] Because the Committee hoped that schools would improve, each school grading was actually a series of gradings over a period of years, so that it was possible for schools to build stronger programs over time. The purpose was to reward good schools and to help poor schools recognize their limitations and correct them. Any reforms were made voluntarily, since the Committee had no enforcing power.

The first report grading was complete in 1929, the second in 1933, and the final survey in 1934. Between the first and second study, most schools improved their standing in 75 percent of the items on the questionnaires. The third survey showed even more improvement which was really promising given the economic depression of the era.[63]

Nursing for the Future (The Brown Report 1948)

The Brown Report, considered to be the third landmark study about the status of nursing in the United States, was prompted by conditions inside and outside the field that had caused shortages of nursing. Over 18,000 copies of Brown's book were sold during the first eight months.[64] Social legislation of the 1930's and World War II gave rise to public demands for quality health care, while nursing schools continued to have difficulty attracting qualified students. Nursing leaders concluded that there was something chronically wrong with the system of nursing education. Findings from the two earlier reports had not been used effectively, and nursing leaders were determined to correct this with the results of a third study.[65]

The Brown Report was funded by a grant to the National Nursing Council from the Carnegie Corporation in 1947. Esther Lucille Brown, a distinguished social anthropologist was appointed as director of the study. The purpose of this study was to learn who should organize, finance, administer, and control professional nursing to meet the needs of the community, not the profession.[66] The committee also considered the probable nature of nursing in the second half of the 20th century, and set the stage for research in nursing itself and in nursing as a part of overall health programs.[67]

Dr. Brown gathered data by making two major trips across the United States, visiting 50 representative schools in all parts of the country; held conferences in Washington, D.C., Chicago, and San Francisco with 1,200 directors of nursing schools; and met with nurses, doctors, administrators, trustees, and university members about the current status and future prospects of nursing.[68]

The Report pointed out the following needs: a study of nursing functions; building integrated nursing service teams; use of nonprofessional teams; mandatory licensing of practical nurses; expanded and improved inservice education; establishment of procedures and standards for state accrediting of nursing schools; establishment of a system for recognizing excellence in nursing practice to raise the status of the profession; and adequate financing of nursing education.[69]

The study recommended: that the term "professional education" be restricted to schools that furnish professional education (universities, colleges, or hospitals with institutions of higher learning), and that the term "professional nurse" be applied only to nurses who graduate from such a school; increasing social contributions of hospitals to nursing education; that financial structure and organization, adequate in facilities and faculties, be distributed to serve the nursing needs of the nation; a variety of other recommendations directed toward reorganizing nursing education and service.

No other publication had aroused such interest, and such alarm from those who felt threatened by the findings and recommendations.

AMERICAN NURSING IN THE TWENTIETH CENTURY

This century has seen the rise of the professional organizations, advances in nursing education, landmark studies, expansion of the nurse's role, the creation of nursing publications, the expansion of sci-

ence and technology, and the women's movement. All of these factors have an enormous positive impact on modern nursing, and promises to do so in the future. In addition, a number of specific historic events had effects on the professional evolution of nursing during this time frame.

World War I (1914–1918)

Wars often provide the impetus for change and growth in science, technology, and medicine. This has been true for nursing as well. World War I began in Europe in 1914. Shortly after the United States became involved in the War, in 1917 members from the American Nurses' Association, and the National League of Nursing Education, met to establish the role that American nurses would take in the war and sent President Woodrow Wilson information about the support of American nurses in the war effort.[70] At the beginning of World War I, about 400 nurses were in the Army Nurse Corps. In the next 1½ years, this number increased to 21,000[71] through recruitment and participation of the reserves from the American Red Cross, under the direction of Jane Delano. Of these, 10,000 served overseas. They did not have military rank as officers, but were subject to military law and had some of the privileges of the military.

During World War I, the United States experienced a shortage of nurses, so the Army opened schools of nursing at all of the major camp hospitals. There, students gained their clinical experiences. Annie Goodrich served as dean of the first school. Because of her philosophy of nursing, the students received more classroom instruction and less clinical experience.[72] By 1921, this program had graduated 500 students. By 1932, these schools were closed due to the financial pressures of the great depression.

The Vassar Training School was another federally funded nursing education program during World War I. Four hundred and thirty college students enrolled in this training program. Stimulated by this interest, another 50 colleges were planning similar programs when the war ended.[73] As the war ended, so did the desire to found such schools.

Another project created by the Red Cross to improve the nursing shortage situation was the training of nurses' aides. Over 2,000 women were recruited, but only 250 of these eventually served overseas.[74] Courses were designed to prepare the average housewife to care for the homebound sick, and teach them hygiene and simple nursing procedures. Nursing organizations were against this program, however, feeling that this reinforced the public's image of nursing as women's work, requiring little education, instead of an emerging profession, requiring extensive education and preparation.

Post-World War I

Nurses began to recognize their impact as a group during the postwar years. Emphasis on health increased, and the field of public health nursing developed. Nursing services were established in the Hospital

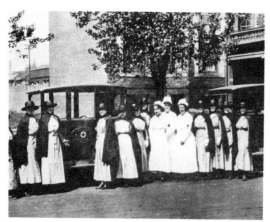

Figure 3-4. Public Health Nursing in Detroit, Michigan in 1918. .

Courtesy American Red Cross

Division of the United States Public Health Service in 1919, the Veterans Bureau in 1922, and the Indian Bureau in 1924. Red Cross nurses also were developing public health projects in areas where local resources were deficient.

Also, because of the war, public attention and interest were directed to nursing. During these years, we see the rise of universities sponsoring nursing courses, the endowment of schools (Yale, Western Reserve), the development of the Association of Collegiate Schools of Nursing, the employment of nurses in industry, nursing service in the federal government, and the landmark studies.

The Depression

The stock market crash of 1929 created widespread unemployment across the nation, and nurses were no exception. Although the need for qualified nurses increased, employers did not have the financial resources to hire them. Up to this time, a great number of nurses had been employed as private duty nurses, but now potential clients no longer had the means to employ them. Hospitals continued to use students for service because they were cheaper to hire than graduate nurses. Consequently, many nurses were without jobs.

Nursing organizations set aside their vested interests and formed the Joint Committee on the Distribution of Nursing Services to find solutions to the problems facing professional nursing. The government, through the establishment of the National Recovery Act (NRA) and the Works Progress Administration (WPA), was able to provide some jobs for nurses.

Nursing organizations decided on several ways to ease the unemployment situation. One strategy was to close small, inferior schools, which reduced the number of graduating nurses each year and stimulated increased interest in standards of care. It also created a need for graduate nurses to fill the positions previously filled by students. Another strategy was to reduce the workday from 12 to 8 hours. In addition, new government health programs were generated.[75,76]

Additional benefits for nurses came with the passage of the Social Security Act in 1935, which provided pensions to the aged, unemployment insurance, payments to the disabled, dependent mothers, and children, and an expanded health program. This newly established program was administered through the U.S. Public Health Service and the Children's Bureau and provided job opportunities in public health for nurses.[77] Another development that occurred simultaneously involved the epidemiology of chronic disease. Chronic illness began to be associated with advanced age and replace communicable diseases as the leading cause of death. This, coupled with the growth of hospital insurance programs, brought more patients into hospitals, which in turn provided many more jobs in nursing and helped to change the focus of professional nursing from private duty to hospital nursing.

World War II

The United States officially entered World War II following the attack on Pearl Harbor on December 7, 1941. Hospital nurses were in great demand as were nurses for the war industry and the military. This was also the time of the baby boom in the United States, and nurses were needed to care for mothers, infants, and children in the community and in the schools. Training of volunteers and teaching refresher courses for inactive nurses, the federal funding (Bolton Nurse Training Act) of nurse scholarship, and the development of the Cadet Nurse Corps[78] all were suggested as solutions to the nursing shortage.

Students admitted into the Cadet Nurse Corps attended one of the 1,125 participating schools and had all of their expenses— tuition, books, maintenance, uniforms, and monthly stipend—paid for by the United States Public Health Service.[79] In order to qualify for the Cadet Corps, candidates had to be between the ages of 17 and 35, in good health, and have good academic records from high school. Once the program ended, they had to work actively in nursing at either civilian health care agencies or in the military.

The Bolton Nurse Training Act, which established the Cadet Nurse Corps, allowed selected nursing programs to graduate students six months earlier than the traditional 36-month-long course. In order to meet state board requirements, however, another six-month period of education was needed. To meet this requirement, three levels of Cadets were established: pre-cadets, junior cadets, and senior cadets. Pre-cadets were those students in the first nine months in school. They spent this time learning the basic sciences and fundamentals of nursing. The next 15 to 21 months were spent as junior cadets, and they advanced through an accelerated curriculum. Senior cadets had finished their formal education and, in order to meet state board requirements, were assigned a practice assignment in a civilian, military, or federal health care agency.[80,81]

The government spent $184 million in direct federal aid from 1942 to 1948. This expenditure allowed for great achievements in nursing. Eighty-seven percent of all nursing schools across the nation participated in the Corps. Student enrollment ranged from 85,000 in 1940, to 129,000 in 1946, and dropped to 89,000 in 1949, as government support was phased out.[82]

Many nurse educators were concerned that the quality of nursing education would suffer because of the acceleration of these educational programs. On the contrary, it turned out that nursing schools were forced to reevaluate and improve nursing curriculum resulting in overall improvement of nursing education.

In addition, the Division of Nursing Education encouraged changes in students' working experience. They saw to it that the students workweek, including classroom education and clinical experience, was reduced to 48 hours per week from 55 to 75 hours per week.

Nursing during World War II was quite different than it had been in other wars. The introduction of more sophisticated firepower increased the number of military and civilian casualties, but improved medical care and transportation reduced mortality associated with injury, infection, and disease.

By the time the war ended, 100,000 nurses had volunteered and 76,000 served in the Army or Navy nurse corps.[83] By the end of the war, nurses had served in 50 countries around the world and had varied experiences. In the Philippines, 66 nurses remained behind after evacuation and became Japanese prisoners; 37 months later they were freed when Americans recaptured the area.[84]

During World War II, military nurses saw both their status and rank change. In 1920, Army nurses had been given equal rank as men, but not equal salary. In 1942, Navy nurses were given equal status and rank, and both Navy and Army nurses were granted equal pay. In 1947, full commissioned status was granted. The segregation of black nurses also ended. Later, in 1954, the last evidence of segregation was dropped by the Army, and male nurses were admitted to the service with full officer rank.[85-88]

The war also lead to more freedom for women. When the men were serving overseas, many women supported the war industry by assuming jobs and roles traditionally held by men. Nurses served at the front and were wounded and killed. Nurses received a great deal of favorable publicity and were heroines.

Civilian nurses at home rose to meet the needs of the country. In some instances, due to lack of adequate staff, they had to assume roles beyond the traditional nursing role. To alleviate this situation, the Red Cross developed a program to train volunteer nurses aides. By the end of 1945, 212,000 women had been certified as aides and contributed millions of hours of service in hospitals.[89] Nurses, in order to effectively use the services of these aides, were forced to define which nursing actions were skilled and which were not.

The Post-World War II Era

Some changes brought about by the war resulted in definite gains for nursing. Schools improved and educators were more highly educated. Federal scholarships were made available for nurses, and salaries were raised. As integration of the races in nursing schools increased, black nurses were commissioned in the armed services. Men and married students were admitted into nursing schools. Use of nonprofessional workers became accepted.

The changes mentioned above were expected to increase the number of nurses practicing in hospitals and in public health, but this was not the case. The nursing shortage grew worse instead of better due to a drop in the number of students entering nursing school, attrition of nurses in the field due to marriage, retirement, etc., and a reduction in the number of nursing aides. Hospitals were forced to reduce their admissions primarily due to the lack of adequate nursing staff. But at the same time, public health needs for medical care were increasing.

Due to the shortage of nurses, practical nurse education and licensing were promoted by the National Association for Practical Nurse Education, formed during World War II with the backing of the public, doctors, and many nurses. By the close of 1947, half of the states had established procedures for licensing practical nurses (LPN). Professional nurses recognized their responsibility for assisting in teaching and supervising LPNs and designed courses and standards for them. Another outcome of the nursing shortage was the hiring of nurses from other countries by some agencies. Use of nursing aides and volunteers also increased during the postwar years.

The concept of team nursing developed as a means of providing nursing care for all patients who required it. Agencies may define the term somewhat differently, but basically, the staff on a health care agency unit is divided into districts. Each team is responsible for the care of the patients in its district, and each team has a designated leader who organizes the work for the rest of the nursing team. Composition of the team depends on agency policy and scheduling but is generally composed of other nurses, LPNs, and nursing assistants. The team members usually do most of the hands-on care, with the leader supervising. This enables fewer professional nurses to be responsible for larger numbers of patients.

Today, there is a trend toward a new concept known as primary nursing. Primary nursing is characterized by one nurse being responsible for a smaller group of patients and assisting them with all of their needs and care.

The shortage of nurses is one that remains with us. Hopefully, with the coming of the 1990s, the organization, definition, and scope of professional nursing will become clearer, and further shifts in societal values and needs will alleviate some of the shortages.

NURSING EDUCATION

As we have seen, in the 1700s and early 1800s, most nurses in America were associated with religious communities. Catholic nursing orders, such as the Ursuline Sisters, based in France, trained their own nurses and established themselves in vari-

ous settlements throughout the New World. In addition to these nursing sisters, other women who provided services to the sick were either family members or hired servants. Guided by practical experience and home remedies, they varied greatly in their abilities and skill. The term "nurse" was applied to anyone hired to care for ill people.[90]

The first organized attempt to train nurses in the United States began in 1839 in Philadelphia.[91] A Philadelphia physician, Dr. Joseph Warrington, organized a number of elementary classes for nurses that included lectures along with medical students and practice on mannequins.[92] In 1862, a training program was organized for nurses at The Women's Hospital of Philadelphia.[93] This six-month program was required of all nurses who were hired to work at the hospital, and although no diploma was awarded, the graduates were recognized as trained nurses.[94] In 1873, Linda Richards was recognized as the first nurse to graduate from a training program in the United States. She attended a yearlong program at the New England Hospital for Women and Children in Boston.[95]

The Civil War (1861–1865) acted as a catalyst in bringing the need for more highly skilled nurses to the attention of society. In 1873, three important schools of nursing were founded: Bellevue Hospital School of Nursing (New York City), Massachusetts General Hospital School of Nursing (Boston), and The Connecticut Training School in New Haven. All were based on the Nightingale model established for nurses in England.[96]

The Hospital Diploma Schools

The Nightingale model was a hospital-based apprenticeship program that provided instruction in scientific principles and practical experience for skills mastery. Lectures were generally given by the hospital medical staff, and there was a contractual agreement between the school and the hospital to ensure teaching facilities.[97,98]

The three early American schools differed from the English model principally in terms of financial backing. The American schools had some independent backing but not the larger endowments afforded to schools in the English system. As a direct consequence of this, the American schools became more dependent on their associated hospital institutions. To offset costs associated with the presence of student nurses, the hospitals required a certain amount of ward work in exchange for room, board, and instruction. As patient care improved with the addition of student nurses, hospitals began to enjoy a better reputation and greater financial rewards. Nursing, too, became more respectable as a working opportunity for women, and many were attracted to the field. Hospital schools of nursing flourished, and by 1890, there were 15 schools; by 1900, over 400.

Compared to conditions during most of the 1800s, these turn of the century diploma schools represented a great deal of change for the status of nursing and certainly for the status of hospitals. The education components of these schools, however, were not given a high priority, and formal instruction was often lacking or nonexistent. There is considerable documentation supporting the view that hospital diploma schools existed primarily for the benefit of the hospital enterprise and not for the education of nurses.[99] Mastery of ward procedures was the emphasis, and it was not unusual for students to staff all areas of the hospital including kitchens, laundries, and supply departments.[100]

Nursing leaders recognized early in the 20th century that this system of nursing education was inadequate to prepare nurses for professional nursing practice.[101] A number of nurse leaders such as Isabel Hampton Robb, Mary Adelaide Nutting, and Annie Goodrich all worked to enlighten both nurses and the public about the need for educational reform. Professional organizations and nursing school alumni groups were formed; many of these became active in calling for changes in nurse training programs and furthering the ideas of licensure and credentialing.

The various Landmark Studies described earlier dealt largely with issues of nursing education. The Goldmark Report, for example, noted that the majority of nursing schools failed to provide an education equivalent to that in other professions and, that a primary reason for this lack was insufficient funds allocated for education by hospitals.[102,103]

Additional studies recommended major changes in nursing education, but there was very little support for implementing any of them. Hospitals were very protective of their nursing schools and were reluctant to support changes that would give them less control. For prospective students, hospital diploma schools offered an attractive arrangement financially. Most students or their families did not have the means to pay for an education. The general public continued to be pleased with the tremendous strides in the quality of hospital care and were not particularly involved with, aware of, or concerned about the status of nursing education. Also, society's attitude toward the role of women and higher education for women was a factor in the inertia.

The diploma model for nursing education continued to predominate for over 60 years. During this time there were educational improvements, and by early 1940, nursing school standards were being enforced by state boards of nurse examiners. Some schools had associations with universities or colleges, and the average length of the programs had increased from one to three years.

The mid-20th century diploma nursing school curriculum was typically 36 months in length and prepared nurses for roles in hospitals and similar inpatient settings. Graduates were skilled in carrying out tasks associated with bedside care and assisting physicians with procedures and other aspects of medical care. Nursing courses followed a disease-oriented framework (the medical model) and many programs offered introductory courses in the social as well as biological sciences. Students continued to rotate clinically through most departments in the hospital, and some schools offered introductory experiences in public health and psychiatric nursing outside the hospital setting. Clinical rotations typically included evening, night, and weekend hours. Students commonly lived in a nurse residence or dormitory within the hospital and were required to meet a number of personal as well as educational qualifications.

COLLEGIATE EDUCATION IN NURSING

The movement of nursing education from hospitals to colleges and universities took a long time. During the period when diploma schools were flourishing, a few early collegiate programs did become established. In 1909, the University of Minnesota established what is considered the first nursing program to be administered wholly within a university setting.[104,105] The Yale School of Nursing was established in 1923 and is considered the first autonomous collegiate school of nursing in the United States. The movement grew slowly, but by 1940 there were 76 baccalaureate nursing programs in the United States.[106] Almost all of these programs were specialized for public health nursing, or for administration, teaching, and supervision in hospitals and schools of nursing.[107]

In the period following World War II, colleges and universities began to expand, and significant gains were made in establishing collegiate nursing programs.[108] The success of the Cadet Nurse Corps, established to meet the nursing needs of the military during the war, also helped associate nursing with higher education. Nurses trained within this program spent their first nine months in a university setting learning the basic sciences and fundamentals of nursing.[109] After the war, many of these nurse veterans took advantage of the G.I. Bill of Rights and continued their education.

At this time, baccalaureate programs in nursing varied significantly in curriculum, content, and quality of faculty. In 1948, the Brown Report called for the stratification of nursing and nursing education into practical and professional, the latter taking place firmly within the collegiate setting. The report further recommended upgrading all present programs and faculty, mandatory inclusion of psychiatric nursing preparation in baccalaureate programs, public financing of nursing education, and instituting a system of accreditation of nursing schools.[110–112]

The recommendations set forth in the Brown Report had far-reaching effects in promoting baccalaureate education for nursing. Efforts to accredit nursing schools were accelerated, and the task of identifying appropriate and acceptable curriculum content was begun.

During the 1950s, two distinct types of baccalaureate nursing programs developed. The first was called the basic degree program and was designed for students who had no previous education in nursing. The second type was usually called a general nursing program and was designed for diploma graduates or nurses who had been trained in other kinds of programs.[113] By 1957 these latter programs had been discontinued, and diploma graduates were admitted to regular college programs with advanced standing.[114] Curricula began to emphasize more liberal arts.

1965 was a landmark year in the history of nursing education. The ANA, after several years of study and research, took a firm public stand on collegiate education for nursing. In an official position paper published in December of 1965, the ANA Committee on Education recommended that the baccalaureate degree be the minimal educational preparation for professional nurses.[115] A distinction was made between professional nursing practice and technical nursing practice. Professional nursing practice was described as theory oriented rather than technique oriented and involved coordination of illness prevention and health maintenance as well as aspects of caring and curing.[116] This type of practice was further described as having a responsibility to supervise, teach, and direct all those who give nursing care.[117] Technical nursing practice was described as centering around specific nursing measures and medically delegated techniques, which were carried out with a high degree of competency and skill. The minimum preparation recommended for technical nursing practice was the associate degree.

Although the issue of collegiate versus diploma education had always been controversial, the ANA paper intensified feelings and heightened conflicts of opinion. Prior to this, the issue had been merely a topic to consider for most nurses. With such a strong statement from the major professional nursing organization, diploma nurses in particular felt threatened and confused. Hospital administrators and many nurse administrators were angry. Instead of fostering collaboration and cooperative planning among nurses, the position paper "became an issue that, to this day, has caused a polarization between nurse educators and nursing service administrators and a divisive force in the profession as a whole."[118]

Despite the stormy controversy and resentment generated by the position paper, it has proved to have profound effects in its proposal to end an age-old conflict. Since 1965, diploma schools have steadily declined and college and university programs have taken their place.

The Lysaught Report

In 1968, the National Commission for the Study of Nursing and Nursing Education (NCSNNE) was founded. Fully supported by the ANA and the National League of Nursing, this Commission launched a comprehensive study to analyze how nursing and nursing education could be improved to meet the health care needs of society.[119] The results of this study, commonly known as the Lysaught Report, was published in 1970 as *An Abstract for Action*. Dr. Jerome P. Lysaught was project director of the study. The Lysaught Report identified three major problems in nursing education: a shortage of qualified faculty, inadequate and outmoded facilities, and a lack of funds and financing for schools of nursing.[120] Final recommendations included increasing research efforts regarding nursing practice and nursing education, improving the educational environment based on findings from this research, and clarifying professional roles.

The Lysaught Report was a credible study, and the majority of nursing organizations, allied health professions, and other public interest groups supported and applauded the recommendations. The commission was funded for three more years for the purpose of attempting to initiate some of the recommendations. In light of a history of commissioned studies and the Landmark studies resulting in little follow-up action, it was clear to nursing leaders that bona fide changes were not only necessary, but were crucial for both nursing and society. A second Lysaught Report, *From Abstract into Action*, was published in 1973, which detailed a number of positive accomplishments, among them the establishment of statewide master planning committees in nine target states to promote nursing education within the mainstream of general education.[121]

In the meantime, and despite the upsurge of two year ADN programs, BSN programs have made significant gains in the periods following the ANA Position Paper and the Lysaught Reports. In 1982 there were 393 BSN programs in the United States. [122] These programs are fully collegiate in the sense that the university or college administration is responsible for creating the major in nursing, overseeing the planning for course selection and faculty appointment, and assigning credit. Educational standards and policies are consistent with other academic programs offered by the institution.

BSN programs are generally four years in length and include courses in the biological, physical, and social sciences, the humanities, and nursing practice.

The general aim of these programs is to prepare nurses as general health care providers and for potential leadership positions in nursing. Graduates are prepared to give nursing care to people of all ages and in all types of settings. Emphasis is placed on health promotion and illness prevention in addition to the clinical nursing care of people who are ill.

Associate Degree Nursing Programs

One of the effects of the 1965 position paper was the proliferation of associate degree nursing programs. The idea for these technically oriented nursing curricula was born in the early 1950s, when small community based junior colleges began to flourish. Mildred Montag proposed the first plan in her doctoral thesis, *Education of Nursing Technicians*, published in 1951. A pilot research study was undertaken in 1952 by Teacher's College, Columbia University, and included seven junior colleges and six hospitals.[123] The study results were released in 1957 and demonstrated that nurses could be educated totally within an academic setting, be technically and competently trained as bedside nurses, and successfully pass the state board licensing examination for registered nurses.

The number of associate degree nursing (ADN) programs expanded rapidly, and by 1980 there were 707 accredited schools.[124] The early ADN curriculum was characterized by a ratio of one general education course to one nursing theory course. More recently the ratio is closer to one general education course to two nursing courses. Some programs require one or two summer sessions, in addition. Associate degree programs now are in the majority. Figure 3-5 provides a comparative view of the three types of nursing programs in 1982.

Type of Program	Number of Schools	Total Enrollment
ADN	726	37,183
BSN	393	24,804
Diploma	303	12,903

Figure 3-5. Enrollments, and Numbers of State—Approved Schools of Nursing in 1982.
Source: National League for Nursing, 1982

Although the concept of ADN nursing education remains controversial, ADN graduates are employed in a wide variety of settings and function in many roles. Much of the conflict and turmoil within nursing today stems from the fact that there are two-year, three-year, and four-year nursing programs, all of which are quite different, and all of which lead to the registered nurse (R.N.) credential. Each type of nursing program sets its academic and clinical goals in line with certain outcomes, i.e., graduates are theoretically prepared to practice within generally defined limits. Regardless of how appropriate these goals are or how successful schools are in meeting them, there is virtually no recognition or differentiation between registered nurses once they enter the job market. It is not uncommon to find nurses from all types of educational backgrounds in the same leadership positions, for example, or nurses being underutilized in strictly supervised technical types of practice.

Associate degree graduates are caught in the middle of all this confusion. Not only is the ADN the newest type of program, but ADNs represent a compromise between the hospital training of the past and the full-fledged collegiate degree. The terminology "technical nurse" and "technical nursing practice" also never has come to be an acceptable title. ADN graduates, as well as many other nurses, feel it has a demeaning quality, and employers feel it is too narrow and restrictive.

The issue of licensed practical nurse education is not addressed within the scope of this textbook but is another important topic when considering ADN programs. Practical nurses always have been "technical nurses," and their educational standards have increased significantly over the years.

ADN programs clearly have filled the need to train more bedside nurses and have been a strong motivating force in moving nursing education out of the hospital and into the college.

Graduate Education

Graduate education for nurses has existed since 1899, when Columbia University Teachers College established a program for nursing leaders.[125] Most of the early programs that followed were highly specialized and generally not consistent. Some were nearly all clinical, and others just the opposite.[126]

In the 1950s a number of attempts were made to organize graduate education. The National League for Nursing sponsored several conferences for the purpose of formulating guidelines for organization, administration, curriculum, and testing in masters education in nursing. In 1955, the master's degree was termed the "second professional degree for nurses," and the National League for Nursing identified specialization and research as its primary focus.[127]

Graduate education on both the master's and doctoral levels has received increasing attention since the 1960s. Programs are available in nearly all areas of the United States for nurses who want to pursue additional education in teaching, administration, research, and specialized practice. Today, programs that lead to a master's degree in nursing provide students with an opportunity to:

- acquire advanced knowledge from the sciences and humanities to support advanced nursing practice and role development.
- expand their knowledge of nursing theory as a basis for advanced nursing practice.
- develop expertise in a specialized area of clinical nursing practice.
- acquire the knowledge and skills related to a specific functional role in nursing, e.g., teaching, administration, management.
- acquire competence in conducting research.
- plan and initiate change in the health care system and in the practice and delivery of health care.
- further develop and implement leadership strategies for the betterment of health care.
- actively engage in collaborative relationships with others for the purpose of improving health care.
- acquire a foundation for doctoral study.[128]

Doctoral programs were slow to develop as they depended on the efforts of nurses who were prepared at the doctoral level in other disciplines. The first doctoral program in nursing was established at Teachers College, Columbia University in 1920, and until 1961 there were only three such programs in the United States.[129] Presently, there are 23 programs that lead to the doctoral degree. These programs offer one of three types of degrees: the Doctor of Nursing Science (DNSc), the Doctor of Education (EdD), and the Doctor of Philosophy (PhD).[130]

Doctoral work is highly specialized, focusing on research and the development of scientific theory in nursing. Many faculties of nursing now require the doctoral degree, and there is increasing recognition that doctoral preparation is necessary for the attainment of true professional status.

Reform in nursing education continues into the 1980s. Although the idea of collegiate education has rooted itself firmly as the emerging entry level to practice, much needs to be done. Having more than one type of basic preparatory program, for example, is confusing to both nurses and the public. In addition, service oriented programs (diploma schools) tend to increase the cost of health care and penalize graduates in terms of educational mobility.

Many influences in today's society point nursing toward a clear and unified approach to education. Various professional, political, and socioeconomic trends, as well as new advances in the health care system, are forcing the related issues of quality care and competence in nursing. The ANA recently has undertaken a study to assess the role of credentialing in nursing (see Chapter 4). As the results of this major study are analyzed and combined with other related efforts, the issue of nursing education will hopefully be placed on a more defined and unified path—one that is acceptable and accessible to both nursing and the needs of society.

CONTEMPORARY NURSING

Episodic Nursing Roles

The image of the nurse in white in the hospital setting, providing care and ministering to the sick, is a worldwide concept.

Traditionally, nurses have been prepared in acute care settings such as hospitals. This type of **episodic care** emphasizes the role of the nurse in the delivery of curative and restorative health services to persons with chronic diseases or acute conditions. Episodic practice has become associated with the cure aspect of nursing.

In the episodic or acute care setting, the role of the nurse is to assess, plan, implement, and evaluate patient care. When patients are not able to meet their own needs, nurses assist them. See Figure 3-6 for examples of typical nursing actions.

As they carry out professional nursing activities, nurses perform many functions that require them to fulfill their professional role in independent, interdependent, and dependent ways. **Independent** nursing actions are those that are performed by nurses based primarily on their assessments, judgments, and knowledge. Nurses carry out these actions without specific orders from health care professionals. Examples of some of these actions include bathing, dressing, mouth care, hair care, supportive care assessment, formulating nursing diagnoses, care planning and charting, and assisting patients to meet other needs. As primary nurses and nurse practitioners, nurses carry out many of their nursing actions in an independent manner.

Interdependent nursing activities are those that nurses perform in collaboration with others on the health care team, such as physicians, therapists, and nutritionists. Generally, patient care decisions are made by this group of professionals, who meet to discuss a patient's problems and needs, set goals, and establish priorities. Increasingly, patients and their families are being asked to participate in the problem solving discussions. Frequently, nurses work interdependently in team nursing or in providing long-term care.

Dependent nursing actions are those ac-

Assessment Nursing Actions
Uses scientific rationale in collection of patient data
Contributes to the patient data base using resources (patient, family, health records, others on the health team)
Identifies changes in patients health state as they occur
Documents patient progress
Assesses health state of patients, families, or groups
Assesses self-care needs of patients
Identifies areas where change of behavior is needed
Formulates nursing diagnoses

Planning Actions
Develops individual plan for patients
Prioritizes needs based on assessment
Incorporates patient, family, and others in the plan
Validates plan with patients
Establishes goals using outcome criteria
Uses research findings and information from the literature
Communicates the plan in writing and verbally

Implementation Actions
Carries out individualized plans
Maintains patients' health state or contributes to a higher state of wellness
Performs technical procedures as necessary
Maintains life support in emergency situations
Uses leadership skills and teaching skills
Serves as a role model for health practices
Collaborates with others to promote health
Accepts responsibility and is accountable for the implementation of the plan

Evaluation Actions
Uses goals and outcome criteria to evaluate the plan
Includes patients and families in the evaluative process
Reassesses
Identifies alternative means of meeting patient needs
Evaluates new literature and research findings
Includes other health team members in the evaluation

Figure 3-6. Patient needs are met through use of the nursing process.

tions nurses carry out following the orders of others on the health team. These usually are written by physicians, but can be written by physical or occupational therapists, for example. Because the nurse is not prescribing but is carrying out the prescription, the nurse is functioning in a dependent role. This does not relieve nurses of accountability and professional responsibility. When acting dependently nurses must:

- have written orders
- understand the orders
- establish their correctness
- question unclear or erroneous orders
- perform the prescribed task appropriately
- assess the outcomes
- evaluate the outcomes

In recent years, the traditional role of the nurse at the bedside has been expanded in scope. Nurses can choose a wide range of areas and specialized roles in the episodic setting. Intensive and coronary care units, kidney dialysis units, and specialized oncology services are specific examples of clinical areas that provide such roles.

The increase in science and technology has required nurses and health care providers to develop expertise in using new machinery and new techniques to gain an understanding of patient responses to them. Figure 3-7 lists some of the speciality areas that nurses can select to work and become expert in.

Many of these new roles require additional training or education. Speciality groups have formed, and many have their own journals and organizations (see Chapter 5). Nurses interested in any of these areas can write to those journals or organizations for further information. Although most of these new roles are still at the bedside, some are in areas such as administration, education, or research. A discussion of selected roles in the episodic setting follows.

EPISODIC NURSING ROLES

Administration
Director of nursing
Supervisor of nursing
Head nurse
Assistant head nurse
Clinical coordinator
Charge nurse

Education
Director of continuing education
Continuing education instructor
Patient education instructor

Research
Principal Investigator
Research Coordinator
Research Assistant

Practice areas
Psychiatric nursing
Medical surgical nursing
Intensive care units
Cardiac or coronary care units
Neonatology
Pediatrics
Rehabilitation nursing
Geriatrics
Dialysis units
Nurse anesthetist
Operating room
Recovery room
Emergency room
Maternity nursing
—Labor and delivery
—Postpartum
—Nursery
Infection control (nurse epidemiologist)
Enterostomal therapists
Oncology
Orthopedics
Thanotology nurse specialist
Patient advocate
Clinical specialist (within any specialty or
    subspeciality practice area)

Figure 3-7. Selected Episodic Nursing Roles and Practice Areas.

Primary nurses coordinate and administer nursing care for patients from the time of their admission to their discharge. These primary nurses are responsible for the care of their patients 24 hours a day during their hospital stay. They develop the plan of care for each of their primary patients, and the plan is followed by other nurses and other nursing service personnel when the primary nurse is off duty. Proponents of this particular role feel that primary nurses have more autonomy and more responsibility and accountability for holistic patient care. There is generally no additional education needed for a general duty primary nurse. Additional training, education, or practice may be required in intensive care or other highly technical areas.

Clinical specialists are leadership positions for nurses who are experts in a specialized area of nursing, for example, gerontology, pediatrics, or medical nursing. Clinical specialists usually have a master's degree in their speciality areas and their functions may vary from institution to institution. A range of functions generally includes such things as providing direct patient care, teaching patients and families, teaching staff new methods of care, and conducting research.

One of the specialty areas that attracts nurses is anesthesia administration. These individuals are called **nurse anesthetists.** Nurse anesthetists are registered nurses who have completed a course of instruction in anesthesia after nursing school. They visit a patient prior to surgery to assess preoperative medications and anesthesia needs, and discuss anesthesia procedures with patients. The duties of anesthetists are similar to physician anestheologists, but the nurses are supervised and supported by physicians. During the surgery they administer the anesthesia and assess the patient's responses to drugs and gases being administered, blood loss, etc. Following surgery, they accompany patients to the recovery room and evaluate their status and progress.

Enterostomal therapy is another specialty area. Enterostomal nurses teach and assist patients who have had surgery for colostomies, ileostomies, or urinary diversions. Their primary role is to teach patients how to care for themselves and help them adjust to their altered body image. Additional training is available for this, usually provided through a hospital or other health care facility sponsored program.

Geriatric nurse specialists provide comprehensive care to older patients in hospitals, nursing homes, and clinics. Some nurses who practice in this area have advanced certificates or degrees in the care of the elderly.

Infection control nurses (or nurse epidemiologists) monitor the hospital or nursing home environment for infection. They assess infections that have been incubating at the time of a patient's admission (community associated) and those that develop after admission. They assess, report, prevent, and control infections in the acute care setting. A good working knowledge of asepsis and microbiology are essential for nurses entering this area.

Oncology nurse specialists work with cancer patients and their families. They provide physical care and emotional support, and some are skilled in administering various types of chemotherapy.

Hospice nurses care for patients who are dying in a hospice. A hospice is a specialized health care facility for the terminally ill. The hospice concept is a relatively new idea in the United States, but has been successfully implemented in some areas of the country. These nurses provide physical care and emotional support for dying patients and their families.

Another new area for nursing is thanatology (the study of death). A nurse **thanotologist** is one who helps to meet the physical and psychological needs of the dying patient and his family. In addition to this, they teach other staff members how to cope more effectively with death and dying and improve their ability to assist patients through this time.

As the diversity in the episodic care field of nursing continues to expand, the job possibilities will be almost endless. Nurses in the future will be able to choose from an even wider variety of specialities in order to meet their personal and professional goals.

Distributive Nursing Roles

Nurses who work outside of the hospital setting usually are engaged in some facet of **distributive health care** as opposed to episodic health care. Distributive health care, in turn, is linked to the *care* aspect of health as opposed to the cure. One of the distinguishing features of distributive care is that it is continuous and doesn't operate within definitive beginnings and endings, such as admission and discharge from a hospital, or declarations of sick and well. In distributive care, the emphasis is on health, and total health needs are planned and assessed in terms of the individual's lifespan. Activities include such things as risk assessment for potential adverse health states and the promotion of healthful living habits. Episodic illnesses and injuries occur intermittently during the lifespan and, in one sense, the care provided (episodic care) can be viewed within the larger framework of distributive care. In actuality, people often have both care and cure needs at the same time. Despite this overlap, the terminology is helpful in explaining career choices and categorizing nursing roles in a logical fashion.

Distributive nursing practice is carried out within the framework of the nursing process, and there is emphasis on health maintenance and disease prevention. Health teaching, counseling, and care of the sick at home and in outpatient facilities are major components. A large portion of distributive nursing care services takes place within the realm of community health nursing. (The reader is referred to the chapters on Community Concepts and Family Concepts for a discussion of many of these nursing roles. In addition, Chapter 5 and Chapter 27 provide further insights into selected distributive nursing roles.) Figure 3-8 presents an overview of selected distributive nursing roles, including a number of community based and additional roles not covered in other chapters.

The Expanded Role in Nursing

The trend in the past two decades has been for nurses to take a more active part in patient care, increase their autonomy on the health team, and become more specialized. The **expanded role** is one of the outcomes of this trend. The expanded role generally refers to nursing practice that employs skills and expertise beyond a nurse's basic educational training program.

A nurse practicing in an expanded role usually has attended a specialized program that leads to a certificate qualifying her as a **nurse practitioner.** Nurse practitioner programs generally are specialized according to age of client (e.g., pediatric, adult, geriatric), or according to a clinical specialty, such as community or family health, college health, or oncology nursing. Major components of these programs are advanced training in health assessment and the delivery of primary care. **Primary care** refers to the care that takes place during the client's initial contact with the health care system or health provider.

Nurse practitioners are able to skillfully elicit a health history and critically evaluate the findings, conduct a physical examination, and evaluate a client's development, maturation, coping ability, emotional well-being, and any presenting complaints. Nurse practitioners are guided, through theory and experience, to discriminate between normal and abnormal findings and between normal variations of development and abnormal deviations. This role clearly includes a number of tasks that heretofore have been the sole province of the physician, particularly those that relate to medical diagnosis and the prescription of therapeutic measures. A critical skill of the nurse practitioner is to use sound judgment in deciding which clients can be cared for by the nurse and which should be referred to physicians or others on the health care team.

Nurse practitioners work in a variety of employment settings including physicians' offices, ambulatory care clinics, nursing homes, and community health settings. In addition to taking health histories and performing physical examinations, they may collect specimens, order laboratory tests and x-rays, make house calls, and prescribe medications.

Since 1971, 30 states have revised their nurse practice acts to accommodate the expanded role for RNs; a number have revised their definitions of nursing to include more autonomous functions within the area of diagnosis and treatment.[131] Only three states presently allow nurse practitioners to prescribe drugs; Idaho law, for example, allows nurses to prescribe from a limited formulary that includes antibiotics, contraceptives, antihistamines, decongestants, and topical ointments.[132] Certified nurse practitioners are perhaps the largest group who practice in expanded roles. As of yet, there are no legal ramifications as far as who can call herself "nurse practitioner," although the American Nurses Association has designed an accreditation process for programs that prepare nurses for this expanded role. The National Board of Pediatric Nurse Practitioners and Associates has initiated efforts to certify practitioners by examination. A growing number of nurse practitioner programs are part of BSN or advanced degree programs; e.g., a program may lead to an MSN *and* a nurse practitioner certificate. It is important to be aware that not all nurses who practice in an expanded role are certified practitioners. Increasingly, nurses are acquiring skills through on-the-job training and continuing education.

International Nursing

Nurses who practice their profession

ROLES AND SETTINGS	CHARACTERISTICS
Community Health Nurse Generalist	• also called public health nurse generalist • most often employed by city or county health departments • BSN preparation usually required • provides general health care to individuals, families, and target populations • functions as health educator, health counselor, coordinator of services, and direct care giver within home of clinic setting
Community Health Nurse Specialist	• also called public health nurse, specialist • master's degree in nursing preferred • responsibilities may include supervision of other nurses, responsibilities for planning and evaluating health and nursing services in the community, and conducting research
Visiting Nurse	• also called home health nurse • may be employed by visiting nurse associations, home health care agencies, public health departments, or be self-employed as a private duty nurse • gives direct care to clients in the home setting, often providing continuous care for chronic disease states and rehabilitation • all levels of nursing preparation are in this role; complex families are preferably cared for by nurses with minimal BSN preparation
Occupational Health Nurse	• sometimes referred to as employee health nurse or industrial nurse • delivers primary care and preventive health services to individuals in the work setting • educational preparation relative to scope of responsibility; may be prepared as nurse practitioner • experience and expertise in specialized areas of health counseling, such as alcoholism, stress management, and family living may be required.
Certified Nurse-Midwife	• registered nurse who has completed a program in nurse-midwifery accredited by the American College of Nurse-Midwives; some of these programs lead to a master's degree as well as a certificate in nurse-midwifery (CNM) • a CNM functions as a highly trained specialist in providing prenatal care to women with uncomplicated pregnancies, obstetric care during labor and delivery and postpartum maternal and infant care; depending on the setting, care may be episodic or continuous throughout the childbearing years • employment may be in group health organizations, private medical offices, hospitals, health departments, or private practice

ROLES AND SETTINGS	CHARACTERISTICS
School Nurse	• may be employed directly by boards of education, by local health departments, or by private schools • scope of responsibility varies greatly but includes emergency care and referral, health screening and testing, counseling, age specific health education, and assisting in the management of health related programs and school policies • educational requirements vary from state to state; special certification is required in some jurisdictions
College Health Nurse	• employed by a college or university health service/health office • delivers primary care to students, faculty, and staff employees; may provide infirmary inpatient care • educational background varies according to scope of responsibility; may be prepared as nurse practitioner • a large portion of care for this age group centers around general health counseling, mental health counseling, and health education
Ambulatory Care Settings — Clinic Nurse — Office Nurse — Outpatient Nurse	• settings may include outpatient departments of hospitals, doctors' offices, neighborhood primary care clinics, specialized clinics such as family planning and child health clinics, or other group health organizations • functions and responsibilities vary tremendously and may be broad or specialized; the delivery of primary care (both episodic and distributive) is usually a major component; the degree of health education and health maintenance activities delivered concurrently are determined by the philosophy of the agency and individual health care provider • registered nurses in these settings may be prepared as nurse practitioners, particularly in pediatrics and in other clinics that perform large numbers of routine physical examinations
Nursing of Specialized Populations	• there are a variety of roles and employment opportunities for nurses in specialized institutions and settings, where care may range from acute episodic to long-term distributive, or a combination of both. Examples include: —nursing in correctional institutions, e.g., prisons —camp nursing —nursing in homes for the mentally retarded or handicapped

ROLES AND SETTINGS	CHARACTERISTICS
	—public buildings or businesses, e.g., department stores, museums, zoos —recreational enterprises, e.g., circuses, rodeos, fairgrounds, sports events

Figure 3-8.   Overview of Selected Distributive Nursing Roles.

outside of their home country can be considered **international nurses.** In most instances this will involve adjusting to a culture different from one's own and delivering nursing care to individuals with different ideas about health and illness, different customs and beliefs, and different ways of relating to others.

Transcultural nursing requires a body of knowledge related to delivering culturally sensitive nursing care. It requires sensitivity to nursing behaviors, practices, values, and beliefs of people from all cultures. Nurses have been working internationally for many years, but the concept of transcultural nursing has emerged only recently as a separate field of study. It is important to note that transcultural nursing is applicable to both international nurses and nurses caring for culturally different people in any setting. (The reader is referred to Chapter 10 for further discussion.)

There are numerous opportunities for registered nurses to work abroad in community health nursing, primary care, acute care, teaching, and general health care administration. Prospective employers include foreign governments and business enterprises, religious missions, universities (both foreign and domestic), U.S. military organizations, U.S. government agencies, and various other national and international organizations. Figure 3-9 lists some of the recognized health organizations and agencies that provide opportunities for the practice of international nursing and sources of information on nursing opportunities overseas.

1. Project Hope
   c/o Hope Center
   Millwood, Virginia 22646
   Tel: 703-837–2100

   Project HOPE (Health Opportunity for People Everywhere) is an American private voluntary organization that functions to improve health conditions throughout the world. Emphasis is on education and the development of existing health care systems.

2. World Health Organization (WHO)
   Avenue Appia
   CH-1211 Geneva 27
   Switzerland

   WHO is the official health agency of the United Nations, and its general purpose is to foster the attainment of the highest possible level of health by all peoples. Functions include quarantine and epidemic intelligence; international standardization services, such as statistics, biologicals, and drugs; direct services to governments in surveying their health problems and strengthening their health services; educational and research assistance related to health matters.

3. Pan American Health Organization (PAHO)
   525 23rd Street, NW
   Washington, D.C. 20037

   PAHO is an intergovernmental public health organization and a specialized agency of the Organization of American States (OAS). It is also the American regional agency for WHO. The purpose of PAHO is to combat disease, lengthen life, and promote the physical and mental health of the peoples of the Americas. It receives and disseminates epidemiologic information, furnishes technical assistance, finances fellowships, promotes cooperation in medical research, and provides professional education in Latin America.

4. U.S. Agency for International Development (USAID)
320 21st Street, NW
Washington, D.C. 20037

An agency of the U.S. government that provides a wide range of technical and educational assistance to foreign governments. Included in this range are the building, staffing, and maintenance of medical facilities, water and sanitation projects, and family planning programs.

5. The U.S. Peace Corps
806 Connecticut Avenue, NW
Washington, D.C. 20525

The Peace Corps is a branch of ACTION, an agency of the U.S. government that coordinates volunteer services and programs. Peace Corps volunteers work in many parts of the world and provide assistance to host governments in economic and social development including nutrition, nursing education, nursing and hospital administration, and public health nursing.

6. International Council of Nurses
BOX 42
CH-1211 Geneva 20
Switzerland

Nurses can write to this organization for their publication, **Nursing Abroad**, which provides a description of the services offered by ICN member associations in arranging salaried employment or study abroad.

7. International Voluntary Services, Inc. (IVS)
1717 Massachusetts Avenue, NW
Washington, D.C. 20036

IVS recruits skilled volunteers to work in developing countries in the broad area of rural development, which includes health.

8. Intercristo
P.O. Box 9323
Seattle, Washington 98109
800-426-0507

An information center on worldwide Christian service. Information on nursing opportunities available on request.

9. Option
P.O. Box 81122
San Diego, California 92138

This agency provides information on volunteer and salaried employment in areas of need, both domestic and international. They publish a monthly newsletter and yearly catalog describing available opportunities.

10. Technical Assistance Information Clearinghouse
200 Park Avenue South
New York, New York 10003

A publication list is available that includes a directory of U.S. organizations in development assistance abroad and reports of development projects by country.

Figure 3-9. Source List of International Nursing Opportunities.

ADAPTED FROM:
VeNeta Masson "International Nursing: What Is It and Who Does It?" **The American Journal of Nursing,** July 1979, p.1245.
Curriculum papers, Undergraduate Program, The Catholic University of America, School of Nursing, Washington, D.C., 1980.

CONTEMPORARY ISSUES IN NURSING

As nursing has grown and changed over the last century, certain dilemmas and problem areas have arisen. The question of nurse shortages, for example, has been a prominent issue that seems to wax and wane over time. More recently the issues of reality shock among newly employed nurses and the burnout syndrome among more experienced nurses have emerged. The remaining discussion on contemporary nursing will address these issues, as well as a very positive issue, that of computer technology in nursing.

Nurse Shortages. A shortage or surplus of nurses is a lack of balance between the number of nursing jobs or positions and the number of qualified nurses available to fill them. From a historic standpoint, a shortage of nurses is characteristic of the profession. The only time in history that an oversupply of nurses existed was during the great economic depression of 1929.

Varying perceptions of the need and demand for nurses, how the supply is estimated and projected, what constitutes a shortage and its causes prevents definitive answers to the questions about shortages. It appears that these issues will continue to be debated. The question of a shortage must be examined in terms of societal conditions, expectations, and values.

The registered nurse resources of the country, the nurses educated and available for nursing positions, are related to a number of major factors. The number of students who enter and graduate from nursing schools and then remain actively engaged in nursing is the primary indicator of the nurse supply. A large number of nurses who maintain a current license practice part-time or do not practice at all. Inactive or part-time employment is related to marital status, sex, age, and family responsibilities. Low pay for available positions, poor working conditions, and few opportunities for career advancement also cause nurses to leave employment or change jobs.

In addition to the number of nurses available for practice, another factor in the adequacy of the nurse supply is the demand for nursing services in the different health care settings. As health care facilities expand, new treatments are developed and new types of care are made available to patients; therefore, more nurses are required. New hospital beds, specialized nursing services, such as intensive care units, kidney dialysis units, and ambulatory care centers, contribute to the demand for nurses.

These characteristics of the nurse supply give rise to the question of a shortage or surplus of nurses. Those who believe there is a surplus of nurses point out that registered nurse resources have grown tremendously and are not fully used. A large number of nurses (about 24 percent) who

maintain a current license do not practice.[133] In addition, 53 percent of employed nurses work part-time.[134] Furthermore, the number of vacant positions for nurses in the health care agencies, and the difficulties in recruiting and filling the positions are highlighted. It is said that nursing staffs are used to their fullest productivity and work considerable overtime. To counter understaffing, health care agencies have to resort to hiring temporary staff from supplemental agencies.

This is only part of the debate. The way the adequacy of the nurse supply is judged is another issue. The nurse supply is the number of registered nurses who are employed or are available for employment. Basic to determining the adequacy of the nurse supply are the concepts of demand and need. **Demand** defines requirements primarily on the basis of economic factors. Demand is assessed by determining how many dollars are available from employers to pay salaries. It is measured by the number of budgeted nursing positions required for the nursing services the population will use, and that can be paid for. **Vacancies,** a measure of shortage, are the number of budgeted positions that are not filled. **Need,** on the other hand, defines requirements by considering the standards of good care and the number of nurses that can be expected to be available as determined by health professionals. Need is assessed by applying criteria considered to produce optimum levels of nursing care or service to the health care needs of the population to be served. Assessment of the nurse supply are interpreted differently depending on need and demand concepts, predictions on the number of nurses in training, and the proportion of trained nurses that practice. It has been proposed that looking at the adequacy of the nurse supply based on the aggregate numbers of nurses in itself leads to perception of a surplus. Relying on the annual output of the nursing educational system to aug-

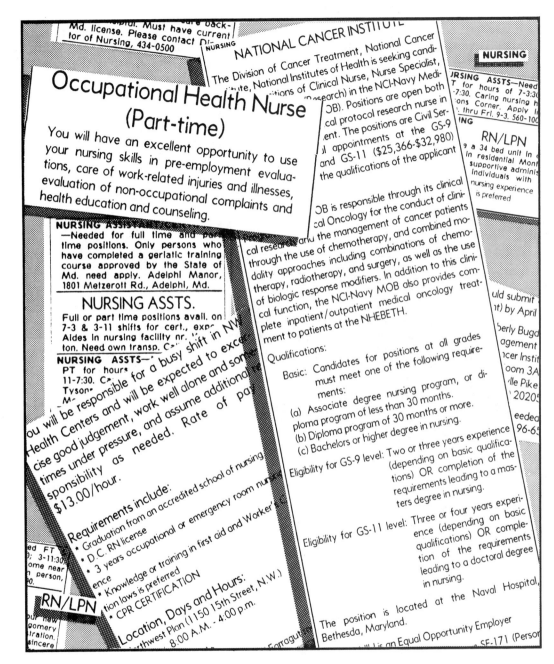

Figure 3-9a. Examples of Temporary Nursing Agency Advertisements.

ment the supply also contributes to a false perception of the balance between supply and demand for nurses. Over the years, the solution to the nurse shortage has been to educate and graduate more nurses, ignoring the fact that a certain proportion of these nurses will be inactive, work part-time, or drop out of the profession. Some believe that the shortage of nurses is not a function of the number of nurses but of their misutilization. They suggest that in the hospital, for example, nurses are frequently expected to assume the responsibilities of other departments. Nurses act as pharmacists, aides, housekeepers, secretaries, and messengers. If they were free to practice nursing, the shortage would be reduced. The solution lies in better management and improved utilization of nurses. In this same regard, another interpretation is that the supply of nurses will never reach demand, unless appropriate responses are made to shortages. Attention needs to be focused on the health care de-

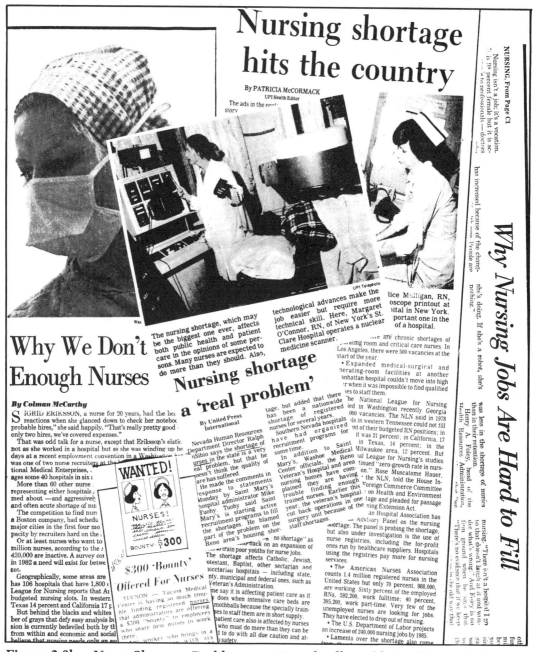

Figure 3-9b.   Nurse Shortage Problems are Periodically Publicized in the U.S.

livery system, the roles and responsibilities of nurses, improved working conditions, career development, and ways to retain nurses in the work force.

Nursing has accumulated a large body of knowledge about its practitioners and has developed and refined methods for determining the number of nurses available and needed for nursing practice. The first counts of the number of registered nurses were made in the states that had laws requiring registration (New Jersey passed its registration law in 1903).[135] Even today, the chief source of data on the nurse supply is the number of nurses licensed by the state nurse licensing boards.

Since the beginning of the century, the number of registered nurses has grown in increasing proportion to the population. These relationships are shown in Figure 3-10. The national average of the number of nurses per 100,000 population climbed from 55 in 1910 to 520 in 1980, an increase of 465 nurses per 100,000 population. The number of nurses per 100,000 is not uni-

form among regions of the country, however.

The northeast tends to have the largest number of nurses per 100,000 population and the south the least number. The growing proportion of nurses to the population is assumed to reflect the increased demand for nurses. But the adequacy of the supply must be addressed in terms of the different areas of the country, the structure of the health services, the needs and demands for services in the area, and their availability. The characteristics of nurses in the area and their work force participation must be analyzed to determine the significance of their numbers versus need or demand.

The 1963 report of the Consultant Group appointed by the Surgeon General of the United States Public Health Service highlighted national nursing shortages both quantitatively and qualitatively. The Consultant Group set goals for the number of nurses required through 1980, including the numbers prepared for particular health care settings, fields of nursing prac-

Year	Number of Nurses in United States	Nurses per 100,000 population				
		United States	North-east	North central	South	West
1910	50,476	55	75	47	34	104
1920	103,879	98	133	87	60	166
1930	214,292	175	239	159	104	262
1940	284,159	216	304	193	134	299
1950	374,584	249	321	233	174	318
1960	525,374	293	349	270	245	340
1970	750,000	368	491	367	281	355
1980	1,272,851	520	620	547	423	529

Sources: 1910–1950 US Department of Health, Education and Welfare, Public Health Service, **Health Manpower Chart Book** PHS Pub. No. 511, Washington, D.C.: U.S. Government Printing Office, 1957, p. 51. 1960—US Department of Health, Education and Welfare, Public Health Service, Health Resources Administration. *Source Books: Nursing Personnel.* DHEW Pub. No. (HRA) 75-43, Washington, D.C.: US Government Printing Office, 1974, p.13. 1970 & 1980 Division of Health Professions Analysis, Bureau of Health Professions: **Supply and Characteristics of Selected Health Personnel.** DHHS Pub. No. (HRA) 81-20. Health Resources Administration, Hyattsville, MD, June 1981, p. 115

Figure 3-10.   Nurse—Population Ratios by Region 1910–1980.

tice, and areas of responsibility. In response, the Nurse Training Act of 1964 was enacted by Congress. Through this and extended legislation, the federal government has supported a broad range of programs designed to increase the quantity and quality of the nurse supply. The Nurse Training Act has provided student aid for basic and postgraduate training and education, funds for construction of nursing schools, institutional aid for operating schools, and grants for improvement of nursing education programs.

With the Nurse Training Act of 1979, Congress authorized a study to determine if there still was a shortage of nurses and a need for continued federal financial assistance to nursing education. The report of a study committee on nursing and nursing education conducted by the Institute of Medicine (IOM), National Academy of Sciences, was issued in January 1983.[136]

It concluded that there was an adequate general supply of nurses through 1990, and no substantial federal support and activities were needed to increase the overall number.

Nursing shortages did exist in certain geographic areas and practice settings, such as inner cities and rural areas. This was seen as a distribution problem. A shortage was seen in the number of nurses with advanced training in administration, teaching, research, and clinical nursing specialities. As the IOM study was published, newspaper and journal articles announced that 37 percent of California hospitals were not hiring registered nurses; 51 percent were reducing weekly work hours; and 17 percent closed patient care units. Unemployment, a decline in patient admissions, and decrease in patient census were cited as reasons.[137] The IOM study analyses of projected supply of registered nurses did take into account the fact that projections were made at a time of economic recession, when there was great concern for cost containment. Changes in demand for health services and nurses would affect changes in output of nurses. Other factors also would influence the supply of nurses, such as the cost of educating them.

The nursing profession, through the ANA, was quick to point out that the late-1970s and early-1980s were a period of depressed economic conditions and less demand for health services. Improved economic conditions could result in more demand for services and the need for more nurses.

It can be concluded that determining the supply and requirements for nurses is not a straightforward definitive process. Both quantitative and qualitative assessments of need and demand involve some subjective judgment and are influenced by personal and professional views of the health care system and nursing.

The supply of nursing and its adequacy for meeting health care needs will require continuous monitoring to detect changing situations. A periodic critical assessment will need to focus on the supply as well as trends in the demand for nurses. The many factors that influence whether there is a shortage or a surplus and their implications will need to be evaluated. A response to the periodic assessments and efforts to keep the supply in balance with needs will continue to be a real challenge to the nursing profession.

There are many popular reasons for the perceived shortage of nurses, even though the supply is increasing. The staff of the Institute of Medicine study on nursing examined some of these assertions in relation to data on the nurse supply.[138]

- **Fewer nurses are employed in nursing.** The proportion of the total registered nurse populations actually employed in nursing has increased from 59.3 percent in 1949 to 76.6 percent in 1980.

- **Nurses are leaving nursing to work in other fields.**

- **Nurses are leaving active employment to pursue further education.**

Reality Shock. Reality shock is another important dilemma facing nurses today. Kramer explains *reality shock* as the feelings inexperienced nurses have when they discover themselves in job situations for which they thought they were prepared, only to find that they are not.[139] For example, many students have their clinical experience 2 to 3 days per week, during an academic year. They are giving care for only 3 or 4 patients at a time, and the clinical experience is structured as a learning experience. Students are closely monitored and assisted by their instructors, and have no ancillary responsibilities on the nursing unit.

According to Kramer, many problems arise from the fact that nurses are educated to believe in professional values but are hired by bureaucratic organizations.[140] Student nurses are taught to provide individualized attention to clients, autonomy in the decisionmaking process, and independence in nursing behavior. Yet many nurses, particularly those in acute episodic settings, are employed by institutions that are organized around the performance of tasks and are based on examples from industry where products and profitable outcomes are the objectives.[141] When new nurses arrive at their jobs, they are expected by the health care agency and by themselves to be competent. The criteria for competency in the work setting is usually far from the type of competency expected in the nursing school experience. In addition to giving direct care to patients, employed nurses are expected to take on their share of the workload in relation to the number of staff on duty, to manage their workload in terms of priorities, and to assist in the supervision of less professional personnel. When they cannot live up to these expectations, they are disappointed and experience feelings ranging from shock and depression to recovery and resolution. Consequently, some nurses do not adapt well and may even drop out of the profession.

To help nurses remain in nursing and not suffer from reality shock, several things need to be done. Student nurses need to be aware that reality shock may occur. Nursing educators need to present the reality of staff nursing to students as well as the ideal. Students should be fully aware that nursing is largely a 24-hour-a-day, 7 day-a-week profession. This is true in all episodic settings and in some distributive settings. Nurses are expected to work evening or night shifts, as well as holidays and weekends. New graduates need to be oriented to each shift and have adequate time to prepare for shift rotation.

Administrators need to be aware that the agency expectations for new graduates may be too high and an adjustment period is needed. Nursing administrators, supervisors, and head nurses also need to identify those nurses experiencing reality shock.

Nurses who reach the resolution stage will find strength in the fact that they experienced reality shock and have coped successfully and will continually be challenged by the complex problems that are very much a part of the real world of nursing.

Burnout Syndrome. Burnout is a term used to describe a syndrome that experienced nurses may develop. Psychologists have found the burnout syndrome to be a common state among nurses, doctors, social workers, teachers, and other professionals, who are so busy helping others that they neglect their own needs. In many instances, they do not even recognize their own needs. Some factors that contribute to nursing burnout include: heavy workloads; low pay; long and diversified hours; lack of autonomy, inability to deliver holistic, individualized patient care; the inability to assist all patients in positive adaptation; and the continual experience of loss when patients die. Burnout rate is particularly high in intensive care units, burn units, and oncology units, where many people are critically or terminally ill. Although burnout can occur in any setting, it appears to be most concentrated in acute care settings, such as hospitals.

Donna Diers summarized the work of nurses in the following way:

> Nurses deal with the most basic human needs: feeding, heartbreak, warmth, elimination, suffering, loneliness, birth, and death. Our hands get dirty, our uniforms stained, and our psyches eroded by daily contact with human beings in need—people crying, immobilized, angry, frightened, depressed, and only occasionally joyful. We live with the outrage of the diagnosis made or missed, the crisis of faith in a higher being or a physician; the knowledge of decline, disability, permanent change, death and the consciousness of our own mortality. We must be graceful over vomitus. . . , dignified as we change the dressing, . . . (or) give out bad news. With our hands and eyes we touch the lives of others and are admitted to the privacy of their inner space without even asking.[142]

With this type of responsibility, it is understandable why nurses cannot always cope with the stress of nursing. Experiencing a stress response can give rise to the syndrome known as **burnout,** which is characterized by fatigue, insomnia, depression, irritability, headaches, stomach distress, susceptability to contagious illnesses, dread of going to work, dehumanization, and exhaustion.

There is no wonder cure or solution to the burnout syndrome, but research has uncovered several approaches that can be used to avoid it or combat it.

To combat burnout and increase job satisfaction, many agencies have increased the nurse to patient ratio, enabling nurses to provide more holistic care. Hospital administrators feel that this increases satisfaction, because nurses have more responsibility for a smaller group of patients and are able to give more comprehensive care. They, consequently, are more likely to stay.

In some agencies, staff members meet with a counselor to discuss their feelings on a more formal basis. Also, many staff nurses serve as their own support group, encouraging other nurses to express their feelings.

Another method of combating the burnout syndrome is rotation out of the high stress area for a time. For example, a staff nurse in the intensive care nursery would rotate through the normal nursery every other month, in order to minimize the stress. It is important for nurses to be aware that burnout exists so that they can recognize the symptoms in themselves and others, and take appropriate action to alleviate it.

Individual nurses, too, can take steps to combat burnout. The first and most important step for nurses to take is to realize that there is a problem. Once the syndrome has been assessed, several other steps can be taken. Establishing a daily "decompression time" has been found to be helpful. This involves some sort of relaxing activity. Jogging, walking, swimming, shopping, and going for a drive are examples of how decompression time can be spent.

Some nurses have found meditation or a specific stress management program to be helpful. Just setting aside some private quiet time may be effective as well. Relaxing in a hot tub or sitting in a lawn chair are other examples.

Another important coping device is for nurses to establish support groups. Sometimes just sharing feelings, frustrations, and problems with other sympathetic nurses is helpful. Because of the symptoms of the burnout syndrome, many nurses are not aware that it is common. Once they are able to talk about their feelings, they are able to generate a plan for change.

Other nurses have found exploring their employment options can be a means of reducing burnout. Lateral job transfers or a completely new job are ways of doing this.

Most professional nurses experience some degree of burnout at some time in their career. Awareness of the symptoms and taking action to reverse the syndrome is the most important means of successfully coping with it.

Computer Technology and Nursing. As science and technology continue to advance, the information generated can be overwhelming. As a result, we are in what some individuals have called an information revolution. In order to effectively organize, store, and retrieve this information, many agencies are turning to computers for support. New roles subsequently have been created for nurses and other health care providers.

As hospitals and community health agencies begin to computerize their services, departments such as nursing are finding many new ways to improve patient care. Computers can be of great advantage to nurses, and some of the ways they are currently being used to assist nursing practice include:

- classification of patients for workload determination and variable staffing in hospitals
- general nurse scheduling in hospitals
- budgeting and other fiscal analysis for nursing service departments
- documentation of patient care data in all phases of the nursing process, including computer generated nursing diagnoses
- patient monitoring applications, such as direct recording of vital signs, stress tolerance levels, and other physiological processes
- patient data analysis to monitor trends in patients' nursing care needs and to assist in research efforts
- provision of communication interface between departments within a health care institution, e.g., laboratory, x-ray, social services, dietary services, pharmacy
- management of supplies; inventory assistance, ordering, crediting
- assistance with patient education and

professional nursing education
- maintenance of reference data for quick access by nurses on-the-job; e.g., adverse effects of drugs, emergency protocols, community referral listings.

The computer eases decisionmaking and communications, and results in the reduction of errors and better use of professional time and effort.

Computers are still a relatively new phenomena in the health care system, but the number of institutions and agencies that employ them is rapidly increasing. There are a number of emerging nursing roles in the field of automated data processing and medical and nursing information systems within health care agencies.

To understand the role of the nurse, several terms need to be introduced and defined. **Automated data processing** (ADP) refers to the operation of identifying pieces of information, converting them into machine-readable formats, and storing them in a coherent way in a computer, for people and organizations to use. An **automated system** is a defined collection of computerized information that is programmed in a precise way to accomplish specified goals. Automated systems may exist for use solely within one organization, such as hospital personnel system, or may be intended for use by the public at large, such as a bibliographic system in a library. **Hospital information systems** (HIS), often referred to as **medical information systems** (MIS), use computer systems to process information needed to deliver patient care within hospitals or other health care institutions.

Nursing information systems provide computer access to nursing information and selected patient information and enable nurses to record, monitor, analyze, and review these data. There are many specific and potential uses of nursing information systems as listed previously in this section. Nursing information systems can be autonomous and exist as single systems within themselves, or they can be integrated as a subsystem to the HIS or MIS in an institution. The latter is more common and provides more flexibility and resource data for delivering patient care. Health related automated systems are moving from institutions into ambulatory care settings such as community health nursing agencies. One of the major contributions of the computer to community health nursing is its ability to rank nursing care needs of clients.

Specific job descriptions for nurses who work with computer technology and nursing information systems are not yet standardized and are specific to the health care institution. The U.S. Department of Health Services and the National Institutes of Health (NIH) have sponsored an annual computer technology and nursing conference since 1981.[143] At the 3rd national conference, an integrated computer model for nursing was presented.

Much of the current literature, along with findings from the First National Computers in Nursing Conference echoes a recurring theme regarding nursing roles and nursing involvement in computer technology: nurses must become committed to and have a stake in the development of computerized nursing systems, and they must establish standards for the data content of these systems and develop a taxonomy of terms representing the nursing process. This is one mandate for assuring the survival of nursing functions and allowing nurses to control their own practice. The future for nurses and the computer undoubtedly will expand rapidly in the next few years. Nurses need to become increasingly familiar with computer technology, understand the roles of computer professionals such as programmers and systems analysts, become involved in the acquisition of computer hardware and software development, and work diligently to clarify and produce a standardized nursing database.

SUMMARY

The concept of nursing is multidimensional. It is a professional discipline that provides health and illness care to individuals, families, and groups within society. The practice of nursing takes place within a structural framework called the nursing process. The nursing process is supported by the application of scientific theory, the mastery of technical and behavioral skills, and a sensitive and humanistic approach to care giving.

Nursing has been defined variously by nursing leaders, health care agencies, and nursing organizations, to name but a few. From these definitions and an understanding of the concepts of health and illness, the nurse develops her own philosophy and definition of nursing.

Health, illness, and wellness are all relative terms that describe a person's state of being. They are viewed on a continuum and are relative to an individual's age, cultural orientation, personal philosophy, and society. Nurses carry out activities that promote and maintain health, prevent illness, and assist ill and injured persons in returning to their potential health states.

The history of nursing goes far back into early civilization, although most accounts begin with Florence Nightingale's work in the 1800s. Miss Nightingale is known as the founder of modern nursing, and through her ideas and efforts the practice of nursing was organized. She laid the groundwork for nursing as a theory-based profession with its own body of knowledge.

It is important for contemporary nurses to understand the influences of Nightingale and the many nurse leaders who followed her. These early nurse leaders gave a richness to the profession that has helped to shape the practice of nursing today.

Over the years, various organizations and groups have undertaken studies on the state of nursing in America. Several of these studies have been characterized as

"Landmark Studies" and they have impacted nursing in numerous ways.

Formalized nursing education began with Florence Nightingale's school in England. The American diploma school of nursing was developed from this model, and it remained the major type of nursing school for over 60 years. Baccalaureate education for nursing had been promoted by various nurse leaders since the 1920s, but it was not until 1965 that a major promotion of it was launched by the American Nurses Association. Currently there are three major educational programs that prepare nurses for the RN license: the two-year associate degree program; the three-year diploma school; and the four-year baccalaureate degree program. Graduate programs leading to the master's and doctoral degrees have expanded in number since the 1950s and research efforts in nursing have increased accordingly.

Contemporary nursing is characterized by diverse opportunities in clinical practice, administration, education, and research. Episodic care roles are available in hospitals and other acute care inpatient facilities. Distributive care roles that emphasize continuous health promotion and illness prevention activities take place in the community and ambulatory care agencies. The expanded role includes nurse practitioners, nurse-midwives, and other nurses prepared to deliver primary care or highly specialized health and nursing services.

A number of dilemmas in modern nursing have emerged along with the advancements. Nurses in acute care settings are subject to the burnout syndrome, for example, and newly employed nurses often experience reality shock. Related to both of these is a chronic nurse shortage problem; a problem that is both complex and dynamic.

The application of computer technology to nursing is one of the exciting trends in modern nursing and promises to enhance working conditions for nurses, provide more research opportunities, and improve nursing and health care in general.

The challenges that face the contemporary nurse are numerous. Nurses are highly educated, and there is an increased interest in research, the development of nursing theory, and the use of professional management techniques. Nurses are gaining more autonomy and exercising more control over their practice.

The setting for nursing practice used to be primarily episodic, and now, along with the health care system in general, there is a trend toward ambulatory care and a greater demand for preventive services. The needs of society are changing, technology is expanding, and competition among health care providers is high. There will always be a need for nursing services. Perhaps the greatest challenge throughout the history of nursing has been the attainment of professional status. Today nursing can look at itself with great pride; its professionalism is at an all time high and nurses are actively engaged in furthering and maintaining excellence in practice. For the nursing profession, the future is now.

STUDY QUESTIONS

1. List several ways in which history affected the development of nursing in America.

2. What were Florence Nightingale's contributions to nursing?

3. Who should define nursing? Why?

4. What are some factors that have helped nursing evolve toward professional status?

5. How did the status of women effect nursing?

6. What is episodic nursing practice? List several episodic nursing roles.

7. What is distributive nursing practice? List several of these roles.

8. Describe the way you feel around final exams. How does this resemble burn-out?

9. Describe your first day in clinical practice. Did your instructor expect more of you than you felt you could deliver?

10. Interview a nurse who is actively engaged in using a computer in her nursing practice. Describe the role the computer plays.

REFERENCE LIST

1. World Health Organization: **Constitution: World Health Organization.** Geneva: World Health Organization, 1971.
2. Halbert L. Dunn, **High Level Wellness.** (Washington, D.C.: Mt. Vernon Publishing Co., Inc., 1961).
3. Patricia Flynn, **Holistic Health,** (Bowie, MD: The Robert J. Brady Co., 1981), p.12.
4. **The Study of Credentialing in Nursing: A New Approach, Vol. 2,** Staff Working Papers, (Kansas City, Mo: The American Nurse's Association, 1979), pp. 388–391.
5. Barbara W. Narrow and Kay Brown Buschle, **Fundamentals of Nursing Practice,** (New York: John Wiley and Sons, 1982), p.29.
6. American Nurse's Association, **Nursing: A Social Policy Statement,** (Kansas City, MO: The American Nurse's Association, 1980), p.9.
7. Deborah M. Jensen, **History and Trends of Professional Nursing,** (St. Louis: The C.V. Mosby Co., 1959).
8. Louise Fitzpatrick, **Prologue to Professionalism,** (Bowie, MD: R.J. Brady, Co., 1983) p.2.
9. Ibid. pp.11, 12.
10. Jensen, **History and Trends,** p.91.
11. M. Adelaide Nutting and Lavinia L. Dock, **A History of Nursing,** Vol. II (New York: G.P. Putnam's Sons, 1907).
12. Isabel M. Stewart and Anne L. Austin, **A History of Nursing: From Ancient Times, A World View.** 5th Ed. (New York: G.P. Putnams' Sons, 1962) p.101.
13. Sr. Charles Marie Frank, **Foundations of Nursing,** (Philadelphia: W.B. Saunders, Co., 1959) pp.98–99.
14. Annie Matheson, **Florence Nightingale** (London: T. Nelson and Sons, 1913), p.137.
15. Cecil Woodham-Smith, **Florence Nightingale, 1820–1910.** (New York: McGraw-Hill Book, Co., 1951), p.66.
16. Ibid., p.63.
17. F.T. Smith, "Florence Nightingale: Early Feminist" **American Journal of Nursing, 81,** No. 5. (May 1981) 1021–1024.
18. Stewart and Austin, **History of Nursing,** p.101.
19. Frank, **Foundations in Nursing,** p.101.
20. J.A. Dolon, **History of Nursing,** 12th Ed., (Philadelphia: W.B. Saunders, 1968), pp.215–216.
21. Frank, **Foundations in Nursing,** p.105.
22. Florence Nightingale, **Notes on Nursing, What It Is and What It Is Not** (New York, Appleton and Co., 1860), p.65
23. Bonnie Bullough and Vern Bullough. **The Emergence of Modern Nursing,** (New York: The Macmillan Co., 1969).
24. Philip A. Kalisch and Beatrice J. Kalisch, **The Advances of American Nursing,** (Boston: Little, Brown, and Co., 1978), p.18.
25. Ibid., p.19.
26. Gerald Joseph Griffin and Joanne King Griffin, **History and Trends of Professional Nursing,** 7th Ed., (St. Louis: The C.V. Mosby Co., 1973) p.84.
27. Kalisch and Kalisch. **Modern Nursing,** p.24.
28. Jensen. **History and Trends,** p.183.
29. Kalisch and Kalisch, **Modern Nursing,** p.62.
30. Ibid., p.87.
31. Ibid., p.102.
32. Lois R. Wiggins, "The Nurse's Cap, Symbol of a Proud Profession" **The Journal of Practical Nursing, 23,** No. 1, (January 1973) 22–23.
33. Kalisch and Kalisch, **Modern Nursing,** p.142.

34. Agnes G. Deans and Anne L. Austin, **The History of the Farrand Training School for Nurses** (Detroit: Alumnae Association of the Farrand Training School for Nurses, 1936), p.58.

35. Griffin and Griffin, **History and Trends,** p.87.

37. E. Ware, **Transcript of Interview** by C. Schofield, (Baltimore: Johns Hopkins Archives, 1939).

37. Teresa E. Christy, "Nurses in American History: The Fateful Decade, 1890–1900" **American Journal of Nursing, 75,** No. 7 (July 1975) p. ? 1163–1165.

38. Fitzpatrick, **Professionalism,** p.223.

39. Teresa E. Christy, "Portrait of a Leader: Isabel Hampton Robb" **Nursing Outlook, 17,** No. 3, (March 1969) 26–29.

40. Jensen, **History and Trends,** p.106.

41. Lillian D. Wald, **The House on Henry Street** (New York: Henry Hall and Co., 1938), pp.4–8.

42. Jensen, **History and Trends,** p.205.

43. Teresa E. Christy, "Portrait of a Leader: Lavinia Lloyd Dock" **Nursing Outlook, 17,** No. 6, (June 1969) 72–75.

44. Lavinia L. Dock, **Textbook on Materia Medica for Nurses,** (New York: G.P. Putnam's Sons, 1890).

45. Mary M. Roberts, "Lavinia Lloyd Dock—Nurse, Feminist, Internationalist" **American Journal of Nursing,** 56, No. 2, (February 1956) 176–179.

46. Frank, **Foundations of Nursing,** p.215

47. Teresa E. Christy, "Portrait of a Leader: Isabel Maitland Stewart" **Nursing Outlook, 17,** No. 10, (October 1969) 44–48.

48. Fitzpatrick, **Prologue to Professionalism,** p.206.

49. Helen L. Bundge, "Research is Every Professional Nurses' Business", **Nursing Research, 7,** (1958) 816.

50. Louise C. Smith, **Helen L. Bundge,** (Madison, Wisconsin: School of Nursing, University of Washington, 1979) pp.1–4.

51. Lois R. Wiggins, "Lydia Hall's Place in the Development of Theory in Nursing" **Image,** 12, No. 1, (February 1980) 10–12.

52. "Progress in Nursing Education", Editorial, **American Journal of Nursing, 19,** (1919) 220–222.

53. Report of the Committee on Nursing Education, Editorial, **American Journal of Nursing, 22,** (1922) 878–880.

54. Lucie Y. Kelly, **Dimensions of Professional Nursing,** 4th Ed., (New York: MacMillan Co., 1981).

55. Josephine Goldmark, **Nursing and Nursing Education in the United States, Report of the Committee for the Study of Nursing.** (New York: The MacMillan Co., 1923).

56. Ibid.

57. Committee on the Grading of Nursing Schools **Nurses, Patients, and Pocketbooks** (New York: Committee on Grading of Nursing Schools, 1928), p.17.

58. Fitzpatrick, **Prologue to Professionalism** p.224.

59. Committee on the Grading of Nursing Schools, **Nurses, Patients, and Pocketbooks,** p.20.

60. "Nurses, Patients, and Pocketbooks", **American Journal of Nursing, 28,** No. 7 (July 1928) 674–676.

61. M.A. Burgess, "The First Grading" **American Journal of Nursing, 29,** (1929) 429–434.

62. Ibid, 429–432.

63. Fitzpatrick, **Prologue to Professionalism,** p.228.

64. Esther Lucille Brown, **Nursing for the Future** (New York: The Russell Sage Foundation, 1948), p.2.

65. Ibid., pp.1–2.

66. Sr. Charles Marie Frank, **The Historical Development of Nursing** (Philadelphia: W.B. Saunders, Co. 1953), pp.339–347.

67. Fitzpatrick, **Prologue to Professionalism,** p.236.

68. **Planning for Nursing Needs and Resources,** (Bethesda, Maryland, Division of Nursing, U.S. Department of Health, Education, and Welfare, Bureau of Health Manpower Education.

69. Ibid.

70. Fitzpatrick, **Prologue to Professionalism,** pp.44–45.

71. Griffin and Griffin, **History and Trends,** pp.166–169.

72. Annie W. Goodrich, "The Contribution of the Army School of Nursing" in the **National League of Nursing Education,** Annual Report, 1919 and **Proceedings of the 25th Convention,** (Baltimore: Wilkins and Wilkins, 1919), pp.146–156.

73. Bullough and Bullough, **Modern Nursing,** p.169.

74. Griffin and Griffin, **History and Trends,** p.168.

75. Fitzpatrick, **Prologue to Professionalism,** p.28.

76. M. Louise Fitzpatrick, "Nursing and the Great Depression," **American Journal of Nursing, 75,** No. 12, (December 1975) 2188–2190.

77. Bullough and Bullough, **Modern Nursing,** p.189.

78. A. Kalisch and Beatrice J. Kalisch, "From Training to Education: The Impact of Federal Aid on Schools of Nursing in the United States During the 1940s, Final Report of NIH, U.S. Public Health Research Grant, N.U. 00443 (Ann Arbor: University of Michigan, 1974).

79. Beatrice J. Kalisch and Philip A. Kalisch, "The Cadet Nurse Corps—in World War II" **American Journal of Nursing, 76,** No. 2 (February 1976) 240–242.

80. Ibid., pp.240–242.

81. Beatrice J. Kalisch and Philip A. Kalisch "Slaves, Servants or Saints" (An Analysis of the System of Nurse Training in The United States, 1873–1948) **Nursing Forum, 14,** No. 3, (1973) 222–263.

82. Ibid, p.242.

83. "The Nurses' Contribution to American Victory Facts and Figures from Pearl Harbor" **American Journal of Nursing, 45,** No. 9, (September 1945) 683–686.

84. A.R. Clarke, "Thirty-seven Months as a Prisoner of War", **American Journal of Nursing, 45,** No. 5, (May 1945) 342–345.

85. Bullough and Bullough, **Modern Nursing** p.190.

86. E.A. Aynes, **From Nightingale to Eagle: An Army Nurse's History,** (Englewood Cliffs, NJ: Prentice-Hall, 1973).

87. J.O. Flikke, **Nurses in Action** (Philadelphia: J.B. Lippincott, 1943).

88. Bonnie Bullough, "The Lasting Impact of World War II on Nursing" **American Journal of Nursing, 76,** No. 1 (January 1976) 116–120.

89. Kalisch and Kalisch, **American Nursing,** pp.192–194.

90. Fitzpatrick, **Prologue to Professionalism,** p.58.

91. Deborah M. Jensen, **A History of Nursing,** (St. Louis: The C.V. Mosby Co., 1943) p.155.

92. Jensen, **A History of Nursing,** 1943, p.155.

93. Fitzpatrick, **Prologue to Professionalism,** p.61, 62.

94. Ibid., p.62.

95. Ibid.

96. Bonnie Bullough and Vern Bullough, "Educational Problems In a Women's Profession," **Journal of Nursing Education,** Vol. 20, No. 7, (September 1981) pp.6–17.

97. Ibid.

98. Joann Ashley, **Hospitals, Paternalism, and the Role of the Nurse,** (New York: Teachers College Press, Columbia University, 1977) pp.8, 9.

99. Ibid.

100. Fitzpatrick, **Prologue to Professionalism.**

101. "American Nurse's Association's First Position on Education for Nursing," **American Journal of Nursing,** Vol. 65, No. 12, (December 1965), p.109.

102. Fitzpatrick, **Prologue to Professionalism,** pp.216–222.

103. Ibid.

104. Lillian DeYoung, **Dynamics of Nursing** (St. Louis: The C.V. Mosby Co., 1981), p.92.

105. Fitzpatrick, **Prologue to Professionalism,** p.71.

106. Bullough and Bullough, "Educational Problems" pp.6–17.

107. DeYoung, **Dynamics of Nursing,** p.95.

108. Bullough and Bullough "Educational Problems," p.6.

109. Fitzpatrick, **Prologue to Professionalism,** p.74.

110. Ibid., p.236.

111. Ibid, p.235–239.

112. Esther L. Brown, **Nursing for the Future,** (New York: The Russell Sage Foundation, 1948).

113. DeYoung, **Dynamics of Nursing,** p.89.

114. **Mosby's Comprehensive Review of Nursing,** 10th Ed. (St. Louis: The C.V. Mosby Co., 1981) p.486.

115. "ANA Position Paper," 1965, p.107.

116. Ibid., p.107.

117. Ibid, p.108.

118. Fitzpatrick, **Prologue to Professionalism,** p.246.

119. Jerome P. Lysaught, **An Abstract for Action** Report of National Commission for the Study of Nursing and Nursing Education (New York: McGraw-Hill, 1970).

120. Ibid.

121. Fitzpatrick, **Prologue to Professionalism,** p.254.

122. National League for Nursing Statistics, 1982.

123. Fitzpatrick, **Prologue to Professionalism** pp.92–94.

124. National League for Nursing Statistics, 1982.

125. Anne Austin and Isabel Stewart, **A History of Nursing** (New York: G.P. Putnam's Sons, 1962) p.205.

126. Janie H. Brown, "Masters Education in Nursing 1945–1969," in **Historical Studies in Nursing** by M. Louise Fitzpatrick,

(New York: Teachers College Press, 1977), p.112.

127. Ibid., p.111.

128. National League for Nursing: **Characteristics of Graduate Education in Nursing Leading to a Masters Degree** (New York, The League, 1978).

129. Fitzpatrick, **Prologue to Professionalism,** p.83.

130. Ibid.

131. Bonnie Bullough, "Nurse Practice Acts," **Nursing 77,** Feb. 1977.

132. Dianne Hales, "A Different Kind of Doctoring," **America's Health,** Vol. 4, No. 2, summer, 1982.

133. Eugene Levine, Ph.D., "The Registered Nurse Supply and Nurse Shortage," **Study of Nursing and Nursing Education Background Paper.** (Washington, D.C.: Institute of Medicine, National Academy of Sciences, January 1983).

134. Linda H. Aiken and Robert J. Blendon, "The National Nurse Shortage" **National Journal,** Washington, D.C.: (May 23, 1981), pp.948–953.

135. Sara Erickson, "Spotlight on History," **New Jersey Nurse,** (January/February 1983), p.9.

136. National Academy Press, **Nursing and Nursing Education: Public Policies and Private Actions,** Division of Health Care Service, Institute of Medicine, Washington, D.C.: The academy, 1983, p.76.

137. "Layoffs Loom as State and Federal Cutbacks Hit California Hospitals," **American Journal of Nursing,** 1983, Vol. 83, No. 2 (February 1983), pp.196 and 204.

138. Margaret D. West, "The Projected Supply of Registered Nurses 1990. Discussion and Methodology," **Study of Nursing and Nursing Education Background Paper,** Washington, D.C.: Institute of Medicine, National Academy of Sciences, January 1983, pp. 19 and 20.

139. Marlene Kramer, **Reality Shock, Why Nurses Leave Nursing,** (St. Louis: The C.V. Mosby Co. 1974), p.viii.

140. Ibid., p.viii.

141. Patricia T. Haase, "Pathways to Practice—Part I," **American Journal of Nursing,** 1976, **76,** No. 5, 806–809.

142. D. Diers and D.L. Evans. "Excellence in Nursing," **Image,** 1980, **12,** No. 2, 27–30.

143. Proceedings for **The First National Conference; Computer Technology in Nursing.** NIH, US Department of Health and Human Services. NIH Publication Number 83-2142.

ANNOTATED BIBLIOGRAPHY

A Nursing 78 Handbook, **A Guide to Nursing Specialties.** Part I (A to M) Nursing 78; 8:10:57–64; October 1978. Part II (N to Z) Nursing 78; 8:10:49–56; November 1978. These two articles list many nursing specialities and the level of nursing education necessary for that specialty. Also listed are selected educational programs, professional organizations, and specialty journals.

Ashley J: **Nurses in American History.** Nursing and Early Feminism. Am J Nurs 75:9:1465–1467; September 1975. This article discusses the effects of paternalism and the role nurses have played in achieving equal rights for women.

Bullough B: **The Lasting Impact of World War II on Nursing.** Am J Nurs 76:1:118 – 120; January 1976. This article discusses long-term implications of wars on the nursing profession.

Christy TE: **Portrait of a Leader.** M. Adelaide Nutting. Nurs Outlook 17:1:20–24; January 1969. This article about Miss Nutting describes her life and role in nursing education, service, and organization.

Christy TE: **Portrait of a Leader. Isabel Hampton Robb.** Nurs Outlook 17:3:26–29; March 1969. Discusses the life and early death of I.H. Robb and describes her unique contribution to nursing.

Christy TE: Portrait of a Leader. **Lavinia Lloyd Dock.** Nurs Outlook 17:6:72–75; June 1969. Reviews Lavinia Dock's impact on modern nursing.

Christy TE: **Portrait of a Leader. Isabel Maitland Stewart.** Nurs Outlook 17:10: 44–48; October 1969. A discussion of the significant contributions to nursing can be found in this brief article about the famous nurse leader.

Dreves KD: **Vassar Training Camp for Nurses.** Am J Nurs 75:11:2000–2003; November 1975. This charming and interesting article is a personal account of one nurse's experience at the Vassar Nursing Camp.

Fitzpatrick ML: **Nursing and the Great Depression.** Am J Nurs 75:12:2188–2190; December 1975. This clearly written article discusses the impact of the depression on nursing and on health care delivery in general.

Goodwin JO, Edwards BS: **Developing a Computer Program to Assist the Nursing Process: Phase I—From System Analysis to Expandable Program.** Nurs Res 24:4:229–305; July–August 1975. This article presents the development of a computer program to formulate nursing diagnoses related to assessment of the integumentary system. The stages of development are clearly outlined, and the reader can gain a good overview of what is involved in planning an automated program, implementing it, and evaluating it.

Kalisch PA, Kalisch BJ: **The Advance of Modern Nursing**. Boston, Little, Brown, and Company, 1978. This excellent text provides a comprehensive analysis of the transition of nursing into a profession. It includes hundreds of photographs and drawings concerning health care and nursing from ancient times to the present.

Nutting MA, Dock LL: **A History of Nursing.** New York, G.P. Putnam's Sons, 1912. This four-volume collection describes the evolution of nursing from prehistory to the early twentieth century. It includes interesting drawings and photographs.

Pocklington DB, Guttman L: **Computer Technology in Nursing: A Comprehensive Bibliography.** Hyattsville, U.S. Department of Health and Human Services HRA 80–65; September 1980. This publication is the result of a comprehensive literature search of books, articles, monographs, and other publications on computers in nursing. All works are either annotated or abstracted and are classified as to their relevance to nursing administration, education, research, and clinical practice. Contains 220 citations.

Richards LAJ: **Reminiscences of Linda Richards, America's First Trained Nurse.** Boston, Whitcomb and Barrows, 1911. This short book describes the experiences of a nurse in the 1800s and gives a fascinating picture of the role of the nurse during this early period of American nursing.

Smith FT: **Florence Nightingale: Early Feminist.** Am J Nurs 81:5:1021–1024; May 1981. This article discusses the life of Florence Nightingale and the evolution of the Nightingale school of nursing.

4

Accountability

Helen Foerst

CHAPTER OUTLINE

OBJECTIVES

After completion of this chapter, the reader will be able to:

- Describe the evaluation and processes of the nursing profession's accountability as society and health care changes.
- Discuss standards development and how standards assure quality of care.
- Relate standards and their application to the nursing process.
- Discuss the purposes of communicating nursing knowledge through written materials.
- Identify the sources of nursing information.
- Describe how technology facilitates literary endeavors.
- Describe the nursing profession's historical perspectives, philosophy, and goals on continuing nursing education.
- Delineate individual, professional, and employer responsibilities for continuing education.
- Discuss the relationship between continuing education and competence in practice.

GLOSSARY

Accreditation—the process by which a voluntary, nongovernmental agency or organization appraises and grants accredited status to institutions, programs, or services that meet predetermined criteria.

Audit—a formal or official examination and verification. A methodological examination and review. A final accounting.

Nursing Audit—the end review of the patient care record to secure measurements of quality of a comprehensive set of components of nursing care.

Certification—a process by which a nongovernmental agency or association certifies that an individual licensed to practice a profession has met certain predetermined standards specified by that profession for specialty practice.

Clinical Practicum—an experiential learning activity under supervision in a clinical setting. It is sometimes referred to as laboratory experience or skill practice.

Contact Hour—a unit of measurement that describes 50 minutes of an approved organized learning experience.

Continuing Education—planned, organized learning experiences designed to augment the knowledge, skills, and attitudes of nurses for the enhancement of nursing practice, education, administration, and research, to improve health care to the public.

Continuing Education Unit (CEU)—ten contact hours of participation in an organized continuing education experience that meets the criteria established by the National Task Force, including sponsorship, capable direction, and qualified instruction.

Criteria—predetermined elements against which aspects of the quality of an activity or service may be compared.

Definition—an arbitrary description that allows common understanding.

Effectiveness—the extent to which pre-established objectives are attained as the result of an activity.

Evaluate—to ascertain or fix the value of, or worth of. To examine and judge, to estimate, appraise, assess, assay, rate.

Factor—any of the component parts instrumental in determining the nature of the complex. Something that actively contributes to the production of a result.

Implement—to carry into effect, fulfill, accomplish. To provide with the means for carrying into effect or fulfilling. To provide a definite plan or procedure to ensure the fulfillment of.

Inservice Education/Staff Development—an educational program planned by an agency to assist employees in becoming increasingly knowledgeable and competent in fulfilling role expectations within that specific agency. The two terms often are used interchangeably, but staff development usually includes out-of-agency activities.

GLOSSARY Continued

Measurement —a comparison of a single phenomenon with a standard. The recorded number or symbol that represents the magnitude of the phenomenon in terms of the magnitude of the standard.

Need—a condition or situation in which something necessary or desirable is required or wanted. Something required or wanted, a requisite.

Norms—numerical or statistical measures of usual observed performance.

Objectives—criteria by which one measures the degree to which the purpose is achieved. The statements are made in terms of results to be achieved rather than methods to be used.

Orientation—the means by which new staff are introduced to the philosophy, goals, policies, procedures, role expectations, physical facilities, and special services in a specific work setting. Orientation is provided at the time of employment and at other times when changes in roles and responsibilities occur in a specific work setting.

Peer—one of equal standing with another.

Peer Review—a process or technique by which people secure observations associated with behaviors of equals.

Nurse Peer Review—a process or technique wherein registered nurses make judgments about the quality of individual components of nursing care in order to secure measurements of that quality.

Quality—the distinguishing characteristics that determine the value, rank, or degree of excellence.

Quality Assurance—in general, to make goodness or excellence certain or secure.

Standard—an agreed upon, established, or expected level of performance or excellence.

Value—a principle or quality that is intrinsically desirable. To rate or scale in usefulness, importance, or general worth. To consider or rate highly, prize, esteem.

INTRODUCTION

Scientific knowledge is being generated, distributed, and assimilated into our technological society with staggering rapidity. The delivery of health care services is becoming an increasingly complex endeavor in a rapidly changing society. A health professional's knowledge base and skills are the result of rigorous preparatory education that must be constantly expanded and updated. Individuals and employers are accountable to the public for the quality of practice offered. This accountability has placed emphasis on the establishment of quality controls, peer review, certification of health professionals, continuing education, and the production of professional literature.

Nursing can point with pride to a long history of growth, development, commitment to quality patient care, and accountability for the services rendered. The record of accomplishment in fulfilling this obligation has kept pace with scientific and technological achievements, changes in health care needs of society, and constantly changing patterns of medical and health care.

This chapter presents an overview of accountability and standards of practice, the professional nursing literature, and aspects of continuing education for nurses. Accountability is examined in terms of the development and implementation of standards of nursing practice and nursing education. The evolutionary processes for assuring accountability are discussed. The nursing literature is discussed in terms of nursing's responsibilty to document its expertise and of the nurse's responsibility to be familiar with the literature. The professional accreditation of programs offering nursing education and agencies offering nursing services and the certification of nursing practitioners are emphasized. Contemporary trends in achieving accountability highlight peer review and quality assurance programs.

Accountability Defined

Accountability is an obligation to reveal, explain, and justify what one does or how one discharges his responsibilities. Within a job or work situation, areas of responsibility include the purposes, principles, procedures, relationships, results, and incomes and expenditures. Applied to nursing, accountability can be defined as the process by which individual or group behavior is explained, analyzed, and justified in relation to established standards.[1] Accountability involves personal and professional responsibility. The individual's and the profession's values are integrated in concepts of accountability. As health care and professional practice have changed, concepts of accountability have expanded. Efficiency and effectiveness were of special

importance in the 1950s. Economical performance and proper productivity were elements of accountability. In the 1960s the concept of appropriateness was emphasized. Goals, policies, values, and the relative benefits of the various health care systems and professional practices were questioned and stressed. Although quality was a basic tenet of the health professions throughout the century, it became the principal conviction and the motivation for refining old and developing new measures of accountability in the mid-1970s. All of the standard measures of accountability that had been developed for assuring quality, such as licensure, accreditation, certification, continuing education, as well as those related to functional performance, were scrutinized. An unprecedented effort was begun to develop definitive measures of quality for establishing standards of care.

STANDARDS OF CARE

Standards of care are the basic framework of accountability. Standards are the attributes of good care. The development of nursing standards and measures of good care can be traced to Florence Nightingale. Standards were implicit in her untiring efforts to provide for better nursing and care of the sick. They also were reflected in her perception of nursing as an art and as a trained profession. The search for indicators and measures of quality care has its origins in the Nightingale systematic evaluation of care and study of the ways in which nursing care was provided.

Webster defines a standard as that which is set up and established by authority as a rule for the measure of quantity, weight, extent, value, or quality.[2] A standard is further defined as an accepted or established rule or model having a recognized and permanent value. A nursing standard measuring quantity, for example, would be the number of nurses that should be available to provide good care. A nursing standard measuring quality would be the training or education essential for those nurses to render care.

Standards have several major characteristics. Two basic elements used in their development are criteria and norms. Criteria are rules for performance and the degree of achievement of the expected outcomes (specified in the criteria of the standard). Norms are predetermined expected levels of performance or achievement, usually the average or median achievement, that can be expected of a large group.

A criterion in the quantitative standard for the number of nurses needed by the nation to provide care would be a ratio of the number of nurses to the population to be served, for example, 560 nurses per 100,000 people. The norm would be a reasonable goal, established by averaging the ratios attained among the several states, that is judged capable of achievement—for example, 300 nurses per 100,000 population. A criterion of the qualitative standard for the training and education of nurses providing care would be the number that ideally should be prepared at the baccalaureate level, for example, one-half of all nurses. The norm would be established by examining the capability of nursing schools to prepare a prescribed number or percentage of nurses with baccalaureate degrees, for example, one-fourth of all nurses. Standards and criteria set objectives and goals for desirable attainment. In addition, they provide a basis for improvement and measurement of the degree to which the goals are met.

Quality, effectiveness, and efficiency are inferred, judged, and measured by established standards and criteria. Different approaches and methods are used for establishing standards. Essentially, they are based on existing good practices that can be used as models. Methods for developing and establishing standards have evolved from basing criteria on the experience and judgment of what constitutes good practice, to conducting surveys and studies of nursing activities to develop measures of good practice. Increasingly, research is being conducted and provides the criteria for standards development. All of the methods have their limitations and can be criticized. Most standards and criteria require and reflect some degree of value judgment and philosophy of the particular group of experts involved in their development.

The earliest standards of care were derived from experience. They were based on policies and procedures and patterns of practice in given situations and institutions that were judged to lead to the provision of good care. They addressed particular aspects of care and nursing activities or the qualifications and functions of the practitioners delivering care. When there were fewer types of services and nurses, and care was less technical, standards were simple measures of quantity, quality, and performance based on concepts of the role of nursing. They were abstract sets of criteria for elements of nursing practice and indicators of competence or quality and guidelines for practice that nursing leaders accepted as attainable. Performance could be evaluated, and progress and achievement measured, by comparison to the recommended standards such as:

- criteria for educational programs
- levels of educational attainment
- the function of each level of nursing personnel
- staffing ratios or number of nurses required for patient care.

One of the primary responsibilities of a profession is to develop and maintain its own standards. The professional nursing organizations assumed responsibility for the development of the standards by which the services of nurses could be evaluated late in the 18th century. The first step was the establishment of the organizations themselves. The first standards were those for membership in the organizations. The criterion was that members be graduates of training schools. One of the major objectives of the early state organizations was legislation for the registration of nurses, which they saw as the first step in the betterment of the nursing profession. The first state law requiring the registration of nurses was passed by North Carolina in 1903, followed by New Jersey in the same year. The New Jersey law stated:

> "any graduate nurse deserving to practice the profession of a trained nurse must first obtain a license (upon presentation of a diploma and 50 cents) from the clerk of the county in which such applicants reside"[3].

The registration acts set standards for the quantity and quality of training for practice. In the New Jersey law the diploma was to be awarded by:

> "a training school connected with a hospital of the state where at least two year's practice and theoretical training is required"[4].

Standards of performance also were embodied in the early permissive licensing statutes. Only registered persons were authorized to use the particular title or official designation specified in the legislation. Unregistered persons were not prohibited from working in the nursing field but could not use the title. The licensing laws were meant to protect the public and the registered nurses from incompetent practitioners.

Between 1903 and 1923 all of the existing 48 states passed nurse practice acts and established state boards of examiners who inspected schools and administered compulsory examinations for graduates of approved schools. The practice acts have been amended as nursing practice changed. Most acts are now mandatory. A mandatory law requires all who nurse for

monetary compensation to be licensed. The nurse practice acts incorporate statements on the function of the nurse or the nature and scope of nursing practice.

The professional associations developed other means for its members or practitioners to judge one another as professionally competent and to evaluate the quality of their services. The evolution of today's standards of care is reflected in definitions of nursing, in statements on the functions and qualifications of nurses, and in manuals and guidelines for practice. A history of *The National Organization for Public Health Nursing 1912–1952 Development of a Practice Field* records one organization's development of standards for nursing services and education and changes in those standards as the practice and education of public health nurses evolved.[5]

In 1916, the National Organization for Public Health Nursing (N.O.P.H.N.) developed and issued its official definitions of public health, district, visiting, school, and industrial nursing. *The Visiting Nurse Manual* was published. It contained daily nursing routines, nursing care techniques, and specific information on the care of medical, surgical, pediatric, maternity, and chronically ill patients. The manual was regarded as the basic standards for public health nursing. Standards for the qualification of nurses in public health work were issued in the same year, to be enforced by 1930. These are recognized as the first official minimum educational qualifications to be set by the professional nursing organizations. These qualifications were: high school graduation, completion of nurse training, state registration, and a minimum of four months of field experience in public health nursing. The standards were waived for those nurses who graduated from training schools before 1920. The N.O.P.H.N. upgraded and revised its statement of the qualifications for public health nurses every five years. The 1935 standards, for example, called for staff nurses with one year's postgraduate education in public health nursing, and the 1950 standards, for baccalaureate preparation.

An official *Public Health Nursing Manual* was published in 1926.[6] It was to serve as a general guide for practice and included procedures and techniques of care and practice in clinics, schools, homes, and industry. The manual was revised in 1932 and 1939 and was recognized as the standards guidebook for public health nurses for 25 years. The development and revision of standards also included periodic redefinitions of public health nursing, official descriptions of the various kinds of public health nursing services, and the functions of public health nursing. The 1931 statements contained objectives and functions based on age, disease, and practice setting. The 1936 and 1941 statements added emphasis on a general approach to care. The independent functioning of nurses and the assessment of health problems, care planning, and evaluation were stressed in the 1949 statements. Changes in definitions and functions were, naturally, related to changes and new developments in nursing practice.

Many of the original and revised definitions of nursing and functions and qualification standards resulted from various studies of nursing. They were views of what was required as recommended in studies of nursing practice and nursing education. Over the years, broad-based studies of nursing, the surveys on nursing activities, and research on elements of patient care have provided knowledge on nursing practice, services, and patient care needs on which standards were based. The purpose of these studies was the improvement of nursing practice. Some examples of these efforts will be described.

The Goldmark Report of 1923—a study of nursing and nursing education—set goals for the educational preparation of nurses in administration, supervision, and instructor positions, and for public health

nurses.[7] Initiated to study the status of public health nursing and propose training for nurses' preparation, the entire fields of nursing service and nursing education were assessed. The work is recognized as the first in which actual observations of nursing practice were made in order to develop recommendations.

The Committee on the Grading of Nursing Schools of the National League of Nursing Education issued two study reports in 1934. One report recommended and set standards for the educational preparation of faculty in nursing schools—that they be registered nurses with special training and experience in particular fields of nursing.[8] Entrance requirements for students—that they meet the entrance requirements of a good college—were also recommended. The second report, *An Activity Analysis of Nursing*, distinguished nursing functions from non-nursing duties.[9] Conclusions on what every nurse should know and do became criteria for judging a competent nurse.

A natural progression in the development of standards was studied in the particular settings where standards are applied. In 1937, the National League for Nursing Education conducted a study in 50 general hospitals to find out how well patients were nursed.[10] The hours of nursing care provided patients by graduate nurses, students, attendants, and ward helpers were obtained. The time provided was analyzed in terms of type of hospital, service, and shift. Recommendations suggested minimum hours of bedside service per patient in each 24 hours for medical, surgical, obstetric, and pediatric units. The number and kinds of personnel needed and their hours of employment were included.

In the mid- and late-1940s, the profession began efforts to rigorously validate its nursing care standards by more indepth studies of nurse staffing and the utilization of nurses. In 1948, the National League of Nursing Education selected 22 hospitals in the New York City area that were reported to be well managed and were providing quality nursing care. An extensive study was made of nurse-patient ratios in these hospitals.[11] It was determined that, on the average, each patient received 3.5 hours of nursing care per day, of which two-thirds was provided by registered nurses and one-third by nursing aides, practical nurses, and others. This ratio, based on existing good practice in hospitals, became a model for the delivery of nursing services and a standard for staffing mix in hospitals for many years.

Another step was the development of techniques and instruments for measuring the nursing care requirements from which levels of patient care and nurse staffing could be determined in acute care settings. Patients in these settings were classified in care groups according to the intensity of illness and need for care. For example, patients who could feed, bathe, and dress themselves would be placed in one group; those who needed to be bathed, dressed, and fed in another. The purpose of the earliest patient classification instruments was to determine the number of nursing personnel required and how staff should be allocated to care for these patients. Patient classification systems provided norms for staffing. Various tools and guidelines for their use were developed to classify patients in hospitals and nursing services.[12–14] More than 40 different methods have been developed.[15] The patient assessment associated with classification provided indications of care needs that helped to strengthen standards development. As patient classification and other assessment tools for appraising patient care needs were developed and refined, they were used in conjunction with and as part of care planning and evaluation. Well defined patient care standards reflect the nursing process.

Many corollary efforts led to the development and refinement of nursing care criteria, models of nursing practice, and nursing practice standards. One effort and source of professional impetus was the American Nurses Association's Code of Ethics.[16] The code was adopted in 1950 and was revised in 1960, 1968, and 1976. It identified acceptable areas of nursing practice, conduct, and relationships. The code of ethical standards supports high quality nursing care and the establishment, maintainence, and improvement of nursing practice and patient care standards. The eighth standard in the code speaks to the nurse's responsibility to participate in standards development: "The nurse participates in the profession's effort to implement and improve standards of nursing." The ANA Code items and interpretative statements can be found in Chapter 8. The ANA Code for nurses and its interpretative statements reflect the concepts of responsibility and accountability as they apply to contemporary nursing theory.

As the professional association for public health nurses from 1912–1952, the N.O.P.H.N. established standards and guidelines for the practice of public health nurses. The ANA, as the professional organization for registered nurses, is concerned with all matters pertaining to their practice. The first standards were developed for private duty nurses in 1916. Since then, the ANA periodically has defined nursing and established, revised, and published new standards. In the 1950s, the ANA conducted a full study on the functions of nursing and issued publications on the functions, standards, and qualifications of various nurse positions, such as general duty nurses, office nurses, and industrial nurses.[17]

In the 1966 reorganization of the ANA, Divisions of Practice were established for the advancement of practice in the fields of medical-surgical nursing, maternal and child health nursing, psychiatric and mental health nursing, geriatric nursing, and community health nursing. These divisions and the Congress of Nursing Practice were charged with establishing standards of nursing practice in their fields of concern.[18] Generic standards and standards developed in the special fields of nursing by the five divisions were published by ANA in 1973 and 1974 in separate booklets. A list of these standards and others in subspeciality areas published later are listed in Figure 4-1. Also see references 19–35 for the source documents. The standards are guidelines for adaptation by individual nurses to clients in particular nursing situations for development of the care plan and to appraise the effectiveness and excellence of care. They were specifically designed to be used as part of the nursing process. The standards outline assessment factors or criteria for:

- Collection of data about the health status of the individual
- Nursing diagnosis derived from the health status data
- Formulating goals for nursing care
- Developing the plan for nursing care to meet the goals
- Implementation of the nursing care plan
- Evaluating the plan and patient response to care
- Reassessment, rediagnosis, setting new goals, revision of plan of care.

The standards provide assessment factors focused on physiological functions, elements of care, and patient goals for the speciality or subspeciality fields of practice. For example, in the standard for cardiovascular nursing practice, the assessment factors on data for health status include pulmonary, vascular, and circulatory criteria.[26] They must be applied to the specific patient with arrythmias, congestive heart failure, or acute myocardial infarction.

ANA Specialty Group	Year Established
Standards of Nursing Practice	1973
Cancer Nursing Practice Outcome Standards	1979
Cardiovascular Nursing Practice	1981
Community Health Nursing Practice	1981
Emergency Nursing Practice	1975
Geriatric Nursing Practice	1973
Gerontological Nursing Practice	1973
Maternal-Child Health Nursing Practice	1973
Medical-Surgical Nursing Practice	1974
Neurological and Neurosurgical Nursing Practice	1977
Orthopedic Nursing Practice	1975
Operating Room Nursing Practice	1975
Pediatric Oncology Nursing Practice	1978
Perioperative Nursing Practice	1981
Psychiatric-Mental Health Nursing Practice	1973
Rehabilitation Nursing Practice	1977
Urological Nursing Practice	1977

Figure 4-1. ANA Specialty Groups with Standards of Practice.

It should be noted that many of the speciality standards were developed in cooperation with the speciality nursing organization concerned. For example, the *Standards of Nursing Practice: Operating Rooms* were joint endeavors of the ANA and Association of Operating Room Nurses (AORN).[30] The AORN prepared and published for its members an implementation case study to interpret the standards and illustrate how they are used, and republished the standards in 1978.[36] Examples from the hypothetical case for each of the seven standards explain how the criteria are applied to the patient situation.

In publishing the generic and speciality standards in 1973–74, the ANA pointed out that the standards were only an initial step toward measuring quality of care. Work was begun immediately on developing a system or model for use with the standards to assure the quality of care rendered. That model has been developed and is being tested. Work in developing standards and means for their application to the actual practice of nursing is never completed. Standards must be continuously refined, modified, and revised. Means for implementation must be explored to keep them relevant to nursing practice and to assist nurses in being accountable for care given.

PROFESSIONAL LITERATURE

Nursing produced and evaluated its own professional literature at an early date. Writing was perceived as a professional responsibility—an obligation inherent in accountability. To share and communicate expertise and valuable information with others was a mark of professionalism and influenced publication productivity. This philosophy pertains today. The professional literature is as diverse as the nursing profession. The topics are inexhaustible. The literature is disseminated through journals, periodicals, books, texts, and reports that speak to nursing theory processes and document its studies and research efforts. To facilitate the use of the literature, nursing has produced reference guides, manuals, handbooks, indexes, dictionaries, and bibliographies.

Purposes

The professional literature serves many purposes. Writing ability and communication through the written media is important in every facet of nursing. In general, nursing publications are used to communicate two types of information focusing on:

- The issues, trends, or beliefs related to nurses and nursing practice
- The clinical or theoretical knowledge basis of nursing and reporting of technical and scientific methods.

The literature is intended to enhance nurses' knowledge in clinical practice, education, administration, and research. It promotes the application of that knowledge in nursing practice. The hope is to effect change and to keep nursing practice relevant to trends in health care. The purpose and effectiveness of the nursing literature are illustrated in the following examples from its development and trends.

The first publications for nurses in the United States were textbooks published in 1878 and 1879 by groups of nurses in the early schools of nursing. These schools were operated mainly to train workers for the parent hospital. The first two textbooks were handbooks written for the graduate practicing nurses and the student apprentices in the Bellevue and Connecticut Training Schools for Nursing. They were small compact manuals or guidebooks covering the complete system of nursing in these institutions.

The *American Journal of Nursing* (AJN) published its first edition in October 1900. The golden anniversary issue credited the journal with exerting great influence on laying the foundations of nursing.[37] As an important media of nursing communication, and unification, the *Journal* furthered the development of professional organizations. It provided a forum for the exchange of nurses' ideas and was a "source of information about the art and technic of nursing care." By nurturing concerted action and concern for the quality of care offered the public, nursing practice was secured and improved.

The impact that the written word and nursing's literary ability can have on the political process in nursing is implied by Kalisch and Kalisch in their book *Politics of Nursing*.[38] Letters, telegrams, and written policy statements on legislative issues of concern to nursing are used to influence the position and action of key lawmakers on pending legislation. The well-written and literate testimony of the professional associations and other nursing pressure groups can be an effective means of influencing the votes of legislators on proposed laws that involve nursing.

Encouraging Accountability

The commitment of the nursing profession to produce its own literature includes responsibility for preparing nurses to write and publish. To encourage literary endeavors benefiting nursing, instruction in developing writing skills and in the publishing process is included in many nursing education programs. Continuing education workshops also offer this instruction. Texts and journal articles address the criteria and pitfalls in manuscript preparation. Hospital nursing services are instituting programs to encourage writing for publication by nurses at the clinical practice level. Authorship promotes nursing excellence through communication and learning across practice settings. In addition to instruction in writing skills, these programs often include a journal club. Journal clubs stimulate writing and publication. Here, the content, writing style, techniques, and professional impact of journal articles are reviewed and critiqued by groups of nurses. Topics for publication are identified and publication goals reinforced. All of these efforts are deliberate means to foster the essential communication of nursing knowledge through the written media.

Efforts to develop the writing skills of nurses and provide knowledge of the publication process, in part, help to assure quality in the nursing literature. But nursing literature is also, in large part, subject to the criteria and standards of publishers. It is generally accepted, in the scientific community, that the most highly valued articles and informational materials are those of publishers that use a refereed process for evaluating the quality of manuscripts. A refereed process usually uses three or more experts and consultants in the subject area or professional field to review manuscripts for acceptance or rejection. It is a professional peer review process that influences and develops excellence in literary endeavors.

Writing also has many recognized values for the author. It requires review of the current literature, keeps one abreast of professional trends, and promotes learning. In addition, in many education programs in institutions of higher education, writing and publishing is a factor in promotion, tenure, and career advancement. One standard to measure the quality of academic activities is the number of articles published in reputable journals.[39] Publishing is seen as a professional responsibility, and the "future of the profession depends on it."[40]

Accessing the Literature

Rapid advances in science and technology and changes in health care delivery quickly outdate current information and knowledge. On the other hand, modern technology facilitates both the preparation of literary materials and their access. Critical reading is essential to maintaining competence and lifelong learning. This assumes an awareness of pertinent journal articles and new nursing literature. Selection of journal and reference materials appropriate to learning needs is equally important. Knowledge of the sources of professional information, the use of library resources and reference services, and the development of discriminate reading and writing habits and skills are of paramount importance.

Knowledge of and access to the literature is important for its ready use by nurses to help improve the quality of their practice. Knowledge and review of the literature is essential to teachers so that they are fully informed about their subject matter and are up-to-date in their field of

instruction. Search and study of the literature is required by researchers to develop
and formulate their research topics and
methods. Nursing theories are generated
from study of recorded and reported nursing information. Nursing also must perpetuate its literature to continuously develop the profession's scientific body of
knowledge.

Recognizing the importance of access to
the literature, the nursing profession has
furthered the development of nursing bibliographies, indexes, abstracting services,
and other library resources. Three excellent examples of library resources for nursing information are the following nursing
indexes. The *International Nursing Index* is
a periodically updated bibliography published quarterly since 1966 with an annual
cumulative edition.[41] Articles in 200 nursing journals are included. Subjects are
classified in accordance with a system developed with the National Library of Medicine (NLM). Libraries across the country
participating with NLM in the dissemination of health and scientific information
use or modify this classification system to
fit their users.[42] Libraries make titles in
the index available through a computerized information retrieval system.

*The Cumulative Index to Nursing Litera-
ture* was first published in 1956 and in-
dexed topics in major English language
nursing periodicals. It was the only nursing literature index from 1960–65. In 1967,
it added indexes from the publications of
the national nurses' associations, and in
1972, those of the state nurses' associations.
Since 1977 it has expanded coverage to
include selected periodicals for certain allied health professions and changed its
name. Today *The Cumulative Index to Nursing and Allied Health Literature* is still a
valuable source of information on topics in
nursing journals and periodicals. In addition, it contains lists of books, films, filmstrips, recordings, and pamphlets.[43]

The *Nursing Studies Index*, prepared by
Virginia Henderson and a Yale University
staff, is recognized as the foremost index
for nursing literature for the period
1900–1959.[44] Its four volumes are an annotated guide to research reports, studies,
biographies, and historical materials
about nurses and nursing reported in English language books, periodicals, and journals for the first 60 years of the 20th century. It is the single most important
resource for locating historical materials
on nursing practice, education, administration and research, and the development
of the nursing profession. Included are
sources of trend data and information on
nursing personnel, services, agencies, institutions, and programs.

Libraries across the country are a valuable resource for obtaining clinical and
health information. The development of
better library resources for nursing has
been promoted by the Interagency Council
on Library Resources, an advisory body of
representatives of 19 agencies and organizations, including the American Nurses Association, the National League for Nursing, the American Hospital Association,
and the U.S. Public Health Service. It has
encouraged improved library services and
makes information on library resources
available to nurses. The major database on
literature in the nursing field is available
from the National Library of Medicine
(NLM). Databases contain information
available in a printed index or in a series of
printed indexes. Through the use of the
computer for storing and retrieving information, libraries have access to vast resources of information. Computerized information and retrieval systems now make
it possible for nurses and other health professionals to obtain reference materials
and current professional literature at their
own location. The most highly developed
international system is that of the NLM.
The databases are searched for subscribing
libraries in two ways: **on-line** and **off-line.**
On-line means that interaction with a com-

puter is direct through the use of a terminal connected by telephone to the computerized document retrieval system. Off-line means that processing is at a computer center, and information is mailed to a patron or library.

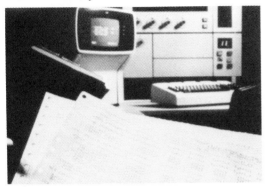

Figure 4-2. On-line computer services allow direct access to reference materials.

The NLM system includes several databases pertinent to nursing. These include the following:[45]

- MEDLINE (Medical literature analysis and retrieval system)
  Covers nursing, medicine, dentistry, and allied health literature since 1978 and some citations since 1975. It includes journals in the *International Nursing Index* and *Hospital Literature* and *Index Medicus*. Available on-line at a subscribing library or institution.

- MEDLARS (Medical Literature Analysis and Retrieval System)
  Covers the same indexes as MEDLINE off-line from 1966 to 1969. MEDLARS went on-line in 1970 and was named MEDLINE.

- AVLINE (Audio Visual Catalog on-line)
  Titles, media type, description, terms, audience level, rating, price, and source of audiovisuals, covering all aspects of health science including nurse patient relations, nurse practitioners, nursing audit, nursing care, nursing staff, legal aspects of nursing, and pediatric nursing, since 1975.

- HISTLINE (History of medicine online)
  Author, title and source of historical information on medicine and other health sciences, individuals, drugs, diseases, institutions, and professions, since 1970.

- CATLINE (Catalog on-Line)
  Author, title, and source of books and serials in the National Library of Medicine's Catalog, covering biomedical, dental, and nursing literature, as well as popular works related to the health sciences by or for laymen.

The NLM system also includes other computerized databases on BIOETHICS (bioethics), CANCERLIT (cancer literature), CANCERPROJ (cancer research projects), and HEALTH (health planning and administration) that have important information of use to nurses.

The NLM retrieval system includes a network of cooperating regional medical libraries that have on-line capability. Eleven major institutions have been designated regional medical libraries (see Figure 4-3). These libraries coordinate requests for on-line accessibility through a communications network. The regional medical libraries also serve as a resource for obtaining other clinical and health information. The approach to the regional medical library system varies from state to state. Materials, documents, and reference services are, preferably, solicited first through the local resource—university, hospital, medical, or health science library. In areas without a local contact point, the regional library may be approached directly.

1. New England Region (Conn., Me., Mass., N.H., R.I., Vt.), Francis A. Countway Library of Medicine, 10 Shattuck St., Boston, Mass. 02115

2. New York and Northern New Jersey Region (New York and the 11 north-

ern counties of New Jersey), New York Academy of Medicine Library, 2 East 103 St., New York, N.Y. 10029

3. Mid-Eastern Region (Pa., Del., and the ten southern counties of New Jersey), Library of the College of Physicians, 19 South 22 St., Philadelphia, Pa. 19103

4. Mid-Atlantic Region (Va., W.Va., Md., D.C., N.C.), National Library of Medicine, 8600 Rockville Pike, Bethesda, Md. 20014

5. East Central Region (Ky., Mich., Ohio), Wayne State University Medical Library, 4325 Brush St., Detroit, Mich. 48201

6. Southeastern Region (Ala., Fla., Ga., Miss., S.C., Tenn., Puerto Rico), A. W. Calhoun Medical Library, Emory University, Atlanta, Georgia 30322

7. Midwest Region (Ill., Ind., Iowa, Minn., N.D., Wis), John Crerar Library, 35 West 33 St., Chicago, Ill. 60616

8. Midcontinental Region (Colo., Kans., Mo., Neb., S.D., Utah, Wyo.), University of Nebraska Medical Center, 42nd St. & Dewey Ave., Omaha, Nebraska 68105

9. South Central Region (Ark., La., N.M., Okla., Tex.), University of Texas Southwestern Medical School at Dallas, 5323 Harry Hines Blvd., Dallas, Texas 75235

10. Pacific Northwest Region (Alaska, Idaho, Mont., Ore., Wash.), University of Washington, Health Sciences Library, Seattle, Washington 98105

11. Pacific Southwest Region (Ariz., Calif., Ha., Nev.), Center for the Health Sciences, University of California, Los Angeles, California 90024

Figure 4-3.   Regional Medical Libraries: Location and Geographic Coverage.

Nurses should be familiar with two im-

portant resources for the reports of government sponsored research and reports by the federal agencies, their contractors or grantees, or special technology groups. The Federal Depository Library System includes some 1,200 libraries nationwide. These libraries receive free and stock federal publications of their choice. Most have the major government publications in the science and health fields. Local libraries have information on the location of the Federal Depository Library in your area.

The National Technical Information Service (NTIS), a component of the U.S. Department of Commerce, is another central, permanent source of scientific and professional literature of government sponsored origin.[46] The NTIS contains a database of 45 files arranged by speciality areas. Of interest to nurses are references to nursing literature in health planning organization and management that includes nurse manpower and nursing services planning. The volumes in the nurse planning information series are shown in Figure 4-4. The NTIS acquires, screens, synthesizes, disseminates, and makes available other specialized documentary material on nursing, as well as methodological information on a wide variety of topics relevant to nursing.

1. **Accountability: Its Meaning and Its Relevance to the Health Care Field**
2. **Nursing Involvement in the Health Planning Process**
3. **The Problem—Oriented System: A Literature Review**
4. **Patient Classification System: A Literature Review**
5. **Nurse Practitioners and the Expanded Role of the Nurse: A Bibliography**
6. **Comparative Analysis of Four Manpower Nursing Requirements Models**
7. **Nursing—Related Data Sources: 1979 Edition**
8. **Relationship between Nursing Education and Performance: A Critical Review**
9. **Nurse Staffing Requirements and Related Topics: A Selected Biography**
10. **Home Health Care Programs: A Selected Bibliography**

11. **Community Health Nursing Models: A Selected Bibliography**
12. **Quality Assurance in Nursing: A Selected Bibliography**
13. **Continuing Education in Nursing: A Selected Bibliography**
14. **A Classification Scheme for Client Problems in Community Health Nursing**
15. **Prospectives for Nursing: A Symposium**
16. **Computer Technology in Nursing**
17. **Factors Affecting Nurse Staffing in Acute Care Hospitals: A Review and Critique of the Literature**

Figure 4-4. Volumes in the Nurse Planning Information Series.

There are, of course, many other reference collections and sources of useful informational materials pertinent to nursing. Only a small number have been discussed for illustrative purposes and to encourage further inquiry. It is important to learn how to access these sources in order to understand the full scope of services available to you for lifelong learning.

Nursing Journals and Periodicals

Nursing journals and periodicals are one excellent resource for keeping abreast of trends in the nursing profession and advancing practice. As the needs for clinical and health information expanded and accelerated, the scope and availability of nursing journals greatly increased. One guide to nursing literature lists 60 major nursing journals alone.[47] If nursing and health related journals are added, the resources number well over 200.[48]

Today, nursing journals reflect the nature of health care, the contemporary knowledge explosion, technical advances, and the need of nurses for information. Between 1900 and 1963, 20 major nursing journals were published. The number increased significantly in the next 20 years, as nursing became more specialized. Nursing journals have a specific audience and

address particular practice interests and specialities. Both the *American Journal of Nursing* (AJN) and *Nursing Research* carry articles for clinical application. The *AJN* articles have a "how to" approach, while the focus in *Nursing Research* is conceptual and scientific.

The professional journals and newsletters are featuring more and more articles on the nursing journals. These articles have primarily addressed publishing opportunities for nurses, journal audiences, and the referee process. A series of articles in *Image*, the journal of Sigma Theta Tau, classified 49 nursing journals in six categories based on their audience and subject content as follows:[49,50]

	Number of Journals
Administration	2
Education	4
General practice	7
Speciality practice	26
Professional development	6
Research	4

The journals devoted to speciality practice were subclassified as follows:

Community/mental health	3
Critical care	7
Gerontology	2
Maternal-child	4
Pediatric nursing	1
Nephrology	2
Oncology	2
Operating room	4
Rehabilitation	1

As can be expected, the survey showed that the journals with the largest circulation were those related to general practice. The three leaders in circulation, with a combined total of more than 1.25 million, were *Nursing '81*, the *American Journal of Nursing*, and *RN Magazine*. The large number of journals in the specialized fields of nursing practice is significant to coverage of major specialities and the scope of the nursing literature.

The American Journal of Nursing, Nursing '84 (the title changes annually to reflect the current year), and the *RN Magazine* offer a broad selection of information on nursing in general. The intended audience differs, however. The *American Journal of Nursing* is the official journal of the American Nurses' Association. It reports, for its membership, important trends, issues, problems, and events of professional concern in the entire spectrum of nursing. It includes important legislation and legal decisions at the federal and state levels, a periodic directory of organizations, a book review section, and articles and programmed instructions in the nursing practice fields. The *RN Magazine* also reports on nursing trends, issues, concerns, and practice. It is directed, however, to the nurse who gives direct patient care and particularly to those nurses who received their basic preparation in the diploma school of nursing. *Nursing '83* whose subject and content areas now include *Nursing Life*, presents easy-to-read selections on clinical practice directed to nurses in direct and acute care settings. It provides excellent surveillance of the perceived practice and employment interests and concerns of staff nurses, such as employee relationships, staff development, and continuing education.

The speciality nursing journals serve as sources of original information on the role and functions of nurses and the art and science of nursing in the particular practice fields. These journals usually feature regular sections devoted to news briefs, book reviews, continuing education programs, trends and issues in the practice fields, and reports on current studies and research with implications for their practice. Those publications that are the official journals of the special professional nursing societies, also feature news on formal organization business, meetings, and members. The organizations' positions on issues and updates on state and federal legislation of interest to the membership also

are included. The journals of the national organizations may carry information and news from or related to their regional or state constituent organizations. The journals focused on the special fields of nursing have value for the specialized information needs of nurses who want to keep abreast of nursing practice, the issues, problems, and conflicts in their fields of practice.

Figure 4-5 illustrates more fully the various focuses of the nursing journals in the four tracts of administration, education, clinical practice, and research. The list is not intended to be all inclusive. *The Lippincott's Guide to Nursing Literature* annotates the contents and subject areas of the current nursing journals.[51] The *Cumulative Index to Nursing and Allied Health Literature*, the *International Nursing Index*, and Henderson's *Nursing Studies Index* help nurses gain access to journal articles on specific subject matter. New journals are still being published periodically and are not included in journal reference lists until they are updated. For example, one of the latest nursing journals is *Nursing Economics Business Perspectives for Nurses*, which published its first issue in July 1983.[52] Anthony J. Jannetti, Inc., who also publishes *Pediatric Nursing, Orthopaedic Nursing, The Pediatric Nurse Practitioner*, and *Occupational Health*, advertises the new journal as meeting an unaddressed need for communicating information about the economics of nursing and the business management aspects of nursing and health care. The audience is nurse executives in middle- and upper-level management positions and nurse consultants who need specific knowledge on the fiscal aspects of nursing service. The regular subject and content areas include: economic issues, markets and marketing, change and innovation, resource management, politics and policy, legal briefs, ethics and values, executive forum, personal finance, and nursing connections. *Nursing Economics* is viewed as a resource for business management skills development and as contributing to the furtherance of the nursing profession in policy and decisionmaking related to the business management, legal and economic aspects of nursing.

Administration
  Journal of Nursing Administration
  The Journal of Nursing Management
  Nursing Administration Quarterly
  Nursing Leadership

Education
  Nurse Education
  Nursing and Health Care
  Nursing Outlook
  Journal of Continuing Education in Nursing
  Journal of Nursing Education

Research
  Advances in Nursing Science
  International Journal of Nursing Studies
  Image
  Nursing Research
  Research in Nursing and Health Care
  Western Journal of Nursing Research

Clinical Practice
  Special
  Cancer Nursing
  Oncology Nursing Forum
  Cardiovascular Nursing
  Critical Care Quarterly
  Critical Care Update
  Focus—American Association of Critical Care
    Nurses
  Heart and Lung
  Journal of Emergency Nursing
  Geriatric Nursing
  Journal of Nurse Midwives
  Maternal Child Nursing Journal
  Pediatric Nursing
  Journal of Neurosurgical Nursing
  Nephrology Nurse

Clinical Practice
  General
  American Journal of Nursing
  Nursing Insights
  Nursing '83
  Nursing Life
  Nurse Practitioner
  Journal of Nursing Care
  RN Magazine
  The Nursing Clinics of North America
  Topics in Clinical Nursing
  Journal of the American Association of
    Nephrology Nurses and Technicians

  Issues in Mental Health Nursing
  Journal of Psychosocial Nursing and Mental
    Health Services
  Occupational Health Nursing
  Orthopedic Nurses Association Journal
  Today's O.R. Nurse
  The School Nurse
  Community Health Nursing
  Rehabilitation Nursing
  Breathline–American Society of Post Anaesthesia Nurses

Figure 4-5. Professional Nursing Journals
Source: Binger, Jane L. and Jensen, Lydia M. **Lippincott's Guide to Nursing Literature**, Philadelphia, PA: J.B. Lippincott Co., 1980, pp. 75–139.

It is imperative that nurses be aware of the current journal sources and become familiar with their subject and content areas in order to select the materials that will best meet their information needs. The need for careful selection of relevant articles and well developed reading habits cannot be overstated. This is an ongoing process of professionalism that can have considerable influence on requirements for changing and improving practice.

CONTINUING EDUCATION

Medical, health care and nursing are no longer static but, continue to change. Competence in practice and individual accountability for the quality of services rendered demands a commitment to continued learning on the part of all health professionals. This commitment implies continuous self development based on periodic review and updating of one's knowledge. Planned appropriate continuing education throughout the professional career is now seen as one assurance of maintaining quality practice.

The terminology **continuing education** came into common use in the past 20 years, and connotes a lifelong learning process that builds on the previously acquired knowledge and skills. Continuing education means continuous updating of knowledge and skills required for practice. The underlying premise is that the quality of health care depends to a large degree on the knowledge, skills, and attitudes of practitioners. The content and structure of continuing education must be flexible in order to meet the practice and career goals of practitioners. Continuing education is defined differently by various health professions. Different concepts of which training or educational activities constitute continuing education stem from the different requirements for basic preparation for general and specialized practice. Continuing education for nurses is broadly defined or interpreted as education of the individual beyond basic preparation for the practice of nursing that promotes the development of nursing knowledge and skills for the continuing enhancement of nursing practice.[53] Continuing education for nurses is directly related to the scope of nursing practice and professional growth. It is most often job related. Nursing does not have one universally accepted approach to basic preparation. Hence, participation in formal degree education is considered as continuing either from diploma or associate degree, to baccalaureate degree, to advanced degree, or to specially designed clinical programs. Included also are programs for advanced preparation in administration, education, and research.

Orientation programs for employment and on-the-job training are not regarded as continuing education unless they fill or update an identified gap in knowledge or skills. For example, if the analysis of nursing audit data identifies a knowledge deficiency among the group of nurses providing care in a given situation, an on-the-job training or in-service education program designed to correct that knowledge deficiency would be considered continuing education. Continuing education for nurses that meets criteria established and recog-

nized by the nursing profession may include:

1. Academic courses, with or without credit, offered by educational institutions, professional associations, or consumer groups
2. In-service education programs offered by the employer
3. Self-directed study or clinical practice based on identified professional nursing needs.

Trends in Continuing Education

The continuous upgrading of professional competence is a priority tenet of the profession of nursing and its organizations. The early role of the professional organizations in continuing education is evidenced in the publication of the nursing journals that contained articles on clinical nursing practice. The *American Journal of Nursing* and the *Public Health Nurse Quarterly*, from their initiation in 1900 and 1913, respectively, were intended to be sources of information about the art and technique of nursing care.[54,55] Signe Cooper and May Hornback, leaders in continuing education in nursing, in their book *Continuing Nursing Education*, trace educational efforts that could be identified as continuing education to the early 1900s.[56] The alumnae associations of the first schools of nursing offered educational programs for their members as early as the 1870s. Hospitals, in the early 1900s, offered postgraduate programs for nurses, such as post-graduate programs in maternity nursing. The early university schools of nursing in the 1920s began to provide credit and noncredit courses for updating knowledge and skills and keeping nurses abreast of practice. The schools of nursing were committed to continuous learning and offered a variety of continuing education programs throughout the 1930s, 1940s, and 1950s.

Continuing education took on national

significance in the 1960s. As the need became more and more evident, federal monies were appropriated for continuing education. The Health Amendments of 1959 included aid for nurses enrolled in short-term courses.[57] The program began in February 1960 and in two years had made 200 grants to institutions for short-term courses and had enrolled approximately 13,000 nurses.

The development of regional medical programs under the Heart Disease, Cancer and Stroke Amendments of 1965 (Public Law 89–239) was a significant impetus for continuing education in the health fields.[58] The purpose of the program was education, research, training, and demonstration in the fields of cancer, stroke, kidney, and related diseases in order to improve the quality of care for patients with these diseases. The intent of the law was to diminish morbidity and mortality associated with these chronic diseases, the "principal killers." This was to be done by disseminating knowledge about them from researcher to practitioner, and by Regional Medical Programs (RMPs) emphasizing continuing education for physicians, nurses, and other health professionals through cooperative arrangements among health agencies and their staffs. The RMPs supported the hiring of a large number of the most competent professionals in heart disease, cancer, and stroke who demonstrated a variety of approaches to health professional training and continuing education and the dissemination of knowledge by telecommunications. Its coronary care training and demonstration projects are credited with training 12,000 nurses in coronary care and expanding the number and effectiveness of coronary care programs.

Continuing education is now well established as a professional responsibility and is supported and provided by educational institutions, the professional societies, and a wide variety of health agencies and commerical interests. Continuing education, today, is not traditional education or the transmission of knowledge from master teacher to learner. It is based on problem solving concepts and approaches for initiating actions that will produce changes required in nursing and health care systems. Continuing nursing education addresses specific learning needs and permits the learner to identify problems. It is intended to provide mechanisms to help the learner solve problems and become more effective and productive in work situations. Continuing education in nursing tends to deal with new roles for nurses, new and innovative health care and services, and the additional knowledge and skills required for specialized areas of practice.

The Continuing Education Unit

In general, continuing education is viewed as an educational offering not awarded academic credit. A system for recognizing credits for continuing education was, therefore, devised. In 1968, more than 30 interested agencies established a national task force to develop a uniform unit to identify, measure, and recognize individual efforts or accomplishments in noncredit continuing education. The task force developed the continuing education unit (CEU), defined standards for continuing education, and set operational procedures and guidelines to implement the CEU mechanism.[59]

The continuing education unit (1.0 CEU) is defined as "10 contact hours of participation in an organized continuing education experience under responsible sponsorship, capable direction and qualified instruction." The CEU provides a common measure for accumulating data on noncredit continuing education training or a universal way of recording completed courses and continuing education activities. Today, the CEU has been adopted by colleges, universities, professional societies, and government and industrial training centers across the country as a basis for award of certificates of continuing education. Licensing boards, certification bodies, professional societies, and other institutions that may require verification of continuing education also use the CEU for recording purposes. The CEU is well suited to computer recording and retrieval of continuing education information. The American Nurses' Association, the National League for Nursing, the Association of Operating Room Nurses, and the State Nurses' Associations have recognized the CEU but tend to use the contact hour as the basic unit, for recording purposes, for their continuing programs.

The criteria and guidelines specified by the National Task Force on the Continuing Education Unit are the essential elements of sound educational programs. They include:

- Sponsoring organization with an identifiable educational unit, to assure that educational objectives are met
- Professional staff qualified to administer, coordinate, and conduct continuing education
- Appropriate educational facilities and instructional aids
- Capability to plan, design, conduct, and evaluate a program or activity in response to the educational needs of a large group
- A system for recording and verifying awarded CEUs.

The CEU is not to be awarded for work experience, orientation courses, community service, publication of articles, committee meetings or assignments, self-study, or research projects.

No organization has authority over another in the awarding of CEUs. It is expected, however, that agencies that choose to use the CEU meet the criteria and guidelines prescribed by the National Task Force

on Continuing Education Units. The CEU does not connote the accreditation of continuing education programs or single offerings. The use of the CEU, rather, implies "approval," meaning that the program or offering has been evaluated by the agencies or institutions concerned as meeting the national task force criteria for awarding CEUs.

The accreditation of sponsors or providers of continuing education is vested with the accrediting bodies of educational institutions. The total nursing program is accredited, not individual courses or separate departments within the nursing program structure, e.g., the Department of Continuing Nursing Education. The National League of Nursing accredits schools of Nursing. The American Nurses' Association accredits providers of continuing education, such as the state nursing associations, military and government services, and commercial providers.

The Professional Associations and Continuing Education

When the need to make opportunities for continuing education available to all types of health personnel became widely recognized in the early 1960s, the professional organizations took the initiative in instilling in their membership the importance of continuing education. The need was discussed at professional meetings, at conferences, and in educational groups. Various programs for furthering continuing education endeavors were developed. The associations have issued statements on continuing education for nurses; developed standards and guidelines for the individual nurse, nursing services, nursing education programs, and the employers of nurses; and established programs for the accreditation of continuing education.

The nursing profession believes and takes the position that the ultimate responsibility for both short- and long-range continuing education rests with the individual nurse. The responsibility is diverse and includes identification of one's continuing education needs, making these needs known to the employer and providers of continuing education, taking the initiative to seek continuing education activities to meet the identified needs, sharing the information obtained from the continuing education activities with the employer and colleagues, and accepting responsibility for an evaluation of continuing education activities.

The professional accountability for continuing education extends to nursing education institutions and programs. Nursing schools are charged with professional responsibility for instilling in students the desire for continuing self-education and for providing continuing education opportunities that meet prescribed educational standards. The standards were developed for all providers of continuing education. They apply the sound principles and criteria for planning, implementing, and evaluating educational courses for the adult learner. The employer's responsibility for continuing education for nurses is seen primarily as accountability to the health care recipient. The employer is expected to facilitate continuing education for nurses through the establishment of policies that stimulate and encourage nurses to participate in continuing education. It is further recommended that employers provide the time and/or finances for appropriate continuing education outside the institution or agency. In addition, employers should hold the participants accountable for the application of learning to the practice situation.

Accreditation of Continuing Education

To help assure quality in continuing education, the American Nurses Association (ANA) developed a voluntary national system of accreditation of continuing education activities in nursing. As defined by the ANA, "accreditation of continuing education in nursing is the process whereby the Association, through designated approving bodies, grants public recognition to continuing education activities which meet certain established educational standards as determined through initial and periodic evaluations."[60] Through the accreditation program, the ANA provides for the implementation of the standards at the national, state, and local levels and encourages sponsors to continually improve the quality of offerings.

The ANA Council on Continuing Education developed specific standards and criteria for continuing education. Through the National Accreditation Board and regional accrediting committees, the criteria are used for accreditation and approval of providers of continuing education. The standards for continuing education provide for a professional nursing judgment as to the quality of continuing education offerings. The standards are based on sound educational principles and include the following factors:[61]

- Assessment of learning needs
- Design of educational offerings
- Implementation of education designs
- Objectives of the educational programs/offerings
- Teaching strategies and methodologies
- Evaluation of outcomes and process
- Record keeping
- Organizational resources/financing.

The ANA accreditation mechanism emphasizes self-regulation and collaboration between all levels of the ANA and other national organizations and agencies that sponsor continuing education activities. Continuing education activities that are approved and conducted by ANA accredited organizations are transferable. Being based on common standards and criteria, all ANA-accredited organizations recognize continuing education programs or offerings of another ANA-accredited organization. This reciprocity is particularly helpful, since continuing education may be acquired from diverse sources and in widely dispersed locations. Most state boards of nursing administering mandatory continuing education licensure regulations and laws also recognize continuing education sponsored by ANA-accredited organizations as meeting their mandatory requirements.

At the beginning of 1982, the ANA reported that 33 state nurses' associations, 5 federal nursing services, and 10 speciality nursing organizations were accredited as providers or approvers of continuing education. Accreditation also was awarded to 20 nondegree granting, expanded role programs in nursing and to the continuing education offerings of 30 individual providers. The ANA periodically publishes a directory of its accredited organizations and approved offerings.[62] This directory is most useful in identifying accredited sponsors of continuing education.

Mandatory Continuing Education

An issue of significant concern to all health professions that generated considerable debate in the early 1970s was that of mandatory versus voluntary continuing education. Mandatory continuing education is prescribed attendance at a set number of practice related courses, or a set number of hours of continuing education within a given period of time, in order to maintain licensure. The contention was that mandated continuing education would maintain and assure professional competence.

As of January 1, 1983, 11 states required mandatory continuing education for nurses. In these states, legislation had designated the State Board of Nursing as the official state agency to control and assure the competence of nurses through continuing education. The underlying rationale is to protect the public by upgrading nursing practice. The premise is that by requiring the nurse to participate in continuing education, learning will result, and practice will be changed and improved. The states' mandating continuing education for relicensure and the particular state requirements are shown in Figure 4-6.

Today, there is little disagreement about the value of continuing nursing education. The technical advances in continuing education for nursing and its increased accessibility in the past 10 years have unlimited potential for assisting in professional growth. Continuing nursing education substantially contributes to expanding knowledge, correcting deficiencies, and promoting excellence. The necessity for completing a required number of hours of attendance at "approved" courses or offerings and submitting the proper forms to assure continuing licensure or certification, however, is still fraught with controversy.

The relative significance and outcome of the process of mandatory continuing education is subject to question and, as yet, has failed to reveal evidence of the usefulness and worth.

The real underlying issue in the value of mandatory continuing education is evaluation of the outcomes of continuing education and the proven effects on nursing practice. "Approved" continuing education offerings, courses, or programs incorporate planned methods of evaluation. The most common evaluation tools are pencil and paper tests on the information learned about each course objective and participants' satisfaction ratings on the methods of course presentation, the learning environment, and the facility or instructors. What is lacking, in terms of mandatory continuing education, is effective ways for

STATE	CE FIRST REQUIRED	HOURS OF CE REQUIRED	LICENSE RENEWAL PERIOD
For all registered nurses			
California	July 1, 1978	30 hrs. (6 hrs. study permitted)	every 2 yrs.
Colorado	January 1, 1984	30 hrs. '79–'81, 30 hrs. thereafter (no limit on home study)	every 2 yrs.
Florida	January 1, 1981	24 hrs. (no limit on home study)	every 2 yrs.
Iowa	July 1, 1980	15 hrs. (5 hrs. home study permitted)	every year
Kansas	July 1, 1980	5 hrs. '78–'80, 15 hrs. '80–'82, 30 hrs. '82–'84 (1,3,6 hrs. home study permitted)	every 2 yrs.
Kentucky	April 30, 1982	5 hrs. '82, 10 hrs. '83, 15 hrs. thereafter (rules not yet complete)	every year
Massachusetts	On birthday 1982	5 hrs. '80–'82, 10 hrs., '82–'84 15 hrs., '84–'86 (5 hrs. home study permitted)	every 2 yrs.
Minnesota	August 1, 1980	5 hrs., '80–'82, 30 hrs. thereafter (no limit on home study)	every 2 yrs.
Nebraska	January 1, 1980	2 hrs. every 5 years (no limit on home study)	every year
Nevada	January 1, 1982	30 hrs. (6 hrs. home study permitted)	every 2 yrs.
New Mexico	January 1, 1981	20 hrs. '79–'81, 30 hrs. thereafter (no limit on home study)	every 2 yrs.
For nurse practitioners			
Alaska	January 13, 1980	30 hours	every 3 yrs.
Mississippi	September 1, 1981	40 hrs. over 2 yrs.	pediatric, anesthetist: every 2 yrs. adult, family, family planning: every year
New Hampshire	1978	20 hours	every 2 yrs.
Oregon	March 31, 1979	100 hours (plus 25 hrs. pharmacological CE if NP prescribes)	every 2 yrs.

Source: **American Journal of Nursing**, June 1980 amended and updated from subsequent Journal articles

Figure 4-6.   Mandatory Continuing Education for Registered Nurses.

evaluating the participants changed behavior and improvements in nursing practice as a result of the learning that may have taken place. Collaborative relationships need to be established between the continuing education and nursing service entities concerned, so that evaluation can take place in the patient care setting. Individual goals in continuing education need to be part of nurses' career development and progression plans and their ongoing performance evaluations. Only then will the question of mandatory continuing education be resolved. Today, however, continuing education remains as a career requirement of every health professional.

SUMMARY

Accountability is assuming responsibility for one's own decisions and actions. In relation to nursing, the concept is not new and, as a mark of a profession, has been a characteristic for two centuries. The evaluation of accountability in nursing has kept pace with the changing society and an increasingly complex health care delivery system. The profession has continually delineated methods for guiding nursing practice and evaluating nursing performance and provided means for changing and improving patterns of practice. Three of these major efforts have been discussed—standards, the nursing literature, and continuing education.

Standards development in nursing began in the early 1900s with the enactment of state nurse practice acts that established criteria for the training of nurses and their performance. The early standards were based on experience and judgments of what constituted good practice and care. Nursing standards were later embodied in manuals and guidelines for practice and statements on the function and qualifications of nurses. In their progressive development, standards were based on studies of nursing practice and nursing education

that provided knowledge on nursing practice, services, and patient care needs. The nursing process began to be reflected in nursing standards in the late 1940s. Today, nursing standards are increasingly derived from research and incorporate means for measuring the quality of care.

The nursing profession has promoted quality in practice and the application of its standards and accountability through the simultaneous development of its nursing literature. The development of nursing's theoretical, clinical, and technical literary materials and media has kept pace with the increasing sophistication in clinical practice, education, administration, and research. Communication expertise has been augmented by deliberate endeavors to encourage and prepare nurses to write and publish. Today, the nursing media is impressive and includes thousands of journals, periodicals, books, texts, reports on practice experiences, and documents on studies and research efforts. The content is as diverse as the nursing profession. To facilitate the use of the literature, nursing has produced reference guides, manuals, handbooks, indexes, dictionaries, and bibliographies. Access to the literature is being made more accessible by computerized storage and retrieval systems. Nursing's literary resources are evidence of its accountability.

A highly emphasized part of nursing's accountability is continuing education for nursing. The enhancement of nurses' knowledge to keep nursing practice relevant to trends in health care has been a long-standing professional goal facilitated by post-basic education and short-term courses. Continuing education and lifelong learning is now viewed as a requirement for maintaining competence in practice. This recognized need has given rise to discrete programs for the continuing education requirements for licensure, and accreditation programs for the sponsors and providers of continuing education.

STUDY QUESTIONS

1. Identify and discuss three ways in which the nursing profession has helped to assure quality of care in a rapidly changing society and increasingly complex health care delivery system.

2. What is the relationship between the ANA's standards for nursing practice and the nursing process?

3. Select a special nursing practice field and develop a care plan for a hypothetical case using the nursing practice standards for that particular field.

4. Name two purposes of the nursing literature and describe how it benefits the nursing profession.

5. Select a nursing topic for a term paper and list three or four library resources you would use to identify literature citations relevant to your topic.

6. Discuss the scope of the nursing journals. What are the major differences and similarities of the journals? Who are the various audiences?

7. List two or more retrieval systems for assessing citations and abstracts from the nursing literature.

8. What is the philosophy and position of the nursing profession on continuing education?

9. Why have states enacted laws requiring mandatory continuing education for the relicensure of nurses? What are the issues and answers?

10. What is the significance of the CEU? How is it used?

REFERENCES

1. Stanley J. Matek: **Accountability: Its Meaning and Its Relevance to the Health Care Field** (Hyattsville, MD: DHEW Pub. No. (HRA) 77–72, September 1977), p.4.
2. Webster's Seventh New Collegiate Dictionary, 1971.
3. Sara Erickson: "Spotlight on History" **New Jersey Nurse** The New Jersey Nurses' Association, (Trenton, New Jersey: The Association, January/February 1983), p.9.
4. Ibid.
5. M. Louise Fitzpatrick: **The National Organization for Public Health Nursing, 1912–1952: Development of a Practice Field** (New York: National League for Nursing, 1975), pp. 48, 53–54, 101–103, 119, 126, 185–186.
6. The National Organization for Public Health Nursing. **Manual of Public Health Nursing, Third Edition** (New York: The Macmillan Co., 1939), 529 pp.
7. Committee on the Study of Nursing. **Nursing and Nursing Education in the United States** (New York: The Macmillan Co., 1923), 584 pp.
8. Committee on the Grading of Nursing Schools. **Nursing Schools Today and Tomorrow, Final Report** (New York: National League for Nursing Education, 1934), 247 pp.
9. Committee on the Grading of Nursing Schools. **An Activity Analysis of Nursing** (New York: National League for Nursing Education, 1934), 214 pp.
10. The National League of Nursing Education. The Committee on Studies. **A Study of Nursing Service in Fifty Selected Hospitals** (New York: The National League, 1937) 74 pp.
11. National League for Nursing Education. Department of Studies. **A Study of Nursing Service.** (New York: The League, 1948), 63 pp.

12. John P. Young: **A Method for Allocation of Nursing Personnel To Meet Inpatient Care Needs** (Baltimore, MD: The Johns Hopkins Hospital, Operations Research Division, 1962), 32 pp.

13. E.W. Jones, B.J. McNitt and E.M. McKnight: **Patient Classification for Long-Term Care: User's Manual.** (Department of Health, Education, and Welfare, Pub. No. (HRA) 74–3107, December 1973), 99pp.

14. Doris E. Roberts and Helen Hudson: **How To Study Patient Progress** U.S. Public Health Service Pub. No. 1169. (Washington, D.C.: Government Printing Office, 1964), p. 121.

15. Myrtle K. Aydelotte, "State of Knowledge Nurse Staffing Methodology" **Research on Nurse Staffing in Hospitals, Report on a Conference.** U.S. Department of Health, Education, and Welfare, Division of Nursing, (Washington, D.C.: U.S. Government Printing Office, 1973), p.11.

16. American Nurses Association, **Code for Nurses with Interpretive Statements,** (Kansas City, Missouri: The Association, Revised 1976), 20 pp.

17. American Nurses' Association. "ANA Statements of Functions, Standards, and Qualifications," **American Journal of Nursing,** Vol. 56 (July 56) p.899.

18. American Nurses' Association. **Bylaws As Amended.** (Kansas City, MO: The Association, June 1974), pp.21–25.

19. American Nurses' Association. **Standards Nursing Practice.** (Kansas City, MO: The Association, 1973), unpaged.

20. American Nurses' Association. **Standards. Maternal-Child Health Nursing Practice.** (Kansas City, MO: The Association, 1973), unpaged.

21. American Nurses' Association. **Standards. Community Health Nursing Practice,** (Kansas City, MO: The Association, 1973), unpaged.

22. American Nurses' Association. **Standards. Psychiatric Mental Health Nursing Practice.** (Kansas City, MO: The Association, 1973), unpaged.

23. American Nurses' Association: **Standards of Medical-Surgical Nursing Practice.** (Kansas City, MO: The Association, 1974), 8 pp.

24. American Nurses' Association: **Standards. Geriatric Nursing Practice,** (Kansas City, MO: The Association, 1973), unpaged.

25. American Nurses' Association: **Standards of Gerontological Nursing Practice,** (Kan-sas City, MO: The Association, 1976), 8 pp.

26. American Heart Association Council on Cardiovascular Nursing and American Nurses' Association Division on Medical-Surgical Nursing Practice. **Standards of Cardiovascular Nursing Practice.** (Kansas City, MO: American Nurses' Association, 1975), 9 pp.

27. American Nurses' Association Division on Medical-Surgical Nursing Practice and Oncology Nursing Society. **Outcome Standards for Cancer Nursing Practice.** (Kansas City, MO: American Nurses' Association, 1979), 14 pp.

28. American Nurses' Association Division on Medical-Surgical Nursing Practice and Emergency Department Nurses' Association. **Standards of Emergency Nursing Practice.** (Kansas City, MO: American Nurses' Association, 1975), 9 pp.

29. American Nurses' Association Division on Medical-Surgical Nursing Practice and Association of Neurosurgical Nurses. **Standards of Neurological and Neurosurgical Nursing Practice.** (Kansas City, MO: American Nurses' Association, 1977), 12 pp.

30. Association of Operating Room Nurses and American Nurses' Association Division on Medical-Surgical Nursing Practice. **Standards of Nursing Practice: Operating Room.** (Kansas City, MO: American Nurses' Association, 1975), 9 pp.

31. Orthopedic Nurses' Association and American Nurses' Association Division on Medical-Surgical Nursing Practice. **Standards of Orthopedic Nursing Practice.** (Kansas City, MO: American Nurses' Association, 1975), 10 pp.

32. American Nurses' Association, Division on Maternal and Child Health: Nursing Practice and the Association of Pediatric Oncology Nurses. **Standards of Pediatric Oncology Nursing Practice.** (Kansas City, MO: 1978), 7 pp.

33. American Nurses' Association Division on Medical-Surgical Nursing Practice and Association of Operating Room Nurses. **Standards of Perioperative Nursing Practice.** (Kansas City, MO: American Nurses' Association, 1981), 9 pp.

34. American Nurses' Association Division of Medical Surgical Nursing and Association of Rehabilitation Nurses. **Standards of Rehabilitation Nursing Practice.** (Kansas City, MO: American Nurses' Association, 1977), 12 pp.

35. American Nurses' Association and Ameri-

can Urological Association. **Standards of Urological Nursing Practice.** (Kansas City, MO: American Nurses' Association, 1977), 12 pp.

36. Association of Operating Room Nurses. "From Standards into Practice" **Association of Operating Room Nurses Journal.** (Denver, Col: Vol 28, No. 4, October 1978), pp. 603–642.

37. Editorials. **The American Journal of Nursing.** Vol. 50, No. 10 (October 1950) pp. 583–585.

38. Beatrice J. Kalisch and Philip A. Kalisch: **Politics of Nursing** (Philadelphia, PA: J.B. Lippincott Company, 1982), pp. 322–336.

39. Elizabeth Swanson and Joanne C. Mc-Claskey: "The Manuscript Review Process of Nursing Journals" **Image,** Vol. 14, No. 3, (October 1982), pp. 72–75.

40. Margretta Styles: "Why Publish" **Image,** Vol. 10, No. 2, (June 1978) p. 29.

41. American Journal of Nursing Co. **International Nursing** Indep. (New York, NY: quarterly and annual circulations 1966 to date).

42. Katina P. Strauch and Dorothy J. Brundage: **Guide to Library Resources for Nursing.** (New York, NY: Appleton-Century-Crofts, 1980), pp. 400–402.

43. Glendale Adventist Medical Center Publications Service. **Cumulative Index to Nursing and Allied Health Literature.** (Glendale, Calif.: bimonthly with yearly cumulation, 1961 to date.)

44. J.B. Lippincott Company, **Nursing Studies Index.** (Philadelphia, PA: Vol. 1—1900–1959; Vol. 2—1900–1929; Vol. 3—1950–1956; Vol. 4—1957–1959.

45. Jane L. Binger and Lydia M. Jensen: **Lippincott's Guide to Nursing Literature. A Handbook for Students, Writers, and Researchers.** (Philadelphia, Pa.: J.B. Lippincott Company, 1980), pp. 209–215.

46. Strauch, **Guide to Library Resources,** p. 27.

47. Binger, **Lippincott's Guide to Nursing Literature,** pp. 267–268.

48. American Journal of Nursing Company. **International Nursing Index.** 1982 Edition.

49. Joanne Comi McClaskey and Elizabeth Swanson: "Publishing Opportunities for Nurses: A Comparison of 100 Journals" **Image** Vol. XIV, No. 2 (June 1982) pp. 50–56.

50. Swanson, Elizabeth and McCloskey, Joanne Connie "The Manuscript Review Process" **Image,** Vol. XIV, No. 3 (October 1983) pp. 72–75.

51. Binger, **Lippincott's Guide to Nursing Literature,** pp. 72, 82, 85, 118, 130–131.

52. Anthony J. Jannette, Inc. **Nursing Economics Business Perspectives for Nurses** Vol. 1, No. 1 (July/August 1983), pp. 1–60.

53. American Nurses Association, Council on Continuing Education. **Continuing Education in Nursing: An Overview.** (Kansas City, MO: The Association, 1979), 16 pp.

54. Fitzpatrick, M. Louise. **The National Organization For Public Health Nursing 1912–1952: Development of a Practice Field.** (New York: National League for Nursing, 1975), p.31

55. Cuneo Eastern Press. "Editorials" **The American Journal of Nursing** Vol. 50. No. 10. (October 1950) p. 5.

56. Cooper, Signe Skott and Harnback, May Shiga. **Continuing Nursing Education.** (New York: McGraw-Hill Book Company, 1973), pp. 19–34.

57. U.S. Department of Health, Education, and Welfare. Public Health Service. **Toward Quality in Nursing Needs and Goals** Report of the Surgeon General's Consultant Group on Nursing. PHS Pub No. 992 (Washington DC: US Government Printing Office, 1963), p. 41.

58. U.S. Department of Health, Education, and Welfare, U.S. Public Health Service, Health Resources Administration. **Health in America** DHEW Pub. No (HRA) 76–616, (Washington, DC: U.S. Government Printing Office, 1976), pp. 111–113.

59. National University Extension Association. **The Continuing Education Unit.** The National Task Force on the Continuing Education Unit, Washington, DC. (The Association, 1974).

60. American Nurses' Association. **Accreditation of Continuing Education in Nursing.** State Nurses' Associations, National Speciality Nursing Organizations, Federal Nursing Services, State Boards of Nursing. (Kansas City, MO: The Association, 1975), p. 2.

61. Ibid. pp. 20–23.

62. American Nurses Association. **Directory of ANA Accredited Organizations, Approved Programs/Offerings, and Accredited Continuing Education Certificate Programs Preparing Nurse Practitioners.** (Kansas City, MO: The Association, periodically updated).

ANNOTATED BIBLIOGRAPHY

Binger JL, Jensen LM: **Lippincott's Guide to Nursing Literature.** A Handbook for Students, Writers, and Researchers. Philadelphia, J.B. Lippincott Co., 1980. This book is a guide to timely nursing journals, relevant nonnursing periodicals, and selected references for nurses unfamiliar with the literature. The format allows students, the practicing nurse, educators, administrators, and researchers quick access and practical step-by-step assistance in identifying pertinent sources and using relevant journals and references more effectively. The guide features use of the library, steps in literature search and surveillance, computerized literature processes, and how to prepare journal articles and manuscripts. It includes a profile of current nursing journals, indexes and abstracts, a list of statistical information resources, and guides and directories on writing and editing. The guide is intended to facilitate the use and dissemination of nursing literature for independent study and continued learning, for instruction, for writing, and for research.

Johnson BC, Dungca CV, Hofmeisler D, Wells SJ: **Standards for Critical Care.** St. Louis, The C.V. Mosby Co., 1981. This text includes concise descriptions of potential problems, assessment factors, expected outcomes, and recommended nursing activities for more than 60 clinical problems. Introductory materials provide a brief rationale for the standards and suggested activities for care plans.

Mason EJ: **How to Write Meaningful Nursing Standards.** New York, John Wiley and Sons, 1978. Designed as a workbook, this text provides step-by-step methods for writing nursing process, outcome, and content standards. Specific examples of actual standards are provided. A design for writing nursing standards for a unit, division, or health care agency is included.

National League for Nursing: **Guide for the Development of Nursing Libraries.** New York, The League, 1981. This guide for the evaluation of the nursing library also may be used for setting up or further developing nursing library resources and services. The characteristics, functions, administration, operation, and evaluation of the nursing library are succinctly outlined and briefly discussed. Topics covered include the library policies, budget, physical environment, collections, and staff, as well as the technical sources—namely, cataloging and classification, indexing, and abstracting, and computerized retrieval. A bibliography is appended.

Strauch KP, Brindage DJ: **Guide to Library Resources for Nursing.** New York, Appleton-Century-Crofts, 1980. This is a guide for all persons involved in nursing on the usefulness of library resources and tools to the nursing profession. It features general information on the library's functions, services, and use, and current library materials in nursing. Included are both general reference sources and annotated lists of books in selected nursing topics as well as a list of periodicals and audiovisual materials in these subject areas. The names of medical, nursing, and allied health publishers are in the appendix.

5

Health Care System

Sr. Rosemary Donley

CHAPTER OUTLINE

OBJECTIVES

After completion of the chapter the reader will be able to:

- Name inputs into the health care system
- Discuss how inputs affect each other
- Name some processes or throughputs in the health care system
- Discuss how health throughputs compete with each other for resources
- Name some health outputs
- Discuss the interrelationships among outputs
- Explain how feedback is used to change health care systems
- Discuss how nursing inputs affect other subsystems within the health care system.

GLOSSARY

Academic health center—a complex of a medical school, a university hospital, and one other health school, usually a school of nursing.

Access to care—Availability and acceptability of services to people.

Accreditors—A group or a professional association that sets criteria, evaluates institutions, and develops a listing of agencies that meet standards.

Certification—Recognition of special competence or education.

Health care team—The group of health professionals that provides care. Physicians and nurses are members on the team.

Health Maintenance Organization (HMO)—Prepaid health plans that encourage outpatient and preventive health services.

High technology medicine—The use of machines to diagnose, monitor, treat, and relay information.

Lobbyists—Individuals who try to influence public policy in behalf of their constituents.

P.L.—Abbreviation for public law.

Planners—Volunteer or public agencies that design and recommend building and program proposals for health care instutitons.

Prospective reimbursement—A system of payment in accord with prearranged policies that are negotiated before services are provided.

Regulators—A group responsible for controlling operations or enforcing standards.

Reimbursement policies—Decisions and agreements that control how health care professionals and institutions are paid.

Secondary care facilities—Institutions that provide routine treatment and inpatient care to moderately and seriously ill people.

Tertiary care facilities—Institutions that admit directly or on referral seriously ill people or people who require highly specialized diagnosis and treatment.

Third party payers—Private and governmental insurers who provide health insurance plans, negotiate rates with hospitals and physicians, and pay approved health care costs.

DEFINITION OF THE HEALTH CARE SYSTEM

Health care systems or health delivery systems are phrases used to describe the method by which health care is given. This chapter will analyze health care patterns using the language of systems theory. It is important to understand the concepts in systems theory; the reader is referred to Chapter 2 in which Heffron notes that input, throughput, output, and feedback are words used to order discussions. The health field is a complex system. There are many inputs, multiple throughputs, serial outputs, and elaborate feedback mechanisms.

HEALTH CARE SYSTEM

INPUTS	THROUGHPUTS	OUTPUTS
Patients and Their Families	Patient Care	Well People
The Public	Patient and Family Education	
The Media	Education of Health Professionals	Health Care Institutions
Lobbyists		Health Professionals
Health Professionals	Research	Standards of Practice
Students of the Health Professionals	Standard Development	Standards of Care
Unions	Regulation	Reimbursement Policies
Health Care Institutions		Law
Technology	Legislation	Health Care Plans
Planners, Regulators, Accreditors		
Insurance Companies (Third Party Payers)		
Legislators		

Figure 5-1. Components of the Health Care System.

Figure 5-1 lists the components of the health care system as they will be presented in this chapter. Some of you may find, as you examine the list that you disagree with this classification system. For example, it may be argued that regulations are "inputs," or that patient care is an "output." Both of these are correct. The task of assigning a label as "input" or "throughput" to components of an open system enables us to discuss their interrelationships. Relationships among parts are significant to goal achievement. In an open system there is a constant exchange of energy, activity, and information. Consequently, the classification system proposed in Figure 5-1 presents one way of understanding how patients, doctors, nurses, and institutions work together to achieve health care.

Each section of the health system operates with different values, goals, and information. Sometimes health systems experience trouble or dysfunction because of these differences. On the other hand, the system usually works to the satisfaction of patients, nurses, and the public. The discussion of the health care system will begin with a close look at the inputs. Health systems need patients, people trained to help them, and a place in which the system can work.

THE HEALTH CARE INPUTS

The Patient as an Input

Who are the patients or clients and how do they enter the health system? Although most patients seek health care because they perceive a lack of well-being, there are various states of health. People can be worried well, mildly ill, moderately ill, acutely ill, chronically ill, or dying when they seek health care.[1] Consequently, one of the first actions to occur is diagnosis. Assessment of well-being is so important that a patient cannot be admitted to an institution or treated by a professional without a diagnosis. The answers to the questions: What is wrong? or Why did you come to the hospital? describe the diagnostic process. Physicians classify patients according to disease states (acute gallbladder attack or myocardial infarction), body systems (cardiovascular or neuromuscular), types of treatment (medical or surgical), and degrees of illness (critical or chronic).

Hospital administrators assess the degree of illness of patients to determine needs for special services and to estimate the costs of care. For example, patients in need of surgery are placed in one section of the hospital. The high cost of hospital care requires that patients, doctors, nurses, and hospital administrators work together from the beginning to determine which treatments are most effective and least costly.

Nurses use the diagnoses of their medical and administrative colleagues. They also make nursing diagnoses.[2] For example, nurses speak about limited mobility, change in body image, or describe the ability to participate in self-care. In practice, however, nurses are bi- or trilingual in that their work requires that they speak the languages of nursing, medicine, and administration. Because nurses spend more time with patients and their families than other health workers, they often translate between patients and health care professionals. This role is important because patients and families often are surprised by diagnoses and plans of treatment. Nurses help patients understand how the health care system works. They help patients express their needs, and they advocate patient rights. Advocacy is an important role in a complex system. Some critics of modern health organizations argue that patients are no longer considered to be important

influences in health care decisions. They suggest that professionals control what happens to patients who are not consulted. To the degree that this description is accurate, the health care system is ineffective. You may wish to conduct an informal survey about patient input in plans of care. Ask your patients how they are consulted about their treatments.

The patient as input can be examined in two ways. Patients enter health care systems to receive treatment. Once diagnosed, they "go through the system" and recover. Another view of the patient as input looks at the patient's input. In this model, patients are defined as partners who contribute actively to the resolution of their illnesses.

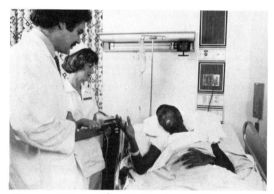

Figure 5-2a.   The Patient as a Partner

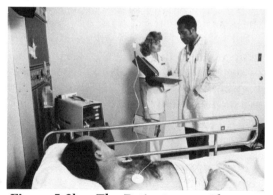

Figure 5-2b.   The Patient as an Observer

Media Input

The media influences the health care system. The press, radio, and television shows, and popular literature portray a typical day in the life of an ordinary patient. Sometimes stories about sophisticated breakthroughs in the treatment of serious illnesses excite the public. Occasionally the media serves as the public's conscience and brings attention to unmet needs. The 1970 articles depicting the shameful treatment of the institutionalized aged shocked and mobilized Americans against scandals in the nursing home industry.[3]

For sociological, psychological, and anthropological perspectives on the roles and lives of patients, families, care givers, and institutions, the interested reader is referred to the works of Talcott Parsons and Erving Goffman. Parson's classic description of "sick role theory" uses a sociological framework to explain what happens to personal, family, peer, and societal expectations when a person is ill.[4] Goffman's illustrations of "sick people" and their professional care givers adds another dimension to the understanding of the complexity of "inputs" in the health care establishments. In analyzing life careers of mental patients, Goffman examines patients' views of their worlds.[5] In a later text, he describes the behavior of one subset of health professionals, surgeons, and their associates.[6]

On a less serious note, each season brings new hospital television dramas to Americans' living rooms. The media provides colorful input into the health care system and reflects public opinion about health care.

The Public as Input

The public contributes to the health care system by its presence on boards of hospitals, health departments, and planning agencies, and by membership in voluntary, civic, or advocacy health groups. Input

from these groups occurs at the levels of planning, program and policy development, and health care financing. For example PL 93–641, the National Planning Act of 1974, and its amendments established public roles in decision making about the allocation of health resources. This federal law proposed a strategy for the development of local and state planning organizations.[7] It is possible to critique the complexity of PL 93–641. However, the underlying concept of the importance of citizen participation in the construction or expansion of hospitals cannot be refuted. In addition to working on planning boards, citizens are members of governing boards of hospitals and community agencies. Each year, people concerned with the treatment of disease, like heart disease or cancer, raise millions of dollars to aid research and to provide patient services. In addition to raising money for health care, or making decisions about the conduct of hospitals, citizens can change specific health practices. For example, public demand for family centered care enabled fathers to participate in childbirth classes and to be present during labor and delivery.[8]

The public exchanges information with the health system. This communication occurs within therapeutic relationships between patients, nurses and doctors. It takes place at board meetings and in fund raising activities. Public views about health care also are presented in newspapers, magazines, and television serials. The information that is generated is fed back into the system and influences future actions and decisions.

Health Professionals as Input

Who are the health professionals and what do they do? In the modern health system, nurses, doctors, and dentists are joined by nutritionists, dieticians, pharmacists, social workers, medical and radiologic technicians, physical and occupational therapists, accountants, medical record librarians, managers, and executives. These individuals are called the health care team.

Some health workers perform public services, such as community oriented nutrition education. Others, like physical therapists, work with specialized groups of patients. Others perform their services away from the clinical area (medical record librarians). The complexity of health care services requires teams of experts. While the hub of health team activity is the hospital, health teams function in school systems, health departments, industrial health centers, home health agencies, specialized institutions for handicapped individuals, and in community based emergency programs.

Health professionals assess, diagnose, triage, treat, refer, care, and cure. They develop or contribute to care plans, record the process and outcome of their work, direct the activities of technicians and assistants, and manage resources.

The input of health professions usually is described by direct care activities. However, health professionals shape and direct the system of care. Earlier in this chapter the public roles of citizens were described. Health professionals also sit on planning boards, hold positions on voluntary health associations, serve on hospital boards, and

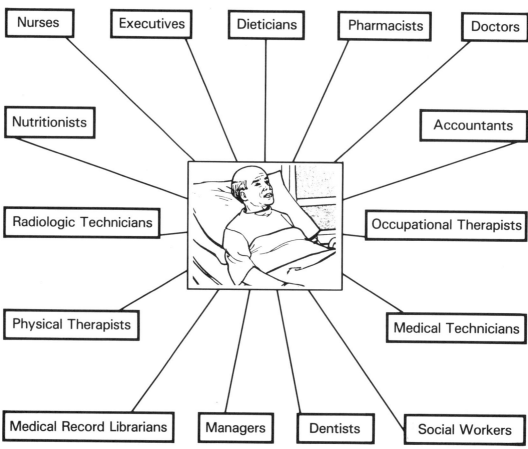

Nurses Executives Dieticians Pharmacists Doctors Nutritionists Accountants Radiologic Technicians Occupational Therapists Physical Therapists Medical Technicians Medical Record Librarians Managers Dentists Social Workers

Figure 5-3. The Health Care Team

head health departments. They order and manage the health system in addition to providing services. They set standards, develop criteria, and participate in peer and institutional evaluation. Health professionals have multiple inputs into the system.

Because there are so many interesting and different career opportunities in the health field, it is not surprising that health careers attract many students.

Students in the various health care professions also contribute input to the system. Recruitment and retention of good students is important for the maintenance and development of the system. Recognizing this, federal and state governments and private foundations have established programs to provide financial assistance. Nursing fortunately has been enriched by program support to schools and financial grants to students. Schools of nursing have used federal dollars to prepare clinical specialists and nurse practitioners and to develop outreach programs of continuing education for registered nurses. Nurses educated for new forms of practice work in rural settings, community hospitals, HMOs, and medical centers. Advanced education has changed the input that nurses have in health care delivery and created expanded and independent nursing roles.

Systems theory suggests that a change in one part of the system affects the whole. Rapid developments in the field of nursing have caused some ripples in the system. You are studying nursing during a period of innovation. You can influence and contribute to the professional dialogue. Major disagreements center around the scope and nature of the "nursing input." Questions are raised: Is the nurse an independent provider of health care? Should nurses work under orders and supervision of physicians? You may wish to study how the changing role of nurses has influenced nursing's input into the health care system.

Recruitment and retention is another important issue related to the input of health professions. Federal investment in the training of health professionals has been based on two premises: health professionals are a national resource, and federal intervention is needed to resolve the shortage of physicians and nurses.[9,10]

Recent national studies suggest that there is no shortage.[11,12] It is too early to determine what impact these studies will have on recruitment, financial support for current students, and innovative education and practice opportunities. There is some evidence, however, that an oversupply of physicians has limited the practice opportunities of nurse practitioners.[13]

Technology as Input

Perhaps the most striking new force in the health system is the rapid growth in the use of technology. Machines and new drugs have enhanced diagnostic and therapeutic capabilities and improved professional communications. Technology has made diagnostic assessment quicker, safer, and easier for patients. For example, CAT (computerized axial tomography) scanners make it possible to visualize the body without intrusion. Artificial kidneys, blood oxygenators, and respirators enable treatment of end stage renal disease, serious cardiac insufficiency, and acute or chronic respiratory failure. Drug research has simplified the treatment of hypertension, depression, and some forms of cancer. Computers have enabled the health team to store and retrieve information about patient care.

Any input this powerful and pervasive has another side. "The technological tiger" is indicted as a culprit in rising health care costs.[14] Over treatment or overuse of technology is always possible in a highly technological society. Concern for privacy, consent, or compassion is sometimes ignored as health professionals work their way through computerized monitors, intravenous lines, respirators, and machines that measure oxygenation and cardiac reserve.[15] High technology care contributes to the complexity of health institutions.

Health Institutions as Input

Lists of health institutions usually include hospitals, skilled care facilities, and ambulatory clinics or centers. However, physicians offices, health clinics in schools or work places, and health departments also offer organized health programs. Health institutions are classifed by:

- size
- sponsorship or ownership
- location
- type of service
- level of care.

Today's health institutions are a far cry from medieval monasteries or inns. Some hospitals span city blocks or cluster in sections of cities. "Pill Hill" in Seattle, Washington, is an example of such a health care complex. In small communities, large hospitals or skilled care facilities employ most of the residents.

Health care institutions develop identities and personalities. Charity Hospital in New Orleans, Louisiana, for example, is intimately associated with the life of the city and with the historical development of the United States. In addition to influencing the lives of patients, their families, friends, and health professionals, health institutions affect the standard and cost of health care. For example, technological sophistication of acute care hospitals and the number of unnecessary hospital beds are cited as factors that have made health care so costly.[16] Because institutions represent a group of interests, their input in the system is more compelling than the influence of small groups of individuals. When efforts are made to change the system, institutions receive most attention. Because

the health care system is an open system, it responds to internal and external pressures. The next section of this chapter examines how groups influence health care delivery.

Unions and Professional Associations as Inputs

Earlier in this chapter, health professionals were grouped in teams. Other organized structures of health workers influence particular institutions or the general system. Typically, health care professionals align themselves with peer groups. These associations provide networks for certification, standard development, continuing education, job and salary information, and professional support.[17] Nursing has developed an impressive list of professional organizations. Figure 5-4 represents an overview of nursing associations.

Academy of Nursing
American Academy of Ambulatory Nursing Administration
American Association for Nursing History
American Association of Colleges of Nursing
American Association of Critical Care
American Association of Nephrology
American Association of Neurosurgical Nurses
American Association of Nurse Anesthetists
American Association of Occupational Health Nurses, Inc.
American College of Nurse Midwives
American Indian/Alaska Native Nurse Association
American Nurses Association
American Society of Opthalmic RN's
American Public Health Association Public Health Nursing
American Society for Nursing Service Administration
American Society of Plastic and Reconstructive Surgical Nurses
American Society of Post Anesthesia
Association of Operating Room Nurses
Association of Pediatric Nursing
Association of Practitioners in Infection Control
Association of Rehabilitation Nurses
American Urological Association

Coalition of Nurse Practitioners

Commission on Graduates of Foreign Nursing Schools (CGFNS)

Dermatology Nurses Association

Emergency Department Nurses Association

International Association for Enterostomal Therapy

MARNA—Mid Atlantic Regional Nurses Association

Midwest Alliance in Nursing

National Association of Hispanic Nurses

National Association of Pediatric Nurse Associates and Practitioners

National Association of Nurse Recruiters

National Association of Orthopedic Nurses

National Association of Physicians' Nurses

National Association of School Nurses

National Black Nurses Association

National Center for Nursing Ethics

National Federation for Specialty Organizations

National Intravenous Therapy Association

National League for Nursing (NLN)

National Nurses Society on Substance Abuse

National Male Nurses Association

North American Nursing Diagnosis Association

Nurses Association of the American College of Obstetrics and Gynecology

Nurse Consultants Association

Nurses House, Inc.

Oncology Nursing Society

Sigma Theta Tau

Society of Otorhinolaryngology and Head and Neck Nurses

Southern Regional Nurses Association

Western Interstate Commission of Higher Education for Nursing

Figure 5-4.   Nursing Has Many Professional Associations
Source: Sigma Theta Tau, 1983

Unions are another group active in health fields. In 1974, the Taft Hartley Act was amended to include workers in nonprofit industries. Since then, labor unions have provided input into hospitals and skilled care facilities. Some unions represent the industrial model of the American Federation of Labor. Others, like the American Nurses Association or the American Federation of Teachers, operate from professional norms. Traditional unions and professional associations compete to represent nonprofessional and professional health workers. Health institutions and unions struggle for patterns that meet the needs of workers and management without losing sight of the special mission of the health industry. When the discussions are successful, salaries and working conditions improve.[18] Hospital unions are controversial. The economic security program is a major platform of the American Nurses Association. However, nurses in management positions express a conflict of interest between the goals of their professional associations and their employing institutions.[19] Some nurses believe that strike clauses should not be written into hospital contracts. Others see striking as a way of informing the public and hospital management about grievances.[20] Management experiences some ambivalence about unions, too. Prior to 1974, unions were allies. Health insurance, negotiated at bargaining tables, increased hospital census and encouraged expansion. Recently labor unions are bargaining with hospitals to improve wage scales and benefits. The Labor movement is a new force in the health system.

Planners, Regulators, and Accreditors as Input

A major direction in health care flows from those who set standards, make plans, or evaluate performance. Some critics of the health system say that planners have had no impact on the system. They argue that the health care industry is unplanned. Usually this point of view is supported by statistics that contrast the number of acute care beds in a community with the number of nursing home beds.[21] The methodology for sophisticated, community based planning developed after the construction of the hospital system. Some reasons for this lie in the history of nonprofit hospitals.

Health care institutions developed in response to the needs of an immigrant people. Religion, social class, ethnicity, and race stimulated hospital construction more than medical need did. The development and expansion of health institutions were influenced by the same motives that brought them into being. Communities' wish "to have their own hospitals" was encouraged by the Hill Burton Act, a federally funded program to build hospitals. By the time health planning came to be taught as a subject in schools of hospital administration, health institutions were built. Recent efforts of the federal government to curb construction and expansion of institutions resulted in a national health planning act.[22] This law mandates public and provider planning for construction, expansions, new programs, and manpower development. While all states have formal health plans, there is not much evidence that state or regional planning has a serious impact on the internal plans and aspirations of institutions.[23]

Health institutions also are subject to review by state health departments and professional accrediting teams. Institutions are licensed by state health departments. They are accredited by the Joint Commission on the Accreditation of Hospitals. Both groups apply standards and criteria to health institutions. Examples of such criteria might be a fixed ratio of professional nurses to patient populations or a minimum amount of emergency equipment at specific locations in the hospital. Efforts to meet these criteria cause institutions to modify procedures or services. Information fed back to institutions following accreditation reviews causes further change. Standards for practitioners or clinical services are set by professional peers. For example many nurses seek certification through the American Nurses Association or one of the specialty organizations.

Health Insurers as Input

Americans have a private/public system for paying for health care. Health insurance is a work related fringe benefit, and private insurers sell health benefits to employers. The major provider of health insurance is Blue Cross, a nonprofit health insurance agency. Multipurpose for-profit insurance companies also offer health insurance. In 1965, the federal government passed two major health insurance bills as amendments to the Social Security Act. **Medicare** (Title 18) and **Medicaid** (Title 19) revolutionized the health field. Initially, because of the opposition of organized medicine, Medicare and Medicaid functioned as traditional insurance carriers. In the 1970s, however, the federal government became the prime financier and standard setter in the health field. Much has been written since the enactment of Titles 18 and 19 about the input of the federal government in the health field. Perhaps the major input of Medicare and Medicaid is explained by studying their beneficiaries. Before 1965, employees lost health insurance benefits upon retirement, and the poor were uninsured. Medicare and Medicaid give the aged and the poor access to the health system. Federal money poured into the health care system since 1965 has caused dramatic increases in health care costs. It is for this reason that health insurers or the health care financing system is seen as a major input into the health care system. Although there has been growing concern about health care costs, Medicare and Medicaid have remained essentially unchanged since 1966. President Reagan's efforts to reduce federal spending, however, resulted in medicare reforms.

In August 1982, President Reagan signed The Tax Equity and Fiscal Responsibility Act of 1982 and altered the way in which Medicare pays its bills.[24] The most significant changes affect the method of payment and the flow of federal dollars into hospitals. To administer this law, it was recommended that hospitals be paid on the basis of diagnostic classification systems (diagnostically related groups). In this way an average cost of treatment is assigned to each diagnostic grouping. Hospitals receive payment based on national average costs, which are adjusted to reflect local wages. The payments are prospective.[25] Medicare will no longer pay hospitals exactly what they spend on the treatment of the aged and disabled.[26] Insurers act as "third parties" that pay for health care. They finance acute health care and support most long-term care centers. Consequently, any change in payment causes an imbalance that must be corrected.

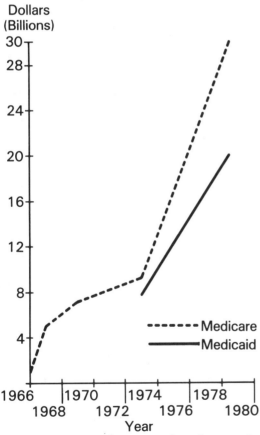

Figure 5-5.   Medicare/Medicaid Growth Care.

As has been evident in the discussion of inputs, the health care system is changing. Major change (expanded roles for nurses, new financing systems) in inputs causes change in the whole system. Today, the health care system is trying to achieve equilibrium and adjust to new inputs, particularly an innovative system of Medicare payments. You have the opportunity to observe how a complex system uses new information and adjusts its methods and goals.

Legislation as Input

Health legislation can be classified in four ways:

- legislation to ensure safety
- legislation to prepare professionals and health workers
- legislation to establish programs of service
- legislation to pay for service delivery.

Safety Legislation. Nurse and physician practice acts are examples of legislation to assure safe health care. Federal and state governments also have statutory authority to license health institutions, set the number of beds, establish programs of immunization and disease control, and enforce food and drug safety laws.

Manpower Legislation. Laws that support students through low interest loans or scholarships are called manpower laws. They help qualified students achieve their career goals. The Health Professions and Nurse Training Act is an example of a comprehensive manpower law.[27] You may wish to study this law and note the programs of study that it supports. Some sections of the manpower law finance the education of medical or nursing students in exchange for a promise of service in a medically underserved area. Other federal laws support professional education for military personnel or veterans.[28]

Health Services Legislation. Public health service laws support a wide range of health programs. Until recently, these programs were established by individual titles in the Public Health Service Act.[29] The Budget Reconciliation Act of 1981 altered the role of the federal government in providing local health services.[30] As a result of this law, 21 federal programs were combined into four block grants. Programs sent to the states included the Maternal Child Health Grant, the Primary Care Grant, the Health, Prevention and Services Grant, and the Mental Health Block Grant. Federal funding for these programs was reduced by 25 percent from fiscal year 1981 to 1982.[31]

Medicare is a two-part, federally administered nationwide health insurance program for the aged and disabled. The payroll tax-financed hospital insurance (HI) program, or part A, provides protection against the cost of in-patient hospital services, post hospital home health services, and post hospital skilled nursing facility services, with specified deductibles and coinsurance amounts. The supplementary medical insurance (SMI) program, or part B, is a voluntary program that provides protection against the cost of physician and certain other medical services.

Health Care Financing Legislation. The most significant health legislation is the set of laws that purchase health care for beneficiaries. Medicare and Medicaid are public health insurance acts.

Medicaid provides matching funds to States to finance medical care for low-income persons who are in families with dependent children or who are aged, blind, or disabled. Federal financial participation in the medicaid program is based on a matching rate according to a State's per capita income. Although the program is governed by a mixture of Federal and State eligibility requirements, the States are responsible for the administration of their respective medicaid programs.[32]

The first section of this chapter has considered inputs into the health care system. Although each input has been discussed individually, it is apparent that energy and information exchange occurs within the input system. Changes in the nature or degree of any component part affect other inputs. For example, physician or nurse shortage has always triggered federal legislation to support professional education. The real test of inputs, however, develops from an examination of the processes or methods within the system.

HEALTH CARE THROUGHPUTS

Patient care, education, research, regulation, standard development, and legislation are processes by which the goals of the health care system are achieved.

Patient Care as Throughput

Texts are written about patient care. It is the major throughput in the health care system. Hospitals are the hub of patient care.

Most hospitals treat adults with medical surgical illnesses. Community hospitals rival university teaching facilities in their capacity to treat acutely ill people in specialized units. Many health care observers believe that the line between secondary and tertiary care facilities is an imaginary one, and that the hospital of the future will be a center for tertiary or most complex care. When a patient is admitted to the hospital, "throughput" begins. The patient, his family, and the professionals begin to look for the source of the patient's difficulties. The modern medical complex is known by its diagnostic capability. Observation, history, intrusive, and nonintrusive examinations of organs, body parts, body fluids, and excretions, are used to identify the cause of the patient's discomfort. Once this is accomplished, the patient is given the appropriate treatment and is discharged. If, however, the cause of the patient's illness is illusive or indefinite, "throughput" continues. When the diagnostic quest is partially or completely unsuccessful, the patient and his family experience repeated emotional and physical conflicts. Sometimes, a diagnostic-therapeutic-diagnostic-therapeutic cycle develops. In these cases, one treatment leads to another test to another treatment. The emphasis on diagnosis and cure is so strong that if an illness cannot be treated, the health team often experiences apathy and a sense of failure. Because of the emphasis on cure, few health professionals or institutions possess the resources to manage treatment failures.

One method of examining throughput within a hospital is to trace the therapeutic course of a patient. Case studies give new insights into inputs and interactions. Patient care has many dimensions. Some common needs for care are summarized below:

- need for acute care
- need for maintenance care
- need for supportive care
- need for rehabilitative care
- need for protective care
- need for hospice care
- need for health education.

Although this chapter focuses on acute care hospitals, patient care is given in long-term, chronic care, or psychiatric hospitals, in ambulatory centers, and in the home. Long-term care is underdeveloped and underfinanced. Patients with chronic conditions have not received attention because acute care modalities emphasize diagnosis and treatment. Recently, several programs have been established to address the needs of the institutionalized aged. In nursing, this program is called the teaching Nursing Home Project. Supported by grants from the Robert Wood Johnson Foundation, this effort is designed to encourage faculty and students to assume clinical decision making in skilled care facilities.[33]

Since the late-1960s, public and private ambulatory clinics and health maintenance organizations have become centers for patient care. **Primary care** is the term used to describe patient care in these centers. Primary care includes:

a person's first contact in any period of illness with a health care system that leads to a decision about the resolution of the problem and the responsibility for the continuum of care, that is, maintenance of health, evaluation and management of symptoms and appropriate referrals.[34]

This definition highlights the important elements of primary care:

- coordinated primary care
- interdisciplinary care
- comprehensive care
- preventive care
- ambulatory care
- continuous care.

An interesting idea about patient care in these settings has been promoted by HMOs. The prototypes of HMOs were occupational health units at construction sites. Some industries had found they could provide better, less expensive health coverage for their employees if they combined work place clinics with general

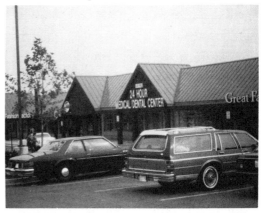

Figure 5-6. The New Health Care Center.

health care programs.[35] The original plan of the HMO supported the use of ambulatory treatment and preventive care for workers and their families. HMOs adopted a new method of paying for health services called prospective reimbursement. Individuals and employers contract for certain benefits and pay a flat fee. Membership entitles people to use HMOs for health education, health assessment, immunizations, and treatments. HMOs operate on an old principle: An ounce of prevention is worth a pound of cure. Another source of ambulatory care is the physician in his office.

A recent study reported that many Americans seek care from their family doctor.[36] However, a physician who practices alone does not seem to be a future oriented model of patient care. New forms of outpatient care are developing. The storefront clinics of the 1960s have been replaced by surgical centers in downtown office complexes and department stores. Some suburban shopping malls provide a "doc in the box"—a drop-in health service similar to 24-hour banking. Innovation in ambulatory care is related to reducing costs and to marketing competitive and convenient health care.

Patient care is also provided in the home by:
- for-profit home care agencies
- voluntary agencies of which the visiting nurse association is a prototype
- hospital based home care programs
- the veterans administration
- hospices—care programs for the terminally ill and their families.

Each home care agency provides patient care as a function of its purpose, philosophy, and sponsorship. Hospice home care programs are designed to help families care for their loved ones at home. The commitment of hospice teams is to support patients and families during dying, death, and bereavement.[37]

Visiting nurse associations operate around a health education model of care. Visiting nurses in the home aim to teach patients and care givers how to care for themselves. Their plans of care always include health education. Freestanding (usu-

ally for-profit) and hospital based programs also give care at home. Their home care goals are similar to therapeutic care offered in hospitals. The significant difference in these programs is concern for cost-effective care. The patient's ability to pay for home care determines the extent and scope of home care services in for-profit and hospital based home care services.

In summary, patient care is given in hospitals, skilled care facilities, physicians' offices, ambulatory clinics, HMOs, and in the home. These programs are sponsored by federal, state, and municipal governments, the military and veterans administration, private corporations that are proprietary or voluntary in structure, and by individuals.

Patient/Family Education as Throughput

Patient/family education is an integral component of patient care. Some organizations (HMOs and visiting nurse home care services) were founded on the belief that health education is basic to patient care. Public health agencies and industrial health programs emphasize health education and personal responsibility for health and safety. Nurses and physicians always have included patient/family teaching in their care plans. However, within the past 20 years, hospitals have developed formal programs for patient, family, and community health education.

Typically, hospitals offer programs in:
- preparation for childbirth
- parenting
- normal and therapeutic nutrition
- stress reduction
- weight control
- living with chronic illnesses (diabetes, arthritis, heart disease, cancer, stroke)
- preoperative and postoperative instruction
- discharge planning.

Many Americans are conscious of their health. Weight control, moderation in the use of alcohol, cessation of smoking, and regular exercise keep healthy people fit. A total culture supports healthy life styles. Personal responsibility for health makes the work of health professionals easier. Public concern with maintaining healthy minds and bodies gives positive feedback to the health care system.

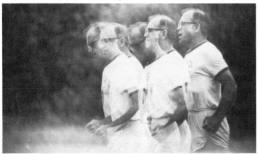

Figure 5-7. Jogging is a National Pastime.

Education of Health Professionals as Throughput

A major responsibility of the health care system is the education of its health professionals. Historically, health care agencies have played critical roles in the education of physicians, nurses, and other members of the health team. Today universities and colleges educate most health workers. Figure 5-7 shows the movement of professional schools of nursing from hospitals to junior and senior colleges and universities.

There are unresolved questions about the balance between theoretical and practical instruction in the fields of health. In the case of nursing, debates continue between advocates for hospital schools and college based programs.[38] At stake is the issue of control of the education of nurses. In medicine, the primary care versus specialist training dialogues express a preference for clinical sites. Will young physicians receive clinical training in community hospitals and ambulatory care centers or in tertiary (highly specialized) hospitals operated by schools of medicine. There are pros and cons to the nursing and medical discussions. Perhaps you and your classmates might stage a debate. Resolved: In the future, all professional nursing education will take place in baccalaureate programs. The education of health care workers is an important throughput. Information learned in discussions about methods of instruction give feedback into the system. This information becomes stimuli for change.

Continuing education for health professionals is a personal, organizational, and public challenge. Professional values and codes address the importance of maintaining and increasing knowledge and skill. The technological and therapeutic advances in biomedical research demand health professionals who like change and value lifelong learning.

Professional associations assist their members by sponsoring continuing education. Review any professional nursing journal. You will see a calendar of continuing education. Hospitals and skilled care facilities play major roles in providing opportunities for professional development through continuing education.

Program type	1970		1980		1981	
	Number	Percent	Number	Percent	Number	Percent
Diploma	22,856	52.4	14,495	19.0	12,903	17.2
Associate	11,678	26.7	36,509	47.8	37,183	49.7
Baccalaureate	9,105	20.9	25,411	33.2	24,804	33.1
TOTAL	43,639	100.0	76,415	100.0	74,890	100.0

Figure 5-8. Educational Pathways for Nursing.

Source: The National League for Nursing, NLN   Nursing Data Book, 1982.

It is possible to group continuing education into three categories:

● orientation

● maintenance and development

● professional advancement.

Orientation programs present the philosophy and purposes of institutions. They acquaint new employees with policies, procedures, and regulations. Some institutions have special programs for new graduate nurses. These internship or preceptor programs continue during the first months of employment. In the early 1970s Kramer described the entry of new graduates into hospitals as reality shock.[39] Today, most orientation programs follow the principles laid out by Kramer. Nurses returning to the work force after a period of absence need orientation, too. Because hospitals are specialized, nurses who change specialties within familiar institutions need to be introduced to new techniques and procedures. Orientation programs address the needs of new, returning, and reassigned nurses. A second type of continuing education recognizes that familiar procedures must be reviewed. Hospitals and skilled care facilities present annual programs on disaster training, fire safety, infection control, and cardiopulmonary resuscitation. Programs also introduce new technology, expanded services, or changes in procedure or policy. The stimulation and development of stable employees is a challenge to health care managers. Growth in the health industry is unparalleled. Consequently, vigorous efforts are needed to keep current employees up to date.

The third type of program promotes career advancement. Sometimes courses are conducted within institutions. On other occasions, employees are sent to workshops or encouraged to enroll in colleges or universities. Health care institutions play significant roles in preservice and continuing education. They also conduct on-the-job training programs for ancillary and technical workers. Today, education is available through correspondence or telecommunication series, as well. The reader is referred to Chapter 4 for further discussion on continuing education.

Research as Throughput

The third component of health care delivery is research.

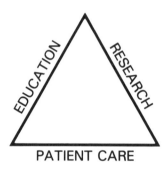

Figure 5-9. The Health Care Triangle

Hospitals and ambulatory care centers connected to schools of medicine (academic health centers) were the first institutions to conduct research. These major institutions conducted:

● clinical trials of drugs

● basic research on disease states

● development and testing of new treatments and technologies.

Research is no longer the domain of medicine or the academic health centers. It is conducted in all sectors of the health community and by all health professionals. In the field of nursing, there have been significant developments in clinical research. For example, nurse researchers have studied preoperative care,[40] comfort measures,[41] care of patients with cancer,[42] infant development[43] and care of the aged.[44] These studies illustrate the research priorities of the American Nurses Association Commission on Nursing Research:[45]

- promoting health, well-being, and competency for personal care for all age groups
- preventing health problems throughout the life span that have the potential to reduce productivity and satisfaction
- decreasing the negative impact of health problems on coping abilities, productivity, and life satisfaction of individuals and families
- ensuring that the care needs of particularly vulnerable groups are met through appropriate strategies
- designing and developing health care systems that are cost effective in meeting the nursing needs of all the populations
- promoting health, well-being, and competency for personal health in all age groups.

Another form of research into health care has developed in the 1970s. Called health services research, it explores the processes and goals of health care delivery. Health services research is conducted by multidisciplinary teams rather than by single investigators. It addresses practical problems, such as access to care and cost of care.[46]

Hospitals and health centers do informal studies about internal organization, operations, market appeal, and management capabilities. They also use data from Medicare and Medicaid reports, Professional Standard Review Organizations (PSRO), records and studies of Health Planning Organizations and Health Systems Agencies (HSA), State Health Planning Agencies (SHPDA), and State Coordinating Councils (SHCC). This information has helped health agencies compare their institutions to others in the region and the country. This information has feedback potential. Informed hospitals and other health agencies compete to make their programs and services most attractive. National data banks have been developed by the federal government and large insurance companies.

Interesting changes have occurred in research. While investigation into the cause of illnesses is still the major research priority, other topics command public attention and public funds. Professionals and health care agencies use the tools of research to study and improve their practices. The federal government's Health Care Financing Administration (HCFA) and other insurance companies that pay hospital bills try to find solutions to growing health care costs.

Standards and Regulations as Throughput

Regulatory, legislative, and standard setting agencies influence practice in complex health organizations in the following ways:

- establishing and enforcing standards of professional practice within states and institutions
- licensing professionals and institutions
- specifying types of service to be given by professionals and institutions
- regulating the growth and expansion of health care agencies
- setting fees for reimbursement for professionals and institutions
- establishing and enforcing safety codes
- establishing and enforcing conditions of participation for federal, state, and municipal programs
- establishing and enforcing criteria for

the certification of health professionals and the accreditation of health care institutions.

The health care system has many lawgivers, regulators, and standard setters. Figure 5-9 lists some agencies with which you should be familiar.

Joint Commission for the Accreditation of Hospitals
State Boards of Nurse Examiners
Health Planning Agencies
State Health Departments
State Legislators
The Congress of the United States
Federal Trade Commission
Specialty Boards of Medicine
American Association of Medical Colleges
National League for Nursing
American Nurses Association and Specialty Nurses Association

Figure 5-10. Selected Agencies that Establish Policies, Regulate Practice, and Set Standards

Several presidents have expressed concern with the complexity and cost of regulatory throughput. President Carter directed federal agencies to simplify regulations. President Reagan proposed deregulation of the health industry. Regulations are mixed blessings. Everyone supported the "straight language" of the Carter administration. However, the application of deregulation in health causes some concern. The popular example given to support deregulation is the airline industry. Deregulation has reduced fares on routes serviced by competitive airlines. Physicians have a monopoly on medical practice and control reimbursement for health services. They are like those airline companies that hold the only franchise to a desired city. The deregulation of nursing homes proposed by the Department of Health and Human Services provoked public and professional outcries.[47] The heat generated by proposed reduction in standards of care caused the Congress of the United States to declare a temporary halt to deregulating nursing homes.[48] The deregulation debate offers an example of feedback in the health system. Those who favor deregulation argue that removal of artificial regulations will free the industry and reduce costs. Those who oppose deregulation say that health care is more a monopoly than a free market and stress the need for regulations to protect the health and safety of captive populations—the institutionalized sick, poor, aged, and retarded. The nature, scope, and extent of regulatory activity is an important issue of the 1980s. Its resolution will impact upon inputs and outputs in the system.

Health care throughputs are processes by which patients receive care, professionals generate new knowledge and receive training, and health institutions interface with society. The study of throughputs opens windows into the health care system.

HEALTH CARE OUTPUTS

Several years ago, the Surgeon General of the United States issued a report entitled *Healthy People*[49]. This study addresses the goals of the health care system and describes personal behavior that leads to health. This American perspective should be read along with the statement of the World Health Organization: *Health for All by the Year 2000.*[50] The report of the World Health Organization balances health care outcomes in first world countries like the United States with health goals of less developed nations.

The statements of the chief of the United States Public Health Service and the World Health Organization set a broad conceptual base for understanding health care outcomes.

When health professionals and managers of health institutions discuss health outcomes, they cite:

• well patients

- well managed institutions
- an adequate number of trained health professionals
- standards of professional practice and institutional care
- adequate reimbursement for health services
- evidence of health planning (accessible health services and health care beds)
- laws and regulations that ensure public safety.

Healthy People as Output

As has been stated many times in this chapter, the major goal of the health system is healthy people. However, when you look within the system for indicators of health, you will uncover indirect measurements. For example, state health departments, hospitals, skilled care facilities, ambulatory centers, and home care agencies record:

- discharge rates by disease
- infection rates
- number of falls in institutions
- number of live births
- number of deaths per disease category
- number of suicides
- number of deaths by accident
- average life expectancy by sex, race, and ethnic origin
- number of maternal deaths
- incidence of certain diseases
- incidence of communicable disease
- number of persons receiving workman's compensation or disability insurance.

Most of these parameters describe absence of disease rather than signs of health. These data confirm the priority that the identification and treatment of disease (medical model) has in the American health care system. It seems illogical to define healthy people as people without significant illness or disability. Yet that definition can be best defended in the American health care system.

Health Professionals as Output

This chapter also records the education of health professions. The development of an adequate number of trained health manpower is a public goal. Assuring their placement throughout the country remains a national priority. Recent studies report that there are enough physicians and nurses. They also note that maldistribution of health personnel persists. The geographic maldistribution of physicians and nurses is related to complex social, professional, and economic forces. There are many reasons to practice in urban and suburban areas. There are few incentives associated with rural and inner city practices. The more important question is: Are there enough of the right types of doctors and nurses? In the field of nursing, the Institute of Medicine (the latest group to study nurse manpower) reports that the 1.33 million nurses in the work force satisfies public need for generalist nursing services. They note, however, a shortage of nurse specialists capable of working in acute care environments.[51]

Health Care Institutions as Output

It is generally accepted that the United States has sufficient health institutions to meet public need. The problems are access to care (overcoming cultural barriers), the balance between acute and long-term care beds, and geographic maldistribution of services. The major concern expressed about institutional care is the cost of inpatient services.[52] Put another way, the United States has developed an enviable system of institutionalized care that is becoming too costly to maintain.

Standards of Care and Practice

Mature organizations set standards. These criteria form the basis for evaluation and training. In the field of health, standards are developed by professional associations and the federal government. You may wish to compare the standards of practice developed by Medicare with those of the American Nurses Association and specialty organizations like the American Association of Critical Care Nurses and the Association of Operating Room Nurses.

Health Care Plans

Health care plans are developed by state and local health departments and by the state health planning and development agencies. Mandated by PL 93-641 and amended by PL 96-79, these plans are statements of policy that provide planning frameworks for improving the health status of area residents. "The intent of these plans is to promote a high level of communication among a diverse constituency involved in health-related activities and to establish a coordinated approach to health policy and program direction."[53]

Read a copy of your state's health plan. It will give you a comprehensive view of the health care system in which you study nursing.

Health Laws as Output

Since President Reagan assumed the presidency, the pattern of health laws has changed. The most complete compilation of current health laws are found in the Budget Reconciliation Act of 1981, which created the block grant program and the Tax Equity and Fiscal Responsibility Act of 1982 that modified Medicare and Medicaid.

At the state level, you may wish to review medical and nursing practice acts to determine the legality of current practice.

Reimbursement Policies as Output

Given the change in Medicare and Medicaid, multiple changes are anticipated in reimbursement policies. It is expected that Blue Cross and other private insurance carriers will follow the direction of the Medicare program. Key concepts of the 1982 tax law—prospective reimbursement, payment for case by diagnostic criteria, targets on reimbursement and ceilings on growth—are expected to stimulate more procompetitive strategies in the private and public sectors.[54] You have the opportunity to watch the evaluation of health care financing output. You also can observe the feedback that follows when fewer dollars are made available to pay health care bills.

SUMMARY

Inputs, throughputs, and outputs are described in this chapter using the language and theoretical frameworks of systems theory. Health systems are dynamic, interacting organizations. They exist as units or subsystems (community mental health ambulatory center), as major systems (mental health centers connected to large academic health centers), and as macro systems (The Hospital Corporation of America).

Every health subsystem provides patient care, participates in the education of its staff, and conducts research into its own operations. Major health systems achieve these goals, too. They also act as specialized hospitals to which patients are referred for sophisticated therapy. They educate health professionals and contribute to scientific knowledge. Macro systems offer and influence patient care, professional education, and research across a geographic region or throughout the country.

In addition to describing the three classic goals of health delivery systems, this chapter identifies political, economic, and social influences.

The demands of a highly mobile "third wave society" are played out in its institutions. Health institutions are not immune to changes in the professions, the economy, and in religious and social values. Because the health care system is a living, dynamic organism, it also contributes to social change. Public expectations about treatment of illness are a testimony to the successful therapy of health care institutions. As students of nursing, you will influence and be affected by health care systems. As professionals, you will be challenged to advance and alter "the system" so that personalized care, informed education, and humanistic research remains a hallmark of the American health care system.

STUDY QUESTIONS

1. Name some inputs into the health care system.

2. Discuss what each "input" contributes to the system.

3. How are patients consulted about their care?

4. What is the most important input that you, a student of nursing, can make in the system?

5. What are some throughputs in the health care system?

6. Can you prioritize the health throughputs?

7. What are the relationships between the throughputs of the health care establishment and its goals?

8. What are some goals of the health care system?

9. Can you prioritize the goals of the systems?

10. Are goals the same in each institution?

11. Do you think system theory is a good model to apply to health care? Why or why not?

REFERENCES

1. Terris, M. Approaches to an Epidemiology of Health. **American Journal of Public Health, 65,** 1975, 1038–1045.
2. Gordon, M. **Nursing Diagnosis.** St. Louis: McGraw-Hill, 1982.
3. Medelson, M. **Tender Loving Greed.** New York: Random House, 1975.
4. Parsons, T. **The Social System.** Glencoe, Ill: Free Press, 1951.
5. Goffman, E. **Asylums.** New York: Doubleday and Company, 1961.
6. Goffman, E. **Encounters.** Indianapolis: Bobbs-Merrill, 1961.
7. PL 93-641. **The National Health Planning and Resource Development Act of 1974.** Washington, D.C.: U.S. Superintendent of Documents, 1974.
8. Moore, M. L. **Newborn, Family and Nurse.** Philadelphia: W. B. Saunders Company, 1981.
9. **Nurse Supply, Distribution and Requirements, Third Report to the Congress. Nurse Training Act of 1975.** Hyattsville, MD: Bureau of Health Professions, Division of Nursing, 1982.
10. Ginzberg, E. "The Future Supply of Physicians: From Pluralism to Policy." **Health Affairs, 1,** 1982, 6–19.
11. Graduate Medical Education National Advisory Committee. **Report of the Graduate**

Medical Education National Advisory Committee to the Secretary. Washington, D.C.: Department of Health and Human Services, 1981.

12. **Nursing and Nursing Education Public Policies and Private Actions.** Washington, D.C.: Institute of Medicine, 1983.

13. Sultz, H., Henry, O. and Sullivan, J. **Nurse Practitioners: USA.** Lexington, MA: Lexington Books, 1979.

14. Schramm, C. "The Teaching Hospital and the Future Role of State Government." **The New England Journal of Medicine, 308,** 1983, 41–45.

15. Blackburn, S. "The Neonatal ICU: A High Risk Environment." **The American Journal of Nursing, 82,** 1982, 1708–1712.

16. **Controlling the Supply of Hospital Beds, No. 2-04602.** Washington, D.C.: Institute of Medicine, 1976.

17. Kelly, L. Y. **Dimensions of Professional Nursing.** New York: Macmillan Co., 1975.

18. "Recent ANA-Negotiated Settlements." **The American Journal of Nursing, 82,** 1982, 1026.

19. Ratkovitch, R. "The Director of Nursing and the Hat of Administration." **Journal of the New York State Nurses Association, 4,** 1973, 40–43.

20. Grand, N. "Nightingalism, Employeeism and Professional Collectivism." **Nursing Forum, 10,** 1971, 289–99.

21. Champion, E., Bang, A., and May, M. "Why Acute Care Hospitals Must Undertake Long-Term Care." **New England Journal of Medicine, 308,** 1983, 71–74.

22. P.L. 93-641 **The National Health Planning and Resources Development Act., op. cit.**

23. Tierney, J., Walters, W., "Evolution of Health Planning." **New England Journal of Medicine, 308,** 1983, 95–97.

24. P.L. 97-248. **The Tax Equity Act of 1983.** Washington, D.C.: The Government Printing Office, 1983.

25. "Play by Number Plan Proposed for Medicare," The Federal Report, **The Washington Post.** February 8, 1983, A-15.

26. **Conference Report to Accompany HR 4961 Equity and Fiscal Responsibility Act of 1982.** Washington, D.C.: Superintendent of Documents, 1982.

27. Smith, K. Reinhardt, U., Andreano, R. "Planning a National Health Manpower Policy: A Critique and a Strategy." **Research in Health Economics I,** Greenwich, CN.: JAI Press, 1979, 1–35.

28. "American Medical Manpower Dilemma: How Many Doctors and Nurses Do We Need?" **Health Affairs, 1,** 1982, 5.

29. **Compilation of Selected Public Health Service Acts.** Washington, D.C.: The Government Printing Office, 1981.

30. P.L. 97-35. **The Omnibus Budget Reconciliation Act of 1981.** Washington, D.C.: U.S. Superintendent of Documents, 1981.

31. P.L. 97-35. **The Omnibus Budget Reconciliation Act of 1981,** op. cit.

32. Special Committee on Aging United States Senate. **The Proposed Fiscal Year 1983 Budget; What It Means for Older Americans: An Information Paper.** Washington, D.C.: U.S. Government Printing Office, 1982.

33. Aiken, L. H. "Nursing Priorities for the 1980s: Hospitals and Nursing Homes." **American Journal of Nursing,** 1981, **81,** 324–30.

34. United States Department of Health, Education and Welfare. **Extending the Scope of Nursing Practice.** Washington, D.C.: U.S. Government Printing Office, 1971.

35. **A Policy Statement: HMOs Toward a Fair Market Test.** Washington, D.C.: The National Academy of Science, 1974.

36. Rogers, D., Aiben, L., Blendon, P. **Personal Medical Care: Its Adaptation to the 1980s.** Washington, D.C.: Institute of Medicine, 1980.

37. Dobihal, S. "Hospice: Enabling a Patient to Die at Home." **The American Journal of Nursing, 80,** 1980, 1448–1451.

38. Lysaught, J. **An Abstract for Action.** New York: McGraw-Hill, 1970.

39. Kramer, M. **Reality Shock: Why Nurses Leave Nursing.** St. Louis: C. V. Mosby, 1974.

40. Lindeman, C. A. and Van Aernam, B. "Nursing Intervention with the Presurgical Patient: The Effects of Structured and Unstructured Preoperative Technology." **Nursing Research,** 1971, 20, 319–332.

41. Padilla, G. et al. "Subjective Distress of Nasogastric Tube Feeding." **Journal of Parenteral and Enteral Nutrition,** 1979, **3,** 53–57.

42. McCorkle, R. Social Support and Symptom Distress in Two Samples with Life Threatening Disease. **Proceedings of the American Cancer Society's Second Conference on Cancer Nursing Research,** 1981.

43. Anderson, G., McBride, M. R., et al. "Development of Sucking in Term Infants from Birth to Four Hours Post Birth." **Research in Nursing and Health,** 1982, **5** (3), 21–27.

44. Wells, T. "Urinary Continence/inconti-

nence: Scope of the Problem." **Geriatric Nursing. 4,** 1980, 236–240.

45. American Nurses Association, Commission on Nursing Research. **Policy Paper on Nursing Research,** Kansas City, MO: The American Nurses Association, 1980.

46. "A Strategy for Evaluating Health Services." **Contrasts in Health Status, No. 2** Washington, D.C.: Institute of Medicine, 1973.

47. "Proposed Rules." **Federal Register,** May 27, 1982.

48. P.L. 97-248, **The Tax Equity and Fiscal Responsibility Act of 1983, op cit.**

49. **Healthy People The Surgeon General's Report on Health Promotion and Disease Prevention.** Washington, D.C.: U.S. Government Printing Office, 1979.

50. Maher, H. "Blueprint for Health for All." **World Health Organization Chronicle, 31,** 1977, 491–8.

51. **Nursing and Nursing Education: Public Policies and Private Actions, op cit.**

52. Hanft, R. "The Impact of Changes in Federal Policy on Academic Health Centers." **Health Affairs, 1,** 1982, 67–82.

53. **District of Columbia State Health Plan, 1981–1983.** Washington, D.C.: District of Columbia State Health Planning and Development Agency, Department of Human Services, 1981.

54. Enright, Sharon. "Procompetition and the Continuing Struggle to Contain Health Care Costs." **American Journal of Hospital Pharmacy. 40** (1983), 282–286.

ANNOTATED BIBLIOGRAPHY

These references are examples of government documents or policy papers developed by private or public groups:

PL 93-641. **The National Health Planning and Resource Development Act of 1974.** Washington, D.C.: U.S. Superintendent of Documents. PL 93-641 illustrates a public law. Available from the local offices of congressmen or senators, it can also be obtained from the Superintendent of Documents in Washington, D.C.

Graduate Medical Education National Advisory Committee. **Report of the Graduate Medical Education National Advisory Committee to the Secretary.** Washington, D.C.: Department of Health and Human Services, 1981. The "GMENAC" report illustrates the work of a specially selected committee that studied medical manpower and filed a report to the Secretary of Health and Human Services. This report was released and became the subject of discussion and debate in the public and professional sector.

Nurse Supply, Distribution and Requirements, Third Report to the Congress. Nurse Training Act of 1975. Hyattsville, MD: Bureau of Health Professions, Division of Nursing, 1982. This report to Congress, mandated by public law, represents the work of a division and bureau within the Department of Health and Human Services.

Special Committee on Aging United States Senate. **The Proposed Fiscal Year 1983 Budget; What It Means for Older Americans: An Information Paper.** Washington, D.C.: U.S. Government Printing Office, 1982. This report, prepared by a staff of a Senate Committee, examines the federal budget and analyzes its impact on a specialized population—the aged.

A Policy Statement: HMOs Toward a Fair Market Test. Washington, D.C.: The National Academy of Science, 1974. Developed by a "think tank" of interdisciplinary professionals, this report illustrates private sector influence on public policy.

Conference Report to Accompany HR 4961, Tax Equity and Fiscal Responsibility Act of 1982. Washington, D.C. Superintendent of Documents, 1982. This document is the official report of the agreements reached by senators and members of Congress who conferred on the 1982 tax law.

Nursing and Nursing Education: Public Policies and Private Actions. Washington, D.C.: Institute of Medicine, 1983. This is a final report of a congressionally mandated two-year study of nursing.

6

The Nursing Process *

Helen Yura
Mary Walsh

CHAPTER OUTLINE

OBJECTIVES

At the completion of this chapter the reader will be able to:

- Define the nursing process.
- Differentiate the nursing process from other processes in nursing.
- Describe the evolution of the nursing process.
- Identify the importance and value of using a systematic process in nursing.
- Describe the value of using a logical framework for performing nursing.
- Draw resources for nursing from multiple theories that provide a base for nursing practice.
- Define, describe, and practice nursing through the use of the nursing process:
  —Assessing—including data collection and data analysis about the client, and arrive at conclusions about the client's strengths and limitations (nursing diagnoses).
  —Planning—including use of client validation, goal setting, and expected outcomes of care.
  —Implementing—including carrying out the plan according to client values, client needs, client abilities, available personnel and their level of preparation.
  —Evaluating—including a review of goals to be achieved and the extent to which client or nurses are able to reach desired outcomes.

---

*Adapted from: Yura, H. and Walsh, M.B. *The Nursing Process* 4th edition, Appleton-Century-Crofts, (E. Norwalk, CT, 1983).

GLOSSARY

Assessing—the act of reviewing a human situation in order to affirm the wellness state and to diagnose potential client problems; to affirm an illness state; diagnose the client's obvious problems, determine the potential for problems, and identify the wellness of the ill client.

Evaluating—the appraisal of changes experienced by the client in relation to goal achievement as a result of actions of the nurse.

Goal—the expected behavioral result of human need fulfillment experienced by a client.

Implementing—the initiation and completion of actions necessary to accomplish the defined goal of optimal fulfillment of human needs.

Nursing diagnosis—the judgment or conclusion reached by the nurse based on assessment data that indicates the potential for or actual human need fulfillment alteration viewed as an excess, an al-

tered pattern in expression, or a deficit, lack, or limitation for the client as person, family, or community.

Nursing process—an orderly, systematic manner of determining the client's problems, making plans to solve them, initiating the plan or assigning others to implement it, and evaluating the extent to which the plan was effective in resolving the problem identified.

Outcome criteria—specific descriptive behavioral expectations stemming from a specified goal with the level of achievement expected and the time interval for measurement of achievement.

Planning—the determination of a plan of action to assist the client toward the goal of optimal wellness based on the highest level of fulfillment of human needs and to resolve potential and obvious nursing diagnoses.

INTRODUCTION

The nursing process is the core and essence of nursing; it is central to all nursing actions; it is applicable in any setting and within any theoretical conceptual reference. It is flexible and adaptable, adjustable to a number of variables, yet sufficiently structured so as to provide a base from which all systematic nursing actions can proceed. . . . There is a basic theme that underlies the process: it is organized, systematic, and deliberate.[1]

The nursing process was not a familiar term in nursing prior to the middle 1960s.

Since then, however, there has been a gradual recognition of the significance and importance of the nursing process. Within a 15-year period (1967–1982), what began as a low rumble has grown to a loud roar in terms of the significance, importance, and impact of using an organized, systematic, and deliberate process when nurses care for clients.

Prior to 1967, a selected few nurses (see Chapter 9) used the term nursing process. These include: Hildegard Peplau,[2] Lydia Hall,[3] Dorothy Johnson,[4] Ida Orlando,[5] and Ernestine Wiedenbach.[6] All these authors touched on what was to become a gold mine of knowledge for professional nursing. The mine was there for many years, but now it is being refined in a more qualitative form as professional nurses see the advantage of proceeding deliberately and with intention rather than intuitively. Identification and deliberate use of a process in nursing has enabled the nursing profession to proceed systematically to carry out the role of nursing and is producing a database on which research can proceed to improve practice and to duplicate nursing actions that are qualitatively developed. The nursing process is further enhanced through theoretical frameworks that give breadth and depth to knowledge about people and their needs. The future of nursing through the use of the nursing process is boundless.

Further dimensions to consider when addressing the nursing process include criteria for a profession, a code for professional nurses, and a definition of nursing.

While many people refer to their occupation as a profession, an occupation should meet certain criteria in order to be viewed, strictly speaking, as a profession. Several sources of criteria are available; for example, A. Flexner,[7] and R. Schein.[8]

Recently, Gail Stuart[9] summarized suggestions of various authors about professionalism in nursing as follows. Nursing as a profession:

- has a history
- has a commitment to the profession
- has a professional organization (American Nurses' Association)
- continues to progress
- provides services for those in need
- is beginning to identify and establish an autonomous practice.

To convince others that nursing is a profession, Stuart suggested that:

- the knowledge base should be expanded to establish nursing science as a recognized body of knowledge
- nursing research should be expanded
- autonomy and power should be used to convince others that nurses can identify and implement independent functions of nursing.

One criterion of a profession suggests that a code of ethics is essential. The most recent revision of the Code for Nurses (see Chapter 8) stresses self-determination of the client, the role of the nurse as client advocate, and the need for quality assurance and peer review.[10]

The struggle to reach universal agreement on one statement to define nursing was evident in the nursing literature for many years. Occasionally in current literature a plea for such a statement appears. For the most part, however, persons who need an accepted statement that defines nursing rely primarily on the definitions suggested by the early nursing leaders. Two of those who proposed definitions of nursing that apply across all ages include Sister Olivia Gowan[11] and Virginia Henderson (see Chapter 3).[12] Embellishment of the definitions they proposed is not necessary; their words of wisdom are as appropriate today as they were when they were written.

Leaders of nursing in the past defined nursing, identified a code for professional nurses, and developed criteria for a profession. These form a mature, professional, and accountable base on which nursing can continue to develop. Two directions are evolving for the present development of nursing and the ultimate specification of the science of nursing:

- identification of theoretical/conceptual frameworks for functioning.
- use of the nursing process for the performance of nursing.

THEORETICAL/CONCEPTUAL FRAMEWORKS

It has been suggested in the philosophy

of science literature that philosophers have experienced false starts and numerous debates among themselves while striving to identify their scientific bases in the development of philosophy of science. It seems important to get on with the work of identifying frameworks for nursing consistent with the underlying philosophies about nursing. It has been suggested that in order to do this:

- the identification of frameworks is important

- definitions and labels are important

- knowing when one is using proposed theories or using jargon without buying into the heart of the theory is important.[13]

During the 1960s and 1970s, a number of nurse authors developed and reported their ideas about nursing including definitions of nursing, views about the human with clear references to beliefs about fellow humans, and perceptions about nursing and the nursing process. Nurse writers of the 1960s who made an impact on the development of a theoretical framework for nursing include: Faye Abdellah,[14] Dorothy Johnson,[15] Myra Levine, [16] Ida Orlando,[17] Joyce Travelbee,[18] and Ernestine Wiedenbach.[19]

In the 1970s, further development of scientific bases for nursing was made by Imogene King,[20] Betty Neuman,[21] Dorothea Orem,[22] Martha Rogers,[23] Sister Callista Roy,[24] Josephine Paterson, and Loretta Zderad.[25] Another development that has had a continuing effect on nursing is the embryonic identification of a classification system for nursing diagnoses. Writers who contributed to this effort were Kristine Gebbie, and Mary Ann Lavin[26], Marjorie Gordon[27] and Phyllis Kritek[28]. Many of these writers, nurses, and theorists are continuing their efforts into the 1980s. Others are joining them by building on their published ideas, applying theories and concepts to practice, and conducting

research to prove the validity, value, and potential of the work accomplished during the 1960s and 1970s.

THEORETICAL BASES FOR PRACTICE

Recent advances in technology have been exciting, stimulating, breathtaking, and potentially overwhelming. It is no longer possible to present all there is to know in one class, one course, one program, or in any one person's educational career, no matter how long. To order available knowledge, it is necessary to establish some means of organizing data. Determining theoretical or conceptual frameworks is one way to organize knowledge.

The multifaceted nature of nursing makes client care in a large variety of settings necessary. The recipient of services (the client) is individual and complex, bringing religious, cultural, economic, educational, sociological, psychological, and physiological dimensions to every encounter. The provider of nursing brings that same variety to each client encounter. To reconcile and consider all these dimensions with reasonable attention, some schema is necessary.

A large variety of theories and concepts that enable the pursuit of quality client care are available to the nurse. Use of a theoretical base by the nurse can facilitate the use of available knowledge and can maximize the quality of care delivered.

Among the various theories that can guide the use of the nursing process are: general systems theory; communication theory; decision theory; problem solving theory; human need theory; and perception theory.* General systems and theories

---

*A more detailed discussion of all theories that underlie the nursing process can be found in Yura, H. and Walsh, M.B.; The Nursing Process, 4th Edition, E. Norwalk, CT, Appleton-Century-Crofts, 1983, Chapter 2: Theoretical Frameworks for the Nursing Process.

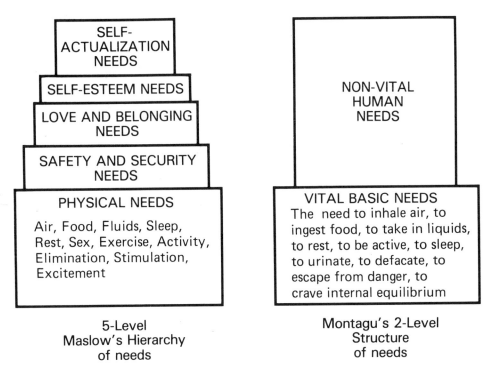

5-Level
Maslow's Hierarchy
of needs

Montagu's 2-Level
Structure
of needs

Figure 6-1. Theoretical Views of Human Needs.

that flow from it are discussed in other chapters in this text. In this chapter, human need and perception theories are discussed.

Human Need Theory

A human need is viewed as an internal tension resulting in an alteration in some part of the person that is expressed in some type of behavior, usually goal directed, and that continues until satisfaction is achieved.[29] A basic or vital human need is one that must be satisfied to sustain life.

Maslow emphasizes the holism of a person, and he states that most needs cannot be isolated, localized, or considered as if they were the only events occurring. Any one desire or need is a need of the whole person.[30] Motivation is stressed as a basis for developing fundamental goals or needs. Rarely is behavior expressive of human motivation except in relation to a situation or to other persons.[31] The character of the

person is an important variable here, as is the degree of intensity of the situation. For example, in responding to situations of great intensity, such as extreme joy, sorrow, fear, or threat, one displays the most unified or completely integrated behavior. If the situation becomes overwhelming, however, disintegration may occur[32] (see Chapter 23).

In order to understand how needs are fulfilled, they should be grouped or classified.

As can be seen from Figure 6-1, fundamental physical needs described by Maslow[33] are strongly similar to those vital human needs identified by Montagu.[34]

Gratification or fulfillment of needs and deprivation or lack of need fulfillment are important concepts. When vital human needs are satisfied, the next higher-level needs emerge and seek gratification or fulfillment. In order to understand and relate to human behavior, it is important to understand the level of need on which a person is functioning at a particular time. Gratification has to do with the power or strength of any one of the human needs. Each level of the hierarchy denotes a group of needs that is less strong or less powerful than the preceding level. For example, safety and security needs are stronger than are needs for love and belonging; unless a person feels safe he will be unable to exhibit love or to demonstrate a healthy state of belonging to another human or group of humans. In like manner, physical needs, those on the lowest level of the hierarchy, are the most powerful, or the strongest. Unless needs for food and sleep are met, persons cannot consider the need for self-esteem. Safety sometimes is completely ignored in an extreme need for food. Therefore, one can conclude that the higher the level of need, the less imperative it is for survival, and the longer gratification can be postponed. This need could disappear permanently, but the pursuit and gratification of higher level needs leads to a healthier person.[35]

Another perspective about human need theory suggests that all humans have a single need in common—a force within each human by which he continually seeks to become more adequate in coping with life.[36] In order for this singular need to be met, there must be a healthy body, because it is the body that is responsible for perceiving the self[37] (see Chapter 15). According to this theory, the goal is to maintain the perceived self as an independent and distinct self, capable of dealing with present and future events of life. Motivation is inherent in each individual and is an internal force that provides direction, drive, and organization for the functioning of each person. The needs as specified by Montagu and Maslow are perceived as the goals, the achievement of which satisfy the need of the person for adequacy. Development of a person's perceptions contributes to the development of his awareness. The need for adequacy is met or there is an effort to meet the need for adequacy based on a person's perception of any one event at any one time. The focus for action becomes the means to achieve its fulfillment.[38]

Perception Theory

What is perceived is determined by each person's unique perceptual field; this field includes more than the direct experience of the senses.[39] A person perceives only what previous experience has made it possible to perceive.[40] Experience suggests that a person sees what he wants to see; what he anticipates as a result of his experience is so firmly established in his thinking that the perceiver may be "blinded" to the real world around him.[41]

Limitations in the functioning of the sense organs, the brain, and the nervous system create limitations in perception.[42] For example, severely brain damaged persons try to maintain organization by avoiding situations that would strain their impaired capacities.[43] In certain situations, however, some positive outcomes may be experienced, such as deaf persons development to a high degree of proficiency in the ability to see.

The process of perception is integrated with those of identification, classification, and coding. These processes are dependent on learning, memory, attention, reasoning, and language. The ability to perceive form, position, and movement of objects in relation to the position and movement of the body is very important in understanding adjustment to normal surroundings.[44] Profound changes in perception can occur when one is exposed to unvarying situations or stimulation over a long period of time (see Chapter 19).

Inferences that a person makes about the nature of objects and events involve knowledge and experiences. Information seldom is derived simply from an instantaneous perception that is immediately forgotten. Impressions last for awhile, and this provides some continuity in perceptions of the environment and enables persons to remember past experiences.[45]

Accurate perception of the environment is essential to preserve life, however, and individual differences are apparent. Persons may perceive and react to stimulation without being fully aware of their percepts. Motivation and emotion have an effect on arousing, directing, facilitating, or inhibiting the perception of situations and events, but differences in knowledge and acquired skill, of intelligence and ability, are of greater importance than motivational influences. For example, witnesses to an accident may give as many and varied reports of the same situation as there are individual witnesses.

The ability to modify immediate perception through reasoning is developed as a person matures; however, experience and learning may have a marked effect on the stage at which it begins to develop.

Persons as perceivers are not always aware of the many aspects of complex situations in the natural environment. Perceptions of form in everyday life may not involve accurate identification of minute detail, although there is the capacity to do this. Generally, there is an overabundance of sensory information, and the observer must select the relevant data to describe objects or events and discard the irrelevant. The observer makes inferences in situations like this.[46] While observers are prone to make inferences from fragments of data, these inferences are influenced by what one expects to perceive; the expectation is that certain stimuli will appear, and perhaps the observer will identify certain stimuli that would have been missed in other situations.[47]

In addition to perceiving form, objects, languages, space, and movement, a dimension of perception involves people, their emotions, and their actions. People perceive other people in a unique manner. Their faces and behavior are integrated into a special scheme by observers. Perceivers are more aware of the intentions, emotions, and personality characteristics (see Chapter 11) of persons than they are aware of the details of physical characteristics.

Perception plays a crucial role in life; it is a major means by which a person gains information about himself, his needs, and the world.

NURSING AND COMPONENTS OF NURSING

By definition, **nursing** is an interpersonal situation in which nurses observe, support, communicate, minister, and teach. Nurses contribute to the maintenance of optimum health and provide care during illness until the client is able to assume responsibility for the fulfillment of his own needs, or when necessary, provide compassionate care/support for the dying person and his family.

To be responsible for client care and to be responsive to the indications of client need, the nurse uses interpersonal, intellectual, and technical skills.

The use of **interpersonal skills** requires initial and continuing contacts with clients, their families, and significant others, as well as an understanding approach and astute insight into each individual who is important or significant in the client situation.

Establishing a situation where clients can trust nurses and the health care team suggests a high degree of interpersonal skill. Especially important is the ability to communicate with clients on their level and about topics in which they are interested. Respect and concern for the perceptions of clients are critical to establishing and maintaining relationships that will permit clients to rely on nurses' skills with the degree of comfort necessary for respite and healing.

The nursing process is an empty structure unless the components of the process are fleshed out with data about the client. A high degree of **intellectual skill** development is necessary in order to recognize the significance of the observations that are made about clients and their situations. Creative approaches to the analysis of the observations are very important, and a rich background of knowledge is critical to the performance of nursing care. Continued development of intellectual skills is inherent in the performance of quality care wherever there is a need for nursing.

Nurses have always been recognized for their **technical skills.** In fact, for many years, the perfection of these skills was the only raison d'etre for nurses. Increased use of technology has made it essential that nurses be able to perform technically; they might need to use sophisticated machinery. Technical skills are important to making the client comfortable. Important in their use, however, is the fact that this is the only **one** of the skills for the nurse to perfect.

The challenge for the nurse is to maintain a blend of interpersonal, intellectual, and technical skills—to neglect none of them—to analyze the needs of the client accurately so that priorities can be set and those skills that can best meet the requirements of each situation can be selected. This aspect of nursing continues to be a major feat and presents a formidable challenge to every conscientious nurse.

PROCESSES IN NURSING

Nurses rely on interpersonal, intellectual, and technical skills to carry out client care. As professionals, they are the leaders of those responsible for providing nursing care for clients and are accountable to the client for providing the care needed and for maintaining a level of skill development that will enable performance of client care in a superlative manner. To fulfill the responsibilities incumbent on a leader, the nurse carries out a **leadership process** that involves decision-making, relating, influencing, and facilitating. The ultimate goal of leadership is to achieve the goals of the group.

One means by which client care can be accommodated is through the **research process.** By systematically examining the various dimensions of nursing care, nurses can gather information about techniques, skills, levels of performance, rationale for care, intellectual decisions, and other phenomena associated with the ministration of nursing measures. Through such activities, nurses are involved in a process of collecting data, analyzing the data that have been gathered, and arriving at conclusions about the data. Ultimately, nurses identify new knowledge about the situation being examined using the research process. Having proceeded through this systematic activity, nurses have a sound basis on which to make decisions and to determine strategies.

The third process that is central to the activity of nursing is the **nursing process,** about which this chapter is written. This process is not unlike the research process in that it is orderly and systematic. It involves assessment—to identify the client's abilities and limitations, planning—to solve identified problems, initiating the plan or assigning others to implement it, and evaluating the extent to which the plan was effective in resolving the identified problem.

THE NURSING PROCESS

A philosophical base provides the foundation for nursing. Each nurse enters a client situation with a set of beliefs and values that directs her activities throughout the client/nurse encounter. Each client holds a set of values and beliefs that the nurse seeks to understand and with which she strives to maintain consistency. In no instance can effective care be planned or carried out unless it is consistent with the client's intentions and wishes. If the client is a family or a community instead of an individual, the determination of values and philosophical principles is equally important and more challenging to define.

Within the philosophical direction of care, determination of a theoretical/conceptual framework is a further component that is an integral part of the nursing process. Just as a building is made of walls that divide the total structure into rooms, so too, the theoretical/conceptual framework for nursing suggests a composite of rooms (concepts) within one structure (theory) where nursing will be performed. Values, beliefs, and philosophies influence the manner in which nursing will be performed and the theoretical/conceptual framework designates the manner by which nursing will be carried out. For example, if the beliefs of Dorothea Orem are followed, the self-care abilities of the client will be recognized and will act as guides for carrying out the nursing process; if Sister Callista Roy's ideas are followed there will be more attention to the client's need for adaptation.

Through the orderly, systematic orientation of the nursing process, the nurse puts herself in close proximity with the client. A "needs orientation" provides the structure and direction needed to plan and carry out the required care. If the nurse can identify client "cues," meticulous analysis of the client data, conscientious planning, implementing, and evaluating will ensure the nurse's accountability for the optimum level of client care. The cyclical process can be repeated as often as necessary depending on the complexity of the client's needs and the extent to which it is necessary to refine the nursing diagnoses (see Figure 6-2). Careful and accurate projection of the goals to be reached (outcome criteria) will help the nurse and the client decide when and how well the needs of the client have been met.

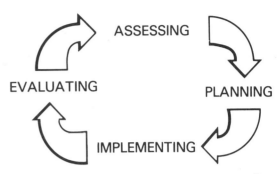

Figure 6-2. The Nursing Process Is Cyclical in Nature.

Assessing

Assessing is the act of reviewing a human situation based on an information database. This is done in order to affirm the wellness state and to diagnose potential client problems; and to affirm an illness state, diagnosing the client's obvious problems, determining the potential for problems, and identifying the wellness aspects of the ill client. The frameworks provide the structure within which the nurse uses the nursing process and fulfills the purpose of nursing, which is the fulfillment of the needs of the identified client.

There are many needs that could be the focus for nurses and clients (see Figure 6-3). These needs provide the framework for all data gathering, nursing diagnoses, goal designation, specification of nursing strategies, and evaluation of goal achievement. The participation of the nurse in the nursing process, within this framework, requires a high level of intellectual, interpersonal, and technical skills.

The assessment phase of the nursing process incorporates all the data gathering efforts and activities of the nurse, including:

- taking the nursing history
- performing the health assessment
- using data gathering tools, for example: thermometer, stethoscope, sphygmomanometer, otoscope, cardiac monitor, and tape measure

air
sleep
nutrition
territoriality
to love and be loved
tenderness
activity
structure, law, & limits
confidence
sexual integrity
spiritual experience
protection from excessive fear, anxiety, & stress
interchange of gases
adaptation, to manage stress
safety
fluids
elimination
rest and leisure
humor
sensory integrity
autonomy, choice
conceptualization, rationality, problem solving
acceptance of self & others
challenge
effective perception of reality
wholesome body image
for self-fulfillment, to be, to become
value system
skin integrity
belonging
freedom from pain
personal recognition, esteem, respect
self-control, self-determination, responsibility
appreciation, attention
beauty & esthetic experiences

Figure 6-3.   Selected Client Needs.

- using the techniques of percussion, auscultation, and palpation
- using all five senses.

These activities provide the information needed to make nursing judgments and diagnoses. The purpose of the assessment phase is to identify and obtain data about the client's needs that enable the nurse and the client or his family to find potential and obvious problems relating to wellness and illness.

In assessing the level of fulfillment of the needs of the client, nurses consider the influence and interrelationship of factors such as age, sex, education, growth and development, and socioeconomic, cultural (see Chapter 10), and religious elements.

Nurses assess the educational level of their clients considering formal and informal education. This includes the use of specialized language related to education or job and special interpretation of terms and phrases used (see Chapter 12). Nurses assess the socioeconomic status of the client as well as his perception of the status and its implication, and the impact of work on the client's perception of himself. They assess the level of fulfillment or alteration in fulfillment of needs for the client.

More specific data are obtained about the client when the nurse performs a health examination that incorporates physical and psychosocial dimensions. A systematic format should be developed and followed by the nurse to assure that the assessment is complete and that no body areas were omitted or forgotten. Additional questions formed from the needs assessment, taken during the nursing history, can be used to obtain more specific data while the physical and psychosocial examinations are in progress. Information and specific inferences about the client's potential and obvious problems related to human need fulfillment are considered (see Chapter 7).

Data about the client and his health status may be gleaned from family members, significant others, neighbors, and teachers, to mention a few. Data about the client and his family may be graphed on a genogram (see Chapter 25), which is a particularly useful tool that provides nurses with a quick visual reference point for the relationship of the client to family members in one or more generations. Such data round out the data provided by the client. Data about living and work environments and about variables that influence the present as well as future health status of the client add to the accuracy of nursing diagnoses and provide information about goal expectations and level of goal achievement.

The time used for data gathering during the assessment phase of the nursing process is time well spent. Not only are data available for nursing diagnoses, but the assessment phase forms the framework for all phases, including goal specification and determination of goal achievement. In other words, the present and immediate health situation for the client is only the first phase of goal directed actions needed to achieve positive health results. Immediate, intermediate, and long-range expectations are specified. These expectations often extend far beyond the immediate status of the client until he is home or back to work. Thus, for hospitalized clients, data gleaned during the assessment phase and subsequent decisions about the data have direct bearing on discharge from the health care agency and the health follow-up expected after discharge.

It is during the assessment phase that the client begins to participate in the nursing process to assure the maintenance of the integrity of need fulfillment where there is an alteration. The nursing process offsets the alteration in an expedient, effective, and economic manner. The client participates in all phases of the nursing process as do his family and significant others. If circumstances temporarily limit the client's involvement in his own care planning, every effort should be made to involve the family as soon as possible.

It is during the assessment phase that the helping relationship is established between the nurse and the client, beginning with the first nurse-client interaction that determines the client's health status. The initial dialogue with the client should be the beginning of a purposeful interaction through all phases of the nursing process. In addition, this beginning interaction initiates the nurse's commitment to the client, a commitment that enhances the holistic view and care of the client.

While the data are being collected, the nurse validates inferences to assure accuracy in interpretation. When the nurse infers the existence of a problem, or assumes a condition or situation from known facts or evidence, she confirms or validates the problem, condition, or situation with the client. The client has the opportunity to corroborate or discount the inferences made by the nurse.

The nurse sorts, organizes, categorizes, synthesizes, groups, compares, and analyzes the data obtained about the client. Then she makes judgments ranging from verifying the absence of a problem to verifying a complicated one that the client or family is successfully handling (e.g., from one that requires mechanical or pharmacological aids or the services of other health team members, to the designation of potential and obvious problems making acute or long-term demands and requiring a multitude of health and nursing care services).

The assessment phase concludes with the designation of potential or obvious nursing diagnoses. The designation of nursing diagnoses draws heavily upon the nurse's intellectual and interpersonal skills and sets the framework for all activities in the remaining process, concluding with evaluation.

Nursing diagnoses can be proposed for each of the needs specified earlier. They can be stated as needs being met excessively, altering the pattern of need fulfillment, or being met in a partial, limited, or totally deprived fashion. The nursing diagnoses can be further specified as acute, chronic, or intermittent, for example, and be qualified with the reason for the alteration in need fulfillment (see Figure 6-4).

When data to support the nursing diagnosis are evident, the potential or obvious nursing diagnosis is specified and the reason for or cause of the alteration is stated. For example, the alteration may be due to or caused by: personal and situational occurrences; environmental affronts; medical, pharmacological, and nursing therapies (commissions and omissions); specific pathological states; specific psychopathological states; physiological miscalculations or nonacceptance; congenital alterations (reparable, irreparable); philosophic, ethical, and religious impositions; social and economic affronts; educational affronts; growth and development affronts, and others. The nurse has logically specified the client's potential and obvious problems based on data. This information is strategic to planning, particularly for goal specification and goal expectation and for prescribing nursing strategies to prevent or offset alterations in need fulfillment. In addition, the nurse will support the fulfillment of those human needs currently met fully or reasonably well.

Human Need	Proposed Nursing Diagnoses
Acceptance of self and others, by others	• Overacceptance of self and others, by others • Alteration in pattern of expression of need for acceptance • Rejection of self and others, by others
Activity	• Excessive activity • Alterations in patterns of expression or fulfillment of the need • Insufficient activity
Adaptation, to manage stress	• Excessive adaptation • Alterations in pattern of expression or fulfillment of the need to adapt • Insufficient adaptation
Air	• Excessive aeration • Alteration in pattern of expression or fulfillment of the need • Insufficient aeration
Appreciation, attention	• Excessive appreciation and attention • Alteration in pattern of expression or fulfillment of the need • Lack of appreciation, attention
Autonomy, choice	• Excessive autonomy, choice • Alteration in pattern of expression or fulfillment of the need • Lack of autonomy, choice
Beauty and esthetic experiences	• Preoccupation with beauty and esthetic experiences • Alteration in pattern of expression or fulfillment of the need • Lack of beauty and esthetic experiences
Belonging	• Excessive belonging • Alteration in pattern of expression or fulfillment of the need • Lack of belonging
Challenge	• Excessive challenge • Alteration in pattern of expression or fulfillment of the need • Lack of challenge

Human Need	Proposed Nursing Diagnoses
Conceptualization, rationality, problem solving	• Preoccupation with conceptualization, rationality, and problem solving • Alteration in pattern of expression or fulfillment of the need • Inability to conceptualize, rationalize, and problem solve
Confidence	• Overconfidence • Alteration in pattern of expression or fulfillment of the need • Lack of confidence
Elimination (end products of metabolism, toxins, poisons, chemicals, drugs)	• Excessive elimination • Alteration in pattern of expression or fulfillment of the need • Lack of or diminished elimination
Fluids (Intake)	• Excessive hydration and electrolytes • Alteration in pattern of expression or fulfillment of the need • Depletion of fluids and electrolytes
Freedom from pain	• Excessive freedom from pain, lack of appropriate pain signals • Alteration in pattern of expression or fulfillment of the need • Inability to experience pain relief
Humor	• Excessive or continuous use of humor, hilarity • Alteration in pattern of expression or fulfillment of the need • Inability to experience humor
Nutrition (Intake)	• Excessive nutritional intake • Alteration in pattern of expression or fulfillment of the need • Insufficient or lack of nutritional intake
Effective perception of reality	• Hypersensitive perception of reality • Alteration in pattern of expression or fulfillment of the need • Ineffective, inaccurate perception of reality
Personal recognition, esteem, respect	• Over-recognition, respect, excessive esteem • Alteration in pattern of expression or fulfillment of the need • Lack of recognition, esteem, respect
Protection from excessive fear	• Excessive fear • Alteration in pattern of expression or fulfillment of the need • Lack of expression of fear, lack of protection
Rest and leisure	• Excessive rest, irresponsible use of leisure • Alteration in pattern of expression or fulfillment of the need • Restlessness, lack of rest, or leisure

Human Need	*Proposed Nursing Diagnoses*
Safety	• Excessive preoccupation with thwarting safety • Alteration in pattern of expression or fulfillment of the need • Diminished or lack of safety
Self-control, self-determination, responsibility	• Excessive control, determination, responsibility • Alteration in pattern of expression or fulfillment of the need • Diminished or lack of self-control, self-determination, responsibility
Self-fulfillment, to be, become	• Independence, preoccupation with becoming • Alteration in pattern of expression or fulfillment of the need • Lack of fulfillment of self, or feeling of becoming, prolonged dependence
Sensory integrity	• Sensory overload • Alteration in pattern of expression or fulfillment of the need • Sensory deprivation
Sexual integrity	• Preoccupation with sexual dimension • Alteration in pattern of expression or fulfillment of the need • Lack of attention to sexual integrity
Skin integrity	• Preoccupation with maintenance of skin integrity • Alteration in pattern of expression or fulfillment of the need • Diminished or lack of skin integrity
Sleep	• Excessive sleep • Alteration in pattern of expression or fulfillment of the need • Insufficient or lack of sleep
Spiritual integrity	• Preoccupation with or excessive spiritual integrity • Alteration in pattern of expression or fulfillment of the need • Ineffective, diminished or lack of spiritual integrity
Structure, law, and limits	• Excessive structure, law, and limits • Alteration in pattern of expression or fulfillment of the need • Diminished or lack of structure, law, limits
Tenderness	• Excessive, smothering tenderness • Alteration in pattern of expression or fulfillment of the need • Diminished or lack of tenderness

Human Need	Proposed Nursing Diagnoses
Territoriality	• Excessive territorial requirement • Alteration in pattern of expression or fulfillment of the need • Diminished or lack of territorial space
To love and be loved	• Excessive expression of love and requirement for love and to be loved • Alteration in pattern of expression or fulfillment of the need • Diminished or lack of ability to love and be loved
Wholesome body image	• Excessive valuation of overall image or of selected body parts • Alteration in pattern of expression or fulfillment of the need • Diminished or poor body image
Value system	• Excessive or rigid application of value system • Alteration in pattern of expression or fulfillment of the need • Diminished or lack of value system

Figure 6-4. Proposed Nursing Diagnoses Based on Needs Assessment

The assessment phase of the nursing process assures that the nurse and client focus on those needs that are reasonably well met by the client or his family in addition to those in which there is evidence of alteration in need fulfillment. Using a framework for nursing provides the client with the best assurance that all dimensions for the person (well and ill) will be recognized. Inherent in this protection is evidence that disease will be prevented and wellness promoted by diagnosing potential problems of the client.

When assessment data verify the human needs that are met, those having a potential to be unmet, or those unmet, and the client supports the judgments made, the planning phase of the nursing process begins. Plans are made to maintain the well state if needs of the client are considered to be met, and potential nursing diagnoses are specified or plans are made to offset an illness state if a few or many needs of the client are considered to be unmet. For the ill client, the needs that are reasonably met and those with a potential to be unmet are also the focus for planning.

Planning

Planning is the phase of the nursing process where a determination of nursing action plans to assist the client toward the goal of optional wellness is made. The purposes of this phase are to:

• signify the priority of the client's potential and obvious problems

• specify the behavioral outcomes or goals for the client and the expected time of achievement of these outcomes

• differentiate client problems and those that could be resolved by nursing intervention from those that could be referred to other members of the health team

- designate the specific actions or nursing strategies, their frequency, and results
- write the client's potential and obvious nursing diagnoses, nursing actions and their frequency, and the expected outcomes on the nursing care plan.

The planning phase terminates with completion of the nursing care plan, which is the blueprint that provides direction for implementing the plan and provides the framework for evaluation.

In terms of priority setting, the more life threatening the client problem, the higher the priority. Nurses use their own judgment but also consider the designations of priorities as viewed by the client. Priorities can be conveniently classified as high, medium, and low. As high-priority problems are resolved, fully or in part, a reordering may be needed. Problems in the medium- and low-priority categories may be considered a high priority at some time. For instance, if constipation is a problem it may receive a place quite high on the priority list if it persists. Each client problem should be so ordered that the integrity and unity of the client can be maintained. If there are differences in the designation of priority among the nurse, the client, and other members of the nursing or health team, collection of additional data usually brings about resolution of the differences. The nursing focus is on preserving the well aspects of the sick person while diminishing ill aspects of the person.

If no obvious problems exist or a potential problem exists, the nurse verifies the client's state of wellness and plans with the client for periodic verification of the state. Information and support services may be provided for the client's use. If, in the interim, symptoms appear or the client feels he has a problem, he is instructed to return to see the nurse immediately. In using the nursing process with the well client, the nurse and client participate in the assessing and planning phases, while the client assumes responsibility in the implementing and evaluating phases.

The expected behavioral results or goals for the client are specified for each obvious or potential nursing diagnosis. This holds true for a family or community nursing diagnosis, as well as for the individual. For example, if the client's nursing diagnosis is overnutrition due to excessive eating, the expected behavioral result of intervention would be attainment of a well balanced nutritional level in accordance with the height, target weight, and life style of the client. The level of human need fulfillment that can be achieved by the client should be realistic considering the reason for the alteration. A date when the behavioral result is expected should be indicated.

Once the determination is made regarding the time when goal achievement is expected and the specific outcome criteria are defined, the nurse designates possible interventions for each nursing diagnosis. Solutions offered by the client should be considered and incorporated. The possible success of each solution is estimated considering the human variables of age, sex, sociocultural background, level of growth and development, for example, and drawing upon scientific principles and sound research results. The best solutions are selected and a judgment is made as to the persons—the nurse, the client, the family, the nursing or team members—who will carry out the action.

The nursing diagnosis and supporting data, the goal descriptions and expectations, the date and time for expected goal achievement, as well as the time interval for measurement of the level of achievement of need fulfillment, and the specific prescribed nursing strategies with frequencies complete the development of the nursing care plan—the blueprint for action. The format for the nursing care plan should flow from the goals of the nursing care plan and draws heavily on the intellectual skills of the nurse. A sample client situation with a developed nursing care plan follows. Note that the format uses the human need theory framework.

Client Situation—Mrs. Martha Bender

Mrs. Martha Bender, age 81, was admitted to the nursing unit of a health care agency with severe headaches. She is a known hypertensive and had been hospitalized four times in the past two years for control of hypertension. She lives alone and manages a two-story, three-bedroom house, which has been the family home for generations. Mrs. Bender's husband died following a stroke four years ago, and her three children are married with families of their own. Each lives within 10 miles of their mother's home. Each of the children had offered Mrs. Bender a home with them, but she refused, stating that she needed to have her own household; she had to be independent and be "her own boss." Close contact was maintained between Mrs. Bender and her children. In fact, her children planned among themselves the personal and phone contact with their mother as well as the availability of one of the children at all times. Mrs. Bender also stated that if she became unable to care for herself, she would go to a nursing home. Years ago, she and her husband made investigations and tours of nursing homes in the area in case a nursing home experience would be necessary. One nursing home was selected on a contingency basis.

The assessment data obtained by the nurse verified a severe headache mainly in the occipital area that diminishes when Mrs. Bender's head is elevated. The sensation of pain is lessened by the use of cold compresses to the temporal area. This intervention was made by Mrs. Bender prior to admission and was continued on admission at her request.

She complained of loss of appetite accompanied by a distaste for food. She is unsteady on her feet and stated she bumped into the bathroom door causing an area of ecchymosis with an abrasion on her left shoulder and leg. Mrs. Bender appears tired and stated she could barely get around and take care of herself since her headache started two days ago. Her blood pressure was $^{210}/_{100}$ on admission; pulse 80, respiration 15. She is 5′ 1″ and weighs 120 pounds. The physician prescribed furosemide (Lasix®) 40 mgm daily, p.o., q day; propranolol (Inderal®) 20 mgm BID to reduce her blood pressure; a low salt diet; activity as tolerated; Acetaminophen (Tylenol®) 650 mgm for headache q 3-4 hours p.r.n., and continuation of cold compresses to head as desired.

Additional data obtained by the nurse through the health assessment of Mrs. Bender included difficulty focusing her eyes and sensitivity to light. She wears eyeglasses for reading. She had some difficulty hearing, especially noted on the left side. She yawned, looked sleepy, and complained that she slept little for the past two nights. She generally sleeps 6 hours a night and gets to bed after an 11:00 p.m. television news report and awakes about 5:30 a.m. She spends the first half hour of bedtime praying and reading the bible. She generally had been taking a one-hour nap after lunch and bathes in the evening.

Upon completion of the nursing history and health assessment, needs that were reasonably well met were verified and those needs found to be partially or fully unmet or with the potential to be unmet were identified. Nursing diagnoses (potentially, partially, and fully unmet human needs) were determined and shared with Mrs. Bender for validation and accuracy. A nursing care plan with goal determination and achievement were prescribed. The following nursing care plan developed for and with Mrs. Bender emerged.*

*The authors are grateful to Patricia Frensky Orfini for reviewing this client situation and nursing care plan. Her thoughtful, useful suggestions have been incorporated and have strengthened the presentation.

Nursing Care Plan—Mrs. Martha Bender—October 1

Client Need	Nursing Diagnosis	Goals with Outcome Criteria	Nursing Strategies with Frequencies
Freedom from pain	Experience of pain related to: • pathological affront of hypertension • injury • ecchymosis • abrasion	Relief of pain as evidenced by: • control of pain within 24 hours • statements regarding absence of pain for 3–4 hours during first 24 hours • verbalizing the absence of pain after 48 hours.	1. Assessment for Mrs. Bender: (to be completed in 18 hours) a) location of headaches b) circumstances or events that impact upon headache—either diminish or increase it c) extent of pain relief with acetaminophen; amount of time needed; interval of recurrence d) character of pain e) sensation and symptoms accompanying pain f) areas for pain, numbness, tingling, and discomfort other than head, i.e., extremities, back, abdomen g) associated symptoms, i.e., weakness, paralysis, etc. 2. Offer and administer acetaminophen for pain — check level of pain relief — plot the onset of and relief of headaches in conjunction with blood pressure recording, acetaminophen (Tylenol®) administration, diuretic action, and look for relationships — do not delay acetaminophen when pain recurs; instruct Mrs. Bender to report onset of headache immediately — look for precipitating events — report failure to obtain pain relief to physician — observe for nausea, vomiting, skin rash 3. Continue the cold compresses to the occipital area while headache persists a) facilitate Mrs. Bender's participation by: — providing cold compress setup within reach — maintaining cold temperature of water/ice solution — providing adequate shoulder covering to prevent chills — arranging for waterproofing of pillows and head covering — supplying additional wash cloths to wipe dripping b) check skin for evidence of irritation, breakdown q 2 hours c) massage neck and shoulders to promote relaxation and pain relief 4. Position Mrs. Bender so that her head is elevated at all times to prevent increased intracranial pressure

Client Need	Nursing Diagnosis	Goals with Outcome Criteria	Nursing Strategies with Frequencies
			— assess what degree of elevation seems most comfortable and record here _____.
			5. Administer furosemide as prescribed by physician at 8 am
			a) check BP q 2 hours
			b) note any headache relief with lowering of blood pressure
			c) look for manifestations of drug allergy to furosemide, i.e., skin rash, hives, itching, nausea, vomiting, diarrhea, dizziness, blurred vision
			— if found, discontinue drug administration and notify physician
			d) look for side effects of furosemide
			— orthostatic hypotension
			— check for ↓ Na., ↓ K, muscle weakness and cramping, confusion, tingling in extremities
			— check for sugar in urine
			— check for confusion, tingling
			6. Administer propanolol (Inderal®) 20 mg before breakfast 7:30 am and before dinner 4:45 pm
			— take apical pulse before giving drug
			— report change in pulse rate rhythm, BP recordings; report pattern to physician
			— check intake/output ratio; record
			— check for adverse drug reaction: dry mouth and eyes, nausea, vomiting, confusion, hair loss, skin changes, profound bradycardia, palpitation
			7. Teach Mrs. Bender relaxation exercises, particularly to face, scalp, neck, shoulders,
			— 15 min p.c. and bedtime (8:30 am–12:30–5:30 and 10:30 pm)
			8. Adjust environment
			— quiet, pleasant surroundings
			— ask Mrs. Bender about number of visitors and length of stay she desires
			— adjust lighting
			— minimize frightening noises
			9. Gently comb her hair
			— avoid hair styles that put traction on scalp
			— avoid tight head covering or bands
			10. Suggest comfortable, loose fitting nightgown, robe, and slippers
			11. Observe for signs of transient ischemic attacks (TIAs)

Client Need	Nursing Diagnosis	Goals with Outcome Criteria	Nursing Strategies with Frequencies
			— weakness, numbness — temporary dizziness and unsteadiness — temporary loss of speech; difficulty understanding speech — diplopia — change in personality or emotional state — sudden loss of vision or temporary dimness 12. Solicit assistance of family members in observing for signs and symptoms noted in #11
Fluids (Intake)	Potential loss of fluid volume and Na & K related to: • pharmacological action of furosemide (Lasix) • fluid loss • Na loss • K loss	Maintenance of adequate fluid volume in three days as evidenced by: • Serum K 3.5–5.0 mEq/L • Serum Na 132–142 mEq/L • Skin, tongue, oral mucosa moist, intact, smooth • 5 lb weight loss with stabilized weight after 48 hours	1. Assess fluid intake and output for Mrs. Bender q shift — record quantity of fluids — record type of fluids — encourage citrus juices, milk, apricot nectar, tomato juice, coffee to maintain adequate K — elicit the assistance of Mrs. Bender in recording intake — check color, concentration of urine 2. Observe for signs of hyperkalemia daily — decreased pulse — orthostatic hypotension — muscle weakness and cramping — confusion — tingling sensation in extremities 3. Observe for signs of hypokalemia — weakness — nausea, vomiting — abdominal distention — rapid, irregular pulse — lethargy — confusion 4. Check the status of skin, tongue and oral mucosa for texture, level of dryness or moisture, integrity of tissue. Check for thirst q shift. 5. Check weight daily before breakfast—7 am 6. Assess electrolyte reports daily
Sensory integrity	Diminished sensory integrity related to: • pathological affront of hypertension • aged state • change in sensory input	Enhanced sensory integrity as evidenced by — improved ability to communicate with staff, using nonverbal techniques, etc. by 48 hours — improved vision and experience of visual comfort within 48 hours — verbalization or im-	1. Complete the assessment of Mrs. Bender within 24 hours — determine if focusing difficulty occurs with near and/or far objects — determine level of light needed to obliterate photosensitivity — determine level and quality of hearing loss 2. Adjust bed position so Mrs. Bender is faced away from window and bright lights

Client Need	Nursing Diagnosis	Goals with Outcome Criteria	Nursing Strategies with Frequencies
		proved skin sensation within one week — expression of improved taste within 3 days	— provide Mrs. Bender with dimmer attachment for bed lights — refrain from shining flashlight into eyes of Mrs. Bender during evening and night hours — if reading, check that eyeglasses are worn 3. Adjust bed position so that Mrs. Bender's right side is accessible to facilitate hearing — stand in front of client when speaking — speak clearly, slowly and distinctly — verify that Mrs. Bender has received the message — instruct nursing and auxiliary staff on position and method of articulation — refer hearing problem to physician for hearing evaluation, audiometer, value of aid appliance — provide for hearing aid mechanism for telephone if feasible and useful 4. Utilize touch and nonverbal communication to convey acceptance and valuing 5. Demonstrate to family members the techniques to maximize the limited communication time (handholding, caressing, articulation, nonverbal communication) 6. Answer call bell in person—do not rely on intercom system 7. Do not chew gum, cover your mouth when speaking 8. Use nonverbal cues to help convey your meaning, facial expressions, hand gestures, writing, pointing 9. Speak slowly and distinctly—do not shout 10. Keep voice at same volume—avoid dropping off at end of each sentence
Nutrition	Potential for alteration in intake of food and fluids secondary to: • pathophysiological affront of hypertension • distaste for food	Maintenance of nutritional state as evidenced by: — eats three well balanced meals with bedtime snack totaling 1500 calories daily — oral fluid intake of no more than 2000 cc daily — verbalizes return to normal energy/activity state within 3 days	1. Assess nutritional status: — ask Mrs. Bender about food preferences — prescribe food selection of high K^+ content, e.g., chicken, fresh fish, milk, sweet potato, bananas, all-bran cereals, beef — weigh daily 2. Check for ability to handle regular meal pattern — order small portions if needed — arrange 4 or 6 meal servings rather than 3 if Mrs. Bender cannot handle usual pattern

Client Need	Nursing Diagnosis	Goals with Outcome Criteria	Nursing Strategies with Frequencies
			— suggest a milk food at bedtime to promote sleep 3. Incorporate activity and exercise with meal plan to assure that she would not be too tired to eat 4. Suggest visit by family members during meal time, because Mrs. Bender may need to solicit assistance of family member's to facilitate eating 5. Explain to Mrs. Bender and family members the basic levels of low salt diet and the need to maintain adequate intake of K^+ 6. Explore with family members their ability to bring in favorite foods 7. Explain to client and family, the relationship between hypertension, sodium, fluid intake and obesity.
Elimination	Potential alteration in urinary and bowel elimination pattern related to: • pharmacological impact of furosemide (Lasix®) diuretic • aged state • loss of appetite	Resumption of usual pattern of bowel elimination within 4 days as evidenced by: — adjustment to current urinary elimination pattern in one week — normal moisture evident for skin, oral mucosa, tongue and lips within 4 days — verbalizes ability to cope with increased frequency	1. Assess the elimination pattern — note time and character of stool — determine level of strength and/or difficulty with defecation — determine level and character of voiding — note any discomfort with voiding—urgency, burning 2. Check voiding pattern q shift (daily) to determine effect of diuretic — expect maximum urine volume 2 hours after furosemide (Lasix®) then gradually diminishing in 6–8 hours—explain to client — contrast output pattern with BP recording q 2 hours during waking hours — note skin turgor condition of oral mucosa and tongue — determine impact on body weight — check for edema; determine location and type and extent 3. Assess ambulatory ability within 1st 12 hours 4. Provide for privacy during voiding and defecation 5. Check for signs of dehydration, and low K 6. Encourage participation in elimination surveillance — note when heaviest voiding occurs — note established pattern of diuretic so that social events and interactions can be planned around elimination schedule 7. Facilitate handwashing and have all toilet articles within easy reach and

Client Need	Nursing Diagnosis	Goals with Outcome Criteria	Nursing Strategies with Frequencies
			in appropriate space, to minimize the necessity of bending over to pick up items and increase intracranial pressure 8. Report to physician signs of excessive fluid loss 9. Encourage walk in hall BID (10 am–4 pm) 10. Assess diet for roughage: — encourage foods high in fiber
Rest and leisure	Diminished rest and leisure related to: ● pathological affront of hypertension with resultant high blood pressure ● aged state ● pharmacological impact of furosemide diuretic ● anxiety	Experience of increased rest and wholesome leisure within a week as evidenced by: — verbalizes return to preillness state	1. Assess usual rest and leisure pattern — determine the level of strength — determine the amount of energy available to accomplish activities of daily living — note the response to exertion, e.g., going to bathroom, sitting in a chair, using the bedpan in bed, assisting with bathing, eating, etc. 2. Plan rest period after each meal and a nap in afternoon (preferably after heaviest voiding period) — instruct client on relaxation exercises — talk about effective ways to experience quiet time — arrange with staff to respect rest periods and quiet times — post sign on door 3. Determine preference for leisure activities. — arrange with family for small radio and guide to programming — suggest phone visits with friends — visit with family members — visit from clergyman 4. Avoid sitting or lying in one position or for prolonged periods of time.
Sleep	Sleep deprivation secondary to: ● pathological state of hypertension with resultant elevated blood pressure ● headache ● hospitalization	Normal sleep pattern resumed as evidenced by: — sleeps 6 hours undisturbed within 24 hours — resumption of afternoon nap and usual sleep pattern in 48 hours	1. Complete assessment of usual sleep pattern within 48 hours (see chapter 20) — record sleep/wake pattern for 48 hours — inquire about client's perception of sleep — determine presleep rituals 2. Arrange room environment so that it is conducive to sleep — eliminate noise — adjust temperature — arrange night light out of direct range of vision 3. Facilitate undisturbed sleep for at least 4 sleep cycles (about 6 hours, 11:30 pm–6 am) during the night — maintain usual time to retire

Client Need	Nursing Diagnosis	Goals with Outcome Criteria	Nursing Strategies with Frequencies
			— provide milk snack (contains tryptophan soporific) — partial bath and soothing back rub at 10 pm — give Tylenol® for headache if needed — assess comfort/discomfort level — allay fears and anxiety if identified — counsel staff on methods of data collection without disturbing client, e.g., taking pulse, observational assessment during sleep stage III & IV 4. Plan for afternoon nap — provide opportunity for am nap to increase REM sleep time — specify the time usually taken — Please Do Not Disturb sign on the door — inform staff — when facilitating afternoon nap, eliminate voiding times and too late hours so that night sleep is not jeopardized 5. Record and analyze all sleep related data.
Skin integrity	Disruption in skin integrity due to: • pathological affront of hypertension resultant in faulty circulation • aged state	Achievement of intact skin within 72 to 90 hours as evidenced by: — decrease in size of abrasions — no evidence of infection	1. Assess the specific reason for the injury, i.e., TIA, dizziness, poor lighting, poor vision, foreign objects in path, inappropriate footwear, etc. 2. Assess texture, quality of skin, tongue, and oral mucosa 3. Check for edema, redness, drainage, change in size of ecchymotic areas — check for signs of allergy to propranol, furosemide, i.e., rashes, hives, itching 4. Avoid excessive bathing, use of soaps, alcohol or any drying agents on skin — use emollients to facilitate skin integrity — protect skin over bony prominences — soft night clothing will protect against roughness of bed linens — mouth care to prevent dryness and cracking 7 am–8:30—12:30–5:30 & 10 on waking & pc & hs & p.r.n. 5. Apply warm soaks to ecchymotic areas three times a day (T.I.D.) 10-2-6. Clean abrasions with soap and water, two times a day (B.I.D.) with morning care and at bedtime 6. Observe fluid intake for adequacy — check excessive output due to diuretic action.

Client Need	Nursing Diagnosis	Goals with Outcome Criteria	Nursing Strategies with Frequencies

Activity	Diminished activity level related to:
	• pathological affront of hypertension
	• aged state
	• hospitalization
		Resumption of preadmission activity regimen within one week as evidenced by:
		— ability to perform selfcare
		— ability to walk length of corridor
		— ability to get out of bed unassisted
			1. Assess Mrs. Bender's preadmission activity pattern within 24 hours. Use family resources
			2. Facilitate activities of daily living (ADL) planned with client
			— plan so that one major activity occurs at a time, i.e., bathing, feeding
			  • 5:30 am—arise; wash face and hands; prayers
			  • 7:30 am—vital signs
			  • 8 am—breakfast
			  • 8:30 am—mouth care, range of motion (ROM), relaxation exercise, leisure activity
			  • 9:30 am—walk
			  • 10:30 am—nap
			  • 12 Noon—lunch, BP
			  • 12:30 pm—mouth care, relaxation exercise, ROM, BP
			  • 2 pm—visitors
			  • 3 pm—nap
			  • 4 pm—walk activity
			  • 5 pm—dinner
			  • 5:30 pm—mouth care, relaxation exercise, ROM, BP
			  • 6 pm—warm soaks, BP
			  • 7 pm—visitors
			  • 9 pm—warm bath, BP, mouth care, relaxation exercise
			— plan a rest period after each activity
			— include walking short distances in the activity schedule; make certain that substantial slippers are worn for walking
			— assess ability to walk on own or necessity of one person accompanying within 24 hrs.
			— refrain from having Mrs. Bender sit or lie for long periods of time
			— adjust activity related to trips to bathroom—offer bedpan in between when frequent voiding is experienced (9 am–12 noon)
			— assess how client bathes (in bed, at sink, etc.) and the portion of the bath she can do
			3. Provide for ROM exercises while in bed 3 times a day. Teach leg exercises
			4. Diminish or increase level of exercise based on degree of strength, blood pressure, and desire
			5. Report to physician any unusual activity or loss of motion, e.g., paralysis, hyperactivity of extremities, momentary loss of consciousness, slurred speech
			6. Encourage family members to par-

Client Need	Nursing Diagnosis	Goals with Outcome Criteria	Nursing Strategies with Frequencies
			ticipate in activities, e.g., ROM, accompany to bathroom, walk in hall.
Safety	Potential and actual alteration in safety related to: • pathological state of hypertension • situational occurrence of hospitalization and living alone • aged state • pharmacological impact of antihypertensive and diuretic	No affronts to safety experienced during hospitalization as evidenced by: • no falls • asking for help when tired	1. Assess the major affronts to Mrs. Bender's safety during hospitalization. Determine: — steadiness of gait — hazards that might cause injury, e.g., chairs, equipment in walking pathway, electrical cords — incompatibilities, allergy related to furosemide, e.g., possible problem with alcohol ingestion — access to call light and appliances to maintain position in electrically operated bed 2. Explain the need for bedrails — check security of bedrails — assist with getting out of bed and accompany on all walking activities 3. Protect from viral and bacterial infection — do not assign staff with colds, coughs, etc., to care for Mrs. Bender 4. Allow sufficient time for eating — position during eating to facilitate swallowing — have staff available during mealtime 5. Assess the immediate environment for irritating sounds, unnecessary noise, noxious odors, drafts — intervene to eliminate same, to maintain airy, odor free, comfortable room 6. Refrain from jolting Mrs. Bender — announce yourself; tap her shoulder to get her attention — take care in handling the bed and bedding; prevent bumping against bed especially when headache pain is evident.
Autonomy	Potential diminution of autonomy, choice related to: • situational occurrence of hospitalization • pathological affront of hypertension • medical, pharmacological, and nursing therapies • aged state	Resumption of autonomy and choice regarding self and environment as evidenced by: • ability to perform activities of daily living • ability to make sound decisions • ability to adequately problem solve	1. Ask Mrs. Bender how she sees herself participating in her care 2. Seek client's advice on timing of caring activities, menu food selections, timing for visitors, etc. 3. Listen to reminiscences of times when client had full control over herself and situation 4. Talk with family members about ways to maximize client's autonomy while yielding to a dependency state until her blood pressure is stabilized — support family members' efforts

Client Need	Nursing Diagnosis	Goals with Outcome Criteria	Nursing Strategies with Frequencies
			to allow autonomy for Mrs. Bender within limits of her health state and their need to intervene to temporarily conduct her affairs as delegated
			5. Facilitate delegation of household affairs to family members while client is hospitalized
			6. Keep Mrs. Bender informed of options in medical and nursing care provided — offer choices whenever possible
			7. Determine with client and family members how emergency health situations will be handled in the future — assist in establishing surveillance system when client returns to her home.
Self-control, self-determination, responsibility	Potential for diminished opportunity for self-control, self-determination, responsibility for self related to: ● hospitalization ● pathological affront of hypertension ● aged state	Maintenance of control over self, self-determination and responsibility as evidenced by: ● continues decision-making regarding care and welfare from onset of hospitalization ● delegates to significant others those specific areas where intervention is appropriate and desired from onset of hospitalization	1. Involve Mrs. Bender in her care as much as is appropriate and safe. — gradually increase involvement as headache subsides and blood pressure is reduced to normal limits 2. Determine how knowledgeable client is about the cause of her headaches and the potential hazard of elevated blood pressure — explore fears related to present and future states of health 3. Compliment Mrs. Bender on her handling of physical crises that resulted in admission to the hospital — review signs and symptoms for which client should be alert, i.e., changes in memory, perception, affect, reasoning, brief periods of loss of consciousness, any weakness or numbness, temporary dizziness, unsteadiness, temporary loss of speech, sudden loss of vision or temporary dimness, recurrence of headache, diplopia — review these signs and symptoms with family members. Ask them to be alert to change in personality or emotional state — plan with Mrs. Bender and family members how this surveillance will be conducted and what should and can be done in the event of occurrence — teach family members to take blood pressure for Mrs. Bender and themselves — check blood pressures of family members to determine baseline

Client Need	Nursing Diagnosis	Goals with Outcome Criteria	Nursing Strategies with Frequencies
			recording. Refer family members to physician if elevated readings found after rest and recheck — provide Mrs. Bender and family members with information on community's electronic medical response systems services for elderly, disabled, or all persons in the home 4. Help client to work through the fact that needing care through the intervention of another person need not diminish her control or responsibility for herself or her situation.

Self-fulfillment	Potential for diminished self-fulfillment related to:
	• situational occurrence of hospitalization
	• pathophysiological state of hypertension
	• aged state
		Experience of enhanced self-fulfillment within one week as evidenced by:
		• expressions of positive views about her condition—feeling neither overwhelmed nor excessively optimistic
		• states that she is not overly concerned about aspect of dependency brought on by her hospitalization and describes how she expects to resume full control over herself·as her situation improves
		• ability to focus on problems outside herself and can muster energy to get involved in these
		• expresses a fresh appreciation for the basic things in life
			1. Assess client's perception of herself
			2. Facilitate fulfillment of usual pattern of activity and contacts with family and friends within the restriction imposed by diminished strength and pain
			— contract visiting times and length
			— arrange communication modality if desired:
			  • phone
			  • letter and note writing materials
			— suggest contacts with neighbor and church groups—particularly those who could be counted on for support.

Personal recognition, esteem, respect	Potential for diminished amount of personal recognition, esteem, respect secondary to: • hospitalization • situational occurrence of potential stigma of hypertension • aged state	Experiences personal recognition, esteem, and respect as evidenced by: • verbalization of these needs	1. Assess the level and quality of communication (verbal and nonverbal) conveying recognition, respect 2. Work with staff to call Mrs. Bender by name with each contact. — maintain client-focused conversation in the environment at all times — listen when Mrs. Bender speaks, noting position, posture, and other nonverbal clues 3. Assist Mrs. Bender gently and firmly when assisting her to bathroom, out or into bed, on short walks 4. Respect need to be slow, need to repeat requests, anecdotes, etc. 5. Ask for clarification to assure mean-

Client Need	Nursing Diagnosis	Goals with Outcome Criteria	Nursing Strategies with Frequencies
			ings are conveyed during conversation 6. Support family members efforts to show respect and build esteem of client — encourage family members to share these feelings with Mrs. Bender 7. Introduce new or different staff members involved in care 8. Explain all procedures thoroughly giving Mrs. Bender enough time to adjust and prepare herself for these 9. Explore further any communication from Mrs. Bender that indicates self-worth feelings. "I'm too old. . ." "I'm not good to anyone." "I'm always in and out for the same sickness."
Appreciation, attention	Potential for diminished amount of appreciation, attention secondary to: • hospitalization • situational occurrence of potential stigma of hypertension • aged state	Experience of appreciation, wholesome attention from onset of hospitalization as evidenced by: • verbalization of these needs	1. Assess the amount and quality of attention received from staff, family, and friends — spend 10 minutes 3 times a day with client 2. Encourage family members to express to Mrs. Bender their appreciation of her efforts to care for herself — encourage client to allow family members to contribute to her welfare by assisting in caring activities, i.e., mealtimes, brief walks — encourage Mrs. Bender to allow family members to look after her home for her while hospitalized — family members voice desire and willingness to do so — family members report what they have done for their mother 3. Convey progress made in recovery to Mrs. Bender and compliment her efforts to comply with nursing and medical strategies.
To love and be loved	Potential for diminished ability to be loved and to love related to: • hospitalization • situational occurrence of potential stigma of hypertension • aged state	Experiences love from significant others and conveys love to others as evidenced by: • many visitors, phone calls, and flowers • verbalization	1. Assess the relationship of family members and staff in conveying love to Mrs. Bender within 5–6 days 2. Assess Mrs. Bender's manner and ability of conveying love to family members and staff within 1 week 3. Point out observations of love shared by family members to client — encourage family members caressing, hand holding, kissing Mrs. Bender if this is their usual pattern — provide privacy for Mrs. Bender

Client Need	Nursing Diagnosis	Goals with Outcome Criteria	Nursing Strategies with Frequencies
			and family members while visiting 4. Encourage client to share anecdotes in which she gave or was the recipient of love by family and friends 5. Allow client an opportunity to express her love needs and strategies to meet these — plan prescribed 15 minute time with Mrs. Bender 3 times a day — use touch to convey caring and love for Mrs. Bender — provide assistance to Mrs. Bender for note writing, thank you notes to generous family and friends 6. Introduce Mrs. Bender to other clients her age when headaches subside and BP is down to facilitate mutual support system.

Figure 6-5. Nursing Care Plan.

Implementing

Implementing is the initiation and completion of actions necessary to accomplish the defined goal of optimal fulfillment of client needs. The implementation phase begins with the development of the nursing care plan. The persons to be involved in the implementation have been identified on the care plan. Participation in this phase requires nurses to have a high level of intellectual, interpersonal, and technical skill. Decision-making, observation, and communication skills are significant enhancements. These skills are used with the client, nursing team members, and health team members.

During this phase, the viability of the nursing care plan is tested. The nurse continues to collect data about the client, the condition, problems, reactions, and feelings. Additional information is gleaned from other health care personnel, family, neighbors, teachers, and medical or health records. The success or failure of the nurs-

ing care plan depends on the nurse's ability to judge the value of new data and her creative ability to make adaptations to account for the uniqueness of the client. For example, the nursing care plan for Mrs. Martha Bender has considerable data along with goal expectations and nursing strategies. New data will emerge as nursing strategies are used and Mrs. Bender responds physically, emotionally, psychologically, and socially to these actions as she proceeds toward the achievement of the goals.

It is strategic that the nurse distinguish and perform the independent nursing functions inherent in the planned actions and those that are interdependent—contributing to the fulfillment of the medical care plan designed by others in the health care team. The amount of time spent with the client may be short or long, but should be goal directed and purposeful.

The nurse may use a specific strategy or action to meet many needs simultaneously. For example, the nurse may plan a caring activity such as a bath, to meet the needs for skin integrity, belonging, and elimination. When the nurse performs a technical action, she continually uses decision-making skills to judge when modification is needed in procedural method, in timing of technical action, and in obtaining consultation and assistance from others to assure safe, effective action.

In each contact with the client, the nurse focuses on the goal of the interaction and continually expands her perceptive ability, gathering data about the client that would indicate the correctness of the planned action. She seeks data that indicate the correctness of the planned strategies or that indicate other problems due to unmet or poorly met human needs. If the nurse is working with other nursing or health team members, efforts should be exerted to maintain a client-centered focus. The client should benefit from the actions rather than be overwhelmed.

The implementation phase concludes with the completion and recording of the planned actions. This includes the results of the actions plus the reactions of the client. All data that give direct evidence of goal achievement should be recorded. This evidence designates the status of problem solving and provides information for the direction of continued problem solving. For example, behavioral data about Mrs. Bender should be recorded in relation to each obvious and potential nursing diagnosis and in relation to goal expectation. These data provide evidence for formalized evaluation, the final phase of the nursing process.

Evaluating

Evaluation, the fourth phase of the nursing process, is the appraisal of client changes as a result of nurse actions or of the client's behavioral changes as these relate to nurse actions. Evaluating, therefore, audits the behavior of the client, consistent with determined goals.

As the final component in the sequence of the nursing process, evaluation was, for many years, a neglected nursing activity. At first, major attention was given to assessment. There was a preoccupation with tool development to assist in data collection. Some tools were long, involved, and so complex that they were impractical. Other tools were so specific and limited to such a small population that they were impractical. Until nurses realized they were collecting information about the client that would contribute to a definition of his needs or problems, nurses were not goal directed in the development of assessment instruments. Gradually, the focus for assessment has been clarified and the data gathered about the client's needs, habits, behavior, strengths, and problems are analyzed in a systematic manner, so that a plan of care for the client can be developed and goals for health can be defined.

It is the plan of care and the goals for health that establish the foundation for evaluation. Based upon the identified problems and needs of the client, the nurse sets goals for care. Validation with the client about his needs or problems is critical. His involvement in goal setting is vital, too. Having specified what the thrust of care will be, the nursing strategies are implemented, and then the nurse asks: How effective were the strategies? What client changes resulted because of nurse actions?

Just as the preoccupation at one time was on tool development for assessment, at present it appears to be on the development of tools for evaluation. These form the **structure** of evaluation and are important; however, the priority in evaluation must be established. To spend all one's time developing a form for evaluation defeats the purpose of evaluation. Structure is important, and guidelines are essential, but these must be developed and decided on so that the nurse can get on with evaluation.

The **process** of evaluation is an important component, too. Whether evaluation is done via direct observation while care is being given, direct observation of the client after care is given, written reports, taped reports, interviews, or various other means, the rationale for determining a process of evaluation is to provide the best means possible for collecting data on which to evaluate client care. A combination of measures may be used to evaluate care. Incorporating the evaluation component within the care plan format is the most efficient way to accomplish evaluation and the most certain way to ensure its completion. In the care plan for Mrs. Bender, the components for evaluation are integral parts of the care plan (see column #5 of the care plan). For example, the nurse plans to provide comfort to Mrs. Bender and identifies when freedom from pain should be achieved; she also records the frequency with which the nurse elicits from Mrs. Bender a report of her comfort or discomfort in order to determine how the client is progressing toward the relief of pain.

When all facets of care have been examined to determine the quality of care rendered, the **outcome** of evaluation is determined, reported, and recorded. Quality of outcomes may vary depending on the **criteria** that were established at the outset of care. A qualitative assessment precisely defines the state of the client when care began. The nurse, in collaboration with the client, when possible, defines how the state of the client should change as a result of nursing care. She specifies what should be the length of time necessary to achieve the ultimate goal or final outcome; periodic time checks are built into the evaluation plan to determine the extent to which, and the rate at which, the planned care is leading to problem resolution. These definitions and specifications of expected client behaviors and physical characteristics are called **outcome criteria.**

In Mrs. Bender's situation, one goal is to relieve her headache within 48 hours; various nursing strategies are defined with the specified goal to relieve the headache entirely. Periodic checks with Mrs. Bender (every 3–4 hours) are made to determine the status of the headache. When the nurse has collected the data about the client and determined the nursing diagnoses and when she sets in place a plan of care to include goals, nursing strategies, and time frame for goal achievement, essential components are in place to manage client care in an efficient and qualitative manner. If it is determined, through evaluation, that goals are accomplished and client problems are resolved (if Mrs. Bender's headache is gone) the role of nursing has been accomplished and nursing care may no longer be necessary—the client may be able to manage her care independently. If it is determined through evaluation that some portion of the care plan needs revision, if more data are necessary, if additional problems have developed, or any other alteration has changed the previously stated goals, then the nurse reassesses, replans, and reevaluates as she proceeds with client care implementation. The cyclic nature of the nursing process and the continual overlapping of all components of the process become obvious when the nurse deliberately examines her actions in the light of client outcomes.

The care plan for Mrs. Bender suggests one way that all components of nursing activity on behalf of the client can be recorded. There are various methods by which client data can be noted for communicating with those persons whose activities are guided by such records. The exact format and specific components of the record can vary from one setting to another, providing the following data about the client are considered:

a. What are the needs?

b. What are the nursing diagnoses (problems, actual and potential)?

c. What are the goals to be achieved?

d. When should the goals be achieved?

e. What is the time interval for determining progress toward goal achievement?

f. What are the nursing strategies?

g. What are the outcomes of care (changes in the state of the client)?

Data about the client, the plan of care, and the rate of progress toward goal achievement are critical to any client situation. Communication between health team members as each works toward client care goals is essential. When there is effective, accurate, and complete communication among those responsible for health care, the care of the client is maximized.

SUMMARY

Within the past two decades, major progress has been made in the identification, development, and use of the nursing process. A number of nurse leaders have written about the science of nursing, and increasing numbers of nurses are using and applying these ideas in the practice of nursing. Guiding these efforts are accepted criteria for a profession, a code for professional nurses, selected definitions of nursing, as well as specification and research about theories and concepts that are viewed as foundations for nursing.

The core and essence of nursing is the nursing process. Although distinct from the leadership and research processes, nurses use both these processes to carry out the nursing process through the use of intellectual, interpersonal, and technical skills. Following the orderly systematic activity of the nursing process enables the nurse to assess client needs; diagnose client problems that are amenable to nursing intervention; and plan, implement, and evaluate the client's care. The deliberate use of this process is the best assurance that the client—individual, family, or community—will receive the nursing care that is needed to maintain wellness or to resolve problems at the appropriate time. The human need framework is a logical framework for the performance of the nursing process and the achievement of the goal of nursing—the maintenance or fulfillment of the human needs of the client.

STUDY QUESTIONS

1. Define nursing.

2. Define the nursing process.

3. Document each cited definition according to the author who proposed the definition.

4. Name and define the elements/phases/ steps of the nursing process.

5. Cite the sources for these labels and definitions.

6. Differentiate the nursing process from the nursing research process.

7. Differentiate the nursing process from the nursing leadership process.

8. Explain the recency of nursing process identification.

9. Cite at least three persons who have contributed to the development of the nursing process:
   —in the 1950s
   —in the 1960s
   —in the 1970s.

10. Specify a theory/concept (or a combination of theories/concepts) that is consistent with your values and beliefs and that you can or do use for providing client care.

11. Explain the way that such a theoretical/conceptual framework enables quality care performance.

12. Cite a specific client situation and illustrate the relationship of the theoretical/conceptual base to the care of that client.

13. Explain the use of assessment in a specific client situation.

14. Present the means by which this client care is planned.

15. Discuss the implementation of this client care.

16. Examine the way by which client care is evaluated.

17. Comment on the value or limitations of using the nursing process in this client situation.

REFERENCES

1. Helen Yura and Mary B. Walsh: **The Nursing Process: Assessing, Planning, Implementing, Evaluating,** 4th Ed., (E. Norwalk, CT: Appleton-Century-Crofts, 1983) p.1.
2. Hildegard Peplau: **Interpersonal Relations in Nursing,** (New York: Putnam, 1952).
3. Lydia E. Hall: "Quality of Nursing Care" **Address at Meeting of Department of Bac-** calaureate and Higher Degree Programs, New Jersey League for Nursing, February 7, 1955, Seton Hall University, Newark, N.J., Public Health News, June 1955.
4. D.E. Johnson: "Philosophy of Nursing" **Nursing Outlook,** 1959, Vol. 7, pp.198–200.
5. Ida J. Orlando: **The Dynamic Nurse—Patient Relationship** (New York: Putnam, 1961).
6. Ernestine Wiedenbach: **Clinical Nursing: A Helping Art** (New York: Springer, 1964).
7. A. Flexner: **Universities** (New York, Oxford University Press, 1930).
8. E. H. Schein: **Professional Education: Some New Directions,** Carnegie Commission on Higher Education (New York: McGraw-Hill, 1972).
9. G.W. Stuart: "How Professional is Nursing?" **Image,** 13 (1981) pp.18–33.
10. American Nurses' Association. "Code for Nurses" **The American Nurse,** 8 (1976) pp. 8,5.
11. M. Olivia Gowan: Administration of College and University Programs in Nursing, from the Viewpoint of Nurse Education. **Report of the Proceedings of the Workshop on Administration of College Programs in Nursing** (Washington, D.C.: The Catholic University of America Press, 1944).
12. Virginia Henderson: **The Nature of Nursing** (New York: Macmillan, 1966) p.15.
13. F. Suppe: "Implications in Recent Developments in Philosophy of Science for Nursing Theory." In **Fifth Biennial Eastern Conference on Nursing Research** (Baltimore, MD: University of Maryland, 1982).
14. Faye Abdellah and E. Levine: **Better Patient Care Through Nursing Research,** 2nd Ed., (New York, Macmillan, 1979).
15. D.E. Johnson: "The Behavioral System Model for Nursing" in J.P. Riehl & C. Roy (Eds.) **Conceptual Models for Nursing Practice** (2nd Ed) (New York: Appleton-Century-Crofts, 1980) pp.207–216.
16. M.E. Levine: "The Four Conservation Principles of Nursing" **Nursing Forum 6** (1967) pp.45–59.
17. Orlando, **Nurse-Patient Relationship,** p.36.
18. Joyce Travelbee: **Interpersonal Aspects of Nursing** (Philadelphia: Davis Co. 1966).
19. Wiedenbach, **Clinical Nursing** p.23.
20. Imogene King: **Toward a Theory for Nursing** (New York: Wiley, 1971).
21. B.M. Neuman and R.J. Young: "A Model for Teaching Total Person Approach to Patient Problems" **Nursing Research,21** (1972).
22. Dorothea E. Orem: **Nursing: Concepts of Practice** (New York: McGraw-Hill, 1971).

23. Martha E. Rogers: **Nursing Science: Introduction to the Theoretical Basis of Nursing** (Philadelphia, Davis, 1970).
24. Sister Callista Roy: **Introduction to Nursing: An Adaptation Model** (Englewood Cliffs, NJ: Prentice-Hall, 1976).
25. J.G. Paterson and L.T. Zderad: **Humanistic Nursing** (New York: Wiley, 1976).
26. K.M. Gebbie and M.A. Lavin: **Classification of Nursing Diagnoses** (St. Louis, Mosby, 1975).
27. M. Gordon: "Nursing Diagnosis and the Diagnostic Process" **American Journal of Nursing, 76** (1976) pp.1298–1300.
28. P.B. Kritek: "The Generation and Classification of Nursing Diagnoses: Toward a Theory of Nursing" **Image, 10** (1978) pp.33–40.
29. Ashley Montagu: **The Direction of Human Development** (New York: Hawthorn, 1970).
30. Abraham Maslow: **Motivation and Personality** (New York: Harper & Row, 1970) p.29.
31. Ibid., pp.26, 28.
32. Ibid., p.29.
33. Ibid., pp.36–38.
34. Ashley Montagu: **On Being Human** (New York: Hawthorn, 1966) p.49.
35. Maslow, **Motivation** pp.97–100.
36. A. Combs, A.C. Richards, and F. Richards: **Perceptual Psychology: A Humanistic Approach to the Study of Persons** (New York: Harper & Row, 1976) p.57.
37. Ibid., p.80.
38. Ibid., p.68.
39. Ibid., p.86.
40. Ibid., p.128.
41. Ibid., p.104.
42. Ibid., p.67.
43. Ibid., p.52.
44. M. Vernon: **Perception Through Experience** (London, Methuen, 1970) p.3.
45. Ibid., pp.4–5.
46. Ibid, p.59.
47. Ibid., p.99.

ANNOTATED BIBLIOGRAPHY

Bower FL: **The Process of Planning Nursing Care: A Model for Nursing Practice** (2nd ed.). St. Louis, The C.V. Mosby Co., 1977. This brief book fully describes the importance of a nursing care plan to organize and direct nursing care.

Inzer F: **Evaluation Patient Actions.** Nurs Outlook 29: 178–179; 1981. This article discusses methods of measuring outcomes of nursing in terms of client behaviors.

Kim M, Moritz DA: **Classification of Nursing Diagnoses.** New York, McGraw-Hill Book Co., 1982. This book presents material presented and developed at the third and fourth National Conferences on the classification of nursing diagnoses in 1976 and 1980. In addition, a development of nursing diagnosis is presented.

Malasanos L, Barkavskos V, Moss M, Stoltenberg-Allen K: **Health Assessment** (2nd ed.). St. Louis, The C.V. Mosby Co., 1981. This excellent and comprehensive text fully explains techniques, from history-taking through integration of assessment. Special areas focus on pregnant clients, assessment of children, and the aging client.

Price MR: **Nursing Diagnosis: Making a Concept Come Alive.** AM J Nurs 80:4:668–671; April 1980. This important article discusses what a nursing diagnosis is, how to develop one, and how to use it.

Rothberg JJ: **Why Nursing Diagnosis.** AM J Nurs 67:5:1040–1042; May 1967. Within this classic article, the author maintains that nursing diagnosis is essential for nursing practice.

Yura H, Walsh MB: **The Nursing Process** (4th ed.). Norwalk, Appleton-Century-Crofts, 1983. This book delineates the steps in the nursing process and uses case studies to demonstrate its usefulness. It also discusses the need for a theoretical framework for nursing practice.

7

Health Assessment

M. Gaie Rubenfeld

Elizabeth A. McFarlane

CHAPTER OUTLINE

OBJECTIVES

At the completion of this chapter the reader will be able to:

- Describe a nursing framework that may be used to guide health assessment.

- Contrast the roles of the nurse, the client, and other health care providers in assessing health.

- Describe the data collection techniques of interviewing, observation, and measurement.

- Use data collection techniques to assess the client's responses within the physiological, psychological, sociocultural, and spiritual dimensions.

- Consider the impact of the client's developmental level on his responses to actual or potential health problems.

GLOSSARY

Aeration—a vital life function of oxygen and carbon dioxide exchange.

Assessment—the collection and analysis of patient data or information leading to the derivation of nursing diagnosis.

Body Maintenance—the restoration and regulation of a balance of functions achieved by the body itself and by the individual person on behalf of his body.

Circulation—the transport of nutrients, oxygen, chemicals, and hormones and the removal of waste products and carbon dioxide from all body tissues.

Cognitive Ability—a composite of a person's capacity to learn, to retain what is learned (memory), and to understand.

Elimination—the output of waste products and indigestible materials from the body.

Emotional Status—mirrored through the overt and covert feelings a person experiences and expresses in his verbal and nonverbal communication.

Health Care Practices—those activities engaged in primarily for the purpose of attaining or maintaining health.

Interviewing—a technique of data collection; a formal or informal process for the purpose of obtaining verbal information about the client's current or past responses to actual or potential health problems.

Life Style—the usual living circumstances and activities in which a person engages.

Measurement—a technique of data collection; the use of a standard to determine capacity, or extent of structures or functions.

Nursing—"the diagnosis and treatment of human responses to actual or potential health problems."*

Nutrition—the intake, assimilation, and use of food for energy, maintenance, and growth of the body.

Observation—a technique of data collection; an identification of the client's physical and behavioral responses by looking or reviewing.

Physiological Dimension—reflected in a person's biological response to alterations in the body's structure and functions.

Psychological Dimension—reflected in a person's cognitive and emotional responses to himself and his environment.

Rest and Activity—the periods that comprise a pattern of movement or exertion and those of repose or rejuvination of the body.

Sensation—the primary means by which a person receives input from his environment.

Sexuality—the characteristic responses of maleness or femaleness of individuals.

Sociocultural Dimension—reflected in a person's noninherited intrapersonal and interpersonal responses to socialization practices learned and transmitted from families and communities.

Spiritual Dimension—reflected in a per-

GLOSSARY Continued

son's personal response to inspirational forces.

Support Networks—family members and significant persons who pro-

vide emotional, physical, or financial support to a person.

*American Nurses' Association. *Nursing A Social Policy Statement.* Kansas City, American Nurses' Association, 1980.

INTRODUCTION

The term health assessment has different meanings to different people. To some, health assessment means an examination of the body's biological systems, to others it may imply health screening for the purpose of detecting a physical impairment, such as hypertension. To the nurse, the term health assessment is more comprehensive—a systematic and continuous collection of data related to a person's health state and his response to that health state.

This chapter presents health assessment from a nursing perspective and provides a framework to guide the collection of data. The focus of the nurse when doing a health assessment is contrasted with the focus of other health care professionals. Ability to apply a framework that ensures a nursing focus and knowledge of the techniques of assessment are skills that are fundamental to a comprehensive health assessment done by a nurse.

HEALTH ASSESSMENT: A NURSING PERSPECTIVE

A Framework for Health Assessment

The nursing process provides the nurse direction in the provision of nursing care that will assist a client in attaining, regaining, or maintaining his optimal health status. Assessment, the first phase of the nursing process, encompasses the collection and analysis of patient data or information

leading to the derivation of nursing diagnoses. The assessment phase can be described as the power or energy source of the process. If the collection of data does not contribute to the identification of actual or potential problems that are amenable to nursing intervention, the planning, implementation, and evaluation phases of the process cannot be operationalized.

The nurse must be concerned with collecting and analyzing client data that will assist in maintaining a nursing focus in the planning and implementation of client care. A nursing focus evolves from awareness and understanding of the purpose of nursing. This purpose is clearly described in the American Nurses' Association's publication *Nursing: A Social Policy Statement*, where nursing is defined as "the diagnosis and treatment of human responses to actual or potential health problems."[1] This definition directs the nurse to collect information about the client that will assist in identifying his response to actual or potential health problems. A comprehensive health assessment provides data that, upon analysis, reflect response patterns related to the client's ability to perform activities contributing to the fulfillment of his needs. Patterns of response that indicate that the client is unable to take independent actions to fulfill his physiological, psychological, sociocultural, and spiritual needs signal a need for nursing care.

The complex nature of the human being and the intricate relationship among his needs and how he seeks to fulfill them lends complexity to the process of health assessment. When analyzing, examining, or assessing a complex phenomenon, such as a human being, an attempt is made to identify, isolate, and study the parts of the whole. Yet understanding of the whole, how and why it responds as it does, is dependent on the integration of the parts.

The nature of the human, the integration of his physiological, psychological, sociocultural, and spiritual dimensions, implies that his responses to a health problem cannot be restricted to one dimension. Thus, when the nurse gathers data to determine a client's responses to real or potential health problems, she cannot limit her assessment to one dimension. Because growth or disruption in one dimension has consequences for the others, she must expand her focus to include all dimensions. The focus of health assessment is presented in Figure 7-1. The wholeness of the human is represented by the circle. The segmented lines separating each dimension within the circle suggest that the dimensions are not separate entities, but rather integrated facets of the human.

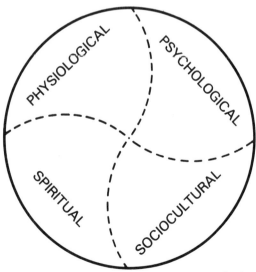

Figure 7-1. The Dimensions of the Human Person

While acknowledging the wholeness and integration of the person, the dimensions provide the means for the nurse to approach the health assessment of the client in an organized manner. She collects data or information relative to each dimension to determine patterns. Each dimension of the person is reflected in his responses. The nurse assesses these through interviews, observation, and measurement. During the health assessment, the nurse evaluates the client's responses in terms of the impact the health problem has had on them. It is, therefore, important for the nurse to determine if an actual or potential health problem has changed the manner in which the client usually responds.

Health assessment by the nurse, then, should include the collection of data related to physiological, psychological, sociocultural, and spiritual responses of the client to a health problem. Analysis of these data will lead to identification of response patterns. If the patterns indicate that the client cannot independently perform activities contributing to the fulfillment of his needs, a nursing diagnosis is made, and the planning phase of the nursing process begins.

The four dimensions of human beings are described as follows:

1. **Physiological**—reflected in a person's biological response to alterations in the body's structure and functions.

2. **Psychological**—reflected in a person's cognitive and emotional responses to himself and his environment.

3. **Sociocultural**—reflected in a person's noninherited intra- and interpersonal responses to socialization practices learned and transmitted from families and communities.

4. **Spiritual**—reflected in a person's personal response to inspirational forces.

The Nurse and Other Health Care Providers

The focus on the physiological, psychological, sociocultural, and spiritual responses of the client to actual or potential health problems distinguishes the health assessment done by the nurse from assessments done by other members of the health team. While the data collected by the various members of the health team may overlap, each member assesses the client with a different purpose in mind. This purpose defines and gives direction to the assessments done by other health care providers, such as physicians, nutritionists, dentists, social workers, and psychologists.

Physicians assess health to determine whether or not a pathology exists and how a client is progressing in his recovery from that pathology. The focus is primarily on the physiological health of the patient. Depending on the area of specialization, a physician may be more concerned with one part of a client's body than with another. Nutritionists are concerned with a person's health as it relates to his dietary patterns. Dentists assess a person's health as it relates to the mouth and teeth. Nutritionists and dentists focus on physiological health. Psychologists are concerned with a person's mental status and emotional development, and therefore focus on psychological health.

Using a person with diabetes as an example, the differences in purpose or focus of the various members of the health team become more apparent. A physician diagnoses the pathology, diabetes, by assessing the client's physical health, including blood glucose levels. A nutritionist would assess the client's dietary intake to determine what changes need to be made to decrease the glucose levels. A dentist assesses the person's mouth and teeth to determine the presence of infections or potential infections, knowing that in a diabetic person infections occur frequently and are detrimental to the person's health. A psychologist might assess the person's emotional state as he attempts to cope with the chronic illness. The social worker would assess, among other things, the person's financial ability to afford the prescribed treatments, and uses that information to assist the client, if necessary, to secure financial assistance.

The nurse is interested in the person's total response to the health problem of diabetes. She assesses the client's physical responses: an indication of a loss or gain in weight; condition of skin, especially at insulin injection sites; condition of feet; and changes in vision. She assesses the client's psychological responses, such as his emotional responses to having diabetes or the amount of psychological stress he experiences (emotional stress can cause an increase in the body's glucose level). She assesses the client's sociocultural responses: the presence or absence of an effective support system, and how the support system influences the client's response to treatment; adherence to social and ethnic dietary patterns that might be inconsistent with a diabetic diet; or language differences that might create misunderstandings about the prescribed treatment. She assesses the client's spiritual responses, the meaning he attaches to his illness, or religious practices that impinge on receiving health care. Each of these dimensions—physiological, psychological, sociocultural, and spiritual—are reflected in the client's responses to his health problem, diabetes.

HUMAN RESOURCES FOR HEALTH ASSESSMENT

The outcome of the health assessment, its comprehensive nature and quality, is dependent on multiple factors. The level to which the nurse has developed her intellectual, interpersonal, and technical skills affect the breadth and depth of the assessment, and therefore the validity of her nursing diagnoses. Sources available for data collection determine the quality of the information found. If the client is conscious and responsive, assessment of his physiological dimension is less complex in terms of searching for information related to his health history and usual physiological responses. Availability of family members or other significant persons as sources of information becomes crucial when the client himself cannot provide the needed data. Other health care providers and their assessments can provide additional perspectives from which the nurse can supplement or verify information she has gathered.

The Nurse

The nurse's expertise in doing health assessments is primarily dependent upon the level of her intellectual, interpersonal, and technical expertise. Her knowledge and understanding of what constitutes adaptive and maladaptive responses to health problems is essential to her decisionmaking regarding the need for further exploration of the dimensions. The ability and ease with which the nurse can establish supportive relationships with clients, family members, and other health care providers influences the quality and validity of the data collected, as well as the opportunities available for collection and verification of data. The nurse's knowledge of and ability to apply the technical skills used in health assessment determines the nature of the data she collects. Effective use of the techniques of observation, interview, and measurement in client assessment is required if the assessment is to be more than the gathering of overt signs and symptoms. The sophistication of the nurse's intellec-

tual, interpersonal, and technical skills determine her ability to effectively use data collection techniques.

The Client

The client's developmental level, physical condition, and intellectual and emotional status determine the information he can provide during the interview and his ability to validate the nurse's findings. If able and willing, the client assumes an active role throughout the health assessment. He provides information during the interview and cooperates when the nurse uses observation and measurement techniques in assessing quantitative responses. The client will be more willing to assume this role if the nurse is able to assure physical and emotional comfort during the assessment. If the client is unable to provide information and validate findings, the family and other significant persons become primary sources of information about the client's health history and the impact the health problem has had on his usual manner of responding to his needs.

Other Health Care Providers

While the health assessment is viewed as a complex process for the nurse, the client can experience complexity in terms of the number of health care professionals who interview him, examine him, and continually observe him. Each health care institution adopts specific forms that must be completed for each client and retained in the client's record. Much of this information overlaps, and the patient feels he is repetitiously interviewed and examined.

The nurse may use the data gathered by other health care providers if it can be validated. This will eliminate some discomfort the patient experiences due to repetitious assessments. Members of the health care team should seek to identify ways to contribute data that supports the focus of other health care professionals. The physical assessment done by the physician, the dietary assessment done by the nutritionist, and the emotional assessment done by the psychologist provide data and findings that can be essential to the nurse's assessment of the client's responses to health problems. Likewise, the nurse can provide information and findings supportive of health assessments done by other health care professionals.

The level to which the nurse has developed her intellectual, interpersonal, and technical skills, the availability of data from the client and family, and the ability to use other health care professionals as resources determine the breadth and depth of the assessment process and influence the validity of findings. Therefore, the nurse must maintain and improve nursing skills, and use all the resources that contribute to a comprehensive health assessment.

TECHNIQUES OF DATA COLLECTION

The nurse uses three broad categories of techniques when collecting data pertinent to assessing the client's responses to health problems. **Interviewing, observation,** and **measurement** provide the means to gather information related to the client's physiological, psychological, sociocultural, and spiritual dimensions. While it is essential to use the three techniques throughout assessment, the types of responses reflected in each dimension determine the extent to which the nurse can use each technique. Physiological responses can best be assessed through measurement complemented by interviews and observation. Information related to the client's psychological, sociocultural, and spiritual dimensions is collected primarily through interview and observation, and may be supplemented by measurement.

Interviewing

Through interviewing, the nurse collects data relevant to the client's general health history, as well as his perceptions of his present health status. A thorough knowledge of therapeutic communication techniques is necessary to be an effective interviewer. The nurse must maintain an open approach to the client so that the client will feel free to respond fully to the questions asked. While a set of guidelines to organize questions is helpful, the nurse must take cues from the client and ask additional questions in areas where gaps appear to exist. The most helpful guidelines, therefore, give broad cues for questions. If the client's response to those broad questions indicates a problem area, then the nurse must branch into more specific inquiries and allow the client to relate necessary details. For example, if the client says yes, he has discomfort, the nurse must ask where it is, how long it has existed, the nature of the discomfort, and what the client has been doing to alleviate it.

Information acquired during an interview can provide the nurse adequate data by which a client's responses to an actual or potential health care problem can be identified or it may provide only clues. In either case, the nurse supplements the interview with other assessment techniques. Observation and measurement could be employed to assist in verifying her findings or to gather additional data to follow up on clues the nurse received during the interview.

The interview can be either formal or informal. When the client enters the health care system, a formal or structured interview is called for, in which the nurse gathers information that could be essential in determining the client's medical and nursing care. A person's allergies to foods or medicines and his usual diet, including sociocultural preferences and religious restrictions, are examples of factors that must be known when planning care. Therefore, factors such as these should be identified early in the client's encounter with the health care system.

Interviews of a less formal nature are appropriate and necessary for the ongoing, comprehensive assessment that is required throughout the nurse/client relationship. It often takes time for the client to feel comfortable enough to reveal information of a personal nature. Here is an example of a situation in which a less structured interview might occur: A nurse is instructing a client on his diet when the client changes the subject and expresses fear about an anticipated diagnostic test. The nurse can use this cue to make further inquiries about the client's feelings toward the health problem and the required tests and therapy.

Another example is the nurse's use of the time when giving a bath to ask the client questions about his skin. Because the skin is observable during that time, questions can be more specific to what is being seen. The client may have a scar on his back to which the nurse can refer; in a more formal situation where the client is dressed, he may forget that he had had surgery there for the removal of a mole. That piece of information may be an important determinant of the nurse further assessing other moles on the client's body.

These examples also illustrate the importance of questioning the client on his past health. Historical questions allow the nurse to see patterns of responses, to identify risk factors due to cumulative conditions, and to understand the client's previous coping mechanisms that may be of value or detrimental to his present condition.

Likewise, questions about the client's family health history will give the nurse clues about possible risk factors for illness in the client. If the nurse knows that a client's parents both died at a young age from heart disease, she will know that the client's circulatory status should be given extra consideration during the assessment.

Observation

Observation is the second data collection technique. Primarily, this means the nurse must be alert, seeing the subtle as well as the obvious aspects of the client's behavior. The nurse must observe the client's nonverbal communication while listening to verbal comments. This is especially important in collecting data on the client's psychological dimensions, which may be difficult for the client to describe in words. Likewise, observing a client's interaction with his family may provide more information than questioning the client about his significant relationships. With observation, however, the nurse must guard against jumping to conclusions. Whenever possible, validate nonverbal behaviors with additional questioning.

Accurate observation is often dependent on the setting of the nurse/client encounter. A darkened room may help the nurse assess pupillary reactions, but it will be a disadvantage when looking at a skin lesion. A chilly room may make a client clench his teeth and hands, which may be wrongly interpreted by the nurse as a symbol of anger or withdrawal.

There are many tools that aid the nurse in observation. Most essential are her own senses of sight and hearing. These senses alone may be used when observing physiological responses, such as rate, rhythm, and depth of respirations, and are essential when observing the client's psychological, sociocultural, and spiritual responses.

Instruments may be used to enhance observations. A flashlight will illuminate a specific area; a tongue depressor may hold the tongue down so that the throat can be seen; a nasal speculum will allow the visualization of the posterior parts of the nose. Likewise, the nurse/client positions will contribute to optimal observations. A nurse must move around to get into the optimal position for observation. Shining a light onto a client's bed at night from a position in the doorway does not put the nurse in a position for accurate observation of the client's respiration.

Above all, the nurse must not be afraid to spend time just looking at something. At times, scheduling pressures and demands made by peers or other clients may tempt the nurse to only glance at some aspect of the client that should be studied carefully. Such actions may have grave consequences. Important signs may be overlooked. However, as with other assessment techniques, practice yields precision of observations in less time.

Measurement

Measurement, the third data collection technique, is the most objective and often the most precise method of assessment. Measurement implies that some kind of standard is used to determine the dimensions, capacity, or extent of something. The standards that are used are as varied and complex as the human body that is being measured. Some structures and functions of the body may be precisely measured quite easily; others can only be measured against a general, nonspecific standard. Therefore, standards may be seen as a continuum of precision, one end having exact measurements and the other, less differentiated gauges.

Measurement has two components—one is the standard of the measuring device or instrument used, the other is the significance of those measurements against a standard of the body's expected range of responses. Each of these components has a continuum of precision. An instrument such as a ruler, tape measure, sphygmomanometer, caliper, or thermometer gives numeric readings that may be compared to precise numeric ranges of normal. Other instruments are indirect measuring devices that allow the examiner to touch, feel, or hear things that then are compared to less distinct ranges of normal. These instruments do not give the examiner a nominal value, as such, and some judgment is required to make the measurements. Such an instrument may be a percussion hammer that, when struck against a tendon, may elicit a reflex that then is judged to be absent, weak, strong, or hyperreflexive. Another example is a stethoscope that can be used to auscultate respiratory sounds that then are compared to a range of normal sounds known by the examiner.

When assessing the client's physiological responses, parts of the examiner's body become the indirect instrument of measurement. Palpation of a client's body allows the examiner to feel with her hands specific organs, muscles, or bones that are not directly measurable with recording devices, such as a tape measure. The amount of mass felt by the hands or fingers is calculated through the examiner's knowledge of sizes within a normal range.

Some precise measuring devices normally are not used as often by nurses as they are by physicians and other health care professionals. Examples are x-rays or measurements that require invasive techniques, such as surgery, or the extraction of blood or body fluids. While nurses usually do not initiate such measurements, they do, however, have access to reports of these measurements, and should use them whenever they would aid in making nursing diagnoses.

Measurements that guide the nurse in assessing physiological responses are more abundant and precise than those available to her when measuring psychological, sociocultural, and spiritual responses. While a variety of inventories, scales, and tests have been developed to measure a client's intelligence, emotional status, and socioeconomic status, these usually are ordered, administered, and interpreted by a psychiatrist or psychologist. The findings from these measurements can provide data that support or dispute information the nurse has obtained by interview and observation. Likewise, the nurse's assessment of responses can assist other health care professionals in the interpretation of these measures.

DIMENSIONS OF HEALTH ASSESSMENT: DATA COLLECTION

The nurse must use a framework to organize and guide her approach to data collection. Using the dimensions of the human being as a framework, the nurse is assisted in maintaining a nursing focus as she seeks to diagnose and treat the client's responses to actual or potential health problems. While the holistic nature of the human person is recognized, each dimension and its specific parameters for assessment are addressed separately in this section. This is done in an attempt to provide the student with an assessment guide that will contribute to the systematic and comprehensive collection of data. Although the nurse is directed to assess parameters of a particular dimension, she is reminded that the dimensions are interrelated, and responses reflective of one dimension may have an impact on other dimensions.

Guidelines for data collection within each dimension and parameters for assessment of data are presented on the following pages. For each parameter, a set of cues for interview, observation, and measurement are given in table format. Within each dimension, the cues are guidelines for first-level data collection; many additional areas could be assessed, some needing more complicated procedures than appropriate for this chapter. Numerous texts on assessment could aid the reader in developing additional skills in other data collection techniques. These guidelines will en-

able the beginning-level nurse to gain an overall picture of the client's responses to an actual or potential health care problem. If abnormal or maladaptive responses are found, the nurse would assess further or refer the client to another health care provider for additional data collection.

The nurse must form questions based on the cues given in the interview guideline tables. The wording used to formulate the questions will depend on the vocabularies of the nurse and the client. Observation cues include non-valued items that should be noted and some that indicate abnormal responses or changes that should be ruled out. The measurement cues include two parts. The first part of the cue is the item to be measured. The second part (in parentheses) is the tool or method commonly used for that measurement.

Physiological Dimension

The physiological dimension is reflected in a person's biological response to alterations in the body's structure and function. To collect data on the physiological responses of a client, the nurse first must decide what parts of the body are of highest priority in a given situation. Because of the complexity of the physiological dimension, some method of dividing the body into units is necessary. The body's physiological systems—heart, lungs, muscles, and so forth—interrelate; an action of one system affects others. The client's physiological response to his health state is dependent upon the structure and functions of these interrelated body parts. In looking for the responses, the nurse must be aware of the interrelationships.

The following parameters will provide a structure for the nurse's assessment of the physiological dimension: sensation, aeration, circulation, nutrition, elimination, rest and activity, sexuality, and body maintenance. The various anatomical and physiological functions of the body are grouped thus so that all aspects of the body can be assessed. A thorough knowledge of anatomy and physiology is a necessary prerequisite for the nurse who is assessing physiological responses. That knowledge tells the examiner what to look for, what is normal, what is abnormal, and how to describe what is found.

Sensation. Sensation, or the use of the senses, is the primary means by which a person receives input from his environment. The skin, eyes, ears, nose, mouth, and their related nerves allow a person to experience physical sensations to which he can respond. The skin receives signals about temperature, humidity, touch, pressure, and pain. It also acts as a safety barrier for the rest of the body. Eyes receive visual stimuli, ears receive sound, the nose receives odors, and the mouth distinguishes tastes.

The nervous system and especially the cranial nerves act as a transmitter of these sensations to the brain, which interprets the various signals. A special aspect of sensation is the body's recognition of pain or discomfort. While this may or may not be directly related to one specific body part, it is included as an important component of the sensation parameter. It is through the sensation of pain or discomfort that alterations in the body's physiological responses are often diagnosed. The individual's level of consciousness and responsiveness is also an important part of sensation.

Collecting information on this parameter is a logical beginning step for the nurse to take in a first-encounter assessment of a client. Determining the level of consciousness, orientation, and the status of the various senses will help the nurse adapt future data collection techniques to that client's responsive abilities. The client's answers to interview questions will predict his ability to accurately answer questions about other parameters. These

answers, along with the observed and measured responses, tell the nurse the client's level of hearing, sight, smell, taste, and touch, and whether or not he is comfortable enough to tolerate subsequent data collection.

Several instruments may aid the observation of certain body parts in this pattern. An ophthalmoscope may be used to see internal eye structures. This instrument is also adapted for use as an otoscope, which allows the examiner to look into the ear canal; it also can be used as a lighted speculum to look into the nose. A full explanation of the use of these instruments is beyond the scope of this text, but a nurse can learn the mechanics of them, and with practice will find these are valuable aids to observation of the eyes, nose, and ears.

Instruments of measurement are less complicated and may be readily usable. A simple ruler, preferably in millimeters and centimeters, allows for measurement and accurate description of skin lesions, if any are observed. A Snellen chart is a commercially available wall poster commonly used to measure visual acuity. The client reads sets of letters at a distance of 20 feet from the chart, which rates levels of vision numerically. Hearing can be measured simply by holding a ticking watch next to each ear, or by the examiner whispering a phrase behind the client's back to test if he can hear. These are imprecise measurements, but are valuable indicators of gross hearing problems. A tuning fork is another simple instrument that, when activated and held against a bone in the skull, can test bone-conducted hearing. It also can be held next to the ear to measure air-conducted hearing.

Smell may be measured by holding a series of distinctively odorous items under each nostril. The client with his eyes closed is asked to identify each odor. Taste is similarly measured by swabbing parts of the tongue with substances that are salty, (table salt), sweet, (sugar), sour, (lemon), or bitter (aspirin).

Table 1.

Guidelines for Assessment of Sensation

Interview: Questions and Areas to Discuss

1. Level of Consciousness—Who is he? Where is he? What day and time is it?

2. Pain or Discomfort—If so, where? When did it begin? When does it occur? Description of intensity, characteristics, treatments tried, and results.

3. Skin—Sensitivity changes, lesions, texture, color, dryness, or moisture.

4. Vision—Corrective lenses; changes such as blurring, double vision, halos around lights, spots; changes in lacrimation.

5. Hearing—Loss; ringing in ears.

6. Smell—Changes in ability, nasal discharge, obstructions, bleeding.

7. Taste—Changes in sensation; unusual odors or tastes.

Observation:

1. Level of Consciousness—Awake, alert, oriented to surroundings.

2. Signs of Pain or Discomfort—Facial expression, body movement.

3. Skin—Color, vascularity, lesions, signs of scratching or rubbing.

4. Vision—Squinting, excessive blinking, tearing, eye movement (lateral, vertical, and oblique), symmetry of eyes. External eye structures: conjunctiva moist, nonirritated; lid closure full or partial; cornea moist and smooth. Internal structures: lens and vitreous clear, retinal structures intact, optic disc defined.

5. Hearing—Hears normal voice tones; leans forward, asking for repetition of words; hearing aid. Outer ear structures: intactness, canal openness (no excessive wax or hair). Inner structures—tympanic membrane intact, canal clear.

6. Smell—Outer nasal structures: nose straight or deviated, nares flare, discharge. Inner

structures: mucosa color, swelling; septum condition; obstructions.

7. Taste—Mouth lesions, breath odor, tongue condition.

Measurement:

1. Skin lesions—Size and character (ruler)

2. Visual Acuity—(Snellen Chart)

3. Hearing Acuity—(Watch tick, whisper, tuning fork)

4. Smell—(Odorous substances)

5. Taste—(Application of salt, sugar, lemon, aspirin on parts of tongue.)

Aeration. Aeration is a vital life function of oxygen and carbon dioxide exchange. The mouth, pharynx, nose, and lungs are the primary structures of this parameter. The mouth, pharynx, and nose allow air to pass to and from the lungs, which provide oxygen to the circulatory system and remove carbon dioxide.

Assessment of aeration is a very important function of the nurse. Persons who are immobilized, such as those hospitalized, have a high risk for respiratory dysfunction. Many environmental factors are hazards to respirations, and upper respiratory infections or allergies are very common. Counting respirations per minute always has been part of the assessment trio of "vital signs," that is, the T.P.R. (temperature, pulse, and respiration). While the respiratory rate is vital, there are other equally important pieces of data for the nurse to collect.

Many clues to aeration responses can be gained through the simple observations and questions listed in Table 2. The measurement techniques are easily learned and applied. Since the lungs are on both sides of the chest cavity, many of the measurements are comparative ones to determine symmetry of functions. **Thoracic expansion** is measured by the examiner's hands being placed posteriorly over the tenth rib area; as the chest expands, the hands should rise equally on both sides. The anterior-posterior diameter of the chest can be estimated visually and compared to the lateral span, or, if indicated, can be measured with a tape measure. **Vocal fremitus** (sound vibrations) is felt by the examiner whose hands are placed on the chest while the client vocalizes "99"; these vibrations are compared side to side for symmetry. **Percussion notes** are sounds heard and vibrations felt when the examiner taps over a part of the body. These notes vary in intensity, pitch, or duration depending on the amount of air in the underlying structures. In measuring these notes the examiner can determine where the air-filled lungs end, that is the diaphragm position during inspiration and expiration; these, therefore, determine the **diaphragmatic excursion.** These bilateral notes also are compared and thus measure symmetry of respiratory functions.

Auscultation, or the listening to breath sounds through a stethoscope, allows for further assessment of respiratory functions. By placing the stethoscope on the chest over lung areas, the sounds of air passing into and out of the lungs can be heard, compared for symmetry on both sides, and a qualitative measurement against known ranges of normal can be determined.

Table 2.

Guidelines for Assessment of Aeration

Interview:

1. Breathing capacity at rest and on exertion.
2. Allergies.
3. Air quality in environment.
4. Coughing—frequency, type, and productivity.
5. Frequency of upper respiratory infections (colds).
6. Smoking habits.

Observation:

1. Respirations—quality and regularity, breathing with mouth or nose.
2. Color—nail beds and lips.
3. Flaring of nostrils.
4. Condition of nasal mucosa, drainage, swelling.
5. Condition of mouth, pharynx, especially tonsillar area.
6. Chest movement—symmetry, use of accessory muscles.

Measurement:

1. Respiratory rate—(counted and timed with watch).
2. Thoracic expansion—(hand measurement during inspiration).
3. Anterior-posterior diameter—(visual estimation or tape measure).
4. Symmetry of vocal fremitus—(hands—estimate symmetry).
5. Symmetry of intensity, pitch, and duration of percussion notes—(fingers, indirect percussion).
6. Diaphragmatic excursion—(percussion, ruler).
7. Symmetry and quality of breath sounds—(auscultation with stethoscope).

Circulation. Circulation is the transport of nutrients, oxygen, chemicals, and hormones and the removal of waste products and carbon dioxide from all body tissues. The heart, blood vessels, and lymph vessels are the primary structures assessed in this parameter.

Because oxygen is a vital substance that is carried throughout the body, circulation responses are linked closely to aeration. If there is an abnormal response in aeration, it is imperative that the nurse collect data on the status of circulation and assess aeration if circulation is abnormal. The pulse and blood pressure are assessed by nurses in almost every client encounter. They are foremost in the measurement category of data collection in this parameter. The usual range of these measurements should be included also as components of questions put to the client. Questions about the condition of the legs, feet, arms, and hands are also important indicators of the circulatory status of the body.

Most of the observations of circulation are done in conjunction with measurement. Some pulsations in various parts of the body can be seen and should be observed, but also should be measured through palpation so that the examiner times and counts their rates. While palpating pulses, measurement of their rhythm and quality should be compared to known ranges of normal and compared for bilateral symmetry. There are many locations on the body where pulses may be felt easily. In most instances, when collecting baseline information on a client who has no actual or potential abnormalities in circulation, a radial pulse is palpated. However, if there is an indication for more precise pulse measurement, all or some of these pulses may be assessed; carotid, temporal, brachial, ulnar, femoral, popliteal, posterior tibial, and dorsalis pedis.

Venous function should be observed over all parts of the body also. Some veins are directly observable; some are not. Any venous area that can be visualized should be checked for discoloration or bulging that might indicate varicosities. The jugular veins are measured for their level of distention or amount of pressure by positioning the patient at certain angles and observing the change in the level of the characteristic pulse wave of the veins. To carry out this measurement, the nurse must study the difference between the carotid pulse and the pulse wave of the jugular vein, because the two can be confused easily.

Auscultation of the heart itself is a valuable data collection technique, allowing for assessment of the sounds and diastolic and systolic phases of the pumping heart. The apical pulse is the most accurate pulse reading, and whenever such precision is indicated, the nurse should listen at the apex of the heart and count the pulse rate there. The nurse should place the stethoscope over the aortic, pulmonic, right ventricular, and apical areas and listen with the bell and diaphragm of the stethoscope so that all ranges of sounds may be heard. With practice and study, the nurse can become more acute in assessing the heart sounds.

Palpation of lymph node areas to determine the size and consistency of these nodes is also an important measurement of circulatory status. Most lymph nodes are in the neck, axilla, and groin, and are not normally palpable. Therefore, if one is palpated, a measurement of its size and consistency is very important. Usually an approximation of size is adequate, but a ruler may be used for more accurate determination.

Finally, any area of the body that appears swollen should be measured. Sometimes, if swelling is unilateral, such as in the extremities, a comparative tape measurement of one side to the other can be made. If it is bilateral, then the pressure of a finger into the swollen area may allow the examiner to approximate "pitting," which usually is recorded on a progressive range of severity from 1 + to 4 + . See Table 3 for further assessment guidelines.

Table 3.
Guidelines for Assessment of Circulation

Interview:

1. Chest pain or discomfort.

2. Known alterations in heart beat.

3. Condition of extremities—temperature changes, vascularity, swelling, cramping.

4. Tolerance for activity.

5. Usual blood pressure measurements.

Observation:

1. Color of extremities, nail beds, and lips.

2. Pulsations over cardiac area, carotid artery area.

3. Quality of vein areas—bulging, surrounding coloration, varicosities.

4. Evidence of swelling, especially of the extremities.

Measurement:

1. Blood pressure—(sphygmomanometer and stethoscope).

2. Pulses—rate, rhythm, quality, symmetry—(fingers and watch).

3. Veins—level of jugular distention—(ruler).

4. Heart—auscultation of rates, rhythm, and quality of heart sounds—(stethoscope with bell and diaphragm).

5. Lymph nodes—(palpation with fingertips).

6. Swelling—(tape measure or finger pressure indentation).

Nutrition. Nutrition is the intake, assimilation, and use of food for energy, maintenance, and growth of the body. The involved body structures are the mouth, teeth, and the abdominal organs. The individual's eating and digestive patterns are critical processes in this parameter.

Assessing nutritional status involves a thorough collection of data regarding: eating patterns; the weight of the person compared to normal ranges for his age and height; and the condition of the body structures used for the intake, assimilation, and use of food. Obtaining a thorough picture of a person's eating patterns can be a long and involved process; one of the most accurate records of food intake can be obtained by having a person record the amount and type of food ingested for one week. This process may not be practical, however, so the nurse must find a more expeditious method of getting the data. One way to do

this is to ask the person to recall exactly what, when, and how much he eats in a typical day. The nurse should be aware of inconsistencies in food measurement among people. She should suggest standard measurements, such as a cupful, to help the client to identify his perceived amounts.

The instruments for measurement of nutritional patterns are used easily by the nurse. Most health care facilities have a scale with a height measurement apparatus attached. These two measurements should always be done simultaneously, since a weight without a corresponding height is not very meaningful. Do not assume that the client knows his correct weight or height. It is helpful to ask the client, before measurement, his perceptions of height and weight. With these data, the nurse gets some idea about the accuracy of the client's perception of his size. A measurement of skin-fold thickness through the use of **calipers** adds another piece of information to the assessment of body size. Although the triceps area is the usual site for such measurement, some persons have an unequal distribution of fat, so it is a good idea to take several readings on various parts of the body and average them.

Measurements of the abdomen are an important part of assessing the structural integrity of the organs involved in digestion. Listening for bowel sounds should be done before the examiner palpates the abdomen. Placing the stethoscope over all four quadrants of the abdomen allows the examiner to determine the degree of activity of the bowels. These are then scaled as inactive, hypoactive, normally active, or hyperactive. Before a conclusion of inactive is made, the examiner should listen at least five minutes. Normally, bowel sounds are heard every 5 to 20 seconds.

Other measurements of the abdomen involve techniques of percussion and palpation in all quadrants. Percussion permits the examiner to listen to variations in dullness and tympany. This allows a fairly accurate determination of borders of organs, such as the liver, the stomach, and the spleen. Borders, when found, can be marked on the abdomen and measured with a tape measure or ruler. Palpating the abdomen also gives the examiner an idea of the size of certain structures and allows for detection of any masses or fluid that normally are not present.

Table 4.

Guidelines for Assessment of Nutrition

Interview:

1. Usual weight, changes in weight.

2. Usual eating patterns, typical day's/week's diet.

3. Condition of teeth and mouth, dentures, and their effect on chewing and swallowing.

4. Food tolerance (abdominal disorders affected by eating).

Observation:

1. Body size and shape.

2. Condition of teeth and mouth.

3. Abdominal shape, symmetry.

Measurement:

1. Height and weight (scales).

2. Triceps skin-fold thickness (calipers).

3. Bowel sounds (stethoscope).

4. Position and size of abdominal organs and detection of any abnormal fluid or mass (percussion, palpation, examiner's hands, and tape measure).

Elimination. Elimination is the output of waste products and indigestable mate-

rials from the body. The renal and urinary structures, the rectum, anus, and sweat glands function as eliminative mechanisms. Maintenance of an overall fluid and electrolyte balance is the goal of elimination.

Because the broad goal of elimination is a balance of fluids and electrolytes in the body, the nurse always must compare the output and input of fluids (data from the nutrition parameter). In some situations, especially with some hospitalized clients, precise measurement of fluid output is indicated. These amounts are compared to the client's intake of fluid or fluid-containing substances. Except for perspiration and formed stool, most body fluid output can be measured precisely in any calibrated container.

In addition to measurements of the amount of fluid output, questioning the client about his elimination patterns will give the examiner baseline information on that person's usual responses. Observations and measurements of the existing elimination, therefore, are more accurate determinants of changes that may be occurring.

Other measurements focus on the qualitative state of the body fluids. Urine can be measured for specific gravity and presence of sugar or acetone without extensive laboratory tests. Of course, these measurements may be found on laboratory reports if these were ordered by the physician. The hydrometer is a simple instrument that, when floated in a liquid, gives a numeric rating of specific gravity. Sugar and acetone in the urine may be determined in several ways; one is through dipping specially treated strips of paper into a liquid and comparing color changes to a preset scale of numbers. Similarly, a test for the presence of blood in stool involves placing a small amount of stool on a specially treated paper and comparing the color change to a specified scale.

Table 5.

Guidelines for Assessment of Elimination

Interview:

1. Usual bowel patterns, color and consistency of stool, frequency of bowel movements.

2. Usual urinary patterns, color and odor of urine, frequency of urination.

3. Usual perspiration patterns, amount, times of increased perspiration.

4. Use of aids to stimulate bowel or urinary elimination.

5. Amount, timing, and frequency of flatus.

Observation:

1. Evidence of perspiration—Appropriateness in relation to environment.

2. Stool—Color, consistency.

3. Urine—Color, odor.

4. Rectal area—Color, intactness.

5. Unusual drainage such as vomitus, tube drainage—Specific observation depends on type of drainage and expected amounts.

Measurement:

1. Urine—Amount, specific gravity, sugar and acetone (calibrated container; hydrometer; Uristix®, Keto-Diastix®, or comparable test.)

2. Stool—Amount, Occult Blood (calibrated container, hemoccult slides).

3. Unusual output, such as vomitus, body drainage (calibrated container).

4. Intake and output balance (calibrated container).

Rest and Activity. Activity and rest are comprised of movement or exertion and repose or rejuvination of the body. The muscular, skeletal, and neurological structures are the primary body parts involved in rest and activity.

Rest and activity are best assessed together, because the balance between the two is crucial to well-being. As with other patterns, questions about rest and activity are important in determining the client's usual pattern. This is especially important if the person has an alteration that is affecting some aspect of his rest or activity capabilities.

Many clues to the status of a person's rest and activity can be gained through careful observation of his movements and facial expressions as he progresses through his daily activities. Specific measurements of the symmetry of the muscular, skeletal, and neurological functions allow for precise data collection. A logical progression through all joints can determine their range of motion, and any that are questionable can be measured with a protractor and compared to normal ranges. Muscle strength should be compared from side to side. The curve of the spine is an important indicator of the symmetrical working ability of the body's bones and muscles. The size of a joint is a critical indicator of its functioning and a valuable clue to detecting abnormalities.

Table 6.

Guidelines for Assessment of Rest and Activity

Interview:

1. Ability to perform activities of daily living.

2. Usual sleep patterns—Timing, amount, interferences, use of aids.

3. Usual activity patterns—Job related, home related, specific exercise program; include amount, type, frequency of activity.

4. Movement of body parts, ability, and limitations.

5. Relaxation—Type, amount, timing.

Observation:

1. Alertness; evidence of restlessness, lethargy.

2. Posture, stance, gait.

3. Symmetry and coordination of body movements.

4. Muscle tone.

Measurements:

1. Hours of sleep, number of interruptions (clock).

2. Range of motion of all joints (protractor).

3. Muscle strength (examiner resistance over body parts, bilateral comparison).

4. Tendon reflexes (reflex hammer).

5. Curvature of spine (estimate from observation and palpation with hands).

6. Joint size (tape measure if indicated).

Sexuality. Sexuality is the characteristic response of maleness or femaleness of individuals. It includes reproductive functions. The genitalia and breasts are the primary physiological structures of sexuality.

Collecting data in the area of sexuality should be approached in the same manner as data collection in the other physiological parameters. Because of the extremely personal nature of sex, it can be an uncomfortable part of assessment. However, it is the nurse's responsibility to approach it with a degree of comfort that communicates reassurance and openness. Interview questions often set the stage for the degree of comfort felt by the client during the observation and measurement phases. A broad opening question is usually an effective introduction to the subject. Such a question might be, "Are you satisfied with your usual pattern of sexual expression?"

The examiner must be careful to maintain a nonjudgmental approach regardless of the types of sex activity reported by the client. This calls for a study of sexual values and beliefs on the part of the examiner prior to assessing the sexual responses of clients.

Observation and measurement of the genitalia require slightly different techniques for men and women. However, observation and measurement of breasts should be included for both, even though the actual breast configuration varies with gender. Breasts should always be palpated to determine the presence of masses, and, if any are felt, an approximation of size and consistency is important.

Because most of the male genital structures are external, the examiner can observe and palpate them without the aid of instruments. The prostate, however, is palpated by the insertion of a finger into the rectum where the prostate can be felt through the rectal wall.

While female external genitalia can be observed easily with no instruments, a speculum is inserted into the vagina to see the internal structures. Palpation of the uterus and ovaries, which are intraabdominal, is accomplished by the examiner inserting two fingers into the vagina while pushing down on the lower abdomen with the other hand. In this way, the uterus and ovaries can be felt through the vaginal wall and an approximate measurement of these internal structures is obtained.

The Papanicolaou test is a measurement that the nurse may do or assist a physician in doing. This is a measurement of the cells in the discharge of the cervical and vaginal area. The methodology for this test may vary from institution to institution, so the specified method should be learned before doing the test. The examiner collects the discharge and applies it to a slide; a laboratory does the analysis of the slide and returns a written report to the nurse or physician.

Table 7.
Guidelines for Assessment of Sexuality

Interview:

1. Usual pattern of sexual expression—satisfac-

tory or unsatisfactory.

2. Changes in desire or activity.

3. Use of birth control, type.

4. Changes in breasts.

5. Women—last menstrual period, number of pregnancies.

6. Men—changes in testicles, evidence of hernia.

Observation:

1. Signs of gender identification (dress, posture, body language).

2. Comfort and openness with the subject of sex.

3. Condition of breasts.

4. Women—external vaginal structures—hair distribution, vaginal discharge (color, odor, consistency); internal structures—condition of vaginal walls and cervix.

5. Men—penis and testicles: hair distribution, color, size, shape, placement of meatus, lesions; femoral regions—scars, lesions, bulging.

Measurement:

1. Any palpable breast lumps—estimate size, shape, consistency (examiner's finger tips).

2. Women—size and shape of cervix and cervical os (estimate by sight using speculum); Papanicolaou Test, "Pap smear," (cotton applicator, wooden cervical spatula, glass slide, fixative agent); size, shape, and consistency of uterus and ovaries (estimate through palpation).

3. Men—presence of hernia (palpate through inguinal ring); size, shape, consistency of testicles (palpate and estimate); size, shape, consistency of prostate (palpate and estimate).

Body Maintenance. Body maintenance is the final parameter of the physiological dimension. This is the restoration and regulation of a balance of functions achieved by the body itself and by the individual on behalf of his body. The endocrine glands, with their hormonal secretions, are a primary regulatory system in the body. The individual person's health maintenance activities, such as preventive immunizations, hygienic activities, and illness treatments are the external balancing functions.

Assessment of body maintenance practices overlaps with the assessment of many other parameters, because it is an indication of how all parts of the body are held intact. Primarily, data are collected through interview questions that focus on the client's perceptions and habits, which are the most important aspects of this pattern.

Special attention is given to the skin and hair because these are critical indicators of the regulating endocrine functions. The thyroid gland is the only endocrine gland easily accessible to examination. Located in the neck, it is not always palpable unless it is enlarged. Its size and consistency should be measured by palpation of the neck area.

Body temperature, easily measured with a thermometer, is an important indicator of the heat regulatory functions of the body. Temperature will usually rise with infective or inflammatory processes.

It is important for the examiner to know what, if any, medications a person is taking, for these may affect many regulatory aspects of the body. A person's preventive health practices, including immunizations, give the nurse an idea of the level of knowledge a person has about his health and an indication of his control over health hazards that might exist. A further indication of health hazards is the condition of the client's home, work, and neighborhood settings.

Table 8.
Guidelines for Assessment of Body Maintenance

Interview:

1. Perception of general health status, i.e., level of wellness.

2. Medications—dosage, frequency, route (include prescribed and over the counter).

3. Immunization record—type, date.

4. Frequency and type of preventive health care practices—dental exams, eye exams, hearing tests, Pap smears, self-breast exams, self-testicular exams.

5. Changes in body temperature, skin condition, hair distribution, energy level.

6. Hygiene practices.

7. Condition of home environment—water, heating, amount of space, refrigerator, sanitation.

8. Hazards of home, work, or neighborhood—crime, pests, physical structure, exposure to noise.

Observations:

1. General body appearance.

2. Hygiene.

3. Skin texture, turgor, color, lesions.

4. Condition and distribution of hair.

Measurement:

1. Temperature (thermometer).

2. Size and consistency of thyroid. (palpation and estimation).

Psychological Dimension

The psychological dimension is reflected in a person's cognitive and emotional responses to himself and his environment. For the purpose of assessment, this description of the psychological dimension directs the nurse to gather data relative to two parameters: the client's cognitive ability and his emotional status. Each of these parameters should be assessed separately, as well as in reference to how the client responds to both the potential or actual health care problem and the treatment and associated therapy that may be required.

The nurse seeks to collect data that will provide information related to the client's cognitive and emotional ability to partici-pate in his health care. She seeks to determine if the client can realistically identify his strengths and limitations, and how these may impact on his ability and willingness to adhere to recommended therapy. Data gathering techniques (interview and observation) are used by the nurse to assess this dimension. Measurements of the parameters are done primarily by other health care providers.

Cognitive Ability. Cognitive ability is a composite of a person's capacity to learn, to retain what is learned (memory), and to comprehend or understand. Level of intelligence, past learning experiences, use of the senses, status of the nervous system, and developmental level contribute to a person's cognitive ability.

During interviews the nurse collects demographic data such as the client's age and educational background. These two factors may provide an indication of the patient's cognitive abilities as related to achievement in a formal learning environment. Questions should be asked about the client's usual style or pattern of learning. This information will assist in determining the client's cognitive developmental level, his use of sight and hearing in the learning process, and his capacity to learn. The client's capacity to understand may be ascertained through the clarity and appropriateness of his verbal responses to the questions asked throughout the interview. If the client does not appear to understand a question, the nurse should reword it and avoid the use of technical terms that may be a source of confusion for the client. Questions related to the health care problem should be asked so that the client's understanding of the problem and its required treatment and therapy can be assessed.

Information about the client's cognitive ability obtained through interviewing often can be validated or supported through observation. If the client has been taught a health care procedure that he, personally, must carry out, his level of comprehension of what has been described and demonstrated to him can be assessed by observing him perform the procedure. Observing the client's nonverbal communication, such as a quizzical facial expression, also can provide a clue that the client is having difficulty comprehending information the nurse is giving.

Measurements obtained on the client's visual and hearing acuity, assessed through the physiological parameter of sensation, may provide evidence that indicates that physiological impairment, rather than impairment of cognition, exists. If results of tests assessing level of developmental cognition or intelligence are available to the nurse, they can serve to validate her findings.

Table 9.

Guidelines for Assessment of Cognitive Status

Interview:

1. Orientation to person, place, time, situation.

2. Ability to express self—Verbal communication skills.

3. Ability to learn—Can he comprehend information given him? Can he read? What knowledge does he have of the health care problem and its required therapy and associated treatment, such as diet, medications, and life style alterations?

Observation:

1. Participation in activities requiring comprehension—Does he read? Does he engage in conversation with others?

2. Performance of self-care activities—If physically able, does he appear to know how to participate in his care? Can he perform an activity (e.g., insulin injection) that has been described and demonstrated?

Emotional Status. Emotional status is mirrored through the overt and covert feel-

ings a person experiences and expresses in his verbal and nonverbal communication. A person's emotional status influences and is influenced by the effectiveness of the coping strategies he uses.

The client's verbal responses that are expressed during the interview and his nonverbal responses as detected through observation are both valuable sources of data in the assessment of the client's emotional status. Questions should be asked that encourage the client to express his feelings about the health care problem and the required treatment. The client's motivation related to his intention to adhere to required therapy or health care practices can be determined through questions that are nonthreatening to the patient. Information about his past and present methods of coping with problems also should be sought.

In assessing emotional status it is important that, during the interview, the nurse is especially alert to and observant of the patient's facial expression, muscular tension, and body movement. For example, a patient asked about how a health care problem will alter his life style may respond, "It's not going to change anything." Yet when he responds, the nurse notes that the patient's facial expression is one of sadness, his body appears tense, and he is wringing his hands. Certainly the nonverbal cues would be in conflict with the verbal response, and more information should be sought.

Table 10.

Guidelines for Assessment of Emotional Status

Interview:

1. Mood—Verbal expressions of feelings, particularly in relation to the health care problem, required treatment and therapy, and alteration of usual lifestyle.

2. Coping Strategies—How does he usually cope with problems? How is he coping now?

Does he perceive this as effective?

3. Perception of Self—Does he perceive himself as sick or well?

4. Motivation—Does he perceive himself as capable or incapable of participating in his health care? Is he willing to participate in his health care? Is he presently adhering to prescribed or recommended therapy?

Observation:

1. Mood—Facial expressions (anxious, sad, depressed), muscle tension, body movement (slow, exaggerated).

2. Performance of Self-Care Activities—If physically able and knowledgeable, does he participate in his care?

Sociocultural Dimension

The sociocultural dimension is reflected in a person's noninherited intrapersonal responses to socialization practices learned and transmitted from families and communities. The responses are influenced by social, political, and economic forces, and are characterized by lifestyle, support networks, and health care practices.

This description of the sociocultural dimension directs the nurse to focus on three parameters that characterize the client's sociocultural response: lifestyle, support networks, and health care practices. These parameters should be assessed in reference to potential or actual health problems and the treatment and associated therapy. The nurse uses interviewing as the primary data collection technique to assess the sociocultural dimension. The relationship of this dimension to the body maintenance parameter of the physiological dimension should be noted.

Lifestyle. Lifestyle incorporates the usual living circumstances and activities in which a person engages. It is influenced by employment status, economic status, and routines that become acceptable practices in the person's life.

Demographic data, such as employment status, occupation, and economic status are collected during the client's initial interview upon entering the health care system. This information provides clues as to the client's ability to afford treatment and associated therapy, (e.g., medications, special diet, required aids—glasses, cane).

The client should be asked about routines, habits, and preferences that could influence his health status. For example, if a client's usual daily routine includes drinking large amounts of regular coffee throughout the day and evening, he may experience an inadequate sleep pattern due to difficulty in falling asleep (side effect of caffeine) and nocturia (frequent urination). Gathering information related to the presence of risk factors, such as cigarette smoking, a sedentary lifestyle, and consistent intake of high-calorie, low-protein foods, is essential. Questions should be asked not only to determine the presence of risk factors, but also to ascertain if and how the client may have tried to overcome them in the past.

Table 11.

Guidelines for Assessment of Lifestyles

Interview:

1. Employment Status—past, present.

2. Occupation—Does it require physical or cognitive abilities that may be altered by the health problems?

3. Economic Status—Does the patient have the financial resources to secure the required treatment and associated therapy? Description of residence.

4. Daily Routines—Activity/Rest Patterns. Personal Hygiene Habits. Nutritional Pattern. Dependence on tobacco, drugs, or alcohol.

Observation:

1. Type of Attire—Appropriate to environment, culturally linked.

2. Habits—Risk factors.

Support Networks. Support networks are made up of family members and significant persons who provide emotional, physical, or financial support to a client. The composition and status of relationships between the client and his significant support systems can influence his response to treatment and therapy.

During the initial interview, questions can be asked about the client's marital status, family composition, and responsibilities for other persons. Information about friends for whom he is responsible and who offer him assistance in meeting his needs helps to identify actual and potential sources of support upon whom he can depend.

The nurse should seek to gather data that provide clues as to: human and material resources already available to and used by the client; resources available but not used by the client; and resources that could be available if certain qualifying criteria for use were met. In the first instance, the client's participation in groups such as Mended Hearts, Alcoholics Anonymous, and Weight Watchers gives evidence of health support networks that are already used. In the second instance, it should be determined whether or not the client is aware of available resources, and if there are specific reasons that influence him not to use them. For example, he may be eligible to use a neighborhood health clinic but has no means to get to and from the clinic. In the final instance, based on the information the client has given, the nurse may discover that he is eligible for assistance (e.g., food stamps), but has not made formal application. In this situation, the nurse would use the social worker as a resource for the client.

Table 12.

Guidelines for Assessment of Support Networks

Interview:

1. Marital status.

2. Family composition.

3. Composition of other supportive systems— Their relationship, support to and interaction with the client.

4. Persons responsible for, dependent upon.

5. Sources of support—Emotional, physical, financial.

Observation:

1. Relationships—If hospitalized, does the client have visitors? If so, who and how often?

   If seen in a clinic, is the client accompanied by others?

   If seen in a home, what is the interaction among the persons living there?

Health Care Practices. Health care practices incorporate those activities engaged in primarily for the purpose of attaining or maintaining health. These activities are influenced by the person's beliefs and values about health care, the health care system, health care providers, and methods of treatment and therapy.

A person's socialization to accepting and using the health care system is influenced primarily by his family and his cultural community. Family and community influence the development of his belief about and values of health care, adherence to therapy, response to illness, and his perception of the health care system. His values and beliefs will determine his willingness to participate in the health care system.

Questions about how he usually seeks to resolve health care problems should be asked. His impressions as to the value of seeking professional care, as well as his patterns of adhering to prescribed and recommended therapy, are indicators of his potential acceptance of support given by health care providers. If the client perceives the health care system only as one that is "out to get my money" or "doesn't care about me," the nurse can deduce that he may be reluctant to use the system.

The client's usual health care practices

should be explored. Does he employ non-traditional health care practices? The use of herbs, excessive intake of vitamins, and reliance on psychic healers are examples of practices that could influence the effectiveness of traditional treatments and therapies.

Table 13.

Guidelines for Assessment of Health Care Practices

Interview:

1. Patterns of Health Care—Usual, present. Does he use a formal health care system? Does he use home remedies or nontraditional health care practices?

2. Illness Response—Previous illnesses and hospitalizations. Attitude toward hospitalization. Meaning attached to role of patient. Previous history of coping with stress and changes in lifestyle.

3. Perceptions of Health Care System—Beliefs about and attitudes toward: health care agency, care givers, treatments, and therapies.

Observation:

1. Participation in Health Care Delivery—Active or passive?

2. Illness Response—Overt or covert?

Spiritual Dimension

The spiritual dimension of the human person is reflected in his personal response to inspirational forces. It is the inspirational forces that have been and are experienced by a person that contribute to the development of his theological, ethical, and spiritual values. One's values influence the meaning and purpose ascribed to life and affect the manner in which the client responds to actual or potential health care problems.

A person's religion and spiritual involvement may affirm the inspirational forces

he experiences and provide a source of inspiration for him. An organized or formal involvement in religious or spiritual activities can provide a system of support. These activities may be an essential aspect of a person's life and must, therefore, be respected as such.

A person who is a member of a religious group may hold specific beliefs that influence his choice of lifestyle and his health care practices. An example of this would be a client whose religious or spiritual beliefs require him to avoid certain foods or to fast on certain days. A person's view of disease and his acceptance or rejection of prescribed treatments or therapies also may be rooted in his spiritual beliefs. The nurse must be aware of these and seek to understand how they affect the client's response to a health care problem. The reader is referred to Chapter 10 for more discussion on cultural/spiritual dimensions of health care.

In assessing the impact that a person's spiritual dimension has on his well-being, it is necessary to consider the way in which a person's spiritual self relates to his physical, psychological, and sociocultural self. Responses assessed in the other dimensions are influenced by the depth and breadth of a person's religious and spiritual beliefs and values. These beliefs and values also provide the parameter for assessing the client's spiritual responses.

Table 14.

Guidelines for Assessment of Spiritual Responses

Interview:

1. Religious Affiliation—Religion. Active or inactive participation. Type of participation.

2. Religious or Spiritual Beliefs Influencing:
   a. Health Care Practices:
      Diet, seeking or receiving medical treatment or therapy, rituals or rites.
   b. Perception of Illness: a punishment, a test of faith.

c. Coping strategies.

3. Religious or Spiritual Values Influencing:
Life's purpose and meaning.
Death's purpose and meaning.
Health and its maintenance.
Relationship with God or a higher being, self, and others.

Observation:

1. Religious or Spiritual Support—Time for personal or group prayer or meditation. Visits from rabbi, minister, priest, or other persons from spiritual support system.

2. Religious or Spiritual Attitude—Hopeful, trusting, peaceful.

SPECIAL CONSIDERATIONS: DEVELOPMENT LEVEL

The information presented in this chapter gives general guidelines for assessment that are applicable to most clients. However, many factors influence the nurse in choosing strategies for data collection in a given client situation. The client's age and developmental level are important considerations that will influence both the type of data that are likely to be found and the techniques used to obtain data.

The nurse must have a sound knowledge of usual behaviors associated with periods of growth and development. There are many theories that present categories of usual developmental behaviors; these are helpful to the nurse as a broad measurement standard. One such theory is Eric Erikson's, who described eight stages of ego development.[2] While this is a psychological and social orientation, these stages can serve as an organizational scheme for some of the age-specific areas of assessment with which physical changes can be considered.

Infancy is characterized by Erikson as a time of "basic trust versus basic mistrust." It is during this time that a person is totally dependent on others, so the nurse must assess parents and their reaction and inter-

actions with the infant as well as observe the infant. Naturally, questions must be directed to the parents. During observation and measurement, the accompanying parent assists the nurse by holding the child whenever possible, so that the infant remains secure.

The rate of development in children is very rapid, and there are several instruments designed to test specific levels of development. One such test is the Denver Developmental Screening Test (DDST), which is widely used to evaluate gross and fine motor skills, communication skills, and personal and social behaviors in children from birth to age six years.[3]

The toddler stage is characterized as a period of "autonomy versus shame and doubt." The nurse must carefully assess safety factors in the child's environment as he begins to walk and explore his increasingly accessible surroundings. It is important to assess his developing autonomy during this time when he is learning to control bodily functions and is beginning to use verbal communication skills.

The preschooler goes through a period of "initiative versus guilt," when he strives to respond to the expectations of those around him while testing out his own initiatives. Information about the child's interactions with other members of his family and with other children are important factors for the nurse to consider. At this age, the nurse can direct questions to the child during some parts of assessment. The child's responses will give the nurse much information about his level of development. It is necessary to determine if the child has a daily routine that fosters a balanced diet, adequate rest, and protection from his environment. Determining the child's level of understanding of dangerous things, like cars on the street or hot stoves, is important to assuring his safety.

The school age years are seen as a period of "industry versus inferiority." In moving outside the home for school, the child begins to develop an identity no longer dependent on his family. His interactions with peers, his abilities to "fit in" and be "normal," and his school accomplishments are critical indicators of health responses. The nurse can rely more heavily on the child himself as a source of information during data collection; he may or may not want his parents actively involved during assessment. The nurse must determine the acuteness of the problem and decide the degree to which parents should be involved.

Adolescence, a period of "identity versus role confusion," is a time when a person makes the transition from childhood to the adult world. This developmental stage is sometimes divided into an early, middle, and late period.[4] During these years, depending on the length of schooling, the person plans for and moves into an occupational role. A sex role identity is very important at this stage, during which puberty matures the body's characteristic male or female functions. When assessing persons in this age group, the nurse must be particularly sensitive to the changes in roles, bodily configuration, and comfort levels of adolescents. While collecting data, the nurse needs to view the client as an adult, but allow the person to involve his parents in his health care if so desired. Adult health habits are formed at this age. Therefore, the nurse must determine the young person's level of knowledge about his physical, psychological, sociocultural, and spiritual responses. Because of adolescents' changing sexual capabilities, there is a need for the nurse to be especially sensitive in assessing sexual responses so that a nonjudgmental, open relationship is established between health care provider and recipient.

Young adulthood is a time of "intimacy versus isolation." In this period, the person's self-image and ego strength should stabilize, allowing the development of close relationships with others, usually with those of the opposite sex. Choices about having a family are determined, and pregnancy and childbirth are important health issues. Careers or jobs and their related financial rewards are determinants of security and lifestyles for these persons. The nurse needs to assess the client for life stressors that may affect health as the young adult copes with a developing family, a beginning career, and his contribution to society.

Middle-aged persons are expected to be concerned with "establishing and guiding the next generation."[5] This period is described as a time of "generativity versus stagnation." This is a time of family changes as children (if the person has any) leave and establish their lives separate from parents. While middle-aged adults usually have well-established jobs or careers, they may become insecure about their age as younger persons enter their work environment. Likewise, intimate relationships, while usually well established at this age, may be influenced by aging changes. Menopause is an important body change experienced by women at this time. Chronic illnesses are more frequently seen in this age group. Persons often will be concerned with aged parents and coping with their parents' deaths. These events may be especially stressful as they plan for their own retirement and maturity.

The final developmental stage, later maturity, is a period of "ego identity versus despair." Retirement from a job or career is often a stressful life event, and it is sometimes accompanied by a change in living arrangements and economic status. The nurse must assess the client as well as his environment to determine physical safety hazards, his ability to care for himself, his relationship with significant others, and his ability to cope with inevitable events, such as the death of peers and spouses. An important spiritual concern at this age is the person's beliefs and feelings about death.

In conclusion, the nurse needs to be aware of developmental changes that occur with aging and be able to relate them to their effects on health. Developmental stages are presented not as finite time periods, but rather as a continuum of life events. Each individual ages and develops in a unique manner. Consequently the nurse must be careful not to categorize persons on the basis of generalizations. Careful data collection will give objective data concerning each individual client's level of development.

SUMMARY

This chapter presented health assessment from a nursing perspective. A framework based upon the physiological, psychological, sociocultural, and spiritual dimensions of the human person provides a guide for data collection. The nurse's health assessment is contrasted with that of other health care providers. The roles of the nurse, the client, and other health care providers are discussed. Interviewing, observation, and measurement are the techniques used by the nurse to establish a comprehensive, objective database. The techniques are described so as to provide a basic understanding of their use.

For the purpose of guiding the collection of data, each dimension and its assessment parameters are delineated. Tables provide cues that the nurse can use when interviewing, observing, and measuring. Developmental stages and their impact on health responses are addressed as important components of health assessment. This chapter provides a foundation for the nurse in the area of health assessment. This first phase of the nursing process is a complex activity. The nurse will add to this foundational level of knowledge through continued practice and the addition of more complex techniques. As the number of client encounters increases, the nurse will sharpen her skills in identifying health assessment priorities for each client. The nurse's job description, health care setting, and the characteristics of the client population will influence the nature of the data that are needed to determine the client's responses to his actual or potential health problems.

STUDY QUESTIONS

1. State how a nursing health assessment differs from a medical health assessment.

2. Describe how the nurse incorporates information from the client and other health care providers.

3. List tools or instruments that can be used for interviewing, observation, and measurement.

4. Define the parameters for assessment within each dimension of the human.

5. Choose a stage of development and describe factors that must be considered when assessing a person at that stage.

REFERENCES

1. American Nurses' Association. **Nursing: A Social Policy Statement.** Kansas City, MO. 1980.
2. Block, Gloria J., Nolan, JoEllen W., and Dempsey, Mary K. **Health Assessment for Professional Nursing A Developmental Approach.** New York, Appleton-Century-Crofts, 1981.
3. Frankenburg, W.K., and Dodds, J.B **Denver Developmental Screening Test,** University of Colorado Medical Center, 1969.
4. Erikson, Eric H. **Childhood and Society,** 2nd

ed. New York, W.W. Norton and Company, Inc., 1963.
5. Ibid., p.267.

ANNOTATED BIBLIOGRAPHY

Block GJ, Nolan JW, Dempsey MK: **Health Assessment for Professional Nursing: A Developmental Approach.** New York, Appleton-Century-Crofts, 1981. Outlined according to physiological body systems, this book presents detailed guidelines for health assessment. It integrates content related to differences of age groups within each chapter and gives guidelines for assessing certain lifestyles and environmental factors. Numerous photographs and diagrams assist the reader in visualizing assessment techniques and body parts.

Fields WL, McGinn-Campball KM: **Introduction to Health Assessment.** Reston, Reston Publishing Company, Inc., 1983. Because this book emphasizes techniques of assessing the healthy individual, it is helpful to beginning students. Abnormal findings are presented in separate tables throughout the chapters. Body systems are the major organizational approach for chapters, but chapters on fluid and electrolyte balance, acid/base balance, and integration of health assessment give additional parameters that are valuable to the nurse.

Malasanos L, Barkauskas V, Moss M, Stoltenberg-Allen K: **Health Assessment** (2nd ed.). St. Louis, The C.V. Mosby Co., 1981. This text presents overviews of the interview, the health history, and developmental assessments. Health assessment incorporating a body systems approach is the focus of this text. Sections on health assessment of the pediatric, prenatal, and aging client assist the student in recognizing how the process of health assessment may be tailored to the developmental level of the client. The tables, figures, and pictures enhance the value of the text.

8

Legal Aspects of Nursing

Cynthia Northrop

CHAPTER OUTLINE

OBJECTIVES

At the completion of this chapter the reader will be able to:

- Discuss sources of law and general legal principles
- Discuss the need for malpractice insurance
- Compare and contrast negligence and malpractice
- Relate to major recordkeeping responsibilities and common recording problems
- Identify different types of orders and legal implications of each
- Describe legal accountability in nursing practice
- Define institutional licensure
- Discuss the status of mandatory continuing education for today's nurse
- Discuss the code of ethics
- List patient rights

GLOSSARY

Ad Litem—for the purposes of litigation.

Administrative law—the branch of law dealing with organs of government.

Adversary—a litigant opponent—The opposing party in a writ or action.

Affidavit—a declaration or statement of facts, made voluntarily and confirmed by oath.

Agency—includes every relationship in which one person acts for or represents another by the latter's authority.

Agent—a person authorized by another to act for him.

Allegation—a charge or assertion.

Appeal—a complaint to a superior court to reverse or correct an injustice done or an alleged error committed by an inferior court.

Assault—threat to do bodily harm.

Battery—committing bodily harm.

Bona Fide—good faith.

Borrowed servant—an employee temporarily under the control of another. The traditional example is that of a nurse employed by a hospital who is "borrowed" by a surgeon in the operating room. The temporary employer of the borrowed servant will be held responsible for the act(s) of the borrowed servant under the doctrine of respondeat superior.

Breach of contract—unjustified failure to perform the terms of a contract as agreed upon or when performance is due.

Captain of the ship doctrine—the person in charge may be held responsible for all those under his supervision and makes final decision.

Case law—decisions by the courts.

Cause of action—averment of allegations or facts sufficient to cause defendant to respond to allegations.

Civil law—concerned with the legal rights and duties of private persons.

Common law—derived from court decisions, judge-made law.

Comparative negligence—doctrine of negligence in which negligence of the plaintiff and defendant is compared and an apportionment of damages is made based on the acts the parties are found to have committed.

Compensatory damages—amounts of money for proven loss.

Confidential communication—communications passing between persons in a fiduciary relationship who have a duty not to reveal the information.

Consent—a voluntary act by which one person agrees to allow someone else to do something.

Constitutional law—branch of law dealing with organization and function of government.

Contract—a promissory agreement between two or more persons that create, modify, or destroy a legal relationship. Also, it is a legally enforceable promise between two or more persons to do or not to do something.

Contributory negligence—an act or

GLOSSARY Continued

omission amounting to want of ordinary care on the part of the complaining party that, concurring with defendant's negligence, is a proximate cause of injury.

Corporate negligence doctrine—the hospital as an entity is negligent. The failure of those entrusted with the task of providing the accommodations and facilities to carry out the purpose of the corporation, and the failure to follow, in a given situation, the established standards of conduct to which the corporation should conform.

Cross examination—examination of a witness given, in chief, to test the truth or credibility of his testimony.

Defendant—in a criminal case, the person accused of committing a crime. In a civil suit, the party against whom suit is brought.

Deposition—an oral interrogation answering all manner of questions relating to the transaction at issue, given under oath, and taken in writing before some judicial officer or attorney.

Due care—that degree of care or concern that would or should be exercised by an ordinary person in the same situation.

Due process—certain procedural requirements to assure fairness.

Employer—the employer selects the employee, pays him a salary or wages, retains the power to dismiss him, and can control his conduct during working hours.

Expert witness—one who has special training, experience, skills, and knowledge in a relevant area, and whose testimony as to his opinion is allowed to be considered as evidence; non-expert opinions usually are not admissible as evidence.

Foreseeability, Doctrine of—an individual is liable for all natural and proximate consequences of any negligent acts to another individual to whom a duty is owed.

Informed consent—consent in which the patient has received sufficient information concerning the health care proposed, its incumbent risks, and the acceptable alternatives.

Invasion of Privacy—invasion of the right to be left alone, to live in seclusion without being subjected to unwarranted or undesired publicity.

Jurisdiction—the court has the authority to hear the case.

Law—the sum total of man-made rules and regulations by which society is governed in a formal and legally binding manner.

Lay witness—one who testifies to what he has seen, heard, or otherwise observed.

Legal—permitted or authorized by law.

Liability—an obligation one has incurred or might incur through any act or failure to act, responsibility for conduct falling below a certain standard that is the causal connection of the plaintiff's injury.

Litigation—a trial in court to determine

GLOSSARY Continued

legal issues and the rights and duties of the parties.

Malpractice—professional negligence, improper discharge of professional duties, or a failure of a professional to meet standard of care that results in harm to another.

Medical record—a written official documentary of what has happened to a particular patient during a specific period of time.

Plaintiff—the party that brings a civil suit seeking damages or other legal relief.

Police power—state power to act in order to protect its citizens' health, safety, and welfare.

Policies—guidelines within which employees of an institution must operate.

Precedent—a previous adjudged decision that serves as authority in a similar case.

Privileged communication—statements made to one in a position of trust—usually an attorney, physician, or spouse. Because of the confidential nature of the information, the law protects it from being revealed, even in court. The term is applied in two distinct situations. First, the communications between certain persons (e.g., physician and patient), cannot be divulged without consent of the patient. Second, in some situations, the law provides an exemption from liability for disclosing information where there is a higher duty to speak, for example, statutory reporting requirements.

Procedures—mode or proceeding by which a legal right is enforced. A series of steps outlined by the institution to accomplish a specific objective or task.

Proximate cause—legal concept of cause and effect; the injury would not have occurred by the particular cause; causal connection.

Reasonable care—the degree of skill and knowledge customarily used by a competent health practitioner or student of similar education and experience in treating and caring for the sick and injured in the community in which the individual is practicing.

Reasonably prudent person doctrine—requires a person of ordinary sense to use ordinary care and skill.

Res ipsa loquitur—"the thing speaks for itself." A doctrine of law applicable to cases where the defendant has exclusive control of the thing that caused the harm, and where the harm ordinarily could not have occurred without negligent conduct. Normally, the plaintiff must prove the defendant's liability, but when this doctrine is found to apply, the defendant must prove himself not responsible for harm.

Respondeat superior—"let the master answer." The employer is responsible for the legal consequences of the acts of the servant or employee while he acts within the scope of his employment.

Right—power, privilege, or faculty in-

GLOSSARY Continued

herent in one person and incident upon another.

Rules and regulations—clear and concise statements mandating or prohibiting certain activity in an institution.

Standard of care—those acts performed or omitted that an ordinary prudent person in the defendant's position would have done or not done; a measure by which the defendant's conduct is compared to ascertain negligence.

Standards—criteria of measuring, and conformity to established practice.

Statute of limitations—a legal limit on the time one has to file suit in civil matters, usually measured from the time of the wrong or when a reasonable person would have discovered the wrong.

Statutes—legislative enactments; act of legislature declaring, commanding, or prohibiting something.

Subpeona—a court order requiring one to come to court to give testimony; failure to appear results in punishment by the court.

Suit—court proceeding where one person seeks damages or other legal remedies from another. The term usually is not used in connection with criminal cases.

Testimony—oral statement of a witness, given under oath at a trial.

Tort—a legal or civil wrong committed by one person against the person or property of another.

Verdict—the formal declaration of the jury of its findings of fact, which is signed by the jury foreman and presented to the court.

INTRODUCTION

Nursing practice is governed by many legal and ethical concepts. Nurses, because of their health care delivery role, are accountable for their professional judgments and behavior. In the past, physicians and agencies assumed much more responsibility for nurses' actions than they do today. This is due partly to the expansion of the nurses' role in the health care system and the increasing professionalism demonstrated by nurses. If nurses are to be responsible for their acts, then they must be accountable as well. This chapter will discuss general legal concepts and the legal and professional responsibilities of the professional nurse.

GENERAL LEGAL CONCEPTS

Many concepts from law have an impact on nursing practice; therefore, it is important for nurses to know the basics of these concepts. Before this can be accomplished, however, the sources of law and how laws affect nursing practice should be understood.

Sources of Law

There are five major sources of law (see Figure 8-1).

In some situations, each of the five sources may be used by a lawyer representing clients in disputes. In others, only one or two sources may be necessary. For ex-

1. **Constitution**—United States, State

2. **Judicial Opinions**—Federal, State, Administrative

3. **Legislation**—Federal, State, City, County

4. **Regulations**—Federal, State

5. **Common Law Principles**—Traditions Principles of Justice, Fairness, Autonomy, Respect, Dignity, Precedent

Figure 8-1. The Sources of Law.

ample, if a nurse was wrongly fired from a job at a hospital and then retained an attorney in order to be reinstated or to correct the wrong, the lawyer could examine the facts of the situation and go to several sources of law to prepare the case. Depending on the situation, similar cases might be found in the judicial opinions or judge-written decisions in that particular jurisdiction. Federal legislation and regulations on employment practices might also be drawn upon. Common law principles of fairness and justice might be argued by the attorney, depending on how and under what circumstances the nurse was fired. Also, if the nurse was not given notice or reasons for the firing, or not given an opportunity to refute the firing, interpretation of the federal or state constitution's due process clause may assist in proving a violation of constitutional rights.

The five sources of law are intertwined. For example, there are judicial opinions that discuss and apply common law principles and interpret the constitution, legislation, or regulations. Courts are bound to follow opinions or previous decisions of their particular jurisdiction. This is the common law principle of precedent. Other judicial opinions may be used to persuade the court, but they need not be followed since they did not originate under that court's jurisdiction. Precedent may not be followed if the court can distinguish the facts before them from the previously de-

cided case. In addition, societal views change over time and this is often reflected in court decisions. The emergent philosophy of an era has an influence on how laws are written. As an era changes, the laws that govern may also change. It is important for nurses to keep up with the status of laws that influence nursing practice. This can be done by reviewing current nursing journals.

The Court System

The federal court system and individual state court systems are the two main court systems in the United States. The federal system has three tiers, as do most state systems (see Figure 8-2). In the lower courts (district and circuit courts), cases are heard for the first time, and evidence is presented. The higher courts are appeal courts, where argument is offered to persuade the judges that certain errors may have been made when the case was tried in the lower court. Only under special circumstances is new evidence introduced in the higher courts.

There are other courts that have been established by Congress or state legislatures for selected and limited purposes. For example, disputes dealing with federal tax issues would be settled in the tax court; custom or patent disputes would be decided in customs and patent courts.

Also established by Congress or state legislatures are administrative law systems that handle certain types of claims. Decisions made in these systems have the force of law and usually may be appealed to a federal or state court system. For example, if nurses are injured on the job, they may be eligible for workers compensation. First, a claim would be filed with the state workers compensation administration. If the claim is denied, the appeal process would have to be exhausted within the administration. Once one exhausted the appeal there, without success, the claim could be filed in the state court system.

Federal	State*
Supreme Court	Court of Appeals or Supreme Court
U.S. Court of Appeals	Circuit Court
U.S. District Court	District Court
*Some states have a 4-tier system; most have a 3-tier system.	

Figure 8-2. The U.S. Court System.

LAWS AFFECTING NURSING PRACTICE

Many laws affect nursing practice because the legal system serves to protect the rights of individuals or groups and determines the responsibilities of individuals in civil and criminal cases.

Law can be classified in a variety of ways, but the major classifications are criminal law and civil law. **Criminal law** involves conduct considered harmful or offensive to society. The punishment for committing the crime ranges from a heavy fine to imprisonment. **Civil law** involves legal rights of individuals.

Most litigation involving nursing to date has been civil and not criminal in nature.

Torts . . . . Negligence and Malpractice
　　　　　　　Defamation, Libel, and
　　　　　　　　　Slander
　　　　　　　Assault and Battery
　　　　　　　False Imprisonment
　　　　　　　Invasion of Privacy

Contracts . . . . . Nurse and Client
　　　　　　　Nurse and Agency
　　　　　　　Agency and Supplemental
　　　　　　　　Staffing Agency
　　　　　　　Agency and Educational
　　　　　　　　Institution
　　　　　　　Nurse and Insurance

Criminal . . . . . . Homocide
　　　　　　　Manslaughter

Constitutional . . Due Process
　　　　　　　Rights

Legislation . . . . . Licensing
　　　　　　　Reporting Statutes
　　　　　　　Good Samaritan Statutes

Figure 8-3. Selected Categories of Laws Affecting Nurses.

Several areas of law affect nursing practice (see Figure 8-3).

Torts

A tort is a general term in civil law that describes a legal wrong committed against the person or property of another. The word tort comes from the Latin word "tortus" meaning twisted. Conduct between private individuals that is wrong or twisted is classified as a tort. Civil wrongs usually take one of two forms:

- simple, direct interference with a person or with property
- disturbances of intangible interests such as one's reputation.

In a civil suit involving a tort, only the injured person can begin and maintain the suit. If the decision in the end is to grant a remedy to the injured person, the remedy is money or discontinuance of the disturbance, which is intended to compensate for the injury. The goal of the remedy is to provide the means (funds) so that the injured person can be placed in a similar position as the situation prior to the injury.

Negligence and malpractice are two examples of torts that deal with clinical practice situations. **Negligence** is an unintended act or failure to act that leads to an injury. Anyone can make a mistake or have an accident that results in injuries to another. Negligence can be defined as carelessness. **Malpractice,** on the other hand, is negligence by a person who is a member of a profession. Individuals are liable for their own negligence. Negligence and malpractice are the torts that most often involves nurses (see Figure 8-4).

1. Personal Liability
2. Duty and Standard of Care
   a. Ordinary Standard
   b. Professional Standard
3. Breach of Duty
4. Causation, Proximate Cause
5. Damage, Injury, and Remedy
6. Vicarious Liability
   a. Physician
   b. Employer
   c. Indemnification
7. Defenses
   a. Contributory Negligence
   b. Comparative Negligence

Figure 8-4. Legal Principles of Negligence and Malpractice

An "ordinary" person (not a member of a profession) is held to an "ordinary" standard, meaning that his action will be judged in light of what any other "ordinary" person would have done under the circumstances. The action of a member of a profession is judged by what a similar member of that profession would have done under the circumstances. The "ordinary" person's duty is not the same as a member of a profession who, because of increased knowledge and a special relationship, owes a higher duty. Employment in an agency establishes a nurse's duty to carry out services in a safe and reasonable manner. In some legal cases, nurses have been held to an ordinary standard, and in other cases they have been held to a professional standard. Which standard applies varies from situation to situation and state to state. When confronted with a practice dilemma, the safest approach is to decide how a similarly prepared nurse would act under the circumstances in question. Other sources may be used in determining how the nurse should have acted under the same circumstances (see Figure 8-5).

The breach of the duty owed and the outcome of that breach relate to the rest of the elements of negligence and malpractice. Nurses can make mistakes, such as medication errors, that lead to no injury,

for example, giving a patient a vitamin when one was not ordered by the physician. Nurses have not committed negligence or malpractice if what they did was not the cause of injury. Injuries are usually physical, actual injuries, however, courts and juries grant remedies for psychological injuries, especially if they are in conjunction with physical injuries.

1. Specific functions assigned to nurses in written manuals and employer's policy and procedure
2. Testimony of others that describes the existing usual and reasonable nursing practices under similar circumstances
3. Education, experience, continuing education
4. Textbooks, journals, other publications in the field
5. Standards of professional organizations (e.g., standards of nursing practice, American Nurses Association)
6. Standards of accrediting or licensing groups (e.g., Joint Commission on Accreditation of Hospitals)
7. Policy Statements of Professional Associations (e.g., ANA **Code for Nurses**)
8. Nurse Practice Act and Regulations

Figure 8-5. Determining the Applicable Standards of Nursing Care

An example of a particular nursing practice situation follows. Examine it in light of the principles discussed thus far and decide whether the nurse who inserted the catheter is negligent.

A patient is to have an abdominal hysterectomy. The surgeon orders that a foley catheter be inserted into her bladder and attached to straight drainage as part of the preoperative preparation for surgery. A nurse mistakenly inserts the foley into the patient's rectum. Never checking for urinary drainage, the nurse then connects the catheter to the drainage bag and sends the patient to surgery.

After the surgery has begun, the surgeon discovers that the patient's bladder is full, but sees the drainage bag hanging at the side of the table, and quickly surmises the catheter must not be in the correct location. "Those nurses!" he shouts, losing his temper. "They never do anything right!" Still scrubbed, he reaches under the drapes, grabs the misplaced catheter and pulls it out. In doing so, the catheter flips into the open surgical wound, thoroughly contaminating it with fecal material. Despite precautionary measures taken in the operating room the patient suffers a severe infection, pain, extended hospital stay, prolonged recovery period, and develops abdominal adhesions. To recover for injuries sustained, the patient sues both the surgeon and the nurse.

The court found only the physician negligent, because placing a catheter in the rectum even though it was the wrong place could not lead to infection, adhesions, and loss of wages. No causal link between the nurse's mistake and the injuries the patient suffered was found to exist.

The following list identifies activities of nurses who have lost legal cases involving allegations of negligence and malpractice.

Some common acts of negligence and malpractice include:

- Failure to count or incorrectly count the number of sponges or instruments where a duty exists to account for them.
- Improper exercise of judgments that bedrails should have been used to safeguard patients.
- Lack of supervision of patients at regular and appropriate intervals.
- Failure to contact or notify the physician of changes in patient's condition.
- Failure to give emergency treatment to a patient in the hospital.
- Failure to recognize adverse signs and symptoms, discontinue treatments, and contact the physician.
- Lack of judgment in evaluating physician orders.

- Failure to administer medications properly (right dose, right route, right patient, right drug, right time).
- Failure to apply appropriate principles regarding application of hot and cold.
- Failure to assist patient with ambulation.
- Failure to evaluate patient complaints and follow up with physician.
- Failure to report to superiors and to physicians changes in patient's condition.
- Failure to monitor vital signs.
- Improper identification of patient for surgery.
- Failure to take reasonable precautions in regard to patient's personal property.
- Lack of sterile technique.
- Failure to administer anesthetics properly (applies to nurse anesthetist).
- Failure to properly remove a foley catheter.
- Failure to administer correct blood type to a patient.
- Refusal to admit a patient to a hospital floor.
- Failure to take a reasonable patient history.
- Failure to refer a patient to a physician for diagnosis and treatment.
- Failure to follow proper physician orders and treatments.

In cases of vicarious liability, someone else is also held responsible for another's negligent acts. For nurses, that is usually a physician or an employer. One type of vicarious liability is respondeat superior or "let the master or employer respond." In order for respondeat superior to exist, a negligent act must occur within a relationship of employment with an employer and within the scope of duties of that employment. The employer shares responsibility with the employee for negligent actions because the employer's responsibilities are to hire reasonable employees and to supervise and evaluate them. A physician who employs a nurse in his office practice has the responsibility for respondeat superior because the physician is the employer.

A physician also may be vicariously liable for a nurse's acts along with the nurse's employer. The physician who writes an erroneous treatment or medication order that any reasonable and prudent nurse would execute shares in the liability incurred. Hence the surgeon was vicariously liable and not the hospital. Recently, this situation has changed greatly, and more often the courts are holding nurses accountable for their actions. In addition, the hospital does more evaluation and supervision of nurses and, therefore, has been held

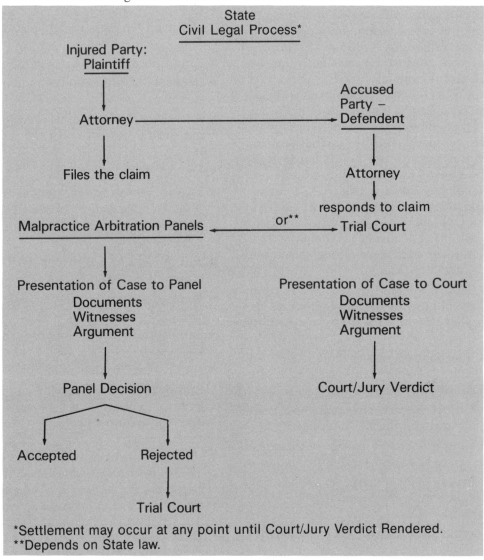

Figure 8-6. The Civil Legal Process.

accountable more often than the physician.

In determining who the injured party sues, two main factors are examined: liability and ability to compensate for the injury suffered. The fact that nurses are not sued very often relates to both of these factors. Nurses may not be liable or may only be liable to a small degree in a given negligence situation. Nurses, because of societal status and salary, are not viewed as ones with monetary means to compensate for injuries. Therefore, in many situations nursing negligence is the topic of lawsuits not against the negligent nurses but against the hospital or other employer. In situations where the employment or insurance contract allows, a hospital may sue the employee for expenses it incurs in defending the employer. Indemnification allows the employer to recover from the employee the monies spent on litigation settlement of a claim where the employer is negligent.

In many states, claims of malpractice against physicians and other health care providers must follow a particular legal process. Each state has unique requirements for beginning a lawsuit where malpractice is the accusation (see Figure 8-6).

The injured person, the plaintiff, first seeks the advice of an attorney. Review of the facts and sources of law may determine that the plaintiff has sufficient evidence and legal support to proceed with a lawsuit. The plaintiff's attorney files the necessary papers to describe the claim with an arbitration panel or with a trial court. The initial choice of forum depends on state law and legal procedure. At the same time, the accused person, the defendant, is served or sent the same papers that are filed with the panel or court. Usually, at this point the defendant needs to retain a lawyer or, if insured against malpractice, the insurance company needs to be contacted in order to provide legal counsel if that is a provision of the insurance agreement.

In some states nurses may or may not be subject to the rules pertaining to malpractice panels. For example, in some states only claims against physicians and hospitals must go to arbitration first; other state rules or procedure require arbitration for all health care providers. The arbitration panel involves 3 to 5 individuals (consumers, lawyers, physicians, or other health providers) and is ideally faster, less formal, and less expensive. The trial court involves a judge, usually 12 jurors, and a longer waiting time before the case is heard. However, several states have abandoned the panel process because their experience with it did not produce the ideal situation.

Documents, primarily agency records about the plaintiff, witnesses, and argument or discussion make up the presentation of the case to the panel or trial court. Both parties may present these items as evidence to either persuade or dissuade the decisionmakers to favor or reject the plaintiff's claim. Settlement outside the forum may occur at any time before the time when the panel judge or jury renders a decision. Either side may reject the panel's decision and file an appeal in the trial court. If a settlement between the parties occurs prior to a final decision, the question of malpractice is never answered. Should the insurance company pay the plaintiff and the plaintiff agree that receipt of payment settled the claim, the plaintiff has waived his right to sue for that particular claim.

An **expert witness,** one who provides an opinion when deemed necessary by the court, often is used by either the plaintiff or defendant in the presentation of the case. This witness usually has no prior connection with the claim and his testimony or consultation with the attorney helps to interpret evidence, clarify questions, or establish what standard should be applied in order to make a decision.

A lay witness is one who can say what happened in a particular situation because he participated in it or observed it. Lay witnesses describe what they saw, smelled, touched, or heard.

Nurses can and have been both lay and expert witnesses in lawsuits that deal with nursing and other situations. A nurse who observed a physician's malpractice may be subpoenaed to testify about what was observed. On the other hand, a nurse may be consulted by an attorney to give advice about how much home nursing care would be necessary to rehabilitate an automobile accident victim. While the lay witness can be subpoenaed, the expert witness cannot. The expert witness enters into a contractual agreement to consult with and provide assistance to an attorney for a fee. The fee for expert services or consultation should never be contingent on the outcome of the case.

Certain lay witnesses subpoenaed by either party may claim that what they are being asked to reveal in court is a **privileged communication.** The legislature and legal rules of procedure determine who may claim this privilege not to divulge the information being requested. In most states, physicians, psychiatrists, psychologists, members of the clergy, and husbands and wives are allowed to claim the privilege. In a small number of states, nurses, social workers, and accountants have the privilege. If the legislature does not include nurses under the privileged communication clause, then nurses in that state must testify and reveal confidential information.

The privilege to keep certain information from a court subpoena is not absolute. For example, if a person decides to sue another and needs to present testimony about his own mental health, the privilege will be waived because the person to whom the obligation is owed to maintain confidentiality is requesting his own psychiatrist to testify. However, the privilege could be claimed if it were the other party's mental health status that is needed in the case and if the other party did not plan to introduce the evidence.

Defamation is a tort involving an action that injures one's reputation in the community. The particular action can be written, called **libel**, or verbal, called **slander**. Both of these torts fall into the category of defamation. Very few cases exist where a nurse has been sued for either libel or slander. However, there are a few cases where a nurse has successfully sued other individuals for defamation. Nurses have sued physicians for accusing them of negligence or malpractice in front of family members or fellow workers. Any statement that injures a person's reputation, verbal or written, published or said to someone other than the person who is the subject of the statement may constitute defamation. The defense to defamation is that the statement is true. The judge or jury must be convinced by the evidence presented that defamation has occurred.

Assault and Battery are two torts involving intentional acts. **Assault** is a threat or an attempt to make bodily contact with another person, without the person's consent. For example, if a patient refused an injection and the nurse then attempted to administer it, this is thought to be assault. If the nurse restrains the patient and administers the shot, she has committed **battery.** Battery is the assault carried out.

Every person has the legal right to consent to treatment. Treatments and procedures cannot be carried out without the patient's permission. Therefore, obtaining the patient's permission before performing nursing care and treatment is an essential part of nursing practice. Without the consent and agreement of the patient, the nurse may commit a battery against the patient.

False imprisonment is a tort that involves intentional placement of someone in an area that has physical barriers; with force of intimidation, someone is kept in a place against his will. The use of restraints or psychiatric isolation rooms as nursing intervention needs careful scrutiny, because it may constitute the tort of false imprisonment. The only acceptable use of restraints is to protect a patient from harm. Restraints should never be used in a punitive manner. Restraints, when necessary, should be used for short time periods and only to safeguard a patient through a crisis. Because of recent lawsuits, many health facilities require that restraints be used only after physician review and treatment order. The order for restraint is good for only a short time, after which reevaluation by a physician is required before the order can continue or be renewed.

Invasion of Privacy is a tort that involves confidential information that is revealed without permission to someone not entitled to know it. Cases involving this tort in the health care area have been successful. For example, pictures of patients have been taken without their permission and then used in texts for medical education. While this is an admirable use, permission must be obtained before displaying part of another's body. Another example of invasion of privacy is telling someone who is not part of the health team details of test results or a patient diagnosis.

Contracts

Contracts are agreements or obligations into which two or more individuals or agencies enter. They are thought of as promises made between consenting individuals or agencies. Contracts have three elements that, if they exist, the law will enforce in order to protect society's interest in having promises performed. The elements are: offer, acceptance of the offer, and consideration.

Contracts can be made verbally as well as in writing. An employment contract, for example, is usually in writing and sets forth the terms of what the employer and employee will do in order to carry out the employment agreement. Terms of contracts can be negotiated before the offer of a job is finalized. Most often, the act of signing an agreement signals the acceptance of an offer by both parties. The most frequent example of consideration in the employment contract is the exchange of services or work for payment. Both parties gain something and both give something that, except for the agreement, they would not have given.

Nurses make contracts with their clients daily when negotiating mutual goals. While most are verbal agreements, nurses make promises to clients and vice versa regarding health care. However, most case law discussing contracts and nurses deals with grievance and employment situations and not agreements between nurses and clients in delivering nursing services within an agency. This is not to say, however, that future litigation involving nurses will not focus on this area.

When a nurse contracts with a supplemental staffing agency to be temporarily assigned to another agency, that assignment is based upon a contract between these two agencies. The most important implication for the nurse involved in these contracts is the sorting out of responsibilities of everyone involved. The nurse is personally liable for her own actions; the responsible employer, however, is the supplemental staffing agency and not the agency in which the nurse actually renders the service. Nurses, prior to agreeing to be temporarily assigned, should review all contracts that exist and in particular should note any terms that relate to malpractice, negligence, or insurance. Be sure to ask questions and understand all the terms of any contract to which you are about to be subjected.

The relationship between a health care agency and an educational institution, in which students will use the agency for learning, is also a contractual one. The agency agrees to allow instructors and students into the agency, and the educational institution is thus provided experiences for its students. Most contracts have a term that states that the health care agency retains responsibility for patient care, and the instructor's responsibility is to supervise the students. Should a student make a mistake and be negligent, the contract helps determine who the responsible parties are.

First and foremost, students are responsible for their own actions. If they commit an act of negligence, they will be measured by what a nurse would have done in a like situation. The instructor and staff of the agency also may be negligent but only if they failed to evaluate or supervise the student. If the instructor knew a student was weak in a particular area and did not take steps to prevent mistakes as a result of the weakness, then the instructor shares liability with the student. Most educational institutions require students and instructors to carry malpractice insurance. In addition, contracts between schools and agencies often require malpractice insurance.

Many nurses hold their own malpractice insurance. Obtaining this type of insurance involves establishing a contract with an insurance company and paying for the coverage. The two basic questions to ask in determining how much coverage to purchase are: What is the area of practice? What personal assets are at stake? If you are practicing in a high risk area of practice, such as critical care, anesthesia, or emergency nursing, or if you have substantial personal assets at risk, you will want to obtain higher amounts of coverage.

After these two areas are settled, the most important area to cover with the insurance agent and the contract are the terms about exclusions, since most insurance for malpractice will cover only that. Therefore, if you are indicted on a criminal charge, legal fees for an attorney will not be covered by your malpractice insurance. Or if you are accused of violating the nurse practice act, your malpractice insurance will not provide legal fees. There are often other exclusions identified in the contract that should be studied carefully.

The other critical point to know about the insurance contract is whether there is a difference in the time it is effective. Some insurance contracts specify that a person will only be covered if the contract is in effect both when the malpractice incident occurred and when the claim of malpractice is made. Other insurance contracts will cover the individual at either of the times mentioned above. Understanding when the contract is effective is important, because the time between an incident of malpractice and when the claim is filed can be a period of several years.

Criminal Law

A **crime** is an offense against the public at large. Distinguished from a civil wrong, where private individuals are the parties involved, a criminal wrong will be prosecuted or brought by the state. The purpose of criminal prosecution is to protect the interests of the public as a whole. The elements of crime and the punishments they carry are usually part of a state's legislation and judicial opinions.

In 1981, Wiley[1] described the experiences of several registered and licensed practical nurses with criminal law. These nurses were employed in intensive care units or medical surgical units of hospitals, and because the patients they had cared for had died in suspicious manners, they were accused of either homicide or murder. The deaths were associated with drugs given by the nurses and their activities involving patient life support mechanisms, such as respirators.

While most of the criminal charges were

overturned or the nurse was acquitted, the nurses' rub with the criminal justice system led Wiley to make three recommendations:

- follow hospital (or agency) policies and procedures
- carry your own malpractice insurance because a nurse's interest is different from a hospital's
- retain a lawyer *early*.[1]

Constitutional Law

Constitutional law already has been mentioned in relation to a source of law. The U.S. Constitution and individual state constitutions set forth the structure and function of the different governments and describe the relationship between government and individual citizens.

The hallmark of constitutional law, which is important to discuss here, is due process rights. Due process is actually two rights in one. Every citizen is entitled to notice, to the opportunity to be heard, and to have the facts stated as they occurred. For example, if a nurse is accused of violating the state nurse practice act, the government (in this case the state government) must notify the nurse of the charges and set up a time for a hearing. At the hearing, the nurse has an opportunity to hear the charges and to refute them; this is best done with the help of a retained attorney. The evidence presented can be challenged by the nurse, the hearing officer, or nursing board, depending on the state. During the hearing, the nurse has a right to cross examine any testimony or other evidence presented.

In the case of a disciplinary action taken by an employer against the nurse, the nurse is entitled to similar due process rights. The nurse is entitled to know why the disciplinary action is being taken and to refute the reason. Because of due process rights, a nurse also can examine her own personnel file and insert a statement denying or supporting its contents. In addition, nurses are entitled to know what appeal procedure can be followed in order to challenge decisions made by their supervisors.

Legislation

Legislation is law made by various governmentally authorized bodies at the local, state, and federal levels. The legislature is made up of elected officials and is one of three branches of government. Legislation is developed in a formal process that includes bill writing, approval with committees and houses of the legislature, passage by the entire legislature, and, usually, signing by the President (federal), governor (state) or mayor (local).

While legislation has an impact on and shapes most of nursing practice, the area of community health nursing has been particularly influenced by public health laws and regulations. Two examples of legislation other than licensing that relates to most nurses are reporting statutes and the Good Samaritan Act.

Reporting statutes are laws that require specified individuals to report to designated authorities events that they have witnessed or suspect to be true. The reporting of suspicions is to be done carefully and in good faith to avoid recklessness and malice. One reporting statute that effects most nurses is one that requires a nurse to report suspected child abuse or neglect. While the particular details—to whom and when to report and a penalty for not reporting— vary among different states, in all states nurses are specifically mentioned as responsible for reporting, along with others.

Good Samaritan Acts are state legislation that is intended to encourage people to render emergency first aid or care that may save someone's life at the scene of an accident. The encouragement comes from the fact that if negligence occurs while attempting to save another's life the person who received the negligent care cannot sue the one responsible for the negligence. In some states, nurses are entitled to immunity under Good Samaritan Acts while in others they are not. The act, however, usually applies only to individuals who do not receive remuneration for what they did and what they did was not gross negligence. Gross negligence is an act that is extremely unreasonable, reckless, or wanton. If a court decides that a nurse acted in a grossly negligent manner, then a lawsuit can be maintained against the nurse. Most states have other legislation that provides immunity from lawsuits for individuals employed by fire departments, rescue squads, or other agencies that deliver emergency medical services.

RECORDKEEPING RESPONSIBILITIES

Regardless of where nurses work or practice, recordkeeping is an important responsibility. Records have many uses in the health care system.

Records used by nurses in their place of employment can be divided into two categories. **Clinical records** are all those documents that pertain to the care of a particular client. **Administrative records** are kept solely for the purpose of administering the agency or facility. The difference between these two major types of records is clearer when one examines selected examples of records used in a health agency.

The patient's individual health record is a clinical record. It contains information about the patient's stay or contact with every health provider that may be involved in his care. From the time of admission to discharge, details of assessment, plans, interventions, and progress are recorded. These records are called patient charts. In most agencies, a patient's chart includes the following information:

- the medical and nursing admission information
- a personal data sheet listing name, address, age, marital status, etc.

- consent or permission sheets (when applicable)
- medical history
- nursing history
- physical examination findings
- medical progress sheets
- nursing progress sheets or nurses notes
- laboratory finding results sheets
- procedure finding sheets (e.g., EKG)
- temperature, pulse, respiration, and blood pressure flow sheets
- physician order sheets
- medicine order sheets
- discharge planning sheet
- utilization review sheet.

Some agencies that deliver services to families, such as community or mental health services, keep family records. These usually contain notes on the family as well as individuals in that family.

Administrative records include documents such as incident reports, valuables lists, or minutes of meetings of different segments of the agency. These records sometimes relate to an individual client but are usually kept separate from the client's clinical record. One purpose, for example, of the incident report is to alert the risk manager, insurance company, or quality assurance director where and what type of mistakes are being made in the institution. Everything that happens to the patient is recorded in that clinical record, and an incident report that, when completed, contains similar information to that recorded in the clinical record, is often required by the agency.

Records reflect the quality of care delivered and serve to organize the care given. Patients and health care providers rely on records' being complete. When patients direct that records be transferred to other agencies or health services, continuity of care can be preserved if records are complete and include a discharge summary.

This summary can provide a synopsis of the care delivered and the patient's reaction to interventions.

Other uses of records include research, data collection, and evaluation of patient care. For the agency's purposes, records can be reviewed to examine many aspects of care and organization. Trends in needs and services can be found in records and agencies often plan future services from them. Conducting clinical record reviews within the agency usually doesn't require the patient's permission. Confidentiality, however, must always be maintained. If the research project involves more than records, laws, rules, and regulations of state and federal governments, then institutional policies must be followed regarding informed consent and other human rights protections.

Another major use of the patient record is as evidence in a legal dispute. Client records are considered business records of the agency and are admissible as such under rules of evidence. Lawsuits often are won and lost based on what is in the record. While testimony is also another form of evidence, the written record is seen as more accurate and reliable, since it was written at the time of the incident in question. Because lawsuits sometimes take years to emerge, one's memory (e.g., testimony at trial) is not as reliable as the written record. Because of the reliability of the clinical record, great emphasis is placed on the completeness of the record by individual health care providers and institutions alike.

Access to Records

A major health care legal issue is the right of access by patients to their own records. Within the health care system a range of positions exists. Patients in the military health care system keep their records with them, for example, while in other health care agencies, patients must get a subpoena to access their records. In the latter situation, the patient often has to be anticipating litigation or suing the agency in order to get a subpoena from a court. However, the majority of state legislatures have passed laws requiring agencies to establish reasonable policies and procedures so that patients may access their own records. A copy of the applicable state law should be part of every agency's policy manual. Policies that have been established often cover when and under what circumstances patients see their records. For example, one policy provides that patients who ask to see their health records may review them between the hours of 9 a.m. and 5 p.m. and only when a medical records technician is present to answer questions.

In the last 15 years, most agencies have established open and flexible policies so that patients are able to access their records easier than in the past. The only remaining area where access is still more restrictive is psychiatric records. Some policies allow physicians to object to patients seeing their psychiatric records, in which case, the policy or even the state legislation may provide that the patient be provided a summary of the record and an appeal mechanism for challenging the physician's decision to withhold the record.

The legal issue of access to patient records has changed dramatically in favor of the patient. The law generally recognizes the patient's control over the information in the record. The patient is the one who holds the right to confidentiality and gives permission for access to the record to those not involved in care in the agency. Permission from the patient must be obtained prior to release or transfer of records to others.

Advances in computer technology and access to records is increasingly a concern for both patients and providers. This situation raises legal issues of access, privacy, and confidentiality. Management of medical records must involve a mandate to maintain and protect the privacy of patients. The use of computers benefits the delivery of health care but increases the risk of loss of confidentiality. Protection of confidentiality in automated systems includes controls and checks on who can access the data. In addition, code numbers and other methods have been developed to guard patient privacy.[2]

Informed Consent

Informed consent indicates that patients have had treatments or procedures explained to them and they have given consent based on that information. Informed consent given prior to medical and surgical intervention is an absolute requirement in nonemergency situations. The per-

---

Date _____ Time _____ P.M.
                                                                            A.M.

Name of Patient _____

I authorize the performance upon _____

_____ of the following
(myself or name of patient)

operation or procedure _____

_____
(state nature and extent of operation)

to be performed by and under the direction of _____
                                               (name of doctor)

I consent to the performance of operations and/or diagnostic or therapeutic procedures in addition to or different from those now contemplated (including, but not limited to, the performance of services involving pathology and radiology), whether or not arising from presently unforeseen conditions that the above named doctor or his associates or assistants may consider necessary or advisable in the course of operation.

I hereby authorize and direct the anesthesiologist and/or his associates or assistants to provide for the administration and maintenance of the anesthesia and such other services as are deemed advisable.

I hereby authorize the hospital pathologist and/or his associates or assistants to use his/their discretion in the disposal of any severed tissue or member.

The doctor has fully explained to me the nature and purpose of the operation, possible alternative methods of treatment, the risks involved, and the possibility of complications. I hereby give an informed and considered consent and no warranty or guarantee has been given by anyone as to cure or as to the results that may be obtained. I understand that the operation to be performed on me or any operations under any type of anesthesia may conceivably result in death or in temporary or permanent total or partial disability.

I understand the terms operation and procedure, as used above, shall include diagnostic and therapeutic operations and procedures.

Signed _____
(Check one:)
☐ Patient
☐ Parent
☐ Guardian
☐ Other or person
   authorized to consent for
_____   patient
witness

Figure 8-7.   Sample Consent Form

son conducting the treatment or surgery (usually a physician) is responsible for obtaining the consent; the person who would be committing the tort of battery by touching someone without expressed consent. That person may also be negligent if the consent is not informed.

The nurse's role in informed consent for interventions by the physician is carrying out an agency policy or administrative function. The nurse is accountable for the agency policy. The usual policy requires the nurse to ask the patient to sign a form (see Figure 8-7) that documents the informed consent given by the physician. The nurse should assess patients for reading ability, and if they cannot read, the form should be read to them.

By getting the form signed, the nurse may be the witness to the patient's signature. If this is the case, it should be stated on the form: witnessing signature only. If the nurse was present when the physician discussed the treatment or surgery and explained the risks, benefits, and alternatives to a coherent, legally competent individual, then the nurse is witnessing the informed consent and the client's acknowledgment of that fact. In the latter situation the nurse, as a more extensively involved witness, can provide better evidence for the physician should the patient later raise the issue of informed consent.

Future thought by the nursing profession will need to be directed to the question of informed consent and consent forms for nursing interventions. The **ANA Code of Ethics**,[3] states that obtaining the prior consent of clients is an ethical obligation of the nurse. The major elements of informed consent are:

a. Consent must be given voluntarily

b. Consent must be given by an individual with the capacity and competence to consent

c. Consent needs to involve enough information so that the client can be the ultimate decisionmaker

In emergency situations, health care providers may intervene to save someone's life without obtaining consent, or if the client is a minor, the guardian or parent is the legally competent individual to consent. In many states, minors may consent themselves for selected and specific types of health care. For example, in most states minors may consent to treatment for mental illness, venereal disease, alcohol and drug addictions, pregnancy, contraception, and abortion.

Common Charting Errors

Despite concerns about the types and uses of records, access to records, and informed consent, major accountability and quality of care of the health provider is reflected in accurate and complete recordkeeping. Most common mistakes in recording include failure to:

- record accurate and complete information
- state objective, factual data
- document concisely and legibly, in chronological order
- alter records according to agency policy
- maintain records in a safe, confidential manner
- sign with legal name and proper identification
- observe agency policy on countersigning
- use accepted abbreviations
- meet other existing agency policies or bylaws.

Most errors are self-explanatory but two are worth further discussion: alterations to records and countersigning. Changes in records become necessary when a mistake has been made in the record. A single line drawn through the mistake with the word "error" printed next to the nurses' initials is an appropriate way of correcting the mistake. White-out, cut and paste, and obliteration of the mistake is not appropriate. These methods only leave a question in a jury's mind about what the writer is trying to hide. The correct information is placed in the record in chronological order and labeled "late entry."

The effect of countersigning is usually governed by agency policy. Generally, if one countersigns, it is as if he observed or participated in what is being documented equally with the person who actually delivered the care. Countersigning alleviates no one from responsibility or accountability for his actions. If an agency requires countersigning, its purpose usually is to ensure close supervision and direction for certain types of employees. For example, the nursing supervisor may countersign receipt of physician orders by the staff nurse who has just started the job. The supervisor and staff nurse are equally accountable for the proper processing of those orders.

MANAGEMENT OF MEDICAL ORDERS

One of the many important contributions nurses make to the care of patients is management of medical orders. Receiving, scrutinizing, implementing, and evaluating the effects of medical orders are critical functions of the nurse. It remains one of the dependent functions of the nurse who, according to state law, is dependent on the physician to prescribe medications before they can be given.

Medical orders must come from a licensed physician. In some states, dentists are allowed to legally prescribe medications, too. The safest way for nurses to receive medication orders is through written communications by the physician on the doctor's order sheet. Extenuating circumstances occasionally lead nurses to accepting verbal orders or telephone orders. If this is the case, orders should come directly from a physician. In the best interest of the patients, nurses, agencies, and physician, once a telephone order has been accepted and written on the doctors order sheet, the physician should sign for it on his or her next visit to the agency. When nurses are preparing to accept a verbal or telephone order, they should have another RN listen to the order as well and cosign the chart. After taking the order, nurses should read it back to the physician to be certain that it has been written on the chart accurately. The person who takes the order down should sign the physician name, her own name, the date, time, and the letters T.O. or V.O. (to represent telephone or verbal order).

Standing orders are predetermined directions for potential patient situations, such as what to do if the patient develops a fever. They need to be approved jointly and equally by the physician writing them and the nurse implementing them. Standing orders are to be used in clearly defined, predetermined situations only. Standing orders are more often used in community settings where access to a physician may be limited or distant.

The purpose of standing orders is to provide the nurse with power to act and to expand her usual role into an area of medical practice. The standing order protects the nurse from charges of practicing medicine without a license. Because of this, nurses should examine their skills, experience, and education in light of the standing order. Nurses should not accept orders they don't feel competent to administer.

The nurse is legally accountable for evaluating physician orders. Nursing judgment must be brought to bear on each order the nurse implements. Appropriate medication, right dose and route must be observed. Any question about an order should be directed to the originator, and all questions should be answered prior to implementing any order.

Since the administration of medications and medical treatments is the area most susceptible to lawsuit, careful scrutiny of orders is essential to eliminating errors and lawsuits involving nurses.

When physician orders involve life sustaining or resuscitation measures, nursing may be caught between agency policy and physician order. A medical order that, if implemented, would force the nurse to violate agency policy is never an appropriate order. The nurse should notify the supervisor or director of nursing who, in turn, should notify the agency administration. For example, if a hospital policy says no resuscitation orders must be in writing and the physician refuses to write the order, yet expects that no resuscitation will be given, the nurse must follow the agency policy, notify the nursing supervisor, and resuscitate the patient. In this situation, the existence of the policy serves to protect the nurse, who, if a resuscitation is given and no written order was recorded, might be liable for negligence or malpractice.

ACCOUNTABILITY FOR PRACTICE

Professional nurses are accountable to many different sources. Nurses relate, report, or account to themselves, others, organizations, and the government. Because nurses must account to such a large variety of sources, sometimes these sources conflict with one another. Nurses also have certain legal duties and responsibilities because of the variety of positions they hold. For example, nurses have a written or verbal contract with their employer; must relate to physician orders in order to give medications and carry out treatment; must

act in their own best interests and in the best interests of their patients; are members of a group of professionals; and are licensed as safe practitioners by the government.

Licensure and Nurse Practice Acts

"Licensure" is a state governmental activity. Each state legislature, through its police power, can take steps to protect the public's health, safety, and welfare. Licensure of nurses is designed to ensure that every nurse in that state can function at a minimum level of performance. In this way the state can be sure that when one uses the initials RN or LPN, the care being received is from someone who is a safe and reasonable practitioner.

State Boards of Nursing. A piece of legislation in each state, the **Nurse Practice Act,** establishes and identifies certain powers to a board or commission of nursing. This licensing board is part of the executive branch of government. In addition to its power to grant nursing licenses, a board usually has the power to deny or revoke licenses, accredit nursing programs, and write regulations on nursing.

While the act lists many reasons why nurses' licenses may be denied or revoked, the main reasons include:

1. abuse of drugs or alcohol that affects patient care
2. impersonating, by using the initials RN or LPN when unlicensed
3. ordinary or gross negligence or unethical conduct
4. conviction of a crime.

Through the regulation power, the board may write further detailed rules to govern nursing in that state. Regulations do have the force of law and must go through a formal process that includes public comment before they become effective. The following are selected topics that state nursing regulations cover:

1. Examination procedures, test development, and fees
2. Requirements for renewal of license
3. Hearing procedures
4. Minimum requirements for approving RN or LPN education programs
5. Practice of Nurse Midwife
6. Practice of Nurse Anesthetist
7. Practice of Nurse Practitioner.

State boards may require nursing education programs in their state to meet minimum standards written in regulations. In some states, nursing schools must obtain the accreditation or approval of the state board as well as the National League for Nursing, which is a private nursing organization that accredits all schools of nursing. In other instances, schools need to meet government and private group requirements.

Another major aspect of nurse practice acts is the definition of what constitutes nursing practice. See Figure 8-8 for examples of state nurse practice acts.

Comparison of practice definitions among and across professional groups is essential for understanding what constitutes nursing and where questions of overlap exist. Nursing has independent as well as dependent functions that are delegated to nursing by physicians, such as administering medications.

There are differences in the laws from state to state. Therefore, it is imperative that every nurse obtain and review a copy of the practice act and regulations to which they are accountable. These are located in the state code of laws and code of regulation in most public libraries or can be obtained by writing to the state nursing board or commission.

Institutional Licensure. As an alternative to the state government licensing

Maryland
Practice registered nursing Health Occupations 7-101 (f)
"Practice registered nursing means the performance of acts requiring substantial specialized knowledge, judgment and skill based on the biological, physiological, behavioral or sociological sciences as the basis for assessment, nursing diagnosis, planning, implementation and evaluation of the practice of nursing in order to: maintain health; prevent illness, or care for or rehabilitate the ill, injured, or infirm.
For these purposes, practice registered nursing includes: administration; teaching; counseling; supervision, delegation and evaluation of nursing practice; execution of therapeutic regimen, including the administration of medication and treatment; independent nursing functions and delegated medical functions; and performance of additional acts authorized by the board under 7-205."

Delaware
Practice of professional nursing Chapter 19 Nursing and Schools of Nursing 1902 (6)
"Practice of professional nursing" means the performance for compensation of any act in the observation, care and counsel of the ill, injured or infirm, or in the maintenance of health or prevention of illness of others, or in the supervision and teaching of other personnel, or the administration of medications and treatments as prescribed by a licensed physician or dentist requiring substantial specialized judgment and skill and based on knowledge and application of the principles of biological, physical and social science. The foregoing shall not be deemed to include acts of diagnosis or prescription of therapeutic or corrective measures."

Figure 8-8. Selected Definition of Registered Nursing Practice: Maryland and Delaware.

nurses, institutional licensure is a controversial idea that has surfaced many times in the literature. While this type of licensure exists presently for some personnel, it does not exist for nursing because of the state practice acts. Institutional licensure means that each employer or institution of employment would be responsible for licensing health workers within rules established by state boards or private accrediting groups that regulated those institutions. For example, hospitals are regulated by state boards and are accredited by the Joint Commission on Accreditation of Hospitals (JCAH). The JCAH is a private group related to the American Hospital Association. Institutional licensure can place in the hands of non-nurses the responsibility for shaping and defining the scope of nursing practice. For this reason, the American Nurses Association, the National Association for Practical Nurse Education, and many other groups and individuals are opposed to institutional licensure. Since most state nursing boards are made up of RNs and LPNs with an occasional consumer or other health care provider member, these organizations prefer that nurses be governed and regulated by nursing rather than the employing institution.

On the other hand, critics, including those who write and make laws, continue to scrutinize the state licensing boards. They often describe them as monopolies of self-interest. Many legislatures in the past few years have passed sunset laws that require that all units of government demonstrate to the legislature that such units are worthy of continuing. This required that boards conduct cost-effectiveness reviews and program evaluation. Recently under a sunset law, the New Hampshire State Board of Nursing almost went out of business. Only through massive rallying of efforts did the New Hampshire nurses maintain their state licensure; otherwise anyone in New Hampshire claiming to be a nurse could attempt to function as one.

Mandatory Continuing Education. Most practice acts specify that renewal of a license requires only the payment of a certain fee. Most fees are nominal and paid annually or every two years. In recent years, the nursing profession has voiced concerns about renewal only requiring the payment of a fee. As an assurance of continuing competency to practice, a handful of states have passed a requirement that in order to renew a license to practice nurs-

ing, every nurse needs to produce evidence of attendance at continuing education programs.

In 1982, the mandatory continuing education (MCE) requirement existed in California, Florida, Iowa, Kansas, Kentucky, Massachusetts, Minnesota, Nevada, and New Mexico. Most of these states began with a 5–10 contact hour requirement and gradually increased the number of contact hours required for renewal. The majority of the states require 30 contact hours every two years and limit self-instruction or home study to 5 or 6 contact hours of the total requirement.

There are many pros and cons to mandatory continuing education. Proponents say MCE will assure the public that licensed nurses will continue to be safe and reasonable practitioners and that they have kept up with medical advances and nursing practice since their initial schooling. Opponents of MCE see it as infringement on the individual nurse's freedoms and make the point that attendence at programs doesn't necessarily lead to safe and reasonable competence to practice. Recently, the state of South Dakota rescinded its MCE requirements, while several other states are studying the issue, and others have prepared legislation to be introduced at future legislative sessions. Other states are considering a broader range of options not limited only to MCE or required continued competency tests.

Self-Regulation and Professional Associations

Activities or programs that private associations or groups of professionals conduct to oversee or regulate themselves are called self-regulatory activities. The major distinction of this type of accountability from other types is that it is done by nongovernmental or private groups. Examples of activities by nursing associations include: writing and implementing a code of ethics, writing and implementing standards of practice, certification, and collective bargaining. Only the last topic involves some governmental regulation. It is included here because a major program of some nurses associations is contract negotiation and collective bargaining.

Self-regulatory activities do have prescribed governmental limits. For example, under antitrust or restraint of trade laws, professional organizations may not prohibit their members from advertising services. An activity that is prohibited is for a professional organization to tell its members how much to charge for services. Called fee setting, this activity creates and builds a monopoly that through the above mentioned laws, the government will act to prevent and prohibit.

Code of Ethics. Several nursing organizations have developed policy statements and codes about what constitutes appropriate and expected nursing behavior. The main association for registered nurses is the American Nurses Association (ANA).

One characteristic of a profession is the existence of a code of ethics. Such a code offers one framework for self-regulation. The *ANA Code for Nurses*[3] (see Figure 8-9) is intended to be a guideline for nurses and nursing organizations. It is used to judge what ethical conduct is and often provides helpful suggestions on how to handle problems nurses may confront in their practice. The ANA has published the code of ethics with interpretive statements that are of particular interest, because it offers nurses suggested ways of dealing with incompetent colleagues or anyone whose behavior may negatively affect the client's or the public's health and safety. Other code items discuss advertising, standards, confidentiality, competence, research, employment conditions, and relationships with others.

The ANA has a Committee on Ethics that serves as a resource to individual nurses and state nursing associations and whose

1. The nurse provides services with respect for human dignity and the uniqueness of the client unrestricted by considerations of social or economic status, personal attributes, or the nature of health problems.
2. The nurse safeguards the client's right to privacy by judiciously protecting information of a confidential nature.
3. The nurse acts to safeguard the client and the public when health care and safety are affected by incompetent, unethical, or illegal practice of any person.
4. The nurse assumes responsibility and accountability for individual nursing judgments and actions.
5. The nurse maintains competence in nursing.
6. The nurse exercises informed judgment and uses individual competence and qualifications as criteria in seeking consultation, accepting responsibilities, and delegating nursing activities to others.
7. The nurse participates in activities that contribute to the ongoing development of the profession's body of knowledge.
8. The nurse participates in the profession's efforts to implement and improve standards of nursing.
9. The nurse participates in the profession's efforts to establish and maintain conditions of employment conducive to high quality nursing care.
10. The nurse participates in the profession's effort to protect the public from misinformation and misrepresentation and to maintain the integrity of nursing.
11. The nurse collaborates with members of the health professions and other citizens in promoting community and national efforts to meet the health needs of the public.

Reprinted with the permission of the American Nurses Association

Figure 8-9. Code for Nurses.

Council on Practice is charged with implementing the *ANA Code*. The Committee has issued *Guidelines for Implementing the Code for Nurses* to be used by state councils when they receive a complaint of unethical conduct by a registered nurse. Other publications on ethical conduct of nurses are available from professional organizations (see annotated bibliography).

Standards of Practice. Another activity that nursing associations are involved in is the development of standards by which nursing practice can be evaluated. The standards of practice issued by the ANA are general statements of the content of nursing practice. Intended to assure the quality of nursing practice, the ANA standards are written by the different practice divisions of the ANA. Many speciality nursing organizations have developed their own standards or have worked with the ANA in the development of the ANA standards. Standards have been used by indi-

vidual nurses and nursing departments of health care agencies as resources for developing nursing audits and peer review systems. Both activities are examples of nurses regulating and evaluating their own practice.

Certification. A third self-regulatory activity by private nursing organizations is certification. One example is ANA certification (see Figure 8-10). Available to individual members of the ANA, certification means that a registered nurse has successfully completed an examination process beyond the state licensure examination

ANA Practice Division*	Certification Offerings**	Certified 1980–82	Total Certified
Community Health Nursing	• Adult Nurse Practitioner	1245	1855
	• Family Nurse Practitioner	1199	1860
	• Community Health Nurse	54	114
	• School Nurse Practitioner	197	197
Gerontological Nursing	• Gerontological Nurse	221	374
	• Gerontological Nurse Practitioner	37	37
Maternal and Child Health Nursing	• Child and Adolescent Nurse	25	25
	• Pediatric Nurse Practitioner	201	285
Medical/Surgical Nursing	• Medical/Surgical Nurse	169	211
	• Medical/Surgical Nurse Specialist	71	86
Psychiatric and Mental Health Nursing	• Psychiatric and Mental Health Nurse	249	364
	• Adult Psychiatric and Mental Health Clinical Nurse Specialist	253	407
	• Child Adolescent Psychiatric and Mental Health Clinical Nurse Specialist	14	25
	Total	3935	5840

*Source: ANA House of Delegates Reports 1980–1982. Kansas City, MO: ANA, 1982, p. 48, 55, 60, 67, 71.
**New certification offerings planned are: Maternal and Child Nurse; High-risk Perinatal Nurse.

Figure 8-10. ANA Generalist and Specialist Certification.

that indicates that the nurse has a higher level of competency of nursing within a speciality area. The ANA House of Delegates biennial report includes information about certification. Information about requirements for taking the examinations can be obtained by writing to the ANA Practice Division that gives the particular exam.

Not only is certification a sign of having passed an advanced competency rating but it also is a sign of having passed the scrutiny and evaluation of peers. In addition, as the trend increases for nurses to receive direct reimbursement for services, certification may be a necessary step for that reimbursement. Insurance companies, the federal government, other third party payors, and private individuals may see certification as a measure of an individual's ability to deliver services and, hence, require it before one would be eligible to receive funding for services provided.

Collective Bargaining. While governmental regulation and law also oversees collective bargaining by nurses, the ANA, through state nurses associations, acts as a bargaining agent and unit for its members. Collective bargaining recently has become a widespread option available for nurses. Nurses should make the decision to participate based on their individual needs. Bargaining and negotiating a contract for nurses as a group usually focuses on benefits for the nurse who works in that particular agency. Improved staffing, increased salary, and other benefits may lead to improved patient care. The process of negotiating a contract ultimately may lead to a decision on whether or not to strike in order to obtain the goals of the group. This is a very controversial question for nurses, and it should be explored through further reading and study of the issue. As seen earlier, the *ANA Code for Nurses* (Item 9) endorses as appropriate a nurse's involvement in collective bargaining.

Despite the availability of most state nurses associations as collective bargaining agents, nurses have chosen to be represented by non-nursing organizations. School nurses, for example, may be represented by the American Federation of Teachers (AFT) or the National Education Association (NEA). Nursing faculty may participate in the American Association of University Professors (AAUP) or the AFT. Other nurses may be members of selected AFL-CIO unions. Some groups of nurses, such as federal or state employees, however, may or may not have the right to collectively bargain or to strike. Still others can belong only to non-nursing unions.

Patient Rights and Responsibilities: Best Interests of Patients

While patients who enter institutions because of illness may be dependent on others for care and assistance, they continue to maintain rights that existed prior to entering such a facility. Patients, on entering an agency, assume responsibilities toward that agency, such as abiding by its rules and regulations or financial obligations.

A general rule is that every adult (defined in most states as at least 18 or 21 years of age) is competent unless, through a formal legal proceeding, it is determined that the individual is not competent. In the latter situation, a guardian usually is appointed to make all decisions for the incompetent person. In addition, a guardian may be appointed to make only medical, financial, or contractual decisions. The guardian or parent of an individual under 18 or 21 years of age sees to the rights and responsibilities of the child and is deemed to act in the best interests of the incompetent or child.

Every individual possesses rights and obligations. All JCAH-accredited hospitals

1. The patient has the right to considerate and respectful care.

2. The patient has the right to obtain from his physician complete current information concerning his diagnosis, treatment, and prognosis in terms the patient can be reasonably expected to understand. When it is not medically advisable to give such information to the patient, the information should be made available to an appropriate person in his behalf. He has the right to know by name, the physician responsible for coordinating his care.

3. The patient has the right to receive from his physician information necessary to give informed consent prior to the start of any procedure and/or treatment. Except in emergencies, such information for informed consent, should include but not necessarily be limited to the specific procedure and/or treatment, the medically significant risks involved, and the probable duration of incapacitation. Where medically significant alternatives for care or treatment exists, or when the patient requests information concerning medical alternatives, the patient has the right to know the name of the person responsible for the procedures and/or treatment.

4. The patient has the right to refuse treatment to the extent permitted by law, and to be informed of the medical consequences of this action.

5. The patient has the right to every consideration of his privacy concerning his own medical care program. Case discussion, consultation, examination, and treatment are confidential and should be conducted discreetly. Those not involved in his care must have the permission of the patient to be present.

6. The patient has the right to expect that all communications and records pertaining to his case should be treated as confidential.

7. The patient has the right to expect that within its capacity a hospital must make reasonable response to the request of a patient for services. The hospital must provide evaluation, service, and/or referral as indicated by the urgency of the case. When medically permissible a patient may be transferred to another facility only after he has received complete information and explanation concerning the needs for and alternatives to such a transfer. The institution to which the patient is to be transferred must first have accepted the patient for transfer.

8. The patient has the right to obtain information as to any relationship of his hospital to other health care and educational institutions insofar as his care is concerned. The patient has the right to obtain information as to the existence of any professional relationships among individuals, by name, who are treating him.

9. The patient has the right to be advised if the hospital proposes to engage in or perform human experimentation affecting his care or treatment. The patient has the right to refuse to participate in such research projects.

10. The patient has the right to expect reasonable continuity of care. He has the right to know in advance what appointment times and physicians are available and where. The patient has the right to expect that the hospital will provide a mechanism whereby he is informed by his physician or a delegate of the physician of the patient's continuing health care requirements following discharge.

11. The patient has the right to examine and receive an explanation of his bill regardless of source of payment.

12. The patient has the right to know what hospital rules and regulations apply to his conduct as a patient.

Figure 8-11. "A Patient's Bill of Rights." ©American Hospital Association, 1975.

are accountable to the American Hospital Association's Bill (see Figure 8-11), therefore nursing is also accountable for seeing that patients' rights are protected.

Most rights in the AHA bill are legally enforceable, meaning that legislation or judicial opinion exists that establishes each right as one that the law will enforce.

Nurses Rights and Responsibilities: Best Interests of Nurses

The delivery of nursing services is not an effort where only one group's interests should be observed. Nurses have rights and responsibilities that balance and complement those of others, including patients.

One bill of nurses' rights and responsibilities was written by the Maryland Nurses Association (MNA) (see Figure 8-12), developed by the MNA Council and Human Rights, and approved by the Board of Directors. This bill describes nursing rights and responsibilities according to different relationships (for example, the nurse and the patient, and the nurse and employer).

We, the Council on Human Rights of the Maryland Nurses Association, in order to promote increased knowledge and understanding of the rights and responsibilities of all registered nurses, have developed The Bill of Rights for Registered Nurses. We propose that this Bill will aid in educating consumers and health care professionals about the rights of registered nurses, as well as their corresponding responsibilities. Therefore, we submit the Bill of Rights for Registered Nurses as a positions statement of the Maryland Nurses Association.

The nurse has a right;	The nurse has a responsibility:
to practice according to the Maryland Nurse Practice Act.	to assume personal accountability for individual nursing judgments and actions which consider the individual value systems and the uniqueness of each patient/client.
to make independent nursing judgments.	
to question any delegated medical order or any plan of care that may cause possible harm to the patient/client or others.	
	to implement the nursing process in providing individualized nursing care.
to refuse to carry out any delegated medical order or any plan of care that may cause possible harm to the patient/client or others.	to safeguard the patient/client and the public from incompetent, unethical or illegal health care practices,
to pursue quality continuing education.	to refuse to perform any nursing action which will jeopardize the patient/client or the public, and the obligation to communicate the rationale to the proper authority.
to teach individuals and groups health care practices that facilitate treatment, prevent illness, and provide optimal wellness.	to avail one's self of opportunities which will broaden knowledge and refine and increase skills.
	to educate the patient/client and the public.

Employment

to competitive hiring and promotion which is based on knowledge and experience and which is unrestricted by consideration of sex, race, age, creed, or national origin.	to maintain competence and prepare one's self adequately for promotion.
to realistic assignments that can assure the patient/client quality care that includes safety, dignity, and comfort.	to evaluate one's own work environment and to communicate and document unrealistic workloads through appropriate channels.
	to make known individual convictions and preferences prior to hiring.
to negotiate salary and individual conditions of employment.	to assess, evaluate, document, and correct unsafe conditions and to communicate such information to the appropriate authority promptly.
to work in a safe and adequately equipped environment.	

to work with qualified, competent nursing personnel.

to periodic, fair, objective evaluations by peers.

to pay increases based on demonstrated performance.

to due process whenever accused of unethical, incompetent, illegal, or unqualified practice or of prejudicial or inappropriate conduct.

to be an advocate for the patient/client and the public when health care and safety may be affected by incompetent, unethical, or illegal practices.

to representation by a negotiator in labor matters.

to objectively document and report to appropriate authorities evidence of competent, as well as incompetent performance and to evaluate, inform, counsel, and teach nursing personnel when indicated.

to participate in the development of reliable and valid evaluation criteria for peer review.

to maintain competence, incorporate new techniques and knowledge, and continuously upgrade the quality of health care.

to participate in the planning, establishment, and implementation of procedures to ensure due process.

to be alert to any instances of incompetent, unethical, or illegal practices by any member of the health care system and to take appropriate action regarding these practices.

to select and utilize a knowledgeable and impartial negotiator.

Professional

to receive support from the nursing profession at all levels.

to belong to an autonomous nursing organization.

to have expert testimony supplied by the nursing organization for both legal actions and legislative issues.

to full and equal representation on all decisionmaking bodies concerned with health care.

to be involved actively in the political decisionmaking process at all levels of the government.

to participate in activities that contribute to the ongoing development of the profession's body of knowledge.

to be an active member and to participate in the nursing organization's effort to implement and improve standards of nursing.

to provide knowledgeable, objective, articulate expert testimony.

to provide knowledge, active, and effective collaborating with members of the health professions.

to be knowledgeable, active, and effective in the legislative process by direct involvement, effective education and selection of representative legislators, lobbying, and creating citizen awareness in promoting local, state, and national efforts to meet the health needs of the public.

Figure 8-12.   The Bill of Rights for Registered Nurses, Maryland Nurses Association.

Reprinted with permission.

Progress in a profession is related to the control of practice and standards within the profession. Nurses, therefore, should take an interest in defining standards of practice, delineating a Code of Ethics, and studying how laws affect the nursing profession.

SUMMARY

Nursing practice is governed by many legal and ethical concepts. Many law concepts have a direct relationship to nursing practice; therefore, it is important for nurses to have some basic knowledge of these laws. There are five major sources of law in the United States and they are intertwined.

Many laws affect nursing practice because the legal system is designed to protect the rights of individuals and groups. Laws are classified into two major areas: criminal and civil law. Criminal law involves conduct considered harmful to society as a whole, while civil law concerns the rights of individuals. Most litigation involving nurses has been civil in nature and in the areas of: torts, negligence and malpractice, defamation, slander, assault and battery, false imprisonment, and invasion of privacy.

Nurses enter into contractual agreements with both patients and agencies, and also are involved with keeping patient records. Nurses should be familiar with charting policies and the importance of keeping accurate and thorough records.

Informed consent is another area that involves nurses. They should be aware of the facets in obtaining this type of consent and specific agency policies regarding informed consent.

Professional nurses are accountable for their practice to state and professional organizations as well as to patients, families, agencies, and themselves. Nurses have many standards by which to judge themselves, for example: licensing exams, continuing education, ANA Standards of Practice, and codes of ethics.

In order for nursing to continue to emerge as a health care profession, nurses must become involved in formulating standards of practice, enforcing codes of ethics, and participating in legislation.

STUDY QUESTIONS

1. List and discuss the specific nursing tasks or functions that carry the greatest legal risks.

2. What is the difference between a nurse's personal liability and her responsibility as an employee of the institution?

3. Discuss the advantages and disadvantages of a professional nurse obtaining professional liability insurance.

4. What is the nurse's role in interpreting and ensuring the patient's bill of rights.

5. Can a nursing student be sued?

6. What should a staff nurse do if she observes a member of the health care team performing what is judged to be an incompetent or unethical activity?

7. Locate your state practice act and regulations. What is the scope of nursing practice under the act?

REFERENCES

1. Loy Wiley, "Liability for Death: Nine Nurses' Legal Ordeals. **Nursing '81,11** No. 9, (September 1981), 34–43
2. Hiller, M. and V. Beyda. "Computers, Medical Records, and the Right to Privacy." **Journal of Health Politics, Policy and Law,** 6, No. 3, (March 1981) 463–487.
3. American Nurses Association. Committee on Ethics. **Guidelines for Implementing the Code for Nurses.** Kansas City, MO: ANA 1982.

ANNOTATED BIBLIOGRAPHY

American Nurses Association. **Code for Nurses.** Kansas City, ANA, 1976. These 11 points with interpretive statements are one example of a profession's self-regulation. Intended as guidelines, their enforcement is the responsibility of the state nurses associations.

Annas G: **The Rights of Hospital Patients.** New York, Avon. 1975. One of a series on individual rights, this book discusses a patient's right to informed consent, refusal of treatment, privacy, and confidentiality. Other topics addressed are organ donation, autopsy, payment of bills, the terminally ill, and human experimentation.

Annas G, Glantz L, Katz B: **The Rights of Doctors, Nurses and Allied Health Professionals.** New York, Avon, 1981. Rights of practice health care, rights in the provider/patient relationship, rights regarding liability and income, and unionization are the major headings of this book. It also includes helpful appendices, especially a listing of major health law periodicals.

Ashley J: **Hospitals, Paternalism and the Role of the Nurse.** New York, Teacher's College Press, 1976. A historic perspective of nursing, Ashley presents implications of this perspective on current trends in nursing. Exploitation of nurses and the domination by the medical profession are only two themes of this book.

Beauchamp T, Childress J: **Principles of Biomedical Ethics (2nd ed.).** New York, Oxford University Press, Inc., 1983. Taking a fresh approach to ethical principles, these authors discuss theory, initially, and each of four principles, autonomy, nonmaleficence, beneficence, and justice. Relationships, ideals, virtues, and integrity also are discussed.

Bernzweig E: **The Nurse's Liability for Malpractice** (3rd ed.). New York, McGraw-Hill Book Co., 1975. This programmed course includes material on general principles of law, rules of liability, legal proof, and consent. A unique aspect of this book is the section on malpractice prevention.

Bullough B: **The Law and the Expanding Nursing Role** (2nd ed.). New York, Appleton-Century-Crofts, 1980. Beginning with the historic development of nurse practice acts, this book relates law on sociological basis to a variety of expanded roles in nursing.

Campazzi BC: **Nurses, Nursing and Malpractice Litigation.** Nurs Adm Q 5:1:1–18; 1981. This article summarizes the content of almost 400 negligence cases involving nursing over a 10-year period.

Creighton H: **Law Every Nurse Should Know** (4th ed.). Philadelphia, W.B. Saunders Co., 1980. In its fourth edition, this classic text is a survey of a variety of laws affecting nursing in the United States and Canada.

Creighton H: **Nurses Charting. Supervisor Nurs** Part I: 42–43; 1980. Part II: 61–62; 1980. These two articles on charting highlight common concerns and give examples of recording and its importance in lawsuits. The ANA standards and its importance in lawsuits. The ANA standards on data collection are discussed.

Curtin L, Flaherty MJ: **Nursing Ethics Theories and Pragmatics.** Bowie , R.J. Brady Co., 1982. Rights and responsibilities of providers, administrators, and patients are discussed in theory and through many case studies. Solutions and analysis are an integral part of the material presented.

Davis A, Aroskar M: **Ethical Dilemmas and Nursing Practice (2nd ed.).** New York, Appleton-Century-Crofts, 1983. This book addresses topics such as abortion, informed consent, dying and death, behavior control, mental retardation, patient rights, and professional ethics. Examples of ethical dilemmas are discussed.

Hemelt M, Mackert M: **Dynamics of Law in Nursing and Health Care (2nd ed.).** Reston, Reston Publishing Co., 1982. This text outlines doctrines and principles of law related to negligence, contracts, defenses, and damages. Over 30 situations are analyzed from legal perspectives.

Hiller M, Beyda V: **Computers, Medical Records, and the Right to Privacy.** J Health Polit Policy Law 6:3:46 3–487; Fall 1981. The future holds new problems in providing confidential and private patient records. Computers have a great impact on this issue. Giving an in-depth examination, this article discusses this impact of this issue.

McCaman B, Hirsh H: **Medical Records— Legal Perspectives.** Primary Care 6:3:681–691; 1979. This excellent article describes medical records used in a courtroom and common problems in dealing with records: changing records, confidentiality, and access to records by patients.

Murchison I, Nichols T, Hanson R: **Legal Accountability in the Nursing Process (2nd ed.).** St. Louis, C.V. Mosby Co., 1982. Placing the discussion of legal accountability in a unique context, that of the nursing process, these authors focus on the nurse practice act, legal grounds for disciplinary action, the reasonably prudent nurse, and rights of patients. Many cases are used as examples.

O'Rourke K, Barton S: **Nurse Power, Unions and the Law.** Bowie, R.J. Brady Co., 1981. This text provides a much needed discussion on collective bargaining and the politics of nursing. Sample contracts and forms are included.

Northrop C, Mech A: **The Nurse as Expert Witness.** Nurs Law Ethics 2:2; March–April 1981. The authors discuss major legal cases involving nurses as expert witnesses. They describe a service that prepares and refers expert nurse witnesses to attorneys. Nurses may testify in court or consult with attorneys in case preparation.

Wiley L: **Liability for Death: Nine Nurses' Legal Ordeals.** Nurs 81 11:9:34–43; September 1981. This article describes the ordeals of nine nurses involved in six criminal cases. The nurses were 24–44 years old and each was accused of a crime while on duty in ICU or general medical/surgical floors. Advice is given on how to deal with similar situations.

9

Theorists in Nursing

Edna M. Fordyce

CHAPTER OUTLINE

OBJECTIVES

At the completion of this chapter the reader will be able to:

- Name the prominent nursing theorists
- Identify the major premise of the perspective of nursing as presented by each of the prominent nurse theorists
- State the definition of nursing presented by each of the prominent nurse theorists
- State the view of nursing process as described by one or more of the prominent nurse theorists
- Identify the dominant influences which have persuaded the nurse theorist to view nursing from the particular perspective advocated by her.

GLOSSARY

Automatic Nursing Action—Orlando's term for activities or tasks carried out by nurses that have been based on reasons other than the patient's immediate needs.

Behavioral System—Johnson identified this as a combination of all the patterned, repetitive, and purposeful ways of behaving that characterize each man's life.

Complementarity—Roger's principle that relates the interaction between the human and environmental energy fields as continuous, mutual, and simultaneous.

Contextual Stimuli—Roy's description of those occurrences as substances in man or his environment that influence patient adaptation other than those most immediate to him; this term is used relative to focal stimuli.

Deliberate Nursing Action—Orlando's term for activities or tasks carried out by the nurse that have been based on an analysis that ascertains or meets the patient's immediate needs.

Focal Stimuli—Roy's description of those occurrences or substances in man or his environment that most immediately influence patient adaptation.

Health-Deviation Self-Care—Orem's category of patient care activities that are necessitated because of illness, injury, or disease.

Helicy—Roger's human development principle that describes the nature as well as the direction of the human and environmental energy fields and their interaction.

Nursology—the study of humanistic nursing practice as defined by Paterson and Zderad.

Residual Stimuli—Roy's terminology for influences of adaptation in man, such as an individual's beliefs, attitudes, or traits.

Resonancy—Roger's principle that describes the human and environmental energy fields according to the pattern and organization of shorter and longer wave patterns.

Self-Care—the central theme of Orem's nursing theory that refers to those activities that individuals personally initiate and perform on their own behalf for the purpose of their health and well-being.

Universal Self-Care—Orem's definition of those activities individuals do in everyday life to meet their basic human needs.

INTRODUCTION

The purpose of this chapter is to identify leading nurse-theorists and their concepts of nursing. A study of nursing literature provides indications of the maturation of nursing. During the last several years the profession of nursing has progressed from developing definitions about nursing and nursing practice to the attempt to identify the theoretical dimensions of what constitutes nursing. Within a relatively few years, a collection of writings of nurse authors suggests many emerging theories of nursing.

The development of definitions of nursing was an important endeavor and was essential, particularly for determining the legal boundaries of nursing for the nurse practice acts of the various states. Another significant historical trend in the development of nursing theory was the identification and definition of concepts that provided a framework for nursing practice and nursing education. Concepts have been referred to as the building blocks of a body of knowledge. Webster's New Collegiate Dictionary defines a concept as an abstract or generic idea generalized from particular instances.

In discussing theory construction in nursing, Jacox defines concepts as "abstract representations of reality."[1] Concepts are symbolic descriptions, and when several are combined in a meaningful way, a theory is developed. Concepts might be characterized as the workhorses that, when harnessed together in a systematized way, become theory. Theory enables the performance of a task or set of tasks. For example, theory guides the practice of nursing.

Theory provides the framework for the analysis of one set of facts in relation to another, and second, a belief, policy, or procedure proposed or followed as the basis of action. Another perspective commonly accepted in describing theory is the grouping of related concepts to describe, explain, or predict some part of reality. When defining theory, Jacox stated, "it is a systematically related set of statements or propositions."[2] Thus, theory in nursing would include a description of nursing, explain nursing practice, and predict the influence of this practice.

One of the prominent nurse authors of contemporary times, Dorothy Johnson, has emphasized the importance of developing a theoretical base for the practice of nursing, if professional stature is our perspective. She stated, "if nursing is indeed an emerging profession, nurses must be able to identify clearly and develop con-

tinually the theoretical body of knowledge upon which practice must rest."[3] In describing the characteristics of a profession, she noted that "a profession's service to society is an intellectual one, and a sound, scientific basis for that service is indispensable."[4] Another nurse author, Myra Levine, advised that a theory of nursing must recognize the importance of unique detail of care for a single patient within an empiric framework that successfully describes the requirements of all patients.[5]

From the early days of nursing, leaders in the profession have sought to identify and describe the functions of nursing as well as its significant components and dimensions. Modern nursing's founder, Florence Nightingale, a nurse-theorist and scientist in her own right, described the knowledge she considered basic to nursing care.[6] Her perspective emphasized fresh air and sanitation. The environment in which the patient was cared for was of paramount concern to her.

In recent times, a number of authors have emerged espousing specific theoretical perspectives about the practice of nursing. Several of these authors have been selected for discussion in the remainder of this chapter. Each author has contributed to the continuing pursuit of the theoretical base for nursing.

The sequence for the discussion of these nursing theorist/authors was made on the basis of the publication years of each person's writings.

SELECTED NURSING THEORISTS

Virginia Henderson

Virginia Henderson is a writer of international influence whose contributions to nursing have been numerous. She believes her greatest contribution to nursing was the preparation of the *Nursing Studies In-*

dex. Dr. Henderson wishes to be remembered as a practitioner,[7] and indeed, her writings focus on the practice of nursing.

In presenting her views of nursing, Henderson proposed a definition of nursing (see page 36) which still has impact upon nursing today. This definition was previously cited, sometimes with minor variations, in other publications.[8–11] The same central theme is present in the definition wherever cited; that of assisting the patient with activities that ordinarily are performed without assistance, and to help the individual regain his performance as soon as he is able. Dr. Henderson viewed the primary function of the nurse as that of "helping the patient with his daily pattern of living. . . ."[12] This helping function was associated with particular activities or the provision of certain conditions that she described as encompassing basic nursing care, and through which the nurse was seen as a substitute for what the patient lacked in physical strength, will, or knowledge.[13,14] Dr. Henderson delineated the following activities and conditions:

1. Breathe normally.
2. Eat and drink adequately.
3. Eliminate body wastes.
4. Move and maintain desirable postures.
5. Sleep and rest.
6. Select suitable clothes—dress and undress.
7. Maintain body temperature within normal range by adjusting clothing and modifying the environment.
8. Keep the body clean and well groomed and protect the integument.
9. Avoid dangers in the environment and avoid injuring others.
10. Communicate with others in expressing emotions, needs, fears, or opinions.
11. Worship according to one's faith.
12. Work in such a way that there is a sense of accomplishment.
13. Play or participate in various forms of recreation.
14. Learn, discover, or satisfy the curiosity that leads to normal development and health and use the available health facilities.[15,16]

Henderson contended that "the nurse is the authority on basic nursing care."[17] Furthermore, Henderson believed that this list of activities and conditions could be used to evaluate nursing, principally by measuring the success attained in helping patients acquire independence in the performance of these functions.[18]

In her 1955 publication,[19] Henderson emphasized the significance of providing and promoting activities that would be life enhancing according to the individual needs of each patient. She further noted the numerous ways that the patient's daily life was disrupted in respect to these ordinary activities through the hospital experience. Consequently, she stated her concerns about "every nursing routine or restriction that is in conflict with the individual's fundamental need for shelter, food, communication with others and the company he loves; for opportunity to win approval, to dominate and be dominated, to learn, to work, to worship, and to play."[20] Henderson was one of the first authors to include responsibilities of the nurse for those who would not recover from injury or illness in her definition of nursing.

Henderson's writings represent her own personal memoirs, and she recounts the many influences that have shaped her perspective of nursing. The view of nursing that she holds is practice-centered. Virginia Henderson's first work in the nursing literature was her authorship of the revision of Bertha Harmer's *Textbook of the Principles and Practice of Nursing* published in 1939.[21] In subsequent writings, a major hallmark of Henderson's perspective of nursing can be found in her definition of nursing and the 14 activities/conditions that constitute, in her opinion, basic nursing care.

Hildegard E. Peplau

Hildegard Peplau authored a textbook, *Interpersonal Relations in Nursing*, that has made a continuing contribution during the 30 years since its publication.[22] The ideas of prominent psychiatrists (particularly Harry Stack Sullivan) and psychologists of that time were translated and presented in terms understandable to nurses. Dr. Peplau espoused the view that nursing was an interpersonal relationship between a person who needed help and a person who, because of her special preparation, could provide the help needed. Psychodynamic nursing was described by Peplau as recognizing, clarifying, and building an understanding of what happens when nurses relate to patients helpfully.

The major themes present in the 1952 publication were the interpersonal relationship with patients and the nurse's self-understanding and developing maturity. Peplau viewed nursing as an interpersonal process. She observed that every nurse/patient relationship is an interpersonal one, where the difficulties of everyday living arise and recur. A significant feature of Dr. Peplau's perspective of nursing was the emphasis on the nurse's own personality growth and maturation, which influenced the kind of nursing care that was given.

Peplau discussed the psychological tasks encountered in the process of learning to live with people. Four major life tasks are emphasized by Peplau (see Figure 9-1). Each of these developmental tasks of life that the patient struggles with indicate the tasks demanded of the nurse in helping the patient complete the unfinished psychological tasks of childhood. These problems

Four life tasks

- Learning to count on others
- Learning to delay satisfactions
- Identifying oneself
- Developing skills, participation, or problem solving

Figure 9-1. Peplau's Four Major Life Tasks.

of everyday life were the concern of the nurse as she endeavored to help patients meet and encounter the various tasks of life. The nurse, according to Dr. Peplau, performed various tasks in facilitating the personal growth of the patient. The phases of the nurse/patient relationship were identified and described as constituting psychodynamic nursing. Peplau identified four interlocking phases of the nurse/patient relationship (see Figure 9-2). Each phase is characterized by overlapping roles or functions of the nurse and defines the nurse's roles and tasks. The various roles associated with the performance of nursing included that of stranger, resource person, teacher, surrogate parent, sibling, counselor, technical expert, and others. She also suggested that nurses had a responsibility for the environment of the patient.

- Orientation phase
- Identification phase
- Exploitation phase
- Resolution phase

Figure 9-2. The Four Phases of the Psychodynamic Nurse/Patient Relationship.

Additionally, Peplau discussed psychobiological experiences (human needs) and factors that interfere with the achievement of discussed goals, such as frustration and subsequent aggression, opposing developmental goals and resultant conflict, and unexplained discomforts—anxiety, guilt, and doubt.

Peplau suggested that observation, communication, and recording are methods for studying nursing as an interpersonal process. She maintained that nursing can be a therapeutic, maturing, educative force in society.

Peplau asserted that her views were a partial theory for the practice of nursing as an interpersonal process. She suggested that nursing was in a unique position for identifying and studying the recurring human problems of everyday living and for studying the skills used by people during these struggles.

She stated that self-understanding and personal maturity determined one's performance in interpersonal relations in nursing situations. Nursing education, thus, had a responsibility to promote personality development and maturation of nursing students.

Ida Orlando

During the mid-1950s, Ida Orlando undertook a study of what nursing is that entailed the examination of numerous nursing situations to determine the outcome of the nursing care provided. Based on her findings she described the process the nurse went through to influence a change in the patient's behavior. From this personal study of verbatim nursing notes, she contended that the "purpose of nursing is to supply the help a patient requires in order for his needs to be met."[23] This purpose is achieved as the nurse initiates the process of finding and meeting the immediate needs of patients for help.

The focus of the perspective of nursing, as presented by Orlando, is the process the nurse undertakes to accomplish the purpose of nursing. In contrast to other descriptions of nursing process presented in nursing literature, Orlando described this process taking place within the nurse.[24,25] Orlando identified three elements present in a nursing situation[26] (see Figure 9-3). Whenever the nurse observes the behavior of the patient, this is done through the nurse's perceptions. These perceptions trigger associated thoughts and feelings in the nurse; in other words, the nurse's reaction to the behavior of the patient. Orlando advised that the nursing action(s) is the sharing of these perceptions and the related thoughts and feelings with the patient, to determine if this is what the patient is experiencing. This action is known as validation. When this process is followed, the purpose can be achieved.

- Behavior of the Patient
- The Reaction of the Nurse
- The Nursing Action Designed for the Patient's Benefit

Figure 9-3.   Orlando's Basic Elements Present in Nursing Situations.

Orlando identified nursing principles that were to guide the nurse in the practice of nursing and these principles represented the theory of effective nursing practice that could be taught to nursing students. Orlando identified four practices that she considered basic to nursing[27] (see Figure 9-4). Orlando stated the principles that guided these practices as:

Any observation shared and explored with the patient is immediately useful in ascertaining and meeting his need or finding out that he is not in need at that time.[28]

The presenting behavior of the patient, regardless of the form in which it appears, may represent a plea for help.[29]

The nurse does not assume that any aspect of her reaction to the patient is correct, helpful or appropriate until she checks the validity of it in exploration with the patient.[30]

These principles guide nurses in their observing, reporting, recording, and responding through nursing action.

- Observing
- Reporting
- Recording
- Carrying out Actions For or With the Patient

Figure 9-4. Orlando's Four Basic Practices in Nursing.

Orlando identified two types of nursing actions. Deliberative actions are those that, when decided on, ascertain or meet the patient's immediate need. These actions constitute the disciplined nursing response. Any other kinds of action are automatic activities that have been decided upon for reasons other than the patient's immediate needs and, consequently, are ineffective.[31]

Orlando stated three requirements for the disciplined nursing process that she described occuring within the nurse. The process must include inclusion in one's thoughts, must ask a question about the thought, and must consider how the nurse states the thought (i.e., the nurse must claim ownership of the thought).[32]

The foundation of the practice of nursing, according to Wiedenbach, is the philosophy that the individual nurse has about nursing and the individual patient. The nurse's philosophy is the unique attitude toward life and reality incorporated in one's beliefs and conduct and is exhibited in "the way" nursing is practiced. Wiedenbach presented three concepts basic to a philosophy of nursing. She suggested these concepts as guiding the choices and decisions of practices. According to Wiedenbach, the nurse's philosophy should include the concepts of:

Ernestine Wiedenbach

After many years of experience in nursing, Ernestine Wiedenbach described clinical nursing as being comprised of four interlocking components that she identified as philosophy, purpose, practice, and art.[33] Her perspective of nursing is embodied in the descriptions she presents of each of these components.

While a faculty member of Yale University, the School of Nursing, Ernestine Wiedenbach was associated with Ida Orlando, Patricia James, and James Dickoff. The influence of these colleagues is observable in Wiedenbach's writings.

Wiedenbach described clinical nursing as a helping art.[34] "It was a deliberate blending of thoughts, feelings, and overt actions, practiced in relation to an individual who is in need of help. [It] is triggered by a behavioral stimulus from the individual, is rooted in an explicit philosophy, and is directed toward fulfillment of a specific purpose."[35]

The foundation of the practice of nursing, according to Wiedenbach, is the philosophy that the individual nurse has about nursing and the individual patient. The nurse's philosophy is the unique attitude toward life and reality incorporated in one's beliefs and conduct and is exhibited in the way nursing is practiced. Wiedenbach presented three concepts basic to a philosophy of nursing. She suggested these concepts as guiding the choices and decisions of practices. According to Wiedenbach, the nurse's philosophy should include the concepts of:

1. Reverence for the gift of life.
2. Respect for the dignity, worth, autonomy, and individuality of each human being.
3. Resolution to act dynamically in relation to one's beliefs.[36]

As a basis for understanding the philosophy of nursing upon which her publication was predicated, Wiedenbach presented four assumptions about human nature that emphasized a respect for individuals.

Intricately intertwined with the nurse's philosophy is the purpose or goal of nursing. The purpose, or the "why" of nursing, according to Wiedenbach, is "to meet the need the individual is experiencing as a need-for-help."[37] Wiedenbach noted that how the patient perceived this need was contingent on the situation and how this was experienced concurrent with the nurse's contact with the patient. She also observed that meaningful help from the nurse was used by the patient "in enhancing or extending his capability."[38]

The practice of nursing is the "what" that is done to attain the purpose of nursing. The focus for the practice of clinical nursing is the patient who is in need of help. Wiedenbach delineated the interrelated and interdependent knowledge, judgment, and skills that are essential attributes of the nurse for effective nursing practice. In addition, Wiedenbach cited four distinct components of practice to be used in meeting the patient's needs. Three components are "directly related to the patient's care" and are:

1. Identification of the patient's experienced need-for-help
2. Ministration of help needed
3. Validation that the help provided was indeed the help needed.[39]

The fourth component is an indirect part of patient care, though an important aspect, and involves the coordination of "resources for help and of help provided."[40]

The art of helping patients includes the identification, ministration, and validation components of practice through the application of nursing knowledge and skill to fulfill the purpose of nursing. This art or the "how" of clinical nursing is a helping process and is action individualized for the patient. Three principles of helping are presented by Wiedenbach as integral to the art of nursing. The principle of inconsistency-consistency alerts the nurse to heed any inconsistencies observed in the situation. The principle of purposeful perseverance requires the use of nursing judgment as to how long to persevere as well as resourcefulness in communication skills. The principle of self-extension enables the nurse to recognize one's own limitations and enlist whatever help is indicated by the situation, including the participation of the patient.[41]

Wiedenbach described the essence of clinical nursing as deliberative action that "holds the key to consistency in obtaining results the nurse seeks to obtain through what she does in giving nursing care to her patients."[42] Wiedenbach has succinctly described the "way, why, what, and how" of clinical nursing in the interlocking components of the philosophy, purpose, practice, and art of nursing.

Dorothy Johnson

Dorothy E. Johnson has developed a behavioral system model for nursing that focuses on "efficient and effective behavioral functioning in the patient to prevent illness, and during and following illness."[43] Johnson stated that "all the patterned, repetitive, and purposeful ways of behaving that characterize each man's life are considered to comprise his behavioral system."[44]

Johnson identified seven behavioral systems (see Figure 9-5) associated with the human. The first, the attachment or affiliative subsystem, is the most critical and is one of the first to develop. The other six subsystems—develop simultaneously or subsequently as part of the total behavioral system. Each subsystem has specialized tasks to be accomplished for the system as a whole.

Each of the subsystems has a structure as well as a function. Johnson has described four structural elements present in each subsystem. The behavior of the person is an observable element. Although not observable, the other three elements—drive, set, and goal—are each essential.

- Attachment/affiliative
- Dependency behavior
- Ingestive
- Eliminative
- Sexual
- Aggressive
- Achievement

Figure 9-5. Johnson's Seven Behavioral Systems.

Nursing, according to Johnson, is "an external regulatory force which acts to preserve the organization and integration of the patient's behavior at an optimal level under those conditions in which the behavior constitutes a threat to physical or social health, or in which illness is found."[45]

For development and maintenance, the subsystems and the system as a whole require protection, nurturance, and stimulation. As the external regulator of the environment, the nurse becomes the source of these functional requirements to meet the patient's basic needs. Consequently, nursing intervention, in accordance with the Johnson model, entails four specific modes of intervention (note the association with the sustenal imperatives). The nurse restricts, defends, inhibits, or facilitates.

In discussing the Johnson model, Grubb describes a four-stage nursing process: a two-level assessment, diagnosis, interventions, and evaluation.[46]

Johnson's model is a systems model. Johnson believes that the human functions according to the laws that govern all systems. The system of man, like other systems, seeks the maintenance of balance and a steady state, and generally there is enough flexibility in the system to attain this. However, there may be times when,

because of a physical illness or a crisis situation, the system balance is disturbed enough that some external assistance may be required. Nursing may be the force that supplies this assistance through the external regulation of the environment.

Johnson believes that nursing is a service complementary to medicine and other health professions but that it also "makes its own distinctive contribution to the health and well-being of people."[47]

Professor Johnson has advanced nursing's progress toward a theoretical perspective through her own behavioral systems model as well as through her academic service and personal challenge to the profession.[48-51] She has influenced further interpretation of her model and the development of new models.

Imogene M. King

Imogene King has developed a view of nursing that incorporates both a general systems theory perspective and the process of human interactions. Dr. King identified aspects of nursing that have endured over time.[52] Then she set out to determine if these aspects continued to comprise the practice of nursing.[53] She also discussed changes in society and nursing.[54] The outcome of King's personal study of nursing has been the development of a conceptual framework that has subsequently emerged and been identified as a theory for goal attainment.[55]

King identified nursing as:

a process of human interactions between nurse and client whereby each perceives the other and the situation; and through communication, they set goals, explore means, and agree on means to achieve goals.[56]

The process of nursing, described by King, is that of human interaction that includes action, reaction, interaction, transaction, and feedback.[57] Consistent with this viewpoint, King affirmed that the focus of nursing is the care of human beings.

- Action
- Reaction
- Interaction
- Transaction
- Feedback

Figure 9-6. King's Process of Nursing.

King clearly stated the place of concepts in the formulation of her theory of nursing, as embodied in the process of human interaction, by identifying and describing the essential concepts upon which the theory was founded. The concepts she specified as central to human interaction were: "interaction, perception, communication, transaction, self, role, stress, growth and development, and time and space."[58]

King differentiated three levels of function for nursing[59] that she later referred to as the domain of nursing.[60] These levels of interacting systems represented the care of individuals (personal systems) and groups (interpersonal systems) within society (social systems). The important concepts for each of the three levels are fully discussed in King's publications. King viewed these concepts as the content of nursing.[61] Readers of this chapter are encouraged to pursue study of these references. The three levels of nursing function, the concepts that constitute a knowledge base for each level, and the implications of the concepts for nursing comprise a noteworthy portion of King's theoretical perspective of nursing. The levels of function and the associated concepts related to each level are presented in the following way:

Personal Systems—Individuals: Perception, self, growth and development, body image, space and time.*

---

*King, I. A Theory for Nursing, (NY: John Wiley and Sons, Inc., 1981)

Interpersonal Systems—Groups: Human interactions, communication, transactions; role and stress.

Social Systems—Society: Organization, authority, power, status, and decision-making.

The concept of health is an integral aspect of King's view of nursing. She succinctly described the goal of nursing as helping "individuals and groups attain, maintain, and restore health."[62]

To facilitate the application of her goal attainment theory, King developed a goal-oriented nursing record based on the problem-oriented medical record.

In developing her systems approach to describing nursing, King systematically clarified the specific concepts basic to her theory. A notable aspect of King's contribution to theory development in nursing is her own research designed to test the ideas set forth as a theory for nursing. Her description of the process of nursing as a human interaction, the levels of nursing functions, and the related concepts central to nursing practice reflect the scholarly dedication that is a hallmark of this author.

Dorothea E. Orem

Dorothea Orem and her formalization of concepts based on the premise of self-care have become a focal point in the development of curricula for numerous schools of nursing. Although her first major publication on concepts of nursing practice was not published until 1971, a definition of nursing and a perspective of nursing were initially published in 1959.[63] The writings of Dorothea Orem reflect some striking similarities to the view of nursing presented by Virginia Henderson. The diagrams depicting the themes in Henderson's and Orem's concept of nursing, prepared by the Nursing Development Conference Group, are a good source for the study of these comparisons.

The central focus of Orem's perspective of nursing is the emphasis on each individual's self-care agency. Self-care, as defined by Orem, "is the practice of activities that individuals personally initiate and perform on their own behalf in maintaining life, health, and well-being."[64] Orem differentiates two types of self-care: universal self-care and health-deviation self-care. Universal self-care is synonymous with those everyday life experiences that are designated as activities of daily living or basic human needs.[65] Orem categorized six components of universal self-care. (See Figure 9-7.) Health-deviation self-care includes all the variations in care necessary because of illness, injury, or disease experienced by individuals throughout their lifetime.[66]

- Air, Water, Food
- Excrements
- Activity and Rest
- Solitude and Social Interaction
- Hazard to Life and Well-being
- Being Normal

Figure 9-7. Orem's Components of Universal Self-Care.

Orem viewed nursing as a human service concerned with "*man's need for self-care action and the provision and management of it on a continuous basis in order to sustain life and health, recover from disease or injury, and cope with their effects.*"[67]

Orem advocated the design of nursing systems that would incorporate the various activities indicated by the extent of deviation in self-care experienced by the potential patient/client and the situation. When the patient is unable to perform self-care actions, a *wholly compensatory* nursing system is indicated. The *partly compensatory* nursing system would be designed when both the nurse and patient perform the self-care. The third nursing system, a *supportive-educative* (or developmental)

system, is used when the patient can learn the required self-care measure(s) with the guidance and support of the nurse. The patient's needs for meeting self-care requisites determine the design of the nursing system and the subsequent variation in role(s) for the nurse and the patient.[68]

According to Orem, nursing practice encompasses social, interpersonal, and technological dimensions. The technological aspect of nursing practice as described by Orem, includes a three-step nursing process. Orem's view of the nursing process is presented as:

Step 1—a determination of whether nursing care is needed

Step 2—the designing of the nursing care system and planning of nursing care according to that system

Step 3—the provision of the indicated nursing actions.[69]

Orem stated that nursing situations had characteristics of helping situations. Orem identified methods of assisting or helping used by the nurse.[70] The five general methods she suggested were viewed as applicable to a variety of situations:

1. Acting for or doing for another
2. Guiding another
3. Supporting another (physically or psychologically)
4. Providing an environment that promotes personal development
5. Teaching another.[71]

Each of these methods of helping are used in conjunction with a specified nursing system according to the appropriate role of nurse and patient.[72]

Dorothea Orem has contributed a unique perspective of nursing using the framework of self-care. She has provided nursing with a new vocabulary to describe the components of nursing practice.

Martha E. Rogers

Martha Rogers has advocated "a science of unitary man" as the focus of her theoretical viewpoint of nursing. She perceives nursing as the science that "seeks to study the nature and direction of unitary human development integral with the environment, and to evolve the descriptive, explanatory, and predictive principles basic to knowledgable practice in nursing."[73] People are at the center of nursing's purpose, according to Rogers, and the science of nursing is directed toward describing the life process in man as well as explaining and predicting the nature and direction of man's development.

Rogers identified "four building blocks" as essential elements in the development of her conceptual system of nursing. The first of these four, **energy fields,** views both the human and the environment as energy fields. The second building block, **openness,** is predicated on a belief in a universe of open systems. **Pattern and organization** are identifying characteristics of the energy field that is undergoing continuous change. Both the human and environmental fields are considered unique and are characterized by the concept of **four-dimensionality**[74] (See Figure 9-8).

- Energy Fields
- Openness
- Pattern and Organization
- Four-Dimensionality

Figure 9-8.   Rogers' Four Building Blocks.

An evolutionary picture of the individual's development as a uni-directional progression through life was emphasized by Rogers. Rogers suggested the "Slinky" walking spring toy (manufactured by James Industries, Pa) demonstrates the rhythmic nature of life progressing through time and space.[75] Simultaneous with this life progression is the continuous interaction of the human energy field with the energy field of the environment.

To describe the nature and direction of the development of unitary man, Rogers has stated and defined three principles:

- the principle of **helicy** which describes the nature as well as the direction of both the human and the environmental fields and their interaction

- the principle of **resonancy** which describes the human and environmental fields according to the pattern and organization of shorter and longer wave patterns

- and the principle of **complementarity** which relates the interaction between the human and environmental fields as continuous, mutual, and simultaneous.[76]

The development of the science of nursing, with a specified body of knowledge, is a critical need, if the goals of nursing are to be accomplished. According to Rogers, "nursing aims to assist people in achieving their maximum health potential."[77] The goals of nursing include the maintenance and promotion of health and the prevention of disease through nursing diagnosis, intervention, and rehabilitation. Rogers contends that her theory, the science of unitary man, has implications for nursing practice in such areas as the aging process, hypertension, and hyperactivity.[78]

Rogers recognizes the constant exchange of energy between the human and environmental fields as integral to the life process.[79] Consequently, Rogers summarized the professional practice of nursing as seeking

to promote symphonic interaction between man and environment, to strengthen the coherence and integrity of the human field, and to direct and redirect patterning of the human and environmental fields for realization of maximum health potential.[80]

The science of nursing proposed by Dr. Rogers "aims to provide a growing body of theoretical knowledge whereby nursing practice can achieve new levels of meaningful service to man."[81] The body of knowledge comprises the science of nursing, which makes possible the application of knowledge that is the art of nursing practice.[82]

The science of nursing proposed by Rogers is one of the most complex of the theories of nursing. Nonetheless, the serious student of nursing will endeavor to master the dimensions of this conceptual framework, which has been adopted as the basis for some nursing curricula and the practice of nursing.

Joyce Travelbee

The interpersonal relationship between the patient and the nurse (the human-to-human relationship) and the existential dimension of life are the distinguishing features of Joyce Travelbee's beliefs about nursing. Travelbee observed that the purpose of nursing was achieved through the establishment of the nurse/patient relationship.[83]

Victor Frankl and Karl Jaspers, notable existential writers, were major influences in Travelbee's perspective of nursing. Joyce Travelbee was a student of Ida J. Orlando, and her influence is evident in Travelbee's emphasis on the disciplined intellectual approach to nursing.

The definition of nursing presented by Travelbee succinctly summarizes the premise on which her approach was formulated. Travelbee described nursing in the following way:

> Nursing is an interpersonal process whereby the professional nurse practitioner assists an individual or family to prevent, or cope with, the experience of illness and suffering and, if necessary, assists the individual or family to find meaning in these experiences.[84]

From this definition, Travelbee derived her statement regarding the purpose of nursing.[85] Travelbee describes this interpersonal process between two human beings, one the patient and the other the nurse, as experienced in four phases culminating with the human-to-human relationship.[86]

Nursing is viewed by Travelbee as a process, an experience, or a happening "between a nurse, an individual, or group of individuals in need of the assistance the nurse can offer."[87] This process is undertaken to meet needs and necessitates observation, validation of inferences, decision-making, and planning of nursing action, as well as evaluation of the extent to which the needs have been met.

Establishment of the human-to-human relationship is preceded by four phases of experience. The initial phase, the original encounter, occurs when the nurse meets the ill person for the first time. The impressions or inferences that develop at this time are significant because they determine the nurse's subsequent behavior toward that person. The task of the nurse in this phase is to recognize the uniqueness of the patient. When this is done, the second phase, emerging identities, is initiated. A bond between the nurse and patient is established during this phase. The identities of each are seen as distinctly separate, and each appreciates the uniqueness of the other. The nursing task of this phase includes becoming aware of one's perception of the other person (the patient) and distinguishing the similarities and differences between oneself and the patient. Then empathy, the third phase, can occur. Empathy is described as an intellectual and emotional comprehension of another person to such an extent that the behavior of that person can be predicted. One's perceptions of the other person's thoughts and feelings are accurate when empathy is present.[88] Empathy is followed by the fourth phase, sympathy. Sympathy is characterized by an urgent desire to respond through action to alleviate the distress perceived in the other person.[89] The task of the nurse in this phase is to provide helpful nursing action.

The outcome of these four phases is experienced as **rapport** and the establishment of the **human-to-human** relationship. Rapport, in Travelbee's view, is synonymous with relatedness, and is expressed in how two persons perceive each other and behave toward one another. Travelbee further described rapport as "a cluster of interrelated thoughts and feelings . . . communicated by one human being to another."[90]

Readers are urged to note the unique definitions and descriptions of empathy, sympathy, and rapport presented by Travelbee, and to refer to her publications for a more complete discussion of these crucial experiences.

Several major concepts are basic to the view of nursing emphasized by Travelbee and are foundations of her perspective of nursing: the human being, patient, nurse, illness, suffering, hope, communication, and therapeutic use of self.

The nurse/patient relationship is a central point in Travelbee's distinctive view of nursing. It is this relationship that enables the nurse to accomplish the purpose of nursing. Travelbee observed that nursing was in danger of losing its caring functions. She suggested that every activity performed by the nurse could be used as a vehicle through which caring could be expressed. This concern was impressively expressed in her own words. "To care for, and in the caring for, to care about is the very heart of nursing."[91]

Sister Callista Roy

Sister Callista Roy describes an approach to nursing based on findings in the study of adaptation. The Roy Adaptation Model was first developed in 1964, when Roy was a graduate student at the University of California. Roy was a student of Dorothy E. Johnson, and the first formulation of this model was developed in association with that experience. Roy stated that her model was both a systems model and an interactionist model.[92]

Roy was persuaded that adaptation could provide a conceptual framework for nursing. Consequently, she adopted the perspective of the psychologist, Dr. Harry Helson, as the theoretical base for her framework.

The view of the person and the adaptation process held are explicitly stated in eight assumptions. A basic premise of the model is the view of the human person as a bio-psycho-social being along a continuum of health—illness. Because of various stimuli which surround the person, some kind of adaptation constantly is required.

Based on this framework, Roy subsequently stated that the function of nursing "is to support and promote patient adaptation." Thus, the practice of nursing based on this model endeavors to facilitate adaptation through whatever activities are indicated.

Roy observed that, both in health and illness, four particular ways of adapting are characteristic of a person. These modes of adaptation were identified by Roy as physiologic needs, self-concept, role function, and interdependence relations.[93]

Derived from her study of Helson, Roy proposed that the individual's adaptation level is influenced by three types of stimuli: focal, contextual, and residual. The stimuli influencing adaptation that is most immediate to the person is referred to as focal. Contextual stimuli includes all stimuli influencing the patient other than that most immediate to him. Though not as readily identifiable as focal or contextual stimuli, residual stimuli, which includes an individual's beliefs, attitudes, or traits, also influences either adaptive or maladaptive behavior in life situations.[94] The nurse becomes concerned with these stimuli both in making assessments and during nursing intervention.

The goal of nursing, as stated by Roy, is "to promote man's adaptation in each of the adaptive modes in situations of health and illness." Roy maintained that a nursing process, using problem solving as its basis, represents a scientific approach to the service that nursing could provide for society. The nursing process that Roy developed for her model entails six specific steps.

Assessment is undertaken at two levels. Initially the nurse acquires information about the individual's behavior in each of the adaptive modes and seeks to determine whether the behavior is adaptive or maladaptive. Subsequently, the second level of assessment is initiated as the nurse undertakes the identification of the various stimuli (focal, contextual, residual) that are influencing the patient's behavior. Data from these first two steps then are used to formulate a statement regarding the patient's adaptive or maladaptive behaviors for the third step, problem identification. This activity is synonymous with making a nursing diagnosis. Roy is actively involved with the ambitious efforts of the National Conference Group endeavoring to establish a diagnostic classification system for nursing. When the problem has been clearly identified, the nurse is ready to embark upon step four, goal setting. Nursing intervention, step five, focuses on adaptation problems through the manipulation of stimuli as the nurse seeks to promote the patient's adaptation. The final step, evaluation, is focused on determining the effectiveness of the nursing interventions undertaken.

The basis of the Roy model is adaptation. The approach described by Roy is explicitly stated in the eight assumptions central to her model and also form the framework for it. The Roy Adaptation Model has become one of the most popular theoretical approaches to nursing during the relatively short time since its inception.

Josephine G. Paterson and Loretta T. Zderad

The publication, *Humanistic Nursing*, coauthored by Paterson and Zderad, describes the nursing situation that can be existentially experienced. The authors state that:

> nursing is a responsible searching, transactional relationship whose meaningfulness demands conceptualization founded on a nurse's existential awareness of self and of other.[95]

Paterson and Zderad emphasized that nursing is "an experience lived between human beings."[96]

They observed that the nurse experiences peak life events with other human beings. Peak life events include: birth, death, separation, and various other crises. It is through these experiences that the nurse can come to know oneself and others as these experiences are reflected on. These experiences must then be described. In presenting this humanistic nursing practice theory, Paterson and Zderad view nursing:

> as the ability to struggle with other men through peak experiences related to health and suffering in which the participants in the nursing situation are and become in accordance with their human potential.[97]

The essence of these human-lived experiences must be described by nurses. Nursing situations warrant description, and only nurses can describe them. As nurses describe these human phenomena of nursing situations, ultimately nursing theory and science will be developed. This endeavor also will affect the nursing situation and the nurse's knowledge of the human capacity for beingness.

Nursology (a term derived by Paterson and Zderad) is the study of humanistic nursing practice. Paterson and Zderad have proposed a methodology that they describe as occurring in four phases. The first phase entails the preparation of the nurse for the **"task of knowing,"** which necessitates an openness to the situations that will be encountered. Knowing the client "intuitively" and how he views his world is the focus of the second phase. This phase requires the nurse to be a part of what is studied. In the third phase, the nurse reflects on the experience and seeks to record as many aspects of the experience as possible. The final and fourth phase allows for greater understanding of the phenomena under study when the nurse takes "an intuitive leap" as the specific ideas and views of many situations are applied to other situations.

The approach to nursing presented by Paterson and Zderad is predicated on the nurse's involvement with the patient and the experience between them as it is lived in the nursing situation. Paterson and Zderad have called this the "active presence" of the nurse. They recognize that in the actual nursing situation, the nurse may not be able to be "wholly present" to every patient to the same degree. However, they encourage nurses to strive toward this difficult goal.

Paterson and Zderad have proposed that nurses consciously and deliberately approach nursing as an existential experience. They view nursing as a lived experience that must be described. Descriptions of these experiences between nurses and patients in the real world must be shared in order to develop a humanistic nursing theory.[98] An understanding of existential terminology and literature is helpful in appreciating the scholarly perspective of nursing set forth by Paterson and Zderad.

Myra E. Levine

Myra E. Levine describes a perspective of nursing that focuses on nursing's responsibility for maintaining or restoring wholeness for patients. She sees nursing as a keeping together function. The individual patient is the central focus for nursing practice. According to Levine, nursing is concerned with the unity and integrity of the individual patient. To achieve the nursing purpose, Levine identified four principles of conservation that are the framework for conserving the wholeness of the patient.[99]

These principles identify the major areas of care and concern of the nurse. The first principle is the **conservation of the individual patient's energy.** Nursing intervention uses this principle when the nurse is attentive to the energy resources of the patient compared to the energy expenditure associated with his response to a situation. Energy depletion is influenced by many factors, for example, the patient's general condition and the demands made upon the individual because of the disease processes existent.

Conservation of structural integrity, the second principle, is predicated on the awareness that structural changes alter function, and pathophysiological processes all threaten structural integrity. Consequently, the nurse incorporates knowledge of bodily structure and function in the application of this principle. A variety of nursing measures can be instituted in daily care to conserve structure and the associated functions. Positioning, care of the patient's skin, and personal hygiene are aspects of daily care that can facilitate conservation of the patient's structural integrity.

The third principle, **conservation of personal integrity,** encompasses concerns for the individual's self-identity and self-respect.[100] Nursing intervention conserves personal integrity when the patient is accepted, valued, and respected as he is. Consideration for the rights and privileges of each patient for privacy, participation in his care, and regard for confidentiality are evidence of this principle.

The fourth principle is **conservation of social integrity.** The social integrity of the patient is conserved when nursing care facilitates the individual's continuing contacts and relationships with family and other important associations that are meaningful to him as a member of society.[101]

According to Levine, nursing is a human interaction. Nursing intervention is therapeutic and supportive. Therapeutic intervention entails influencing the individual's adaptation favorably or toward renewed social well-being.[102] Intervention is supportive when the course of adaptation cannot be altered, or the status quo is maintained. Nursing intervention, according to Levine, must be designed so that it fosters successful adaptation.

Nursing intervention is a conservation of wholeness for the individual patient. The conservation principles embody the major areas of care in which nursing can fulfill this conservation function. Levine has succinctly summarized her perspective of nursing in describing the task of nursing as recognizing "the value and wondrous variety of all mankind while offering ministrations that conserve the unique and special integrity of every man."[102]

Betty Neuman

Betty Neuman conceptualized a model of health care that she proposed could be used by various disciplines of health care providers, including nurses. The Neuman perspective of health care focuses on the individual and his environment, with particular emphasis on his relationship to stress. Though the model is referred to as a "total person approach to patient problems" it is recommended for use with families and groups, as well as for individuals. The purpose of the model is to provide a framework for health care givers to assist in attaining and maintaining a maximum level of wellness through purposeful interventions.

Nine assumptions are presented by Neuman as basic to the development of her model. These assumptions identify beliefs about the individual and characteristic responses to stress that man develops during his lifetime. The relationship of primary, secondary, and tertiary prevention are noted and defined in the context of this model.

The individual is viewed by Neuman as an open system and is represented in the model diagram by a series of concentric circles. The basic structure of the individual is envisioned as the core. This core is bounded by lines of resistance, a normal line of defense, and a flexible line of defense, which represents the individual's response to stressors that impact upon the individual throughout his life.

Intervention by the health care provider may be instituted at whatever level indicated in respect to primary, secondary, and tertiary prevention levels. The identification of the stressors and the subsequent impact upon the physiological, psychological, sociocultural, and developmental influences as variables affecting the individual determine the timing and locus of interventions.

The application of this model by the nurse (or care givers of whatever discipline) can be facilitated through use of the Assessment/Intervention Tool developed by Neuman. The tool is an interview guide to obtain data essential to determining and providing appropriate care. Neuman emphasized the importance of incorporating the individual client's perception of his condition in developing the goals for care.[103]

Neuman has endeavored to describe a framework for health care that includes many possible dimensions. It is recommended for the care of individuals, families and groups by care givers in any health care setting. Stress and the individual's response to stressors is the basic phenomenon emphasized.

SUMMARY

The perspective of nursing held by selected nurse-authors was briefly presented in this chapter. Each of these authors has contributed to the building of a theoretical foundation for the practice of nursing.

Historical evidence of efforts to state a theoretical premise for the practice of nursing can be found in the writings of Florence Nightingale. During the past three decades, the writings of a growing number of nurses reflect their attempts to enlarge the scientific dimensions of nursing care and state a perspective that is commensurate with those recognized as distinguishing a professional discipline. Several of these authors were selected for presentation in this chapter as representative nursing theorists with whom nurses should be familiar.

In viewing these authors from a historical perspective, it is evident that personal, cultural, environmental, and theoretical forces influenced the focus heralded by each of these nurse-theorists.

Though there are notable differences between these authors, there are also some similarities. One common factor is the inclusion of the needs of the patient as an important component in determining the role of the nurse as well as the focus of nursing practice. The interpersonal relationship between the nurse and the patient is noted as a central focus by many of the authors. The variations observed in the perspective of each author are expressed in the components of nursing practice that are emphasized as well as the conceptual frameworks on which the ideas are centered.

A chart, Comparison of Selected Nurse Author/Theories, highlighting the basic premises of authors presented in this chapter, follows (inside back cover). It is hoped that this comparison of authors according to a specified list of variables will aid in the understanding of the noteworthy contributions of those selected for discussion.

STUDY QUESTIONS

1. Name three nursing author/theorists.

2. For each of the individuals named in question one identify and briefly state
   a. the definition of nursing given by the author
   b. the view of the nursing process described by the author.

3. Describe the perspective of nursing held by each nurse-author discussed in this chapter.

4. State the historic progression of the development of nursing theory.

5. Discuss the factors that have been influential for each nurse-author identified in this chapter.

REFERENCES

1. A. Jacox, "Theory Construction in Nursing: An Overview," **Nursing Research, 23** (1974) No. 1, p.4–13.
2. Ibid., p.8.
3. Dorothy E. Johnson, "The Development of Theory: A Requisite for Nursing as a Primary Health Profession," **Nursing Research, 23** (1974) p.372.
4. Ibid., p.372.
5. M.E. Levine, "Adaptation and Assessment: A Rationale for Nursing Intervention." **American Journal of Nursing, 66** (1966), pp.2451–2454.
6. Florence Nightingale, **Notes on Nursing: What It Is, and What It is Not.** (New York: D. Appleton and Co., 1879)
7. G. Safier. **Contemporary American Leaders in Nursing.** (New York: McGraw-Hill Book Co., 1977).
8. Virginia Henderson. **The Nature of Nursing.** (New York: The MacMillan Co., 1966) p.15.
9. V. Henderson. "Research in Nursing Practice—When?" **Nursing Research 4** (1975) p.4.

10. V. Henderson, "The Nature of Nursing," **American Journal of Nursing. 66** (1966) p.63.

11. Virginia Henderson and Gladys Nite, **The Principles and Practice of Nursing.** 6th ed. (New York: The MacMillan Publishing Co., Inc., 1978) p.34.

12. V. Henderson. **Nursing Research** 1955, p.5.

13. Ibid., p.5.

14. Virginia Henderson, **The Nature of Nursing.** (New York: The MacMillan Co., 1966) p.16.

15. V. Henderson, "The Nature of Nursing," **American Journal of Nursing, 64** (1964) p.65.

16. V. Henderson. **The Nature of Nursing,** 1966, pp.16–17.

17. Ibid, p.16.

18. Ibid.

19. V. Henderson, "Research" 1955, p.6.

20. V. Henderson, "The Nature of Nursing," 1964, p.65.

21. Bertha Harmer and Virginia Henderson. **Textbook of the Principles and Practice of Nursing.** 4th ed. (New York: The MacMillan Co., 1939).

22. Hildegard E. Peplau, **Interpersonal Relations in Nursing** (New York: G.P. Putnam's Sons, 1952).

23. Ida J. Orlando, **Dynamic Nurse-Patient Relationships** (New York: G.P. Putnam's Sons, 1961).

24. Ibid.

25. Ida J. Orlando Pelletier. "The Dynamic Nurse-Patient Relationship" Talk presented by Ida Orlando Pelletier. (Walter Reed Army Medical Center, Department of Nursing, Washington, D.C., October 1980).

26. I. J. Orlando. **Nurse-Patient Relationships,** p.36.

27. Ibid., p.31.

28. Ibid., pp.35–36.

29. Ibid., p.10.

30. Ibid., p.56.

31. Ibid., p.60.

32. I. J. Orlando. Talk, 1980.

33. Ernestine Wiedenbach, **Clinical Nursing: A Helping Art.** (New York: Springer Publishing Co., Inc., 1964) p.12.

34. Ibid., p.2.

35. Ibid., p.11.

36. Ibid., p.16.

37. Ibid., p.15.

38. Ibid., p.15.

39. Ibid., p.31.

40. Ibid., p.31.

41. Ibid., pp.36–52.

42. Ibid., p.107.

43. D.E. Johnson, "The Behavioral System Model for Nursing," in Joan P. Riehl and Sr. Callista Roy, **Conceptual Models for Nursing Practice.** 2nd Ed. (New York: Appleton-Century-Crofts. 1980) p.207.

44. Ibid., p.209.

45. Ibid., pp.212–214.

46. J. Grubbs, "An Interpretation of the Johnson Behavioral Systems Model for Nursing Practice" in Joan Riehl and Sr. Callista Roy, **Conceptual Models for Nursing Practice.** 2nd Ed. New York: Appleton-Century-Crofts 1980. p.231.

47. D. Johnson, "Behavioral System Model." p.207.

48. D.E. Johnson, "A Philosophy of Nursing," **Nursing Outlook, 7,** (1959).

49. D.E. Johnson, "The Significance of Nursing Care," **American Journal of Nursing, 61** (1961).

50. D.E. Johnson, "Tonight's Action Will Determine Tomorrow's Nursing." **Nursing Outlook, 13** (1965).

51. D.E. Johnson, "Development of Theory: A Requisite." Nursing Research, **23** (1974) p.372.

52. Imogene M. King. **Toward a Theory for Nursing.** (New York: John Wiley and Sons, Inc., 1971) p.X; 119.

53. Imogene M. King. **A Theory for Nursing.** (New York: John Wiley and Sons, Inc., 1981) p.150.

54. I.M. King. **Toward a Theory for Nursing,** 1971, pp.107–118.

55. I.M. King. **A Theory for Nursing,** 1981, p.144.

56. Ibid., p.144.

57. I.M. King, **A Theory for Nursing,** p.145.

58. Ibid., pp.10; 13.

59. Ibid., p.145.

60. I.M. King. **A Theory for Nursing,** p.13.

61. Ibid., p.142.

62. Ibid., p.13.

63. Nursing Development Conference Group.**Concept Formalization in Nursing.** 2nd Ed. Dorothea E. Orem (Ed.) (Boston: Little Brown, and Co., 1979) pp.69–70.

64. Dorothea E. Orem. **Nursing: Concepts in Practice.** 1st Ed. (New York: McGraw-Hill Book Co., 1971) p.13.

65. Ibid., p.21.

66. Ibid., pp.21–28.

67. Ibid., pp.1–2.

68. Dorothea E. Orem, **Nursing: Concepts in Practice.** 2nd Ed. (New York: McGraw-

Hill Book Co., 1980) pp.94–102.

69. Ibid., pp.200–203.
70. D. Orem. **Concepts in Practice** 2nd Ed. p.95.
71. Ibid., pp.94–95.
72. M.E. Rogers, "Nursing: A Science of Unitary Man" in Joan Riehl and Sr. Callista Roy **Conceptual Models for Nursing Practice,** 2nd Ed. (New York: Appleton-Century-Crofts, 1980). p.329.
73. Ibid., p.330.
74. Ibid., pp.330–332.
75. Martha E. Rogers, **An Introduction to the Theoretical Basis of Nursing** (Philadelphia: F.A. Davis Co., 1970) pp.90–92.
76. M.E. Rogers. "Nursing: Science of Unitary Man." p.330.
77. M.E. Rogers. **Theoretical Basis in Nursing,** p.86.
78. M.E. Rogers. "Nursing: Science of Unitary Man." p.336.
79. M.E. Rogers, **Theoretical Basis in Nursing,** p.92.
80. Ibid., p.122.
81. Ibid., p.88.
82. Ibid., p.121.
83. Joyce Travelbee. **Interpersonal Aspects of Nursing** (Philadelphia: F. A. Davis Co., 1966) p.121.
84. Ibid., pp.5–6.
85. Ibid., p.13.
86. Joyce Travelbee. **Interpersonal Aspects of Nursing** 2nd Ed. (Philadelphia: F. A. Davis Co., 1971) p.123.
87. Ibid., p.8.
88. J. Travelbee, "What's Wrong with Sympathy?" **American Journal of Nursing, 64** (1964) p.68.
89. Ibid., pp.68–69.
90. J. Travelbee. **Interpersonal Aspects** 2nd ed. pp.149–150.
91. J. Travelbee. **Interpersonal Aspects** 1st Ed. p.2.
92. Sr. Callista Roy "Adaptation: A Conceptual Framework for Nursing" **Nursing Outlook,** 18 (1970) pp.42–45.
93. Sr. Callista Roy, **Introduction to Nursing: An Adaptation Model.** (Englewood Cliffs, NJ, Prentice-Hall Inc., 1976) pp.30–33.
94. Ibid., pp.18–37.
95. Josephine G. Paterson and Loretta T. Zderad. **Humanistic Nursing** (New York: John Wiley and Sons, Inc., 1976) pp.3–7.
96. Ibid., p.3.
97. Ibid., p.4.
98. Ibid., pp.76–83.
99. M.E. Levine, "Holistic Nursing," **Nursing Clinics of North America** (1971) p.258.
100. M.E. Levine, "The Four Conservation Principles of Nursing," **Nursing Forum,** 6 (1967) pp.50–54.
101. Myra E. Levine. **Introduction to Clinical Nursing.** 2nd Ed. (Philadelphia: F. A. Davis Co., 1973)
102. Myra E. Levine, "Adaptation and Assessment: A Rationale for Nursing Intervention." **American Journal of Nursing 66** (1966) p.2452.
103. B. Neuman, "The Betty Neuman Health-Care Systems Model: A Total Person Approach to Patient Problems" in Joan Reihl and Sr. Callista Roy, **Conceptual Models for Nursing Practice** 2nd Ed. (New York: Appleton-Century-Crofts, 1980).

ANNOTATED BIBLIOGRAPHY

Henderson V: **The Nature of Nursing.** MacMillan Co., 1966. Dr. Henderson presents her professional memoirs in this reference. She has included not only her view of nursing, but identifies the individuals and experiences that have been most influential in her professional life and have contributed to the perspective of nursing she holds. Her views on nursing practice, nursing education, and nursing research also are presented.

Johnson DE: **The Behavioral System Model for Nursing.** In Riehl and Roy: Conceptual Models for Nursing Practice, 2nd ed. 1980. Dr. Johnson presents a concise overview of her view of nursing in this chapter. She includes descriptions of the components of her model with a documented explanation of each of the behavioral subsystems she identified as comprising man's behavioral system.

King IM: **A Theory for Nursing.** Wiley and Sons, 1981. An update of Dr. King's perspective of nursing with findings from her personal research are presented. The concepts she has identified as basic to her theory are thoroughly discussed with substantial documentation of related literature included. The progression of Dr. King's view of nursing is evident when this reference is compared with her previous publications.

Levine ME: **Introduction to Clinical Nursing,** 2nd ed. Davis, 1973. This reference was written for the beginning nursing student. Levine's view of nursing is presented within a conceptual framework and emphasizes a patient-centered approach. The holistic approach of nursing held by this author is described including the application of conservation principles that she has identified and described in this and previous publications.

Neuman B: **The Betty Neuman Health-Care Systems Model.** In Riehl and Roy: Conceptual Models for Nursing Practice, 2nd ed. 1980. Betty Neuman described and illustrated her model for nursing incorporating a total person approach. The assessment/intervention tool associated with the model is presented and explained. The diagram of the model (first published in *Nursing Research* in 1972) provides the reader with an excellent road map of the components of the model.

Orem DE: **Nursing Concepts in Practice,** 2nd ed. McGraw-Hill, 1980. This second edition expands the self-care conceptual view of nursing developed by Orem and described in the 1st edition (1971). This reference, like its forerunner, includes a comprehensive guide to this author's perspective of nursing.

Orlando IJ: **Dynamic Nurse-Patient Relationship.** Putnam, 1961. A vanguard view of nursing and the nursing process. This author's description of the nursing process was one of the first publications to use this terminology and explain its place in nursing practice. This publication is a classic of

nursing theory development literature. It is noteworthy to observe that the research findings of this author were obtained in the practice setting and influenced the view of nursing that she developed.

Paterson JG, Zderad LT: **Humanistic Nursing.** Wiley, 1976. A scholarly perspective of nursing as an existential experience lived between a nurse and other human beings. The process of developing a humanistic nursing theory is described by the authors.

Peplau HE: **Interpersonal Relations in Nursing.** Putnam's, 1952. A classic in psychiatric nursing. Dr. Peplau translated the ideas of prominent psychiatrists, especially Harry Stack Sullivan, M.D., and psychologists of that time period into an understandable language for nurses. Her application of this knowledge base for nursing practice included identifying phases in the nurse/patient relationship and the roles, functions, and tasks of the nurse in facilitating the personal growth of the patient.

Rogers ME: **An Introduction to the Theoretical Basis of Nursing.** Davis, 1970. Dr. Roger's theoretical view of nursing science and unitary man is presented in this reference. Though this reference may appear to be complex to the readers' initial study of nurse-author theorists, it is a comprehensive description of the view of nursing advocated by this influential nurse-author.

Roy Sr.C: **Introduction to Nursing: An Adaptation Model.** Prentice-Hall, 1976. The adaptation model of Sr. Callista is presented by its author and her nursing colleagues in this reference. The application of the model is demonstrated throughout the publication. Both beginning nursing students and experienced nurses will find material helpful to their practice in this publication.

Travelbee J: **Intervention in Psychiatric Nursing: Processes in the One-to-One Relationship.** Davis, 1959. This classic book presents Travelbee's beliefs about interpersonal relationships between patients and nurses. It uses an existential framework based on the writings of Frankl and Jaspers. Travelbee's application of this knowledge to nursing culminated with her description of nursing as a human-to-human relationship.

Wiedenbach E: **Clinical Nursing: A Helping Art.** Springer, 1964. The components of nursing and their application to practice are emphasized in this historic reference. Wiedenbach was one of the first nurse-authors to develop a theoretical framework for nursing practice incorporating the personal philosophy of the nurse as an important element. In this reference she presents three concepts she considers basic to a philosophy of nursing.

Section 2

Concepts Related to the Process of Communication

This section presents concepts related to developing a nurse-patient relationship. These concepts include ethnicity, communication, patient-teaching, and change. Since communication is vital to the formation of the nurse-patient relationship and the nursing process, it is essential that these concepts be considered carefully.

Cultural variability and ethnicity are discussed in this section as broad areas that may require unique knowledge in order to carry out the nursing process. Communication as a component of culture is addressed and examples of nursing actions are highlighted as they have implications on establishing a nurse-patient relationship. Methods of establishing a means of communication are discussed in this chapter as well.

Communication has a theoretical basis and the chapter on communication introduces the reader to several models and then focuses on how to use the nursing process to communicate effectively.

The chapters on patient-teaching and change discuss aspects of communication used by nurses to influence the health behaviors and health status of individuals, families, and groups within the context of the health care system.

Selected clinical applications are given in these chapters, to provide examples of how the nursing process is used in each concept area.

In order for nurses to effectively interact with patients, families, and groups, they must know how to communicate first, and then use that knowledge to provide holistic nursing care.

10

Culture, Health and Illness

Joan M. Roche

Janet-Beth Flynn

CHAPTER OUTLINE

OBJECTIVES

At the completion of this chapter, the reader will be able to:

- Define the terms in the glossary.
- Describe the relationship of culture to prevalence of disease and illness.
- Describe the differences between culture and cultures.
- Identify and discuss American core values which serve as standards for behavior.
- Describe the relationship of culture to health behaviors, beliefs, and practices.
- Discuss the concept of culture shock.
- Describe a cultural assessment.
- Incorporate the cultural assessment in the nursing care plan.

GLOSSARY

Core Values—Values that are central to a specific culture.

Cultural Relativism—A perspective through which cultures are viewed as different and acceptable. There is no attempt to define inferior or superior cultures.

Culture—A set of standards for perception, belief, evaluation, communication, and action (Goodenough: 1970).

Culture Shock—A state of anxiety precipitated by the loss of familiar signs and symbols of social intercourse when one is suddenly immersed into a cultural system markedly different from his home or familiar culture.

Cultures—Groups of people who share similar beliefs, attitudes, values, and practices. There may be more variability with cultural groups (intracultural) than between groups (intercultural).

Ethnocentrism—The judging of other cultures by the standards of one's own cultural heritage. There is an implicit or explicit tendency to view one's own culture as the superior one.

Intercultural Variability—Differences between cultures.

Intracultural Variability—Differences within a culture.

Sick Role—A set of behaviors expected of people who are ill.

Social Roles—A series of expected behaviors that are culturally acceptable.

Stereotyping—Assuming the presence of a particular characteristic or set of characteristics in a member or members of a group without consideration of individual traits. Stereotyping is not based on objective assessment and is frequently derogatory.

Subcultures—Groups within a larger society sharing the overall culture but each with many of its own distinctive lifestyles, beliefs, and values. In the United States, teenagers are often considered as a subculture.

INTRODUCTION

All groups of people confront similar issues in adapting to their environments. These issues are fundamental to the maintenance of the group and of its individual members. They include providing for nutrition, shelter, care, and education of children, division of labor, social organization, health maintenance, and control of disease. Man is characterized by the ability to devise cultural solutions to meet these needs, and it is this ability to adapt to varying environments using cultural means that is responsible for his success as a species.

Our understanding of the cultural dimension of man is derived from the field of anthropology. Cultural anthropologists use a comparative approach in studying groups of people through which they attempt to understand both similarities and differences among human groups. This knowledge, in turn, contributes to our understanding of humanity as a whole. Anthropology also is characterized by a holistic view of both culture and man. Cultures are very complex, consisting of facets covering all aspects of life (see Figure 10-1). Cultures are seen as systems in which all parts are interrelated. Events in the system do not occur in isolation. Changes in one part of the system result in changes in other parts. The wholeness of man is emphasized in the awareness that human interaction is with a total physical and social environment. Man's behavior has meaning in the context of the environments with which he interacts.

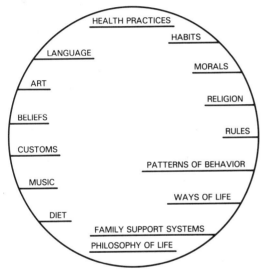

Figure 10-1.   Components of a Culture.

The cultural basis of human behavior has great importance for the practice of nursing. With anthropology, nursing shares a holistic view of man. Almost all facets of culture have an impact on nursing practice. Some of these facets have more weight than others, however. (See Figure 10-2.)

Both anthropology and nursing are concerned with adaptation. Anthropologists seek to understand the process of adaptation and the role of culture in adaptation. Roy has defined the purpose of nursing as that of fostering client adaptation.[1] In attempting to achieve this purpose, "the system of the person and his interaction with the environment are the units of analysis of nursing assessment . . . manipulation of parts of the system or the environment is the mode of nursing intervention."[2] While anthropologists focus on understanding culture in terms of a group of people, nurses use cultural information to understand and assist individual clients, their families, or groups in achieving optimum health.

BIOCULTURAL PERSPECTIVES

Over millions of years, man has demonstrated that he can adapt successfully to a number of environments. Through the mechanism of culture, man has lived in natural environments that are hospitable and inhospitable, in diverse settings, such as mountains, deserts, islands, fertile plains, and, more recently, complex industrial settings. Temperate, hot, and cold climates require different strategies for living, and man has devised them.

Man shapes and, to some extent, is shaped by his environment. The occurrence of specific genotypes (genetic makeup) and phenotypes (visible traits) result from both biological and cultural adaptation. An example of this is an individual who receives genetic instructions for blood type O from one parent and for blood type A from another. The individual will show a visible trait of blood A (his phenotype) and genetic instructions for both A and O (his genotype).

Through time, and in all environments, man has coped with disease and illness. The fossil remains of prehistoric man show the presence of arthritis, trauma, and tooth decay. In the historic record, there is evidence of epidemics of smallpox, bubonic plague, and influenza. There is a staggering array of health problems around the world today. Diseases of poverty and malnutrition persist in industrialized as well as in nonindustrialized countries. Famines and droughts still take an enormous toll in human life and health.

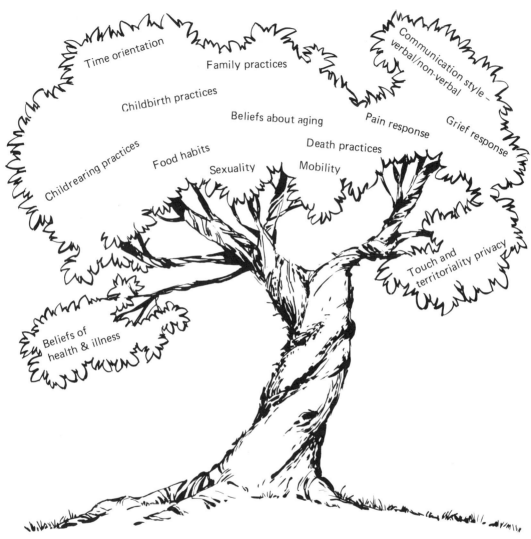

Time orientation

Family practices

Communication style - verbal/non-verbal

Childbirth practices

Beliefs about aging

Pain response

Grief response

Death practices

Childrearing practices

Food habits

Sexuality

Mobility

Touch and territoriality privacy

Beliefs of health & illness

Figure 10-2.   Selected Aspects of Culture That Have an Impact on Nursing.

The absence, presence, and severity of disease in a population are indicators of human adaptation. Through a process of long-term adaptation, the occurrence of selected genes can provide an advantage where specific health threats exist. One of the most striking examples of this process is seen where malaria occurs. Malaria continues to be a life threatening disease in large areas of the world. Populations that inhabit these regions are at continuous risk for the disease. In many of these popula-tions, biological adaptation has taken place with the appearance of the sickle cell trait in recessive form. A proportion of such populations will be disabled or die due to inheriting these genes from both parents; others will suffer similar conse-quences due to malaria. Individuals carry-ing this trait, however, have some protec-tion from the disease and can live to produce another generation. Under en-vironmental conditions in which the threat of malaria does not exist, the adap-

ROY'S MODEL OF ADAPTATION IS BASED ON A SERIES OF EIGHT ASSUMPTIONS THAT RELATE BOTH TO THE CONCEPT OF THE PERSON AND THE PROCESS OF ADAPTATION. THESE ASSUMPTIONS ARE OF PARTICULAR RELEVANCE WITHIN THE CONTEXT OF CULTURE.

Assumptions	*Cultural Context*
The person is a bio-psycho-social being.	Man lives and develops in sociocultural settings.
The person is in constant interaction with a changing environment.	Culture provides the individual with options for adapting to changes in both his physical and social environment.
To cope with a changing world, the person uses both innate and acquired mechanisms which are biologic, physiologic, and social in origin.	Man assesses the cultural options and adopts or creates responses to these changes.
Health and illness are one inevitable dimension of the person's life.	Each society develops and refines cultural strategies for alleviating suffering and for promoting health.
To respond positively to environmental changes, the person must adapt.	Each culture seeks strategies needed to maintain the well-being of its members.
The person's adaptation is a function of the stimulus he is exposed to and his adaptation.	Cultural rules, norms of behavior, and attitudes provide man with a possible range of adaptations.
The person's adaptation level is such that it comprises a zone indicating the range of stimulation that will lead to a positive response.	Culture content may or may not be useful in all environmental situations.
The person is conceptualized as having four modes of adaptation: physiologic, self-concept, role function, interdependent relations.	Culture influences each of the adaptive modes in some way.

Figure 10-3. Assumptions relating adaptation to relevant cultural factors.

Adapted from: Joan P. Reihl and Sr. Callista Roy (Eds.), **Conceptual Models for Nursing Practice,** 2nd edition. (New York: Appleton-Century-Crofts, 1980), pp. 179–188.

tive significance of the trait is overlooked, and the problem of transmission of sickle cell disease becomes highly visible.

In the United States and other industrialized nations, the health picture has changed considerably in the last 50 years. Advances in both the prevention and treatment of disease have almost eradicated certain disease or disease outcomes. Smallpox, for example, has been eliminated. Improvements in sanitation, the discovery of antibiotics, and a wide variety of public health programs are 20th century accomplishments that have had an impact on the infectious diseases. Polio, diptheria, and pertussis rates decreased dramatically as vaccination programs were implemented. The pneumonias and other bacterial diseases have become more manageable with antibiotic therapy. With all of these improvements, however, new health threats have emerged. Legionnaire's Disease, Acquired Immune Deficiency Syndrome (AIDS), Reye's Syndrome, and other "new"

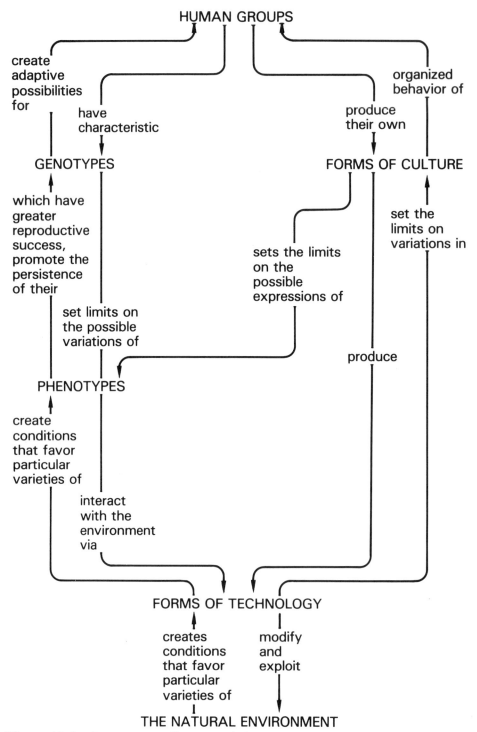

Figure 10-4.   Interaction of man with his environment.

Reproduced with permission of Phillip Whitten. David E. Hunter and Phillip Whitten, eds. **Encyclopedia of Anthropology.** (New York: Harper and Row, Publishers, 1976), pp. 4–5.

diseases continue to appear, indicating that the process of man's adaptation to his environment is an ongoing one.

As many of the infectious diseases of the past have yielded to modern science, new health problems have emerged. Acute illness still ranks as a significant factor in the demand for health and medical services, but there has been a shift toward an increase in the incidence and prevalence of chronic diseases and chronic illness.

These are long-term processes, in which therapeutic goals are aimed at the control of symptoms and disease rather than at cure. Diabetes, hypertension, cardiac, and pulmonary disease are among those health problems identified as chronic. Chronic diseases are most apparent in industrialized countries and can be considered a pattern of disease for those environmental settings. In general, these problems seem to be linked to cultural and social factors, such as stress, lack of exercise, smoking, overcrowding, and overeating. All of these are thought to lead to altered health states.

AMERICAN VALUES

The United States is a land of diversity. Geographically, the area is large with vast differences in climate and terrain. The people represent a variety of lifestyles and ethnic traditions. There are differences in foods, accents, values, and forms of work and play. Some of the differences are obvious; others are subtle and less easily recognized.

All inhabitants of the United States have, even if in distant generations, ancestors who migrated to this country from other parts of the world. Areas from which people have migrated have changed over the centuries. While earlier groups came primarily from the European countries, more recent populations have come from Latin America, Africa, and Asia. They have come as immigrants, refugees, and so-called "illegal aliens." In the early years of this century, the United States was described as a **melting pot**. This term implies that immigrants, by assimilation and acculturation, somehow became American and lost their cultural identity. However, the popular notion has been challenged, as the reality of our cultural pluralism has been recognized. The 1960s and 1970s were decades of increasing awareness of ethnic identity and pride.

Ethnic groups share characteristics, such as language, dialect, values, food habits, customs, and a sense of distinctiveness as a group. Recent census data indicate that 5.4 percent of the people in this country were born outside the United States, and 10.9 percent claim another ethnic heritage along with their American one.[3] At a minimum, 106 ethnic groups have been identified within the United States.[4]

According to Murray and Zentner, many different orientations and value systems operate in a society at one time, but only one orientation dominates in any given period. Currently in the United States, middle class orientation and values are dominant.[5] Examples of these values can be seen in Figure 10.5.

1. Speed, change, progress, activity, and efficiency.
2. Personal achievement, occupational, financial, and social status, self-reliance.
3. Youth, beauty, health.
4. Science and technology.
5. Materialism and consumerism.
6. Group conformity.
7. Competitive and aggressive behavior.
8. Mobility.
9. Pursuit of leisure.
10. Equality.

Figure 10-5. Examples of the dominant middle-class values in the United States.

Source: Ruth Beckmann Murray and Judith Proctor Zentner, **Nursing Concepts for Health Promotion**, 2nd Ed. (Englewood Cliffs, NJ: Prentice-Hall, Inc., 1979), p. 342.

Within this rich diversity, **core values** are central to the American culture. Self-reliance has been identified as a core value with which all other values are connected. This does not mean that any or all individuals are, or can be, totally self-reliant. However, it is the ideal by which people evaluate and are evaluated. Self-reliance manifests itself, in part, in a fear of dependence on others and in the belief in individual freedom.[6] In everyday life, expressions like "pulling one's self up by one's bootstraps" indicate the importance of individual achievement.

The belief that individuals should work for a living is another American core value. Individuals believe that hard work and industry will lead to the "good life." Many immigrants also hold this value, since one of the reasons they came to America was to have a better life. They work hard at menial jobs and struggle to learn the language and, educate themselves and their families.

American culture is characterized by a vast array of manufactured products, a concentration of populations in urban settings, and high-level technology. Values associated with American culture have been described as those of the middle class. There is an emphasis on material goods and on systems that support comfort in life. These include electricity, central air-conditioning and heating, and ease of transportation. The success of individuals and groups is, to a great extent, measured by the possession of material goods and a comfortable lifestyle. Success and achievement also are measured by level of education and by occupation, although to a lesser extent; these alone do not always guarantee high status.[7]

The belief in opportunities for all persons is an American ideal. The value of equality for all, or **egalitarianism,** is one that has not become a reality for some individuals or groups. Ethnic minorities, women, and handicapped persons have had limited access to paths that traditionally have brought material success. This commitment to equality is often expressed in an informal approach to others, overlooking differences in age or prestige. For Americans, there is frequently an attempt to establish relationships on a first-name basis almost immediately.[8]

Another American core value is the value of romantic love and free choice of spouse. Building on this value is the value of each married pair to establish its own household in which to raise children. Owning one's own home is an American dream.

The health care system reflects the norms and values of American culture. There is an emphasis on cleanliness and efficiency. The technology is sophisticated, encompassing diagnostic, monitoring, and treatment aspects of care. The orientation to time is defined by the clock, and routines are established for specific hours of the day and night. Clients are seen by appointment during specified times. In inpatient facilities routines for physical care, medications, and treatments are scheduled by the clock. Meals are served according to a schedule rather than when individuals are hungry and may not conform to individual preferences for eating. Visiting hours are regulated, and there are restrictions on children's visits. In some instances, only immediate family members, such as spouse or parents, may visit. This is particularly true in traditional post partum maternity units and intensive care units. There is much variation in these patterns, however, and not all agencies reflect the same degree of efficiency and technology.

Values are a part of a pattern of living, and because of this, they change slowly. Values are meaningful for those who hold them, and they are accepted without question. Others are expected to respect, if not accept, another person's values. Nurses cannot change a patient's values quickly. Any open attack on an individual's value system is likely to be deeply resented, and the lines of communication may be cut.

We are not always aware of what our values are. What values do you hold? Are some of them different from your parents' and friends'? Probably, because life experiences help shape each individual's value system. Since everyone's experience is different, it is easy to see how patterns can differ. Nurses need to understand the influence of their own values and culture, when working with patients, in order to be more aware of the value systems of others.

All individuals, regardless of their cultural orientation, tend to view their own values as superior to those of others and may even attempt to have others accept their value systems. In nursing, it is important to respect patients' values and to use a sensitive, diplomatic approach if it is necessary to present them with other values. The decision to incorporate new values into an existing set of values should be worked out mutually and ultimately left to the individual involved.

CULTURE AND CULTURES

Man is characterized by his need to live in social groups. **Culture,** used in a very broad sense, is a people's way of living, or a design shared by a group or groups of people. Culture, however, does not exist in and of itself, but can be inferred only from the behavior of people. Culture has been defined as a set of standards for perception, belief, evaluation, communication, and action.[9] While man has the inherent capacity for culture, the specific cultural standards differ from group to group. In every society, culture is learned through both explicit and implicit means. It is shared by the members and is transmitted from one generation to another.

Culture has material and symbolic aspects. Material dimensions include objects, clothing, tools, and forms of technology. The symbolic realm consists of language, ritual, values, norms of behavior, religion, kinship systems, and other nonmaterial content.

Symbolic systems help to organize one's life and social relations. Material aspects of culture would be the importance of a car to a teenager; the object itself carries with it implications of power, adulthood, and freedom. The symbolic domain of ritual allows for culturally prescribed approaches to life passages. Events such as marriage, childbirth, and death typically are surrounded with culturally appropriate rituals. Culture provides solutions for everyday life situations and problems. While the repertoire of solutions varies from culture to culture, there is a regularity to human existence in every society, to which humans respond with culturally defined behavior.

Anthropologists make a distinction between **culture,** the design for living, and **cultures. Cultures** are groups of people who share similar beliefs, attitudes, values, and practices, that form a common design for living. Where groups occupy territories spread over a wide geographic area, there may or may not be continuity of a particular culture. Boundaries between cultural groups may be difficult to identify, and what appears to be all one culture may, in fact, be several. Native Americans often are presumed to be one culture but are actually a number of cultures. There are differences in language, in customs, and in means of using the environment for life sustaining needs. These are known as **intercultural variability;** that is, differences between cultures.

There may be differences within any one culture. Individuals or groups of individuals do not consistently conform to cultural norms and standards in the same manner. Childrearing may vary from family to family in matters of expressions of affection, discipline, play, and other aspects of child care. Adherence to religion and religious practices may vary within groups. Food preferences and eating patterns also may differ. Reasons for such differences include individual preferences, economic status, religious beliefs, role, social standing, age, and sex. Each member can and does choose options for behavior from the whole of the existing cultural content. In any culture, the options may be limited or broad, but social sanctions are used for behavior that is perceived to fall outside the norms of the culture. Differences within a culture are called **intracultural variability.**

In every cultural group, members are socialized with the expectation of participation in the life of the group. Individuals are exposed to the norms, values, and behaviors appropriate for the particular culture of which they are members and for their specific roles within that culture. In every culture, there are expectations of what is appropriate. For instance, the roles of women vary from culture to culture, but in each, there is a role or roles appropriate within the context of that culture. Roles appropriate for one culture do not readily transfer to others. Some adaptation on the part of individuals and groups is necessary in situations of culture change or migration to other environments.

Many times when individuals move to another country, community, or neighborhood, or are admitted to the hospital, they experience a phenomena known as culture shock. Kramer defines **culture shock** as a state of anxiety precipitated by the loss of familiar signs and symbols of social intercourse, when one is suddenly immersed in a cultural system markedly different from his own.[10] Verbal and nonverbal cues in the environment are misleading, because they are misinterpreted by the individual. Responses may be wrong, inappropriate, or totally lacking.

When individuals enter a different culture, whether foreign or a subculture, they experience culture shock. Research in this area has found that individuals suffering from culture shock undergo several stages of behavior as they progress through it. The first phase has been called the **"honeymoon phase."** In this phase, individuals are frequently fascinated with the new culture. Friends and family often act as buffers or translators for the newcomer, and he has no real interaction with the new environment. The newcomer is excited and desires to learn more about the new culture. In this sheltered cocoon, the new culture looks interesting and rosy. Soon, however, the reality of the situation emerges. Familiar cues, such as rewards, sanctions, and role behaviors, are lost, and the honeymoon phase terminates. The individual becomes disenchanted.

The **disenchantment** phase begins when individuals come "into daily contact with conflicting values and ways of doing things for which appropriate skills, interpersonal cues, and responses are lacking."[11] Minor details that did not bother the individual earlier may cause him to lash out bitterly at the causing culture. Rejection of the culture and regression of behavior can be observed during this phase. The home environment, family, and friends suddenly assume enormous proportions. Individuals feel the need to be nurtured and protected in an environment in which they have some control. Preoccupation with the past and an idealization of the home culture is also common. Loneliness is experienced, and contact and extra reassurance from friends and family are required. Contact by means of telephone and mail become central to the individual. If this phase continues, it can become maladaptive, because it arrests the progress of self-discovery and growth. The individual in this second phase of culture shock may begin to reject himself. He may feel that he is a failure, that he cannot cope, and that he should not have made a move into a different culture. He may blame himself for every mistake that occurs and may feel defeated when imminent success is not evident. Behavior may be aggressive or hostile, and the person may feel depressed or extremely fatigued. As this phase burns out, individuals experiencing culture shock enter the third phase.

The **resolution or recovery phase** is the beginning of a positive adaptation. There is a marked reduction in tension, individuals are able to see the lighter side of the situation, and are capable of objectively evaluating the new culture. Individuals then are able to interpret the verbal and nonverbal cues of others more accurately in the host culture.

Effective function is the last phase in the culture shock process. This is the highest level of adaptation, and not all individuals reach this stage. In this phase, individuals become as comfortable in the new culture as in the old. Responses can be made in appropriate ways, and there is a high degree of understanding of the new culture. The old ways are not forgotten or abdicated, but are adapted to meet the new environmental requirements. Individuals are able to grow and change in a healthy, meaningful way.

Not all aspects of a culture are shared with all members. Age and sex influences exposure to cultural content, and specialized knowledge, such as healing practices, may be known to only a few members. Partly as a result of differing participation in the overall culture, **subcultures** may emerge. These are groups within the larger culture that, while sharing the overall culture, have distinctive beliefs, values, and in some instances, lifestyles. They also may have a specialized language that facilitates communication within the group. As an example, the hospital has been described as a subculture. It demonstrates a system of values, a belief system regarding care for the sick, a specialized language, and norms of behavior for its various members including its patient population. Other subcultures in the American culture might include teenagers, professional athletes, the entertainment industry, and the military.

One's own culture, because it is familiar, seems right to its members. It defines the ways to perceive, to act, and to assign meaning and value to one's actions and the actions of others. Behaviors, communication styles, and person-to-person interaction styles observed in other cultures often seem strange, as might actual encounters with individuals from other cultures. Encounters with individuals from other cultures provide an opportunity for appreciating the variety of responses in human situations. Because one's cultural standards seem right and others seem strange, there is the possibility of misunderstanding. Other cultures may be perceived negatively and thought to be inferior to one's own. The judging of other cultures by one's own standards is known as **ethnocentrism.**

Stereotyping is another form of cultural misunderstanding. It occurs when people assume the presence or absence of characteristics in members of other cultural groups. They may be labeled "lazy," "stoic," "dirty," or as having various other traits. Stereotyping is not based on objective assessment of others, but rather, results from preconceived notions. In order to provide holistic, individualized care to patients, families, or groups, nurses must take care not to stereotype patients on the basis of cultural orientation.

One anthropological perspective for understanding human behavior in various cultures is known as **cultural relativism.** This approach is different from ethnocentrism, in that norms and behavior are viewed in relation to their specific cultural contexts. The approach emphasizes that cultures cannot be evaluated as better or worse; cultures are just different. It assumes that differences are an adaptation to specific physical, cultural, or social environments. For instance, in Western civilizations the preferred form of marriage is monogamy. This is not so in some areas of the world, where polygamy is the norm. In these societies, there are economic, cultural, and social factors that support and encourage polygamy's continuation. It is as difficult for an individual coming from such a heritage to understand the western custom as it is for westerners to appreciate polygamy.

FAMILY, GROUP, AND THE LIFECYCLE

The pattern of living in every culture has a regularity of its own. Human beings everywhere order their social relations so that they can live together effectively. Mutually understood behaviors are a necessary part of this. A series of **social roles,** i.e., expected behaviors that are culturally acceptable, is found in every society. Only when these reciprocal behaviors are understood and respected can the purposes of the society be carried out. Individuals are socialized into the role behaviors appropriate for membership in the group. In every society, for example, there are culturally approved role expectations for men and women. Role expectations also differ based on age and social status and, even in the so-called primitive cultures, can be extremely complex.

The basic unit of organization in every society is the family. In its simplest form, this is composed of mother and child; in most societies the father is the male individual who socially fulfills the role but he need not be the biological father of the child or children. In some societies, the mother's brother is responsible for the upbringing of the children, and the mother's husband (who may be the biological father) has the same responsibility for his sister's children. In all societies, the mother-child unit is part of a larger group through which economic, educational, and affective needs are met.

In all cultures, kinship systems determine the relatedness of people. These systems are part of the larger design for living and include ties of marriage and descent. Kinship may be based on biological ties, which are culturally determined to be important, and on social ties, in which no biological tie is present or necessary. Kinship may be reckoned along the maternal line only, the paternal only, or along both lines. Residence patterns often reflect the larger kinship systems, with married children living with either the wife's family or the husband's family or establishing independent households.

In Western culture we consider the nuclear family, mother-father-children, to be the standard. Cross-culturally, however, this is not the most usual arrangement, and family structures take many forms. (The reader is referred to Chapter 25, The Family As a System, for further discussion on family structures.)

All human groups note the biological processes of life with culturally acceptable behaviors. The **lifecycle**—representing stages in the process of maturation starting with birth and ending with death—is a universal human experience. Progress through the various stages—infancy, childhood, puberty, adulthood, and old age—involves role changes that are significant for the individual and the group. Not all cultures identify stages in the same way, and there may be specific distinctions within stages. For instance, in the United States, we separate the stages of childhood into infancy, toddler, preschool, and school age. In some cultures, where breastfeeding lasts up to two years, infants are defined as children when they are weaned. Cultural definitions of adulthood—when it is achieved and how it is socially recognized—also vary cross-culturally.

Movements from role to role through the lifecycle are accompanied by rituals that emphasize the importance of these changes. **Rites of passage** serve to separate the individual from his earlier status, allow for a transitional period before moving to another, and finally, become incorporated into his new status.[12] In many cultures, progress from adolescence to adulthood occurs at the time of marriage, i.e., a permanent economic and social arrangement between male and female. Culturally prescribed methods, such as an engagement period that concludes with marriage, surround these events in most societies.

Through infancy, childhood, and adolescence, the individual is being prepared to become a competent adult in his own culture. The process of **enculturation,** the transmission of cultural knowledge from one generation to the next, is the means through which this is accomplished. Childhood is a time of intense learning. Children are expected to learn language, appropriate behaviors toward parents, relatives, other societal members and the opposite sex, social norms, systems of values, beliefs, and religion, and a view of self, group, and the world. Positive and negative sanctions are used by parents, other caretakers, and the peer group to ensure conformity to cultural standards. Both the natural social sanctions of ridicule and gossip and supernatural sanctions, in the form of roots and ancestors, are used.

With the onset of puberty, another turning point in social development is reached. Roles change as the child moves toward adulthood. Rituals and ceremonies mark this step in the lifecycle. The ritual confirms to the group and to the individual that this stage in social development has occurred. While it usually coincides with the physiological changes associated with puberty, there is some variation among cultures in this regard.

Frequently, socially recognized adulthood comes with parenthood. Everywhere there is considerable attention given to matters of pregnancy and birth. In societies where diets are inadequate and health care is poor or lacking altogether, miscarriages and high infant mortality are common. Everywhere there are limits on

the behavior of pregnant women and on newly delivered women. Taboos related to food, sexual activity, bathing, and a variety of other behaviors are culturally developed ways of ensuring a successful outcome of pregnancy—a healthy infant and mother. With miscarriages, stillborns, or fetal death, a violation of taboos may be identified as the reason for these occurrences, and the unfortunate woman may be subject to anger or scorn from her family and group members. Labor and childbirth are processes that, in all cultures, demand the support and presence of designated people. In some cultures, the midwife and the woman's relatives assist her. In professional health care systems, physicians, nurses, and technical staff assist in delivery, and family are only rarely present. In the United States in recent years there has been movement away from a depersonalized approach to labor and delivery, and the inclusion of the father and sometimes the siblings is encouraged, in the events surrounding childbirth. Professional nurse midwives are increasingly in demand, and some hospitals have homelike "birthing" rooms in addition to the traditional delivery room.

Adulthood also can be divided into stages, and these vary among cultures. Chronological age may indicate the stages. Events such as the marriage of children or the birth of grandchildren can note passage from one stage to another. Old age is only one of these stages. In some cultures, old age carries considerable weight and is recognized and rewarded. The elderly are honored members of the group. In the dominant American culture, with its emphasis on youth, many people go to considerable pains to conceal their increasing years, by undergoing face and body lifts, and using makeup and hair dye.

Death is a biological fact. It is, for the living, primarily a social fact that requires some major readjustments. Man has devised many rites, ceremonies, and rules for prescribed and prohibited behaviors concerning the inevitability of death. Death separates the living from the dead. In societies where the dead are respected as ancestors, they continue to exist, but in a changed relationship to the group. Almost universally, there is a belief in some form of continuation of the person. Expected behaviors surrounding death define how mourners should behave and how others in society relate to the dead individual's kin. Mourning periods are culturally defined in terms of length, and ritual acts announce their termination. Funeral customs, despite their variations in form, must be suited to two goals: appropriate disposal of the body and assistance to the mourners in reordering their lives and relationships. Cross-culturally, funeral rites reflect the status of the dead person; those of higher status are accorded more elaborate rites, and the period of mourning may be extended.

FOOD

One of the main tasks facing all social groups is that of providing adequate nourishment for its members. The survival and continuation of the group and of its individual members depends, to a great extent, on successful strategies for meeting this need. Cultures around the world have met this need in a variety of ways. There are hunters and gatherers who feed themselves successfully from the plants and animals in their environments. In these societies, most individuals have some role in the acquisition or preparation of food. Other societies depend on subsistence farming in addition to relying on naturally occurring foods. In the industrialized nations, such as the United States, relatively few individuals are involved directly in the production or distribution of food, and only a small portion of the land is used in the production of food for the majority of the people. In these countries, most food is acquired by means of a cash economy, and a large variety of foods is usually available.

Human nutritional needs are those of adequate calories, protein, carbohydrates, fats, vitamins, and minerals. **Nourishment** is a physiological need. **Food** is a cultural definition, and from the environment in which he lives, man selects substances for use as food. Only a portion of all the available nutritional possibilities are defined as edible. What is considered to be edible is defined differently in cultures around the world. Substances considered to be edible in one culture may be inedible in others. Examples of this are numerous. Shellfish is avoided by some cultural groups but is routinely consumed in others. In India, cattle are considered to be sacred and are never slaughtered for food; in American culture, beef is one of our principal meats. Other substances, such as insects, snakes, cats, and horses, are used as food in many cultures but are rejected by Westerners.

Within the category of edible food, there are many distinctions. Food may be considered fit for animal consumption but not human. Foods may be acceptable for adults, but not for children. Conversely, foods may be thought necessary or suitable for children but partially or totally avoided by adults. For instance, in American culture, milk is seen as a requirement for children, but most adults do not routinely drink it. This is largely the result of culturally learned attitudes. However, adults in some cultures, including some Native American Indians and Oriental people, are deficient in lactase, an enzyme necessary in the digestion of milk, and are unable to tolerate it.

Food taboos are common throughout the world. Some are the result of religious dogma, but the origin of many is unknown. Taboos associated with animal flesh and animal products are numerous. Muslims and Jews do not eat pork; other groups avoid beef. Food taboos often are associated with pregnancy and the post partum period. Some cultural prohibitions on certain foods during pregnancy are based on notions that the child will be marked or harmed in some way, e.g., eating strawberries will result in red birthmarks on the baby. Where food taboos involve foods for which no comparable nutritional substitutes exist, the consequences for health can be severe. Kwashiorkor, for example, is a disease that occurs when young children do not receive adequate proteins, in both quantity and quality, to meet their maintenance and growth needs. The disease results in a lack of normal development. Called the "second child disease," it is frequently seen in children who have been weaned because of a second pregnancy of the mother. The word Kwashiorkor comes from the Ghan language and, literally translated, means "the sickness the older child gets when the baby is born."[13] In some African societies with dietary taboos on milk and meat, Kwashiorkor in children is common. Even in the United States, each year a number of cases of this condition are reported.

Beliefs and customs about food differ from culture to culture but exist in some form in every culture. Foods may be described as "good for you" in that they promote or maintain health. In some cultures specific foods are of enormous importance and are consumed at all or most meals. Among these are rice in the Orient and yams in parts of Africa. In areas where Western culture has been introduced into tribal cultures, foods such as white bread and refined sugars have prestige value and are often consumed in place of traditional foods. The replacement of breastfeeding with bottlefeeding in many societies for infant nutrition (often with disastrous consequences) is one example of recent influences of prestige in changing traditional practices.

There are many social and symbolic aspects of food and food habits. Eating is a

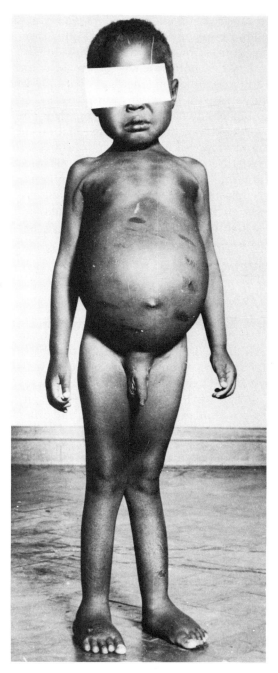

Figure 10-6. Child with Kwashiorkor. Symptoms include: dry, scaly skin with areas of depigmentation; dermatoses; blindness; thin dry hair; alopecia; loss of weight; edema; muscular atrophy, diarrhea; and behavior changes.

social behavior, and it involves prescribed rules all over the world. For example, timing, content of meals and norms for who eats with whom in each society. In some cultures, women and men eat separately. In industralized countries, employers and employees do not usually eat together. The sharing of food has expressive functions in maintaining social ties. Celebrations and feasts are activities in which food, often elaborate and in great amounts, enhances group solidarity. Important events and rituals, such as marriages and funerals, are frequently accompanied by food.

RELIGION

All human societies have some set of beliefs that can be defined, in a broad sense, as religious. No one definition of the term "religion" can be used in all cultures. Religion is the means man uses to deal with forces and beings that are not visible in his material world. These include gods, spirits, good and evil, angels, ghosts, and other unknown powers. In some cultures, invisible beings are part of the "real" or natural world, and in others they are assigned to the realm of the supernatural.

Religion functions to help man deal with life events and situations that are beyond his control. Problems of disease and illness are commonly handled in religions. It offers an explanation of why things happen, as well as culturally prescribed religious behaviors to manage them. Religion defines the natures of good and evil. For many cultures, the term **magicoreligious** is a useful one. These systems include aspects of magic that can be used for good and evil, and witchcraft, which is always seen as harmful.

Religious rituals may be quite simple or extremely elaborate. Rituals contribute to group solidarity and, at the same time, reinforce the beliefs of the systems. Beliefs also are reinforced by trances, visions, or dreams. Systems of religion reflect and are embedded in the larger cultural system. Sacred myths describe the origin of man and how human life came to be. In all cultures, even simple tribal societies, religious systems are complex sets of beliefs.

The great religions of the world today, e.g., Buddhism, Christianity, Judaism, are institutionalized. They are characterized by unique buildings, writings, and ritual specialists. However, religion, whatever its external aspects, serves as a universal solution for fundamental human problems.

DISEASE AND ILLNESS IN CULTURAL CONTEXT

In every society, illness is a matter of concern. It disrupts social relationships and threatens the overall functioning of society. All cultures are similar in that they have some systematic approach to treating disease and caring for the sick. They are different in the specific ways in which disease and illness are caused, diagnosed, and treated. The health beliefs and practices of any society are an integral part of the total cultural system. Illnesses found in one culture cannot always be understood in another cultural system. For example, **susto,** an illness caused by fright, is widely recognized among Latin American peoples. It is a cultural reality for which causes and treatment can be identified, but it has no counterpart in Western medicine.

Western medicine is one system of health beliefs and practices. It is a biomedical approach in which disease is identified primarily through objective measurements. Identification of disease-causing organisms and abnormal laboratory values are a major part of the system. Disease may not be synonymous with illness and may be present without the knowledge of the individual or other societal members. For example, essential hypertension, often called a silent disease, is an example of these distinctions, and an individual may be hypertensive, on the basis of elevated systolic and diastolic readings, without being aware of it. He is "diseased" by biomedical criteria. However, it is likely that the individual will present no disturbance in his work, family, or social life; he will not exhibit behaviors associated with being "ill." Illness is a cultural and social definition describing an inability to function in usual roles and activities.

Non-Western cultures have other beliefs regarding causes of disease and illness. One view is a personal one, in which the affected individual perceives himself and is perceived as a victim. His illness results from the actions of human or supernatural beings and is intended for him alone. These beings may be sorcerers, evil spirits, ancestors, gods, or other beings whose existence is acceptable in the cultural context. Another view is based on notions of equilibrium. Health is maintained under conditions of equilibrium between opposite elements; illness results when equilibrium is disturbed. Balances of heat and cold figure prominently in these systems. The definition of hot and cold is primarily symbolic rather than physical. In Latin America "hot" causes of disease include emotional upsets, such as anger or exposure to the sun; they are treated with "cold." A similar distinction appears in traditional Chinese medicine, in which the forces of **yin** and **yang** interact. Yin represents the positive, which includes heat; yang represents the negative, which includes cold. In both cultural systems, it is believed that treatment with the substances containing the opposite element restores equilibrium and cures the individual.[14]

Sick Role

Every culture has ways of caring for those members who are, by their cultural definition, ill. Persons who are ill and those who care for them reflect role expectations and behaviors. One way of describing these expectations is the sick role. Based on Western cultural norms, it is not known whether or not this model can be useful in cross-cultural understanding of illness as a universal human experience. The role has four components:

- The sick person is exempted from his usual responsibilities
- The sick person is unable to return to health through his own efforts and must seek assistance
- The sick person should wish to recover
- The sick person must cooperate with treatment.[15]

The ill person and the healing and caring persons are involved in a set of reciprocal behaviors. The situation of providing nursing care is one in which role behaviors can be illustrated. The nurse assesses the patient on the basis of behavioral cues provided by the patient. These behaviors may include those related to physical activity, verbalization, eating, interaction with family members and health professionals, and health maintaining and promoting behaviors exhibited by the patient and his family. Similarly, the nurse's evaluation of patient responses to nursing intervention is based on changes or alterations in these behaviors that indicate the effectiveness of the intervention. When behavioral norms are rooted in the nurse's cultural background, the standard of measurement may not be culturally appropriate for the individual patient.

Commonalities and differences were identified when sick role expectations were examined in the United States and India. Both American and Indian nurses believed their patients should trust them, should be cooperative, and should ask questions about their care. However, there were differences in the degree and timing of independence that was expected of their respective patients. The American cultural emphasis on independence and self-help was evident in an expectation of early independence. The Indian cultural orientation toward interdependence and destiny led to a different set of norms for behavior. Indian nurses expected their patients to take a less active role in treatment than did the American nurses. Expected patient behaviors in each culture were norms held by both nurses and patients, not by either group alone.[16] These, then, are implicit and reciprocal understandings that guide both care givers and sick individuals in therapeutic situations.

Healers and Healing

The professional health system of the Western world is characterized by a variety of specialized roles. The roles include those of nurse, physician, dietitian, social worker, and an array of other therapeutic and technical roles. These are usually full-time professional roles for which lengthy training is required. Practitioners generally wear clothing that defines their roles and the types of tasks they accomplish, for example, scrub outfits required in operating rooms. The system is large, complex, and usually, depersonalized. Treatment is privately done in offices, clinics and/or hospital rooms.

In both Western and non-Western societies, traditional systems and traditional healers exist. Traditional healers are often called indigenous curers or indigenous healers. Other titles include shaman, medicine men or women, and among the Navajo, "singers." In these systems, and in the various folk traditions, religion and medicine often are blended. They are systems of belief and practice that have their own internal logic and are imbedded in the larger culture of which they are a part. Herbs, rituals, massage, and medicines are some of the therapeutic tools. Culturally defined

diseases, such as the "evil eye," are known to be outside the curing ability of professional health practitioners and are referred to traditional healers. Conversely, diabetes and other chronic diseases usually are not referred to traditional healers.

In many nonliterate societies, today, as in the past, the traditional healer carries out vital functions in curing disease and in maintaining social solidarity. The healer acts as a judge where illness is caused by

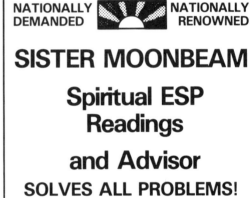

Figure 10-7.   Spiritualists offer one alternative to health care.

the breaking of taboos or other socially unacceptable behavior. Illnesses caused by the supernatural or by witchcraft are also within the realm of the healer's power. Healing rituals are generally performed before the patient's family or the whole community. They serve to cure disease and to correct the life events that led to the illness, thereby reestablishing social stability. The body/mind distinction, so apparent in Western thought, is not reflected in traditional systems.

In the United States today, there are many folk systems and healers. Native American Indian systems, the Black folk tradition with its "root" medicine, and Spanish-American folk medicine are only a few of those routinely used. Spiritualists, faith healers, herbalists, and local curers offer alternative approaches. These jobs are not full-time occupations, as in the case of professional practitioners, and are frequently based on a calling from a higher power.

In order for nurses to work effectively with individuals, families, and groups of different cultural orientations, cultural concepts must be assessed and incorporated into the nursing process.

THE NURSING PROCESS

Because of the great ethnic diversity in the United States, the cultural aspects of patient care have always been an important part of health care delivery. There is even a diversity within the society, as identified health needs may be quite different in New England and in southern California. Some of this diversity is due to the underlying philosophy of the individuals living in each area, and some may be due to the types of ethnic groups present in the area. Today, cultural aspects of health care are even more important, due to the ease of transportation and the high level of technology in modern society. Mobility, pover-

ty, and world turmoil bring more immigrants to America every day in search of a new life. These immigrants need to be channeled into the health care system for illness prevention, immunization, health teaching, health maintenance, and medical care. No other country in the world has so many different cultural groups, each with its own beliefs, values, practices, and lifestyle. Many of these are congruent with the dominant society, but some are not. In order to provide comprehensive patient care, nurses need to be knowledgeable about each of the components of culture and how these components affect behavior and adaptation. Knowledge about many cultures is desirable, but it is especially important to learn about those that are prominent locally.

Nurses are able to provide comprehensive care through use of the nursing process. The nursing process is composed of four interdependent steps: assessment, planning, implementation, and evaluation, but it is heavily dependent upon the assessment phase. Nurses need to be aware that cultural heritage may influence behavior related to health and illness practices, and therefore, make a careful assessment of their patients' cultural background and needs.

Assessment

Although each culture has unique features, some cultural universals can be identified and specifically assessed. These include language, religion, rituals, health perceptions and practices, nutrition, family systems, birth and death practices, time orientation, privacy, territoriality, and touch. Cultural assessments and planning strategies are essential to providing comprehensive nursing care. In assessing the patient holistically, the nurse should systematically gather information regarding each patient's cultural orientation. The assessment tool shown in Figure 10-8 was

Name _____ Age _____ Sex _____ Marital Status _____

Address _____ Phone _____

Religion (specify denomination) _____ Clergyman _____

Educational level _____ Occupation _____

Communication
Language spoken at home _____ Does patient speak English? Yes _____ No _____
If yes, how much? Few words _____ Basic vocabulary _____ Speaks fluently _____
Does patient understand English? Yes _____ No _____ If yes, how much? _____
Can a family member (or friend) speak English? Yes _____ No _____
Can that person stay with the patient to interpret? Yes _____ No _____
If yes, when? (hours) Sun _____ M _____ T _____ W _____ Th _____ F _____ S _____
Can another person act as translator? Yes _____ No _____ Who _____ Phone _____
Does patient reach out to touch? Yes _____ No _____
Do family members touch each other? Yes _____ No _____
Would any common gestures assist in understanding the patient? _____
Does the patient pull away when touched? Yes _____ No _____
Does the patient touch health care givers? Yes _____ No _____

Religious Beliefs
Is Baptism permitted? Yes _____ No _____ Is so, by whom? _____
Under what circumstances? _____
Will the patient permit blood transfusion? Yes _____ No _____
Will the patient accept medications? Yes _____ No _____
If only specific types, which types? _____
Do religious leaders have a role in prevention or treatment? _____
What rituals are necessary? _____ Circumcision? Yes _____ No _____
How are religious artifacts disposed of? _____

Health Perception
Prevention—Related to religion? Yes _____ No _____
Do any beliefs contradict those of health care agency? Yes _____ No _____
If yes, what? _____
Do any beliefs coincide with health care agency? Yes _____ No _____ If yes, what? _____
How is health care system perceived? _____
Illness—Will of God? Yes _____ No _____ Predestined? Yes _____ No _____
  Evil spirits? Yes _____ No _____ Evil eye? Yes _____ No _____
What rituals or practices are necessary to restore health? _____

Health-Illness Practices
What medications and folk medicine treatments, regimens, etc., is patient using? _____

Where are these purchased? _____
Who prepares them? _____ Who administers them? _____
Is the patient permitted by his physician to continue taking these preparations?
  Yes _____ No _____
Who treats the sick in the patient's family? Grandmother _____ Faith healer _____
  Medicine Man _____
Does patient ask for pain medicine or exhibit stoicism? _____
What are cultural beliefs about the experience of pain? _____
Belief as to what caused the disease process the patient is exhibiting? _____
What is the patient's outlook for the future? _____
Disposal of amputated limbs _____
Physical care and comfort—Skin care _____ Hair care _____ Bathing _____
What are practices concerning prevention of illness? _____

Nutrition
Ethnic preference _____ Cultural/Religious taboos _____
Holiday and festive occasions _____ Who prepares food at home? _____
If necessary can someone bring special foods? Yes ____ No ____ Who _____ Phone _____
Has diet been modified by illness? Yes ____ No ____
Likes _____ Dislikes _____

Time Orientation
Does patient need to be reminded of appointments? Yes ____ No ____

Territoriality
Does patient stand close to others? Yes ____ No ____ Far away? Yes ____ No ____
Does patient retreat to room ____ bed ____ for privacy?
Does patient pull covers over face ____ turn away ____ draw curtains ____?

Privacy
Will patient allow physical examination? Yes ____ No ____
  By person of opposite sex? Yes ____ No ____
Will patient remove his/her clothes? Yes ____ No ____
Does another family member have to be present? Yes ____ No ____
Any special considerations of personal belongings? _____

Family
Who makes decisions? _____ Relationship _____
Who makes health decisions? _____ Relationship _____
Can patient make own health decisions? Yes ____ No ____
Does patient have to consult with the decisionmakers? Yes ____ No ____
Do family health beliefs or practices conflict with hospital/clinic health teaching and practices?
  Yes ____ No ____ If yes, describe _____

Effects of illness or hospitalization on other members of household _____

What hours are best for various family members to visit? _____

Death (optional)
What are dominant practices? _____
Deathbed confession? Yes ____ No ____ Last rites? Yes ____ No ____
Who is to be called? Family ____ Clergy ____
Will bedside ritual be required? Yes ____ No ____
Are there measures to ward off death? Yes ____ No ____
Where does patient/family want the patient to die? Home ____ Hospital ____ Other ____
Who should be with patient at the time of death? _____
What is the role of the family members in the death of patient? _____
What are the preparations for burial? _____
Who performs these? _____
Additional comments, observations, and assessments _____

©1980 Janet-Beth McCann Flynn

Figure 10-8. Cultural Assessment Tool.

developed to facilitate individual cultural assessment. This tool can be reproduced and placed on the patient's chart, care plan, or Kardex. When using this tool, it is suggested that the data be gathered by the primary nurse assigned to the patient rather than as a routine admission procedure. The nurse may wish to proceed slowly with the data gathering, perhaps in two or three sessions over several days. In this way, the information gathering is not as threatening to the patient, and the data may be more accurate. The tool may be used selectively along with other assessments, and some parts may be omitted totally.

Communication. When patients do not speak English well enough to express their needs or to understand what is said to them, they can become highly stressed and anxious. Alternate means of communication need to be established including: flash cards, nonverbal behavior, use of translator, or printed material, such as pamphlets or booklets. These printed materials can be obtained from a number of agencies, such as the American Diabetes Association, the American Cancer Association, and others. Translations on flash cards can be made in most high school or college language departments. Frequently, the nursing service office has a list of people who can act as translators. In large cities, embassy offices may be contacted for a reference list of translators. Family members also can be asked to visit at specific times to act as translators. It is important to keep three things in mind when dealing with patients who do not speak English:

- Assess how much English the patient knows.
- Speak to the patient in English, since communication is a natural process.
- Use nonverbal communication.

Inability to communicate also complicates the teaching-learning process. It is impossible to teach a patient, family, or group if a common language cannot be found, or if literature in the patient's language cannot be found. An interpreter will be necessary in situations like this. When this situation arises, it is important to locate an interpreter who will interpret what is said literally by both the patient and the nurse. If it is not tactful to ask a patient

certain types of questions, for example, about birth control, the nurse needs an interpreter who will tell her so and ask her to rephrase the questions to be interpreted in an acceptable way.

Another issue related to culture and language involves asking the patient, "Do you understand?" rather than assessing a change in behavior or evaluating learning in a more concrete manner. In some cultures, it is considered rude to say "no," so the patient may respond "yes," even though he doesn't understand. Later, he may be too embarrassed to ask for further information or to question nurses on other aspects of their health data.

Cultural aspects are extremely important for the nurse to consider. They often are overlooked, due to lack of knowledge, or not viewed as having a key role in the way some patients behave. If the special needs of culturally divergent individuals are not met, then the effectiveness of the nursing process is compromised.

Religion. Religion is another aspect of culture that needs to be assessed, since it can play an important role and have an impact on many aspects of patient's lives. Brownlee writes, "Health workers who come from cultures where religion receives very minimal attention may not fully realize the profound effect religion may have on the lives of patients from strongly religious backgrounds. Religion may affect a people's values, beliefs, practices . . . a . . . whole concept of health and illness and influence the health care that they receive."[17]

Health Perception. "Some cultures view illness as a punishment from God for sinful acts. Others may regard illness as the work of malevolent persons who want to see them suffer . . . others are convinced that illness is caused by evil spirits, and as a result they can receive help only from spiritualists or witch doctors."[18] Prevention and cure are often closely related to the way that the cause of the illness is perceived, and therefore, need to be carefully assessed. If the cause is perceived as punishment, cure and comfort measures may be refused. Other steps may be taken, such as lighting candles, bargaining with God, saints, or spirits, fasting, or using traditional items. Patients may prefer a faith healer or shaman to deal with their illness in a holistic way.

Health-Illness Practices. Another important factor to be considered in a cultural assessment is health-illness practices. It is important to find out the individual's perception of health. Many times it means not the absence of disease but the ability to work in the face of pain or illness. Patients who believe that illness is caused by God as punishment may be difficult to educate to health prevention means.

Further illness behaviors may include self-diagnosis, self-medication and medication exchange with friends. If these do not produce a cure, a physician may be seen. Many cultural groups feel that the health care system will not be helpful for them and they seek alternatives, such as folk medicine, herbs, and folk healers.

Many diseases are also culturally centered. Mexican Americans, for example, suffer from the following conditions:

- **Susto**—(fright), which is caused by a frightening experience. Symptoms include insomnia, tension, and loss of appetite.
- **Empacho**—which is caused by poorly digested foods. Symptoms include: fever, diarrhea, vomiting, stomach aches, and restlessness.
- **Mal de ojo**—(evil eye) caused by magic. Symptoms include fever, headache, irritability, loss of appetite, and restlessness.

Many of these culturally defined illnesses are cured by a knowledgeable adult in the family, a close friend, or a curandero, or curandera (persons who practice folk

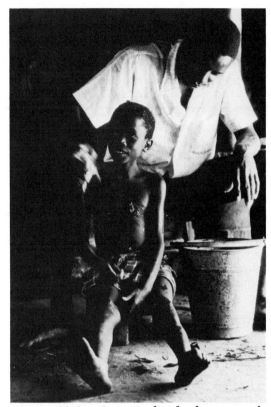

Figure 10-9. Some individuals may seek out herbs and folk medicines as cures.

medicine). At this point, no Western medical cures have been identified.

The Native American also has culturally related illness practices. Prevention or curative rituals may be performed in order to restore the body's harmony with nature. Medicine men or women traditionally fill this role. Curative rituals may include sprinkling cornmeal, singing, dancing, and sand painting.

For the Chinese, health is defined as a normal flow of energy. This life energy is kept in balance by the forces of yin and yang, and when an imbalance occurs, there is illness.

Nutrition. Nutrition is another function of culture that has an impact on nursing and health care. Many nutritional habits are based on religious beliefs. For example, the orthodox Jewish diet forbids shellfish, pork, and meat and dairy products during the same meal, and there are special requirements for handling dishes, utensils, and pots. The heads of men are covered when eating. These beliefs stem from the time of Moses and are still held today.

Diets in other cultures are chosen for their health maintenance quality. If these diets are not followed, it is believed that a disequilibrium will occur and result in sickness. If hot foods and cold foods are not balanced, the individual may become sick. Examples of these cultures include Mexicans, Native Americans, and Chinese. What makes a food hot or cold is not its temperature, but is defined by beliefs about the food themselves. Other diets are based on tradition, for example, some black diets are highly spiced and use ham and pork a great deal.

Food produces "feelings of security and happiness . . . used as a link to friendship, . . . pleasure . . . and as a symbol of religious belief."[19] In the assessment phase of the nursing process, nurses should be aware of the holistic effect of food on patients and the relationship of food, religion, and ritual.

Time Orientation. Most middle class Americans tend to be future oriented. Some cultural groups may appear to be present oriented, although there is some discussion in the literature about the relevance of this component of culture. It is important to recognize this, especially when planning future care, clinic visits, and other health-oriented activities such as immunizations. Time orientation within a 24-hour period is also important to assess. Americans tend to "live by the clock" and instructions to take a pill at 8 am and at 8 pm are meaningful. In other cultures, other timed events, such as bedtime or sunrise, may be more meaningful.

Territoriality. Territories are fixed areas around individuals that are defended against others. There areas are unconsciously learned, are a form of nonverbal behavior, and are generally influenced by culture. E. T. Hall, an anthropologist who studied the use of personal space, divided space individuals use into four measurable distances: intimate, personal, social, and public.

Entering a person's intimate or personal space can be disturbing. One's territory is a culturally defined area, and special distances vary with patient's culture. Individuals in some groups stand very close while others do not. Territoriality should be assessed in a holistic assessment because of the many opportunities health workers have for violating this cultural norm.

Touch. Americans are not a group who touch a great deal or who like to be touched. Many patients, however, touch and like to be touched. Greeting persons without touching them may be interpreted as dislike or rejection in some cultures.

Privacy/Modesty. In many cultures, modesty and privacy are supremely guarded. Nurses and other health care workers often are preoccupied with "getting a job done" and may overlook the patient's need in this regard. Some cultures are extremely modest, especially women. The Mexican-American, Arab, and Gypsy women are some examples of this, as are Orientals and other Easterners. Violations of a person's need for privacy can generate anger and resentment, as well as noncompliance with treatments and therapy. It is, therefore, very important that nurses identify and respect the need for privacy and modesty.

Family. Another cultural facet to be explored is the family structure and role definition. The family is important to all patients. In some cultures, the kin network is extensive, and individuals have close emotional ties to family. In most cultures a specific member of the family is designated as the decisionmaker. It may be the breadwinning male or the oldest female, depending upon the culture. Also, the decisionmaker for family matters may differ from the individual who makes the health related decisions. The person who decides if the sick child will return to the clinic for follow-up should be identified and included in the teaching plan. If that person is not involved, follow-up may not be carried out. Because the person who makes decisions about health is the person who influences the health practices of the family or group, it is very important for the nurse to identify this person.

If the patient is terminally ill, cultural variations of death and dying should be assessed. This may be done by questioning the patient, the family, religious persons, or consulting the literature. In some cultures, death is never directly discussed, so assessment of this culture facet should be done with the utmost sensitivity, and maybe not at all.

At the conclusion of the nursing process, nursing diagnoses are formulated. Some examples of nursing diagnoses based on a cultural assessment might be:

- Limited communication patterns related to a language barrier.
- Inability to eat hospital food related to religious beliefs.
- Divergent health decisionmaking power related to family structure.

After the nursing diagnoses have been prepared and written on the care plan, the planning phase of the nursing process begins.

Planning

The nursing care plan is based on the data gathered during the assessment phase. As it is developed it is written on the patient's chart or Kardex. Concepts related to the cultural orientation of patients should be incorporated into the plan in order for the plan to be individualized, holistic, and comprehensive.

When using the cultural assessment as a guide to prepare the plan, several things need to be considered. If the patient does not understand English, planning for a good interpreter is essential. If the patient is literate in his own language, written materials in his language can be gathered at this time. Also, some of the major drug companies have small booklets providing translations of medical/nursing terms in several languages.[20,21] These may be obtained by writing to the various companies or consulting a patient education specialist.

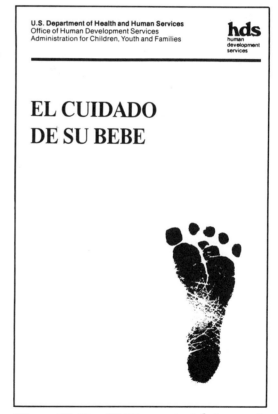

U.S. Department of Health and Human Services
Office of Human Development Services
Administration for Children, Youth and Families

hds
human development services

EL CUIDADO DE SU BEBE

Figure 10-10.   Written materials in a variety of languages can be obtained from voluntary and other types of agencies.

If religious leaders have a role in rituals or services, they need to be incorporated into the plan. For example, if an American Indian medicine man is planning a sing, then arrangements need to be made with him and a schedule established. Also, a room that is at the end of a hall or sound-proof may be necessary, so that other patients will not be disturbed.

Knowing the patient's perception of disease causality is essential in planning care. Any behaviors associated with this perception should be incorporated. If pain and disease are viewed as punishment, providing information regarding the disease process and pain medication may be required.

Planning for health and illness practices is also helpful. The health care team needs to be consulted in planning in this area. If patients wish to take folk medicines or herbs, the physician should be consulted to establish the origin of the medicine or herb in the event that it may be contraindicated. If these alternative herbs and folk medicines are to be incorporated, then a source must be established.

If rituals are performed at the bedside using materials held in high regard to peoples of ethnic groups, it should be determined who should handle and remove them. Many times, it is the person or persons who placed them around the patient, but in some instances the nurse or the housekeeping department may remove any materials. This aspect should be confirmed by the patient and the persons performing the service and incorporated in the plan.

Nutritional aspects of culture need to be taken into account when planning patient care. This is generally an interdisciplinary plan with the agency nutritionist acting as the consultant. Many times, institutional foods can be adapted for special requirements. Most hospitals, for example, have TV style Kosher dinners with disposable dishes and utensils to meet Kosher patients' requirements. Family and friends can be consulted, and plans to bring food from home can be made.

If time orientation appears to be present, nurses should plan to contact patients in advance to remind them of impending immunizations, checkups, or clinic visits. When this is done, there is a greater incidence of follow-through for patients.

In terms of space, touch, and privacy, steps can be planned so as not to violate the patient's sense of territory or privacy. If nurses are aware that this is a real problem, extra time can be allotted to allow for more privacy. Privacy also should be assured if the patient is to have a religious ceremony or folk healing ritual.

Finally, patients' families should be incorporated into the plan. Times for visiting can be scheduled so that nurses have time to interact, assess, and teach them. If appropriate, the family decisionmaker should be sought out and asked to participate in the care and planning as well as in the decisionmaking.

During the planning phase, time limited goals, objectives, and outcome criteria should be formulated and written on the care plan (see Teaching and Learning Chapter 12). These, too, should reflect the cultural components of health and illness.

Once the plan, with goals, objectives, and outcome criteria, has been formulated, the third phase of the nursing process can begin.

Implementation

Implementation is the dynamic process of carrying out the plan. The first step is establishing a trusting relationship with the patient, family, or group. This requires taking the patient, family, or group at face value, without judging them based on ethnocentric standards. In order to begin the nurse/patient relationship, a means of communication must be established. If language is a problem, the assessment tool and the nursing care plan should be consulted for interpreters or material resources. Nonverbal and verbal communication can be used, too.

Patients' folk medicines and herbs can be prepared by the nurse if necessary and administered with other medicines ordered by the physician. Folk healers may wish to assist during the phase of the plan implementation, and when possible, should be encouraged to do so. Traditional beliefs can be supported in this manner and incorporated into the Western mode of health care.

Nurses need to be culturally sensitive to all aspects of the nursing care plan as they work with the wide variety of patients from many ethnic groups seen in the health care system today. During the implementation phase, evaluative data are gathered regarding the effectiveness of the plan. This leads to the fourth and final step of the nursing process, the evaluation of the plan and care.

Evaluation

Evaluation is an ongoing process that weighs the outcomes of the plan. Patient behaviors are measured and evaluated using the goals, objectives, and outcome criteria that were formulated during the planning phase. If the plan is good and the objective and outcome criteria realistic, then the plan is usually effective. If some aspects are not working, then a reassessment of the patient situation is in order. It is important to note that many cultural differences between people are extremely subtle and not easily identified. When these cultural nuances take the form of attitudes and feelings rather than overt behaviors, the nurse may have difficulty evaluating and pinpointing specific causes of the problem. The cause of the problem may be a global mistrust of nurses or the whole health care system, for example, and this fact may never be isolated—particularly in the hospital setting, where contact is episodic and brief. Consultation with family and friends is very helpful in the evaluation phase and can provide the nurse with further assessment information. The nursing care plan then can be revised according to the new findings.

CONCLUSIONS

Culture is man's primary strategy in adapting to his physical and social environment. The presence or absence of disease is a measure of adaptive success to specific environmental situations. In all cultures, human beings have sought solutions to disease and illness.

The inclusion of cultural concepts in the knowledge base of the nurse is needed for effective nursing care. It broadens the nurse's understanding, not only of the significance of cultural traditions in regard to health and illness, but of human behavior itself. It leads to a recognition of both the uniformity and diversity found in cultures and of how man seeks solutions to universal human experiences and problems.

Nurses need to become culturally sensitive when delivering health care and should promote this awareness in other health care professionals. In order to do this, there are several things nurses can do:

- become knowledgeable about individual cultures
- examine their own beliefs, values, and practices
- indicate interest in the patient's culture
- show respect for patient values and beliefs
- avoid ethnocentrism
- avoid stereotyping
- base nursing actions on a cultural as well as a physical assessment.

The challenge for all nurses who seek to provide quality, holistic nursing care is to increase their knowledge of cultures and to use the nursing process accordingly. In order to promote health, nurses must care. In order to care, nurses must continue to learn. Many times, patients themselves can be the best teachers. Nurses need to open their hearts and their minds to all patients in order to be culturally sensitive and, through a mutual sharing, the best possible care can be provided.

SUMMARY

The cultural basis of human behavior has great importance for the practice of nursing. Nurses use cultural information to understand and assist individuals, families, and groups in achieving optimum health.

With the exception of Native American Indians, all inhabitants of the United States have ancestors who migrated to this country from other parts of the world. Areas from which people have migrated have changed over the centuries. While earlier groups came primarily from the European countries, more recent populations have come from Latin America, Africa, and Asia. They have come as immigrants, refugees, and illegal aliens. In the early years of the century, the United States was described as the melting pot. This term implies that immigrants, by assimilation and acculturation, became American and lost their cultural identity. The 1960s and 1970s brought increasing awareness and pride in ethnic identity.

Ethnic groups share cultural characteristics, such as language, values, food habits, customs, and many others. Values play a central role in any cultural group and are defined by that group. Many authors feel that in the United States today, middle-class values are dominant. A few examples of these include change, progress, achievement, youth, cleanliness, beauty, technology, materialism, and equality.

Values are meaningful for those who hold them, and they are generally accepted without question. It is crucial for nurses to identify and respect patients' value systems.

Culture is defined as people's way of living, or a design for living shared by a group of people. Cultures are groups of people that share similar beliefs, attitudes, values, and practices.

Many times, when individuals move to another country, they experience a phenomena known as culture shock. Culture shock has four phases: honeymoon, disenchantment, resolution or recovery, and effective functioning.

Ethnocentrism and stereotyping are types of cultural misunderstandings. These behaviors should be avoided by health care providers, or holistic care will not be possible.

The fundamental and basic unit of any culture is the family. How the family is defined and oriented is dependent on cultural orientation. An accurate view of the role of the family in the life of the patient is important information for the nursing process.

Food plays an important role in all cultural groups serving to nourish and sustain the group. Food has many social and religious functions as well. Many groups avoid certain types of foods, and these are culturally defined.

All groups have some type of religion that helps man deal with life events and situations that are beyond his control. Problems of disease and illness are commonly handled within a religious context. Religion offers an explanation of why things happen, as well as culturally prescribed religious behaviors to manage these events.

Cross-culturally, in every society, illness is a matter of concern. All cultures are similar in that they have some systematic approach to treating disease and caring for the sick. They are different in the specific ways in which disease and illnesses are defined, caused, diagnosed, and treated. Within the framework of illness, all cultures have an expectation of the way the ill behave. This is called the sick role, and it is culturally defined.

Many cultures have persons who care for the sick in traditional fashions. They may be shamans, medicine men or women, curers, or singers.

Inclusion of cultural concepts in the nursing knowledge base is essential for carrying out the nursing process. Cultural sensitivity is largely a learned behavior, and learning resources include the patient, his family and friends, other professionals, and the general and scientific literature.

STUDY QUESTIONS

1. Discuss the meaning of culture and cultures.

2. How does culture relate to adaptation?

3. Define and discuss culture shock. How might it affect patient behavior?

4. List several American core values.

5. Why is stereotyping a hazard to the nurse/patient relationship?

6. Interview a person from another culture, using the assessment tool.

7. Describe several potential patient problems related to cultural heritage.

REFERENCES

1. Sr. Callista Roy, "The Roy Adaptation Model" in Joan P. Reihl and Sr. Callista Roy (Eds.) **Conceptual Models for Nursing Practice,** 2nd Ed. (New York: Appleton-Century-Crofts, 1980), p.183.

2. Ibid., p.179.

3. U.S. Bureau of the Census, **Statistical Abstract of the United States,** 1982–1983 (103rd Ed) Washington, D.C.: Government Printing Office, 1982.

4. Stephen Theernstrom, Ann Orlor, and Oscar Handlin, Eds. **Harvard Encyclopedia of American Ethnic Groups** (Cambridge, Mass.: Belknap Press of Harvard University Press, 1980), xi–ix.

5. Ruth Beckmann Murray and Judith Proctor Zentner, **Nursing Concepts for Health Promotion,** 3rd Ed. (Englewood, NJ: Prentice-Hall, Inc., 1979), p.342.

6. Francis L. K. Hsu. "American Core Values and National Character" in Francis L. K. Hsu (ed) **Psychological Anthropology** (Cambridge, Mass.: Schenkman Publishing Co., Inc.), pp.248–250.

7. Conrad M. Arensberg and Arthur Neihoff, "American Cultural Values" in James P. Spradley and Michael A. Rynkewich (eds.) **The Nacirema** (Boston: Little, Brown, and Co., 1975), pp.364–365.

8. Ibid.

9. Ward Goodenough, **Description and Comparison in Cultural Anthropology,** (Chicago: Aldine Press, 1970) p.98.

10. Marlene Kramer, **Reality Shock,** (St. Louis: The C.V. Mosby Co., 1974), p.4.

11. Ibid, p.5.

12. Arnold Van Gennep, **The Rights of Passage,** (Chicago: University of Chicago Press, 1960, originally published in 1908).

13. Lucille F. Whaley and Donna L. Wong, **Nursing Care of Infants and Children,** (St. Louis: The C.V. Mosby Co., 1979), p.476.

14. George M. Foster and Barbara Gallatin Anderson, **Medical Anthropology,** (New York: John Wiley and Sons, 1978), pp.53–65.

15. Talcott Parsons, **The Social System,** (New York: Free Press, 1951).

16. Patinhara Pokkiarath Bhanumathi, "Nurses Conceptions of 'Sick Role' and 'Good Patient' Behavior: A Cross-Cultural Comparison" **International Nursing Review, 24,** (Jan/Feb 1977), 20–24.

17. Ann Templeton Brownlee, **Community, Culture, and Care,** (St. Louis: The C.V. Mosby Co., 1978), p.156.

18. Barbara Kozier and Glenora Erb. **Fundamentals of Nursing,** (Menlo-Park, Calif.: Addison-Wesley Publishing Co., 1979), p.143.

19. Maric Branch and P. P. Paxton **Providing Safe Nursing Care for Ethnic People of Culture,** (New York: Appleton-Century-Crofts, 1976), p.174.

20. **A Language Guide for Patient and Nurse,** (Indianapolis, Indiana: Eli Lilly and Company).
21. **Breaking the Language Barrier,** (Morris Plains, NJ: Warner-Chilcott).

ANNOTATED BIBLIOGRAPHY

Brink PJ (ed): **Transcultural Nursing: A Book of Readings.** Englewood Cliffs, Prentice-Hall, 1976. A selection of readings intended to raise the consciousness of nurses on cultural aspects of patient care in relation to childrearing, value systems, research methods, and language.

Brownlee AT: **Community, Culture, and Care.** St. Louis, The C.V. Mosby Co., 1978. This book approaches cultural concepts from a community framework.

Campbell T, Chang B: **Health Care of the Chinese in America.** Nurs Outlook 21:4:245–249; April 1973. This article briefly describes the immigration of the Chinese, their beliefs, and habits. It suggests several unique nursing interventions for caring for Chinese patients.

Clark AL: **Culture, Childbearing, Health Professionals.** Philadelphia, F.A. Davis Co., 1978. This book presents an overview of the childbearing practices for persons from nine selected cultures. Also presented are cultural reviews for the selected cultures.

Clark AL: **Culture and Childrearing.** Philadelphia, F.A. Davis Co., 1981. This book focuses on nine selected cultural groups, one of which is the Native American culture. The other chapters include a brief description of other selected cultures and describes the childrearing practices of that group.

DeGracia RT: **Cultural Influences on Filipino Patients.** Am J Nurs 79:8:1412–1414; August 1979. This article discusses Filipino culture and suggest implications for health care delivers.

Foster GM, Anderson BG: **Medical Anthropology.** New York, John Wiley and Sons, 1978. A comprehensive overview of a number of themes related to a cultural dimension of health and illness. A central perspective is that all health-related behavior is an adaptive strategy in all cultures.

Grasska MA, McFarlane T: **Overcoming the Language Barrier Problems and Solutions.** Am J Nurs 89:9:1376–1379; September 1982. This excellent article discusses some of the pitfalls of using translators to ease communication and offers solutions.

Grosso C, Barden M, Henry C, Vieau MG: **The Vietnamese American Family . . . and Grandma Makes Three.** MCN 6:177–180; May–June 1981. A case study is presented and solutions to the patient problems are suggested.

Harwood A: **Ethnicity and Medical Care.** Cambridge, Harvard University Press, 1981. This book presents several cultural orientations and provides guidelines for culturally appropriate health care.

James SM: **When Your Patient is a Black West Indian.** Am J Nurs 78:11:1908–1909: November 1978. Cultural patterns of the West Indians are discussed in this article. Appropriate nursing actions are presented.

Melesis AI: **The Arab American in the Health Care System.** Am J Nurs 81:6: 1180–1183; June 1978. Expectations of health care are quite different for the Arab Americans who do not so much expect personal care as an effective cure. This article describes the origin of the Arab culture and how it affects behavior. Relevant nursing interventions are offered.

Powers BA: **The Use of Orthodox and Black American Folk Medicine.** Adv Nurs Sci 4:3:35–47; April 1982. A case study is used throughout this article to illustrate many facets in Black American health behaviors.

Primeaux M: **Caring for the American Indian Patient.** Am J Nurs 77:1:91–94; January 1977. A Cherokee nurse explains Indian values in this article and relates them to health care. It clarifies that each tribe has its own customs, but that there is a core set of cultural beliefs held by all Native American Indians.

Rosenberg FH: **Lactose Intolerance.** Am J Nurs 77:5:823–824; May 1977. In the United States, over two thirds of adult blacks, Mexican Americans, American Indians, Ashenazi Jews, and Orientals are lactose intolerant. Many interesting facts regarding lactose intolerance are also discussed in this brief article.

Spradley JP, Rynkiewich MA: **The Nacirema.** Boston, Little, Brown and Co., 1975. A collection of readings of American culture describing values, social life, customs, and acculturation.

Theernstrom S, Orlov A, Handlin O (eds.): **Harvard Encyclopedia of American Ethnic Groups.** Cambridge, Belknap Press of the Harvard University Press, 1980. An extensively researched work containing essays, maps, and detailed information on 106 ethnic groups.

Wood CS: **Human Sickness and Health.** Palo Alto, Mayfield Publishing Co., 1979. A biocultural perspective of human societies in which disease is viewed as a critical element in environmental stress and adaptation. Topical areas include nutrition, malaria, syphilis, and women and reproduction.

11

Communication

Rose K. Cringle

CHAPTER OUTLINE

OBJECTIVES

At the completion of this chapter, the reader will be able to:

- Describe the elements of the communication process.
- Describe the ingredients in the Berlo human communication model.
- Describe the characteristics of effective communication.
- Identify selected communication techniques used by others that facilitate communication.
- Identify selected communication behaviors that inhibit communication.
- Explain the concept of a helping relationship.
- Describe the phases of the professional nurse/patient relationship.
- Describe the significance of communications skills in the nursing process.

GLOSSARY

Attitude—a consistent response to a particular set of circumstances or individuals that has both an intellectual and an affective component.

Consummatory communications—communication that is intended solely to fill time.

Dysfunctional communication—communication that interferes with the development of a meaningful relationship because it is either unclear or deliberately disrespectful of the receiver.

Effective communication—communication that is understood by the receiver as it was intended by the sender.

Empathy—the capacity of one individual to share the feelings of another at the moment the feelings are experienced.

Instrumental communication—communication that is intended to assist with the accomplishment of a goal.

Kinesics—communication through the use of body movement.

Language—a systematic means of communicating ideas using signs, sounds, gestures, and marks that have agreed upon meanings.

Linguistics—the scientific study of languages.

Sign—a motion, mark or other representation that announces a situation or event.

Symbol—a motion, mark, or object that represents some other motion, mark, or object.

Sympathy—the quality of being affected by a situation that involves others.

Therapeutic communication—communication that is intended to assist another person to change his way of communicating.

INTRODUCTION

Modern civilization has evolved as a result of activities undertaken by human beings working together. Human beings are able to work together because they can communicate. The word **communication** symbolizes the process by which information, feelings, and ideas are transmitted to other organisms. All living things communicate because communication is essential for survival.

Plants and animals have a system of communication that enables them to survive by adapting to the environment. The buzzing of the bee communicates its presence to other animals and serves as a warning to them to avoid its painful sting. The odor of flowers in the spring signals to the bee the presence of the nectar and the pollen that the bee needs as food to survive. The plant that bears the flower needs to have its pollen distributed in order to perpetuate itself. These types of communication are called signs. A **sign** is a discrete motion, action, or mark that indicates a presence or condition. Human beings, as well as plants and animals, use signs in their communication with each other.

Some types of animals have developed a

variety of sounds to communicate various messages. The meow of an angry cat has a different tone and intensity from the meow of a cat signaling its plan to jump on its owner's lap. This is known as **presymbolic communication.** In addition, human beings have developed a complex system of symbolic language. A **symbol** is something chosen to represent something else. It is an object used to typify an abstract idea. It may be a concrete object such as the cross, which is a symbol of Christianity, or the Star of David, which symbolizes Judaism. The symbol itself may be abstract. Words are abstract. They represent reality in a conceptual way.

Prehistoric man communicated with pictures and diagrams. We do not know exactly how and when these pictures were converted to sounds. The development of the alphabet enabled man to represent these pictures with combinations of letters and to attach specific sounds to specific combinations of letters. This is how word symbols developed. Man's unique ability to store these symbols in memory and to recall them has enabled him to develop an efficient means of communication.

The spelling of words and the way they are organized into thoughts is **language.** In different parts of the world, the alphabet and methods of spelling and organizing words differ, thus, we have **languages.** Human beings use language to interact with one another in a way that has enabled them not only to master the environment, as animals have, but to alter it. To an English speaking individual, the word "rain" symbolizes moisture falling from the sky. The ability to store this word in the brain and to recall it when it is not raining has enabled human beings to alter what happens to the environment as a result of rain. They have built shelters to protect themselves from rain. They have built cisterns to save rain. They have built dams as a protection from flooding caused by too much rain, and they have learned to use the energy of flood water to create hydro-electric power. None of this could have occurred if humans were only aware of rain while it was happening, as is the case with lower animals.

Pictures and symbolic objects are still an important part of human communication. The ease with which people travel to different parts of the world where different languages are used has increased the importance of picture symbols in the modern world. The outline of a man or a woman on a door in a public building communicates the presence of sanitary facilities for men and women regardless of the language. The outline of a wheelchair at a parking spot indicates it is reserved for the handicapped.

Playing the "Star Spangled Banner" at public events in the United States symbolizes loyalty and pride in our country. Flying the flag in front of a house is a way the owners express patriotism. The U.S. flag is an example of an object that can be either a symbol or a sign depending on the context. The U.S. flag flying on a warship symbolizes that the ship is part of the U.S. Navy. If the flag is flown upside down, that is a sign that the ship is in distress. In the first instance, the flag represents the abstract idea of ownership. In the second instance it announces the concrete need for help.

Human communication is a dynamic process that has no starting or ending point. It is so much a part of all aspects of modern life that any method of separating out a particular aspect for study is necessarily artificial. The three broad categories described by Bordon[1] will be used in this chapter. These are intrapersonal, interpersonal, and public communication.

Intrapersonal communication includes all the activities within the person related to communication. These are the way he receives messages, decodes, and synthesizes them, and the way he uses this information to encode and transmit a response. To do this requires the use of all the senses and thinking mechanisms of the brain.

Interpersonal communication refers to all of the situations in which individuals communicate directly with each other. Individuals communicate with each other through the use of verbal and nonverbal messages. **Verbal messages** are the words we hear or see in writing. **Nonverbal messages** are the sounds, sights, and odors that we see, hear, touch, or smell.

Interpersonal communication, occurs in one-to-one or group situations, as in a classroom, a committee meeting, or at a party. It does not occur in situations where individuals are in direct contact but cannot respond to each other, such as occurs between the clergy and the congregation in a church service, or the lecturer and the audience at a public lecture. These latter two would be classified as **public communication.** In addition to the above, public communication includes the impersonal dissemination of information through the media. The distribution of notices in a hospital or of educational materials through the mail are further examples of public communication.

Nurses are concerned primarily with intrapersonal and interpersonal communication. The effectiveness of the nursing process is dependent on the nurses' ability to communicate with other people. She must be able to make herself understood and to understand what the client is communicating through verbal communication and the observation of nonverbal communication. As a care giver, she must be able to communicate with the recipients of her care. During even the simplest procedures, the patient needs to know what may be expected. In the use of highly specialized technology, the patient's cooperation is equally important. If the patient is unconscious, the nurse must be able to communicate effectively with other members of the health team in order to plan and implement care. The nurse's function as a health teacher also requires a wide range of communication skills. If the nurse becomes a nursing educator, she will communicate with students, patients, and co-workers. The nurse in management has a broader range of individuals with whom to communicate. She will communicate vertically with workers that she supervises and administrators who supervise her. She will communicate horizontally with her peers and with representatives from other departments or agencies. In all of these situations, the nurse may be involved in one-to-one communication or in small group communication.

HUMAN COMMUNICATION THEORY

The study of human communication blends theory and knowledge from psychology, sociology, anthropology, mathematics, and linguistics.

Relationship to Behavioral Science Theory

Prior to World War II, inquiry into human communication occurred in academic speech and language departments where attention was directed at the structure of communication. At the same time, psychologists were studying the meaning of behavior. Human communication is the process that gives meaning to behavior. Thus, the understanding of human communication requires a blend of knowledge from these two disciplines.

Two concepts from Freudian psychoanalytic theory continue to be relevant to the understanding of communication theory.[2] One is the concept of levels of awareness. The other is the concept of the agencies of the mind.

According to Freud's theory, mental activity occurs at three levels of awareness. The **conscious** level is the level where the least amount of activity occurs. It, nonetheless, includes all of the mental activity in the awareness of the individual at the moment. The second level is the only **preconscious.** This level contains all the information an individual can recall at will. Two old friends reminiscing will find themselves recalling events that neither has thought about in years. This is an example of mental activity stored at the preconscious level. The third level of awareness is the **unconscious** level. This level stores all the events and relationships from the past that shape a person's behavior. Mental activity in the unconscious mind continuously influences the individual's conscious behavior, even though he cannot bring the actual material into his consciousness. For example, most people have had the experience of feeling uneasy or frightened when summoned to see someone of authority, such as a school principal or a supervisor at work. If the individual does not recall an immediate reason for the summons, the reaction may be motivated by previous misdeeds and their consequences, which are stored in the unconscious mind.

The agencies of the mind are the **id,** the **ego,** and the **super-ego.** The id is the reservoir for all the instinctual, uninhibited urges. It operates completely at the unconscious level. Instinctual urges satisfy needs such as hunger without regard to any other conditions. Totally uncontrolled rage when frustrated is an example of an urge experienced in the id.

The opposing counterpart to this agency is the super-ego. The super-ego consists of all the acquired socially sanctioned attitudes and behaviors. These include the desire to be considered lovable, the feeling of obligation to those who care for us and of responsibility to those who are dependent upon us. The super-ego operates at the conscious and the preconscious level. The id and superego are constantly tugging at each other. It is the ego that serves the function of mediating between these two extremes and produces the behaviors that constitute the compromise. The ego becomes that part of the personality that is revealed to others. It operates at both the conscious and preconscious levels and is the person with whom others communicate. The concept of the ego has been greatly expanded by recent theorists, but the term continues to be used with its original meaning.

Theories of gestalt psychologists also have contributed to the understanding of human communication. Gestalt is a German word meaning pattern or configuration. This school of psychological thought developed in the early-20th century in opposition to the mainstream psychological inquiry at the time. Psychological study then was concerned with the structure of the mind and the location of various mental processes. The gestalt psychologists insisted that to understand any phenomenon, it must be examined as a whole. The parts may be separated and analyzed, but the total determines how a phenomenon is perceived. A simple way to say this is, "The whole is different from the sum of the parts."

In the field of human communication, the significance of any one interaction cannot be determined by analyzing each ingredient individually. Each interaction, like the following, must be examined as a gestalt.

A bereaved widow recalled a card she received from a friend that simply stated, "What can I say?" If one analyzes just the language content of that message it clearly doesn't say much. The legibility of the handwriting, the quality of the paper, the reason for using the mail rather than a face-to-face communication could all be examined, but these analyses would not explain the significance of the communication. The significance is that it was perceived as a very kind expression of sympathy.

Gestalt psychologists were concerned

with the individual and his mental activity. Systems theorists have expanded upon gestalt concepts to apply to all living things.

The process of intrapersonal communication follows very closely the systems theory model described in Chapter 2. The messages an individual receives can be considered the input. The throughput includes all of the components involved in processing that message. The responses the individual makes become the output. The concept of feedback in systems theory is an essential component of the communication process. Each individual needs feedback to determine if his communication has reached its destination and been perceived in the manner he intended. Only in this manner does he know if his communication system is working effectively.

In a larger system, consisting of groups of living things, communication is the process by which an essential element, information, enters the system. Communication between the elements must occur if transformation is to take place. Thus, the communication process may be a system and a subsystem, an element of a larger system.

Communication is a dynamic process. It has no starting or ending point and no single objective. A young woman talking to a small group at a party may have several objectives: to help the hostess keep the party moving, to find out if anyone needs additional refreshments, and to come to the attention of a young man in a nearby group. Responses may come from her immediate group or from outside that group. The young woman who is the source, or initiator, of the communication may use responses in the situation as messages for the hostess or for the individuals who are served, the guests. If the young women succeeds in any of her objectives, she may become the content of messages sent the following day from several different sources. Similarly, a nurse talking with two pa-

tients in a semiprivate room may be interested in helping them become acquainted, gathering data about the patients to include in a care conference, and determining their self-care level. The output of this conversation may influence two separate additional groups: the nurse in her communication **network** in the hospital, and the patients in their communication **networks.** The characteristics of a network are:[3] every unit in a network does not interact with every other unit, the units do not have clear boundaries, the only common characteristic is the relationship to the ego or pivotal center around which the network exists. From the two examples above, the application of network theory to the communication process is evident.

Communication Models

A model that can be applied to any form of communication is the Shannon Weaver Model[4] shown in Figure 11-1. This model was developed by two mathematicians. The basic components are essential to the process of communication in plants and lower animals, in human beings, and even in electronic equipment.

The simple example of the wish to communicate disapproval can be used to demonstrate how the model applies to human communication. The wish originates in the human being represented as information source. That person will decide which channel to use to transmit the message. The channel will determine the form of the message. A verbal signal "Please Stop" may be used, or facial muscles may be used to transmit a nonverbal message. The information source encodes the message and sends it out from the transmitter. The message becomes the signal that must get past the noise source to the receiver. The noise source may be any type of outside interference with the signal reaching the receiver. In human communication it may be a visual distraction that causes the receiver

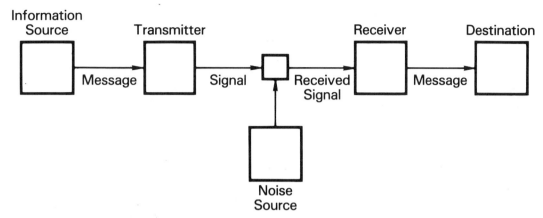

Figure 11-1. General Communication System.

Shannon, Claude & Weaver, Warren; **The Mathematical Theory of Communication**, Urbana, Ill. The University of Illinois Press 1949 p. 5. Reprinted with permission of the publisher.

to look away and not see the nonverbal signal. It may be loud sounds that interfere with hearing, or it may be an overwhelming emotion, such as fear, that interferes with comprehension. In an electronic system, just as with people, it could be a failure at the energy source or it could be static, literally. In the print media, noise could take the form of a failure of the press to reproduce some words, blurring of print, or even large colorful illustrations that distract from the content. For communication to occur, the message must get past the noise source to the receiver. The receiver must be capable of decoding the message so that it can be understood at its destination.

Through the process of communication, human beings reveal themselves to one another. How much is revealed, to whom, when and why are determined by the uniqueness of the individual and the context in which the communication occurs. The sender, message, channel, receiver model (SMCR) is an attempt to develop a comprehensive model that includes all the ingredients that influence each single act of communication.[5]

In this model, the source is the person who originates the idea for the message. The characteristics of the person that influence the message are his communication skills, attitudes, knowledge, the social system in which he exists, and the culture in which the communication occurs.

Communication skills are the tools for transmitting the message. These include: speaking, writing, preverbal uttering, gesturing, and moving. The specific tools selected by the source will be determined by any special abilities he possesses or deficiencies he may have. An individual with an extensive vocabulary will have choices of words to use. A person who is just learning the language may have to use gestures to supplement a limited vocabulary.

Attitudes have both cognitive and affective components. They are formed by a combination of something a person believes and how he feels about that belief. As the individual matures, he develops attitudes about himself, other people, and abstract concepts. A person's attitude toward himself is an integral part of his behavior and will be reflected in his communications with others. Attitudes towards other people may be individualized to a particular person or they may be generalized to a group or class. Generalized attitudes toward people are called stereotypes or prejudices. An example is "poor people are lazy." A person with that attitude will sure-

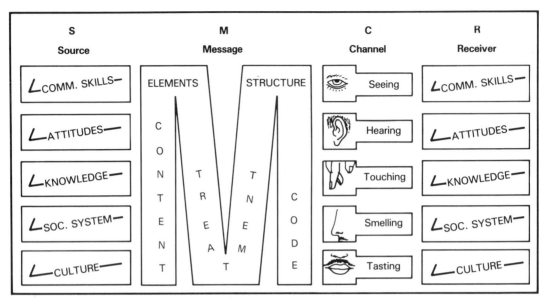

Figure 11-2. A Model of the Ingredients in Communication.

Source: David Berlo, **The Process of Communi-
cation,** (New York: Rinehart & Winston, 1960) p. 72. Reprinted with permission of the publisher.

ly find that it influences his communication with poor people. Attitudes about abstract concepts may have developed as a
result of personal experiences with the
concept or as the result of absence of personal experiences. For example, many people in the United States have attitudes
about different political systems, even
though they have only had personal experience with one. These people cannot believe
that any form of government other than
our own is acceptable. The more a person
can learn about the basis of his attitudes,
the more able he will be to change those
that interfere with effective communication.

The amount of **knowledge** the source has
about the subject of a communication will
influence how he communicates. When he
wishes to make the other person understand something he knows, a thorough understanding will aid in the process. If the
source is seeking additional information,
his communication will be different than if
he is trying to hide his lack of information.

Social systems have developed to provide the structure and order human beings
need to work together harmoniously. These
systems develop around defined goals. In
the family, for example, one goal is the care
and nurturing of children. In the health
care system, the goal is the provision of
services needed to maintain or restore the
health of numerous subsystems of the population. Within each system, roles are assigned to the members of the system, and
norms of behavior are established. The
norms of behavior and the assigned roles
both determine communication patterns.
New members learn these patterns
through the process of communication.
Communication is essential for the social
system to function.

In the health care system, the nurse's assigned role influences how she communicates with her clients. It also influences
how that communication differs from her
communication with the physician.
Norms of behavior influence such things as
the appropriate use of slang or the appropriate time to lower one's voice.

The **culture** from which the individual

originates determines the system of symbols he uses to communicate. Alphabets and language differ between cultures. The use of sign language in the form of gestures and facial expressions varies in different cultures. People of oriental extraction are often considered "inscrutable" because of their apparently unchanging facial expression. It is easier for us to comprehend the words of someone from a western culture whose "eyes flash with anger" or "eyes light up with joy." Each culture also has its own norms of behavior or customs. For example, in some cultures a women does not speak unless she is specifically addressed. In the North American culture, men greet each other by shaking hands. In some other cultures, men embrace.

All five of these ingredients—communication skills, attitudes, knowledge, social system, and culture—are influencing the source simultaneously as the desired message is encoded.

The **message** exists as the concrete product of the communication process. Everything that exists is composed of elements and structure. These are present in every system. The elements are the parts; the structure is the manner in which they are assembled. Because it exists, the message must be composed of elements and structure. Three other factors involved in the message are the content, code, and treatment. The content and code form the legs of the **M.** Both content and code must receive treatment in order for a message to be formed. The content of the message is the idea the source wishes to communicate. The content consists of elements. The code is a way of organizing symbols to make them meaningful. Language is one form of code. Nonverbal communications, such as facial expressions, are another. Different expressions, such as a raised eyebrow, communicate different things. The decisions the sender makes about which codes to use constitute the treatment of the message and determines the message's fi-

nal structure. A young mother communicating with her baby wishes to show her love for her baby. The message is encoded for the sense of sight (the smiling face) and touch (the encircling arms). The hug and the smile are the treatment of the message. A kiss could have been used, instead. The final structure of this message is a young woman smiling with her arms encircling her baby.

The **channels** for receiving messages are the five senses. Most human communication is received by the eyes and the ears. Animals rely more heavily on their senses of smell and taste. Dogs are used to help track lost people and retrieve the hunter's quarry because of their highly developed sense of smell. Human beings use their senses of smell and taste together with other senses. A person may notice a distinctive odor but be unable to identify it until he knows the source. Nurses need to use their sense of smell when they are assessing a patient. Problems such as alcohol intoxication or the presence of infection are communicated by a distinctive odor.

Apparently, the human sense of sight is the dominant one. An individual frequently makes decisions based on what he sees. He looks at vegetables in the market and decides how they will taste. He looks at another person and makes a judgment about that person's personality on the basis of what he sees. The sense of sight is strong enough to distort the sense of hearing and touch. A person may assume a rumbling noise comes from a truck he sees, when in fact it is thunder.

The sense of touch is used less often as a means of communication than are seeing and hearing. In interpersonal communication, it is used primarily to express emotions. Individuals use touch to increase their knowledge of an object, an animal, or person's body. Nurses use their sense of touch to learn about a patient's body during the assessment phase of the nursing process. Touch is also used in the implementation of nursing care. Touch may be used to identify the site for an injection. Touch in the form of massage has a healing effect on sore or stiff muscles. The psychological effects of touch are an important therapeutic tool of the nurse.

Perception, or how the message becomes encoded in the brain of the receiver, starts with the neurophysiological equipment of the individual involved. The relative health of the sensory organs will influence the perception of a message. The physiological structure is a combination of inherited tendency, general nutritional state, and the presence or absence of diseases that may have resulted in impairment. Myopia, or nearsightedness, is an example of an inherited perceptual impairment. A diet that is insufficient in Vitamin A also can result in visual impairment. Scar tissue in the middle ear, as the result of childhood infections, can cause hearing impairment.

Past experiences also influence perception. People are much more likely to perceive what they expect to perceive, based on their past experiences. An individual who has been watching boats sail gracefully past may not immediately realize it when one of the boats overturns. When a person is told than an elderly friend who has been seriously ill has died, she will perceive the message accurately. If she is told that an apparently healthy elderly friend has died in an accident, she may need to have that message repeated.

The physical and psychological state of both the source and the receiver influence the perception of the message. A headache or fever can interfere with perception. Angry feelings not dissipated after a heated argument can interfere with perception of new stimuli. Perception is the most accurate in a physically healthy, relaxed individual who is able to focus his entire attention on the message.

Receiver: The same five factors that influence the source influence the receiver.

These are communication skills, attitude, knowledge, social system, and culture. Similarity between the source and the receiver in these areas will improve communication. Sensitivity to differences in these ingredients will improve communication.

A nurse who is the daughter of first-generation Americans and who grew up in an ethnic neighborhood in a city in the Northeastern United States will differ primarily **in knowledge** from a patient who grew up in the same type of community. Similarities in communication skills, attitudes, and culture will help overcome the communications barrier created by the social system. A nurse from a middle class suburb of a southern city, whose family has been in this country for several generations, will come from a very different culture with different attitudes and different communication skills. Sensitivity on her part to the differences between herself and the patient will improve her communication with the patient. Sensitivity on the part of the patient to these differences will increase the chances for effective communication between them.

Types of Communication

Verbal and Nonverbal: Human communication is both verbal and nonverbal. Verbal communication includes any expression in a common language. These expressions are made through speech, writing, or their counterparts, listening and reading. Ability to articulate and to understand the language is essential to interaction in human society. Without the ability to use language communication, a person cannot acquire knowledge, work, or socialize. Factual information is usually transmitted verbally. We also use words to transmit emotional information, but the affective or feeling component of an emotional message is usually transmitted nonverbally.

Thus, the full meaning of any communication is not grasped if the nonverbal elements are ignored. Nonverbal communication includes preverbal sounds, body movement, facial expression, physiological activities, and the use of space and time.

Preverbal sounds are used to express the range of human emotions. A scream for help and a shout for joy are both preverbal sounds. The ability to communicate in this manner precedes the ability to form language and is thus considered more primitive. It is the language of the id in Freudian theory.

Body movement is a significant form of communication. The way a person stands or sits and the movements of his hands and feet as he stands or sits all communicate something about him and his message to the person with whom he is interacting. A rigid posture with muscles in a continuous semiflexed state is used to communicate fear or physical discomfort. It also may be used to convey anger or respect. Hand and foot movements can be used to enhance a verbal message. A slouching, careless stance can communicate boredom, disrespect, or low self-esteem. Leaning toward the other person conveys interest in his communication. These concepts are illustrated in Figure 11-3.

The use of structure and movement in the form of dance as a means of communication began in primitive times. It may have preceded the development of language. As human beings perfected the use of language, less attention was paid to nonverbal methods of communication. In recent years, interest has rekindled for the study of body movement as a form of communication. The term used to describe this form of communication is **kinesics**.[6]

Facial expressions are usually in harmony with body movement. They are listed as a separate category because they can change when changes in the individual's body movement may be imperceptible. Both body movement and facial ex-

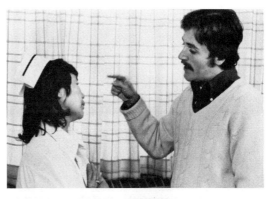
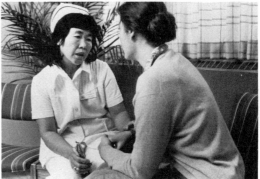

Figure 11-3. Body posture and movement are ingredients of communication in both these pictures.

pression are less under the conscious control of the individual and, therefore, more likely to be the authentic message when not consistent with the verbal message. A person who scowls as he says, "Everything is O.K.," is communicating that everything is not O.K.

Physiological activities such as rumbling sounds from the abdomen or coughing communicate information about the health state of the individual.

The way individuals use **space and time** in their interactions with others is a form of communication. When a person returns a telephone call as soon as he receives the message, he is communicating a wish to be involved with the caller. The reason for the involvement may be positive or negative. Allowing time to elapse before returning the call indicates that the caller has a low priority in the receiver's frame of reference.

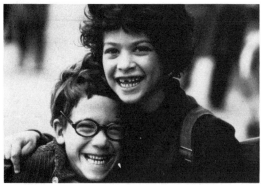

A. Intimate Distance: Touching to 18 Inches.

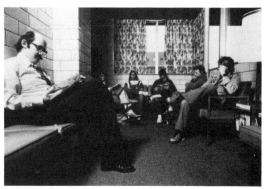

C. Social Distance: 4 feet to 12 feet.

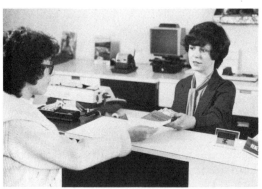

B. Personal Distance: 18 inches to 4 feet.

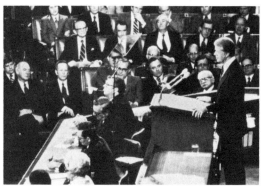

D. Public Distance: 12 feet and more.

Figure 11-4.   Hall's Spatial Relationships.

Hall, an anthropologist, studied the significance of how individuals use space and distance to communicate with others.[7] He described four relationships that can be identified by the actual physical space maintained between the participants. These are in order of closeness: intimate, personal, social, and public. These relationships are depicted in Figure 11-4.

Though actual distances vary within the context, some average figures have been developed. Intimate distance is the distance between two individuals involved in intimate activities. These are the activities related to affection, anger, and the maintenance of body integrity. The distance between two individuals in intimate communication begins with body contact and extends about 18 inches. Nurses in their care giving role often invade the intimate space of a total stranger. Whenever two individuals are close enough to achieve body contact, the possibility exists for one person to gain control over the other. Most people become uncomfortable when a stranger invades their intimate space, because of concern that they may lose control.

Personal distance is from 18 inches to 4 feet. At this distance, subjects of a personal nature can be discussed without concern that the other individual will gain physical control. The expression, "keeping a person at arm's length," is used to convey the wish to avoid being controlled. This is the distance usually maintained between individuals in an interview situation.

Social space is the distance from 4 to 12 feet from the individual. From this distance, one-to-one communication is possible, but business of a private nature cannot be transacted. Most casual social and business transactions occur at this distance.

Public distance begins about 12 feet away from the individual, and precludes the possibility for meaningful one-to-one interaction. One individual may look at and listen to the other and may receive a clear message. It is, however, difficult to make a clear response.

The uses of time and distance, because they are measurable, are easier to assess than other forms of nonverbal communication. In an evaluation of communication difficulties, the way time and space have been used can provide data to clarify the problem. However, communication difficulties cannot be understood and corrected unless all aspects of the situation are included.

Instrumental and Consummatory Communication[8]

Communication can be categorized according to purpose. Communication that is directed toward achieving a specific goal is **instrumental** communication. The goal may be transacting business with the bank teller or it may be comforting a friend who is ill. Social norms will dictate differences in the use of voice tone, choice of vocabulary, and body movement in these two examples, but in both situations, communication becomes the instrument to accomplish the goal. Communication that is the goal in itself is called **consummatory.** This may be in combination with some other activity, such as eating and drinking. It may be during the introductory phase of a relationship, when each party is deciding how much of himself to reveal, or it may be during an unavoidable "waiting" time, such as in a supermarket line. Americans

are reputed to be skilled at this form of communication. An American woman who was living in another English speaking country reported several occasions when she felt rebuffed as she attempted to converse with someone at a bus stop or in a supermarket line. Since both of these were familiar institutions, and the language was familiar, it was the lack of response to her conversational overtures that reminded her she was in another culture. Social "chit-chat" or consummatory communication with strangers was not the practice in that country.

Dysfunctional and Therapeutic Communication

Dysfunctional is the term used to describe the type of communication that interferes with the establishment or maintenance of meaningful interpersonal relationships. It is characteristic of individuals in our society who are lonely and withdrawn. The individuals are often described as neurotic or mentally ill. In some forms of mental illness, such as schizophrenia, dysfunctional communication is considered symptomatic of a thought disorder. In other individuals, it may be both the cause and effect of a lifetime of experiences of feeling misunderstood and rejected. Individuals with these types of communication problems also may have physical illnesses. Thus, such a person may be a nurse's client, regardless of the specific field of nursing she chooses. This is one of the reasons it is important for all nursing students to experience communicating with clients who have dysfunctional communication patterns. Much of the early scientific inquiry in the field of human communication focused on the dysfunctional communications of the mentally ill. Ruesch,[9] a psychiatrist developed the concept of **therapeutic communication.** He describes it as communication that has, as its purpose, changing another person's manner of communicating. Techniques of therapeutic communication are important for the nurse to be helpful to the client with dysfunctional communication. These techniques usually are taught in advanced nursing courses. This chapter addresses the problem of communicating effectively with clients who do not have dysfunctional communication patterns, since this group comprises the majority of people.

Effective Communication

Effective communication is perceived by the receiver as it was intended by the source. The message from the source does not need to be pleasant or positive, it simply needs to be understood as intended. Communication that enables a terminally ill person and his family to understand the nature of his illness and the expected consequences is effective, however heartbreaking it may be. An instructor who tells her class she would like to have the term papers by Thursday and then penalizes the students who deliver them on Friday has not communicated effectively. Her message was not as precise as she apparently intended. If the papers were due Thursday and there was to be a penalty for lateness, the teacher should have said that. What one would like and what one expects are not necessarily the same.

Because of the dynamic nature of the communication process and the constantly shifting settings in which communication occurs, an individual can never achieve closure on the ability to communicate effectively. It is a goal toward which people can continually strive. Some individuals, because of a high degree of sensitivity to other people, and some special talent in organizing and transmitting their ideas, seem particularly gifted in effective communication. Even they may have lapses. Everyone with motivation and practice can learn to improve the effectiveness of his communication.

COMMUNICATION AND THE NURSING PROCESS

Factors Facilitating Communication

No nurse can fulfill her professional role without communicating with clients. There are some rather simple guidelines to facilitating the communications process in any setting. Focusing attention on the other individual is one important part of the process. The freedom of both parties to focus attention on each other is influenced by distractions in the environment—the "noise" of the Shannon Weaver Communication Model. Physical discomfort may be one of the distractions. Two individuals outside in a blizzard will probably limit their communication to messages that assist in finding shelter. Those same two people in a crowded elevator will be distracted by the presence of other people. A quiet, well-ventilated space with comfortable seating arrangements is the physical environment that will be most conducive to their communication.

Intuitive attraction to the other person is an important facilitator of effective communication. There are some people who are instinctively drawn to each other without being able to explain why. However, in both a social and a professional role, it is sometimes necessary to communicate with people to whom one is not especially attracted. When this situation occurs, it is necessary to work harder to establish effective communication.

The social field, or **life space**,[10] in which it occurs influences the effectiveness of the communication. An individual's life space is that individual's perception of his environment at the moment. This includes physical structures and objects, other people, and psychological factors. Lewin specifies these factors as the individual's goals at the moment, perceived obstacles to achieving those goals, perceived facilitators to attaining those goals, and the route he feels obliged to use.

The following example illustrates this concept:

A young woman was alone in the city at 10 o'clock at night. Her physical environment included a lighted city street, some automobiles, and a subway station. The only people in the environment were strangers. Her goal was to return to her place of lodging. She could either take a taxi or the subway. Her finances were limited, so she felt she must use the subway. The obstacles to her taking the subway included a phobia of heights, which results in her becoming dizzy, a very steep escalator, no police officer or woman she might approach to ask for directions to an elevator, and a lifetime of being warned about speaking to strange men. The factors facilitating her goal attainment were a strong desire to get off the street and safely to her lodging, a good command of the language spoken in that city, a knowledge of the city, and the appearance of a pleasant looking young man who walked with a slight limp.

She perceived him as someone who might have some understanding of her distress. She approached him and asked if he could direct her to the elevator. He told her he did not know the location of the elevator in this particular subway station. When she explained her plight he suggested she ride beside him on the escalator, facing him rather than looking down. She did this and safely arrived at the bottom of the escalator. Within a few moments she was on the subway enroute to her lodging.

Each individual involved in an interaction is part of two different lifespaces: her own and the other individual's. If the young man in the example above had just concluded an argument with a jealous girlfriend, he may not have appeared approachable. If the young woman had not appeared genuinely distressed, he might not have responded positively to her need for help. Sensitivity to what is happening in the life space of the other individual is an important contributor to effective communication.

Clients whose ability to communicate is impaired by some physical disability, such as blindness or deafness, present special problems, but there are specific nursing techniques that can be learned to foster communication with the sight or hearing impaired client.

Specific Communication Techniques

There are specific modes of expression and linguistic techniques that can be learned that contribute to the effectiveness of the communications process. Some people resist learning these techniques because they think it is unnatural and will impede communication. With practice, these techniques can become part of the person's natural speech pattern. In fact, individuals who do a great deal of counseling or teaching are often accused by their families of using communication techniques in casual conversation. In most instances, these techniques have become so much a part of the individual's communication pattern that he is not aware he is using them. The small grandson of a college professor recognized this when he remarked: "Everytime I ask Granddad a question, he teaches me a lesson."

In the previous section, the importance of focusing attention on the other party in an interaction was discussed. This requires both observation and listening. Listening requires concentrating on what the other person is saying while formulating a response. One must also observe nonverbal messages simultaneously. It is not a simple task. The nurse who continues to make the bed while she is talking to the patient may be listening to what the patient is saying, but by not observing the patient closely, she may be missing nonverbal cues. Some nurses become skillful at apparently doing both things at the same time. That takes a great deal of practice and a high level of sensitivity to the other person's feelings.

Along with listening and observing, the nurse needs to learn the appropriate use of silence. Nurses often feel they must be doing something for the patient all the time. They even view sitting and talking with the patient as a waste of time. The mere presence of another human being can be helpful. Filling time with idle chatter or meaningless activity may temporarily divert attention from stress, but it will not alter the source of the stress. Silence can be used to think about what is occurring and to devise suggestions for coping. If it appears that silence is being used to avoid a subject of conversation, there are gestures and preverbal sounds that can be used to encourage the discussion to continue. Some people nod their head, others use sounds such as: "Um" or "Uh huh."

The **giving of information** either as an opening to a conversation or in answer to a client's question will assist the flow of conversation. A genuine need for information can be met at the same time that respect for the client's right to question is acknowledged. Conversely, withholding information can impede communication. Refusing to answer a question can imply that the question was inappropriate or that the nurse is not interested in the client's concerns. Introducing oneself and stating one's purpose is more than a social amenity. It is an important communication that gives recognition to the other person as an individual, and it clarifies the reason for the interaction. Individuals with health problems are usually concerned about themselves and anxious to acquire information about their condition. Legislation in recent years has protected the right of the client to know about his condition and at the same time protected his right to privacy. This protection prevents information from a health care agency about a person's physical condition being sent to his employer without his permission. In each health care agency, how and by whom information is transmitted to the client is determined by agency policy. If a patient asks a nurse for information about his condition that she is

not authorized to transmit, the nurse can answer the question by telling the patient she is not authorized to give him the information and telling him who is.

There are many specific techniques for structuring language to encourage meaningful communication. A few of the more distinct types are discussed here. Statements or questions that are **open ended** will encourage the client to express himself fully. For example, if someone is asked for the location of the pain in his foot, the answer will probably relate only to the location. If the person is asked to **tell you about the pain,** he may give information about the location, intensity, and duration. Verbally expressing what is perceived as the nonverbal communication encourages verbalization. Statements such as, "You appeared angry when your visitor left," will make it easier for the patient to discuss the situation. **Broad openings** allow the other persons to determine the direction of the conversation. "How are you?" has, unfortunately, become a stereotyped greeting with a stereotyped response, but it is an example of a broad opening. Broad openings are questions such as, "How did things go at work today?" or statements such as, "I wonder what you're thinking." **Restating** what the other person has said can be used both to clarify and to encourage continuation of the topic. This is a particularly useful technique when the subject may be anxiety producing for both parties. If someone says, "I lost my job," the response, "You lost your job," enables conversation to continue without passing judgment on the content. It also provides feedback to the first speaker that his message has been understood. **Reflection** is the directing of the question back to the questioner. It encourages the individual to find his own solution to his problem. This indicates respect for the individual's ability and relieves the nurse of the responsibility for making the decision. If the patient says, "Do you think this new medicine will help me?" the nurse can reply, "Do **you** think it will?"

There are choices of words and types of statements that are not only not helpful, but to the extent that they make the patient feel rejected or belittled, they can be harmful.

The use of cliches is one example. "Keep your chin up," and "Better days are ahead," are two rather useless statements. "Everyone feels that way sometime," may be interpreted as belittling of the patient's feelings. Direct rejection of the topic with a statement like, "Let's not talk about that," will usually end that conversation. Indirect rejection by changing the subject communicates unwillingness on the nurse's part to pursue the topic. Questions that begin with why, how, or what can be interpreted as a demand for a short answer.[11] They should be used sparingly. "Why did you let the doctor upset you?" does have a coercive quality. An **exploratory statement** such as, "Can we piece together the events that are upsetting you?" will enable the patient to gather the data to answer **why** or **how** he is upset without pressuring him for a specific answer.

A persistent series of short answer questions creates the impression that the questioner is only interested in the facts, not in the person providing the facts. "Did you drink all the juice?" "Did you take your medicine?" "Do you need anything for pain?" in rapid succession will probably make the patient wish the nurse would just leave. It certainly will not encourage him to tell her about a problem he may be experiencing.

The following case report demonstrates how the use of these techniques enabled one nursing student to improve her communication with one client. In this case, improved communication enabled the student to make effective use of the nursing process.

Sarah Jones was a nursing student enrolled in a freshman nursing course. A major objective of this course was to enable the student to develop beginning skills in communicating with clients in different age groups and from different socioeconomic levels. For their laboratory experience, a group of students went with their instructor one afternoon a week to a sheltered housing facility for the elderly. Each student was assigned to a client to identify health problems and to plan and implement assistance with these problems within the limited scope of her own nursing knowledge.

Sarah Jones' client was Mrs. Smith, a frail, 74-year-old women living alone in an efficiency apartment. She had no seriously incapacitating health problems at the time. She had arthritis and mild hypertension. Her apartment was simply, but comfortably, furnished. It was both neat and clean.

The following is taken from a process recording the student made immediately following her second visit with Mrs. Smith.

Student: (observing a plate on the kitchen sink containing chicken bones) "Did you enjoy your lunch?"

Mrs. Smith: "Yes."

Student: "Does the management send your lunch to you?"

Mrs. Smith: "Yes."

(Pause)

Student: "Did you go to church yesterday?"

Mrs. Smith: "No, it was too cold."

Student: "Did visitors from the church come like they usually do on Sunday?"

Mrs. Smith: "Yes."

Student: "Oh, who came?"

Mrs. Smith: (sighs) "I don't remember, some people."

Student: "What did you do?"

Mrs. Smith: "We prayed."

(Long pause)

Student: "Remember you said you were afraid to get in the tub alone? I told you I could help you with a tub bath when I was here. Would you like to do that now?"

Mrs. Smith: "Yes."

Student: "I'll go fix your tub."

(Student goes into bathroom. Starts the water in the tub and locates necessary equipment. She returns to living room.)

Student: "Do you want to put on clean clothes after your bath?"

Mrs. Smith: "Yes."

(Student walks toward dresser.)

Student: "Where will I find your clean underwear?"

Mrs. Smith: "In the middle drawer."

(Student selects clean underwear, then turns to Mrs. Smith.)

Student: "Is this okay?"

(Mrs. Smith nods her head. Student returns to Mrs. Smith's side.)

Student: "I'll help you to the bathroom now."

(Mrs. Smith gets up without speaking. They walk together to the bathroom. Student helps Mrs. Smith undress and get into tub.)

Student: "You have nice new underwear."

Mrs. Smith: "Uh huh."

Student: "Where did you get the underwear?"

Mrs. Smith: "From my daughter-in-law."

Student: "That's nice."

(The conversation continued in this manner while Mrs. Smith bathed and dressed in clean clothing.)

When the student discussed the interaction with her instructor, she reported feeling very tired. She felt burdened with the responsibility to learn more about Mrs. Smith. Her assessment was that Mrs. Smith had lived a financially and socially

deprived life and it was not realistic to think she could engage in meaningful dialogue. The instructor pointed out that Mrs. Smith had given her fragments of information that she had not pursued. They also discussed the student's almost complete reliance on short answer questions.

Role playing was used to recreate the situation. The student assumed the role of Mrs. Smith. The instructor used a very simple vocabulary to structure broad openings and to restate and explore conversational cues. The student observed the instructor's ability to be relaxed during silences and to use the silence to think about the interaction. After this experience the student was willing to try a different approach during her next visit with Mrs. Smith. She planned a broad opening to use during her next visit. She would begin the interaction by saying, "Last week you mentioned your daughter-in-law. Can you tell me more about your family?"

When the student arrived at Mrs. Smith's apartment she found her lying on her bed apparently staring into space. She sat beside Mrs. Smith's bed and smiled in silence. After a few moments she said, "You look worried."

Mrs. Smith: (after a long pause) "I don't know what I'm going to do."

Student: "Can you tell me what's bothering you?"

Mrs. Smith: "It won't do no good."

Student: "If I knew what was wrong, I might be able to help."

Mrs. Smith: (after a long pause) "You can't do nothing."

Student: "I would like to try to help."

(Another long pause. The student was beginning to feel uncomfortable. She resisted the urge to suggest she prepare Mrs. Smith's bath.)

Mrs. Smith: "They told me there's not going to be any hot lunches on Saturday and Sunday." (another pause) "What can I do? I don't have much appetite, but I got to eat a little something."

Student:	"They told you they were going to stop the hot lunches on Saturday and Sunday. What reason did they give?"
Mrs. Smith:	"I don't know. That got me upset, I didn't hear the rest."
Student:	"How did you find this out?"
Mrs. Smith:	"The lady that manages the building, she came to the door." (long pause)
Student:	"She came to the door."
Mrs. Smith:	"Yes, she said there wasn't going to be anymore hot lunches in the apartments on Saturday and Sunday."
Student:	"What else did she say? Can you remember now?"
Mrs. Smith:	"She said we have to come downstairs for hot lunches. You know I can't walk that far. I'm so afraid I'll fall. I used to have one of those canes with three feet on it, but it is broke."

The first thing the student pursued was the information about the lunches. She helped Mrs. Smith call the manager's office. From this phone call, Mrs. Smith learned that a cold lunch of sandwich, fruit, and milk could be sent to the apartments of those residents unable to come downstairs. She became more relaxed when she learned this.

Next, they located the broken cane. Mrs. Smith told the student that her son or some member of his family called her every evening. They decided to leave the cane by the telephone, so that Mrs. Smith would remember to ask if they could arrange to have it repaired.

When the student left, Mrs. Smith was in a pleasant mood, and so was she: Improved communication had resulted in assessment of problems with which she could help. She had done some on-the-spot planning and implemented her plans. She was eager to evaluate the experience with her instructor.

Nurse/Patient Relationship

The nurse/patient relationship is a helping relationship, similar to the relationships members of other helping professions, such as social workers and psychiatrists, establish with their clients. The nurse/patient relationship differs in function from other helping professions because of the specific functions of the nurse in society.

Initial investigations into the use of the nurse/patient relationship were done in the psychiatric setting. Distinctions were drawn between the interpersonal skills needed in psychiatric nursing and the psychomotor skills needed to carry out procedures such as irrigating a wound used in general nursing. Modern technological advances have placed machinery to monitor the patient and administer treatments between the patient and the nurse in acute care settings. The nurse has had to acquire new skills to interpret and regulate the machinery. The machinery has not replaced the patient's need for comfort, emotional support, and knowledge about his health state. In order to provide this, the nurse needs to be able to establish a meaningful nurse/patient relationship. When nurse and patient are able to move beyond the stereotyped concept that each has of the other, a relationship can start to develop.[12] The nurse must be able to stop interacting with the client as though he is simply a patient with a nursing need to be met. She must be able to perceive him as a unique human being with a unique clustering of needs. The nurse alone cannot establish a relationship with a patient who continues to perceive her as the efficient, impersonal dispenser of care. The patient must be able to alter his perception of the nurse, also.

In a helping relationship, the nurse uses her knowledge of human behavior, along with her ability to care about and share the psychological experience of the client, to help the client. Each relationship develops in stages. These are the **introduction,** including the development of trust, **empathy, sympathy, involvement,** and **termination.** Because of the uniqueness of individuals and of each situation, these stages do not necessarily follow an orderly progression. They may seem to occur all together in a very short time span. They may occur in different overlapping combinations. They are discussed separately to facilitate understanding of the process.

In the **introductory** stage, each individual gathers data about the other person's uniqueness. It is during this time that expectations are relinquished that the other person will behave in a certain way because he is young or old, a man or a woman, a nurse or a patient. At this time, each individual should clarify for the other his expectation of the interaction. The beginnings can be very simple statements, such as, "I am Mary Jones, the nurse assigned to your care this evening." In that statement the nurse acknowledges her own and the patient's personhood. If the nurse simply stood at the bedside and said, "Your call light is on," she would be maintaining the stereotyped expectations that each held. These two examples are pictured in Figures 5 and 6. Notice the different use of space, facial expressions, body movement, as well as words in each situation.

During this introductory stage, each individual also will make some decision about the trustworthiness of the other. In order to reveal himself to another human being, the individual must be able to trust that other human being. Trust in this context means the feeling that one will not be subjected to ridicule or exposure if one reveals very private information about himself.

Empathy is defined as the capacity to feel the psychological experience of another person as though it were his own. It is uniquely human. It is not something that one can decide in advance to do, or a skill

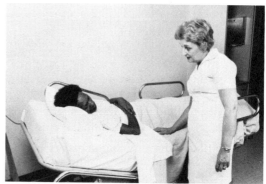

Figure 11-5. "I'm Miss Jones, the nurse assigned to your care today. I saw you had turned on the call light."

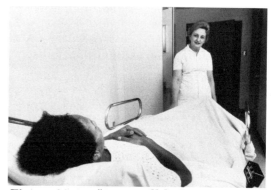

Figure 11-6. "Your call light is on."

one can practice. When empathy occurs, both parties know it instinctively and feel closer as a result. Some individuals seem to have a greater capacity to develop empathy than others. Psychologists speculate that the ability to feel empathy develops in the anterior frontal lobes, and that this section of the brain is more highly developed in some individuals than in others.[13] It seems important that there be some similarity of experiences between people for empathy to develop. Many social support groups in our society are based on the empathetic understanding that can develop among individuals with similar problems. Alcoholics Anonymous is a well known example. The experiences do not need to be identical. A person who has felt pride in any major accomplishment can use that feeling to empathize with the feelings of pride, for example, that a new parent experiences.

Sympathy is defined as the quality of being affected by the state of another. It is this experience that motivates one individual to help another. It can occur without empathy, and empathy can occur without sympathy. A person can wish to help someone because she knows intellectually that he is suffering. Donations to international agencies to provide relief for victims of earthquakes or floods are expressions of sympathy. If the individual does not know the victim personally, he cannot feel empathy. Nurses can best fulfill the nurse/patient relationship when they are able to experience both empathy and sympathy for the client. An individual cannot experience trust, empathy, or sympathy without being emotionally involved. The nurse who is meeting the needs of the patient in a way that permits them both to grow and change is involved.

Involvement occurs when the emotional investment essential to being helpful has been made. There are two other ways in which a nurse may be involved that do not have a helpful outcome. These two types of involvement give the word a negative connotation. One is the solicitous involvement, which may protect the patient from hurt, but also prevents growth. A nurse who will continue to spoonfeed a patient with a paralyzed right arm to spare him the struggle of learning to eat with his left hand is an example of this. The other is a distorted involvement that focuses on meeting the nurse's needs. The nurse may try to fill an emptiness in her life away from work through a relationship with a patient. The patient may be the same sex as the nurse, but is usually someone who lacks family or funds. The nurse may purchase needed toilet articles or clothing for the patient. She may even take the patient to her home at the time of discharge. The relationship becomes a social relationship, and the nurse no longer is able to maintain the objectivity required in a professional helping relationship.

In the mistaken notion that these two types of behavior must be avoided at all costs, nurses used to be and are still sometimes advised to remain aloof. A nurse cannot effectively carry out the nursing process, however, by remaining aloof from her clients. If she has personal problems that interfere with her ability to establish a helpful nurse/patient relationship, she should be encouraged to identify these problems and find appropriate solutions. A nurse whose mother is terminally ill may find herself identifying with other terminally ill patients. A discussion of this with co-workers and arrangement of her assignments to avoid caring for terminally ill patients at that time may be all that is necessary. A nurse who cannot handle her emotions while caring for the terminally ill five years after her mother has died may have serious emotional problems that require psychiatric help.

The nurse/patient relationship has an end. Closure must occur. The purpose of establishing the relationship is to facilitate the identification of patient needs and the planning of strategies to meet those needs. Once those needs have been met by the nurse or alternative arrangements have been made to meet the needs, the nurse/patient relationship should terminate. The effects of the relationship upon the two people will not be cancelled by the **termination.** If real growth has occurred as a result of the relationship, that growth will continue. If the patient returns to the same nurse at a later time, the relationship may be much more quickly reestablished. Another hoped for result of any nurse/patient relationship is that the patient will feel freer to enter into a relationship with other nurses in subsequent health care experiences.

Human beings do not like to say "goodbye." This is especially true when it means giving up a rewarding experience. In most of the major languages in the world today, there are expressions that can be used to avoid saying goodbye. In English, the expression is, "So long," or "See you around." In Spanish, the expression, "Hasta la vista" means "Until I see you again." Saying goodbye is an essential stage of a professional nurse/patient relationship. A nurse may think she can avoid it if the patient is discharged when she is off duty. This type of behavior on the part of the nurse indicates that she did not understand the responsibility she assumed when she began the relationship. She needs to say goodbye the last time she expects to see the patient.

The termination stage is an essential part of the relationship. It is a time to summarize what has been accomplished and to confirm that appropriate followup activities have been planned. It is also a time to reaffirm positive feelings. The nurse can help the patient terminate if she can say openly, "I wish you luck," "I have enjoyed our time together," or even, "I will miss you."

THE NURSING PROCESS

Throughout this chapter, reference has been made to the use of communication skills in the assessment of clients, the planning of nursing care, the implementation of nursing care, and the evaluation of care that has been given. These are the four steps of the nursing process that are described in detail in Chapter 6.

Assessment

The first step of the process, assessment, involves a determination of the client's health state. Assessment includes obtaining a health history, gathering information about the client's subjective complaints, and identifying objective problems. To obtain an accurate health history, the nurse must be skillful in verbal communication. She must use a vocabulary the patient understands, and she must ask the right questions. She must be able to listen attentively to what the patient says. Observation of the patient includes using the senses of sight, hearing, smell, and touch. It includes being alert to the patient's facial expression and body movement. Specialized physical assessment measures require the use of touch to palpate parts of the body, hearing through a stethoscope, and reading gauges on instruments. The mental status of the patient is obtained through observation and the use of a set of interview questions. All of the assessment data needs to be recorded accurately for use in the next step of the process, planning.

Planning

Planning is the preparation of a detailed program of actions to be taken. In nursing, this program of action is called the nursing care plan. After the initial assessment, the nurse formulates a nursing care plan that is put in writing. This plan is used by all the nursing staff caring for the patient and is modified as the patient's needs change. The written plan becomes a tool for communication among the staff. It must be legible and in language that everyone understands.

Implementation

The next step of the nursing process, implementation, involves putting the nursing plan into action. Whether the nurse does the actual implementation herself or delegates it to someone else, she must communicate verbally. If she delegates the action to someone else, she must make sure they understand what they are to do. She must communicate with the patient to allay anxiety when new treatments are introduced.

Even if the treatment procedure has been done before, step-by-step instructions are still necessary as the procedure is carried out. In addition to interpersonal communication skills, the nurse may use public communication materials to teach the patient about his condition and how to assume responsibility for his own care.

All the nurse's observations must be recorded as treatment progresses. These written records are a means of communication with other members of the health team caring for the patient, such as the physician and the nutritionist.

Evaluation

In the final stage of the nursing process, evaluation, the nurse must reassess the patient, using all the communication skills used in the initial assessment of the patient. By comparing the two sets of data, an evaluation of the effectiveness of care given can be made. An evaluation of a particular treatment technique may be done by communicating with a number of patients on whom it was used. This is often done through use of a written questionnaire. The ability to express oneself clearly in writing is essential to the development of a questionnaire.

The nursing process is a continuous process. As stated in the paragraph above, evaluation and reassessment occur simultaneously as the process begins again. The use of communication skills is a continuous element of the nursing process.

Communication skills improve with experience. The nurse/patient relationship can be learned only through experience. The material in this chapter hopefully will encourage nursing students to take the risks involved in developing relationships with patients. Experience, with guidance from an experienced teacher, is how everyone learns to establish mutually beneficial relationships.

SUMMARY

This chapter began with a brief review of the historic development of human communication and a description of the universality of the concept. Major contributions of the social sciences to the understanding of communication are included. Two communication models are presented. The Shannon-Weaver Model presents the components of the communication process as the source, the transmitter, the message itself, the receiver, and the destination. All outside interference in this process is considered noise. Berlo expanded on this model to describe the ingredients that influence each of the components. The source and the receiver are both influenced by their communication skills, attitudes, knowledge, social system, and culture, when they send or receive a message. The channels that are chosen for the communication determine the structure of the message. The channels are the five senses: sight, hearing, touch, smell, and taste. The message itself is composed of elements and structure. The content of the message, the code, and the treatment interact with both elements and structure.

The structure of the communication may be verbal or nonverbal. Verbal communication is the spoken and written word. Nonverbal communication includes preverbal sounds, sights, taste, odor, and body language. The purpose of communication may be instrumental, that is to accomplish a specific goal, or it may be consummatory, to fill time. Individuals whose communication is described as dysfunctional are those whose methods of communication interfere with the development of meaningful relationships. The term therapeutic communication describes the technique used by health care professionals to assist an individual whose communication is dysfunctional. Effective communication, communication that is perceived the way it is intended, is the goal towards which all health care workers should strive.

Factors in the environment that influence communication are discussed. These include noise level, comfort, and timing. Specific interview techniques, such as the use of broad openings, reflection, and silence, are explained. The importance of the use of space, distance, and body language are elaborated upon. There is a comprehensive example of the successful use by a nursing student of these techniques with a client.

The nurse/patient relationship is defined as the nurse's use of her knowledge of human behavior, along with her ability to care about and share the psychological experience of the client, to help the client. The three phases of the relationship—introduction, working phase, and termination—are described as phases of any relationship, regardless of the length of time involved.

The use of communication skills and the nurse/patient relationship are elements of the nursing process. The success of the nursing process depends largely on the nurse's ability to communicate with the patient verbally and nonverbally, and to use written and verbal communication skills with other health team members.

STUDY QUESTIONS

1. What are the five basic ingredients in the communication process according to the Shannon-Weaver Model?

2. How does systems theory relate to human communication?

3. What is meant by the term "effective communication?"

4. How many facilitative communications techniques can you identify?

5. Who are the various categories of people with whom the nurse must communicate while carrying out the nursing process?

6. How does a professional helping relationship differ from a friendship? Give an example.

7. What are the general characteristics according to the Berlo Model that influence the manner in which an individual communicates?

REFERENCES

1. George A. Borden; Richard B. Gregg and Theodore G. Grove: **Speech Behavior and Human Interaction** (Englewood Cliffs, NJ: Prentice-Hall, Inc. 1969) p.5.
2. A.A. Brill: **The Basic Writings of Sigmund Freud** (New York: Random House, Inc., 1938).
3. Seymour Sarason, et al: **Human Services and Resource Networks** (San Francisco: Jossey-Bass Publishers, 1977) p.128.
4. Claude Shannon and Warren Weaver: **The Mathematical Theory of Communication** (Urbana, Ill.: The University of Illinois Press, 1949) p.5.
5. David Berlo: **The Process of Communication: An Introduction to Theory and Practice** (New York: Holt, Rinehart and Winston, Inc., 1960) p.72.
6. Ray L. Birdwhistell: **Kinesics and Context** (Philadelphia: University of Pennsylvania Press, 1970) pp.128–143.
7. Edward T. Hall: **The Hidden Dimension** (New York: Doubleday and Co., Inc., 1966) pp.110–122.
8. William Brooks: **Speech Communication,** (Dubuque, Iowa: Wm. C. Brown Co., Publ., 1971) p.121.
9. Jurgen Ruesch: **Therapeutic Communication** (New York: W. W. Norton & Co., Inc., 1961) p.460.
10. Kurt Lewin: **Field Theory in Social Science** (New York: Harper and Row, Publ., 1951) pp.56–59.
11. Hildegard Peplau: "Talking with Patients"

American Journal of Nursing 60, No. 7 (July 1960) pp.964–966.

12. Sidney Jourard: **The Transparent Self** (2nd Ed.) (New York: Van Nostrand, Reinhold Co., 1971) pp.179–207.

13. Kenneth Clark: "Empathy, A Neglected Topic in Psychological Research" **American Psychologist** 35, No. 2, (February 1980) pp.187–189.

ANNOTATED BIBLIOGRAPHY

Brown B: **An Innovative Approach to Health Care for the Elderly: An Approach of Hope.** J Psychiatr Nurs 15:10:27–35; October 1977. A warmly written description of one nurse's experience helping clients set realistic goals for themselves. The nurse was able to help the clients identify attainable goals. This enabled the clients to feel more self-confident and, thus, willing to make changes in their patterns of living that resulted in an improvement in their health status.

DeVillers L: **What to do When You Just Can't Communicate.** Nurs Life 2:2:34–39; March-April 1982. A helpful guide for the nurse to examine her own communication behavior when she experiences problems in communication.

Garant C: **Stalls in the Therapeutic Process.** Am J Nurs 80: 12:2166–2169; December 1980. Discusses the problems that arise because of controlling the client, rather than letting him develop his own agenda. Stresses the importance of open communication between care giver and client in the development of a therapeutic alliance.

Goldborough J: **Involvement.** Am J Nurs 69:1:39–41; January 1969. The nurse's willingness to reveal herself to the client encourages the client to discuss important emotional experiences with the nurse.

Jourard S: **The Transparent Self, Part Six: A Human Way of Being Nurses** (revised ed.). New York, Van Nostrand, Reinhold Co., 1971. Disrobes members of the helping professions who use their profession to maintain distance from their clients.

Kesler A: **Pitfalls to Avoid in Interviewing Outpatients.** Nurs 7:9:70–73; September 1977. Common communication problems are described. To overcome the problems, easy-to-learn techniques are suggested.

Littlefield N: **A Brief Encounter.** Am J Nurs 82:9:1395–1399; September 1982. Describes how a very skilled nurse with adequate supervision entered into a therapeutic relationship. A useful article for group discussion to explore physical contact, gift giving, and relating while performing treatment procedures. Techniques used by the author would not be suitable for everyone.

Peplau H: **Talking with Patients.** Am J Nurs 60:7:964–966; July 1960. A classic that contains many suggestions to aid the beginning nursing student in the development of meaningful dialogue with her clients.

Rogers C: **The Characteristics of a Helping Relationship.** In Bennis W et al (eds): Interpersonal Dynamics, 3rd ed. Homewood, The Dorsey Press, 1973. Dr. Rogers raises questions that members of the helping professions must ask themselves. As he answers these, he describes the attributes of the "helping professional."

Stewart LM, Dawson DF: **Blind Client Sighted Therapist: The Interface.** J Psychiatr Nurs 17:11:31–35; November 1979. A description of the increased sensitivity to sound, touch, and smell as forms of communication for individuals who cannot see. Ways the sighted individual must modify communication patterns to accommodate the needs of those who cannot see are described.

Travelbee J: **Interpersonal Aspects of Nursing, Chapter IX: Concept: Communication, Chapter X The Human-to-Human Relationship,** 2nd ed. Philadelphia, F.A. Davis Co., 1971. Aids and barriers to effective communication are described in Chapter IX. Chapter X contains a clearly written, comprehensive discussion of the nurse/patient relationship drawing heavily on existential philosophy.

12

Teaching and Learning

Janet-Beth Flynn

CHAPTER OUTLINE

LEARNING OBJECTIVES

After completion of this chapter the reader will be able to:

- Define the terms in the glossary.
- Describe the teaching process.
- List methods of teaching.
- Compare and contrast teaching methods for adults and children.
- Compare and contrast barriers and facilitators to learning.
- Discuss educational aids.
- Discuss the role of the nurse in the teaching process.

GLOSSARY

Affective Domain—the area of learning that involves beliefs, attitudes, and values.

Barriers to Learning—blocks that prevent learning.

Change agent—one who facilitates change.

Cognitive domain—the area of learning that involves the acquisition of factual information.

Facilitators of learning—factors that aid learning.

Goal—a general statement of intent or outcome that is derived from needs identified by the nurse and the patient together.

Learning—a permanent change in behavior that results from a meaningful learning experience.

Objectives—narrow statements of intent that are derived from the goals.

Philosophy—an underlying system of beliefs that focuses an individual's thoughts and actions.

Principles of learning—rules under which learning occurs.

Psychomotor domain—the area of learning that involves physical performance of skills.

Teaching—a purposeful activity based on goals and objectives in which one or more individuals provide information to one or more persons.

INTRODUCTION

Patient teaching is one of the most important roles performed by professional nurses today. Although teaching has always been a part of the nurse's role, only in the last two decades was this role more clearly defined. These clarifications developed largely from nursing theories and the nursing process approach to patient care. Other factors influencing the nurse's teaching role include: the American Nurses Association's *Standards of Nursing Practice*, which describes the role of teaching as a function for all nurses[1]; *The Patient's Bill of Rights*, which indicates the patient's right to know and to understand his diagnosis and his treatment[2]; and in general, the ever-increasing base of knowledge from the biological, and social sciences, education, and other fields that provide the nurse with tools and concepts that were not formerly at her disposal—theories of how people learn, for example.

Nurses have been identified as the health care providers who are most frequently involved in the assessment, planning, and implementation of the patient teaching process.[3] Educating patients is extremely important in all aspects of the health care process. Increasing a patient's knowledge base about a particular illness, surgery, or preventable disease care, helps reduce anxiety and assists the person to gain some control of the situation. The patient's ability to care for himself is then increased and he has a better chance to stay healthy. Since one of the major goals of nursing is to assist patients to achieve and maintain the highest health state possible, knowledge of the teaching-learning process is a valuable tool.

The teaching-learning process obviously has two components: teaching and learning. Redmond states that "teaching is a special form of structured sequenced communication by which the one teaching helps another to learn."[4] Learning is defined as a change in behavior. These changes can be shifts in performance, knowledge, or attitudes.[5] Nurses teach by providing information, and promoting adaptation required in alterations of health states. In order to carry out this awesome task of patient teaching, nurses need to know how to apply the concepts of teaching and learning.

The purpose of this chapter is to identify concepts pertinent to teaching and learning and to provide a framework for their application within the structure of the nursing process.

LEARNING

Theories

In order to examine the teaching-learning process, we must examine how people learn. The process of human learning is the concern of philosophers, psychologists, and educators. Writings show concern for how man learns as far back as Aristotle.[6] Current theories of learning have evolved to explain how people learn, what they learn, and why they learn. In order to teach, nurses first have to be able to answer these questions and explore some of the theories of learning.

In the early days of learning theory, philosophers theorized about how man learns. These early theories were based on reflection, not on experimental data. Thomas Hobbs and John Locke[7] were two early philosophers whose writings reflected the notion that man learns of the world through his senses and his experiences with the environment.

With the birth of psychology came clinical research designed to test learning theories. Early scientific researchers included John Watson (1875–1958) and Ivan Pavlov (1849–1936).[8] Working independently, each formulated a theory of learning now called "behaviorism," which is the study of observable behavior. Behaviorist theory was founded on the premise that learning is based on conditioning, and could be changed through careful manipulation of the environment.

Edward L. Thorndike[9] (1874–1949) advanced the idea that human behavior could be changed by careful manipulation of the environment. He viewed the learner as passive within the environment. He felt that learning could be transferred to new situations and was concerned with the transfer of academic learning to everyday practice. He proposed that learning should be based on a careful assessment of the learner's behavior. This is an important concept and one quite relevant for nurses.

Another theorist whose work can readily be applied to nursing is John Dewey[10] (1858–1952). He believed that the outcome of learning should be clear to the learner at the beginning of the educational experience. He also developed the idea that the aim of education should be the growth of individuals toward independence. This idea, too, is congruent with the ultimate goal of nursing.

Stimulus-response learning theory was advanced by the psychologist B. F. Skinner[11] (1904–   ) whose work is based on objective laboratory observation of experimental animals. He views the causes of behavior as due to both the environment and the genetic heritage unique to each individual. Skinner feels that most human learning is caused by environmental experiences. Within this framework, the learner is viewed as passive, reacting to stimuli, and controlled by the environment in which he lives. Teaching, according to Skinner, is simply the arrangement of the environment in which the individual learns.

Jerome Bruner[12] (1915–   ) is another current theorist who has written about how individuals learn. His theory adds an interesting dimension to the study of learning, because it considers how values and cultural differences affect learning. He views learners as persons active within their environment, not simply reactors to it, as Skinner believes.

Robert Gagné[13] (1916–   ) defines learning as a change in human capability that cannot be accounted for by maturation, growth, or development. He writes of learning hierarchies that go from simple to complex. One must master the lower part of the hierarchy to be able to grasp the more difficult, abstract concepts and problem solving skills at the top of the hierarchy.

No one theory explains how people learn. Each theory has strengths and weaknesses, so nurses must select the most relevant features of each, in order to assist them in writing a comprehensive teaching plan.

Principles of Learning

The teaching-learning process is based on many principles or rules of learning that are drawn from the theories of learning. The nurse's ability to design a good teaching plan can be greatly enhanced if she keeps these principles in mind. (See Figure 12-1.) In order for patients to learn, each principle of learning and its effect on the particular needs of the patient must be considered.

Domains of Learning

Psychologists[14,15] have grouped learning into three distinct areas that are called the domains of learning. The **cognitive** domain deals with knowledge, facts, and other types of information that require the

INTERNAL PRINCIPLES (THOSE WITHIN EACH PERSON)

Principle	Explanation	Nursing/Teaching Intervention
Attitude	Accepting attitude	Assess the patient's attitude. Is the patient accepting or hostile and rejecting.
Values	A personal way of evaluating a situation, based on a lifetime of experiences.	Material should be presented in a way that is congruent with the values of the learner.
Maturation	The patient must be developmentally able to learn. He must have the appropriate cognitive and psychomotor skills.	Careful assessment of growth and development *throughout* the lifespan should be conducted to determine motor skill ability as well as psychosocial ability.
Motivation	The patient must want to learn the information.	Assess the cues the patient is giving. Is he questioning? Interested?
Readiness to learn	The patient must be ready and willing to learn.	Assess the acceptance of the health state. Is the client ready to discuss relevant factors of illness?
Meaningfulness	The information must have meaning for the patient. He must be able to understand it and relate it to previous learning or behavior.	Does the patient understand the information and is he able to transfer it to his life situation?

**EXTERNAL PRINCIPLES
(THOSE WHICH EFFECT INDIVIDUALS FROM WITHOUT)**

Principle	*Explanation*	*Nursing/Teaching Intervention*
Participation	The patient should be an active participant in the learning process.	Encourage involvement through manipulation of the environment and materials.
Repetition	Material is more likely to be retained if it is repeated.	Use a variety of teaching materials to present the same information over a period of time.
Feedback	The patient will learn more effectively with continuous and prompt feedback.	Provide comments, assurance, and other information about his performance promptly and objectively.
Action	The patient retains information longer if he is able to use it.	Provide opportunities for patients to use new information. For example, discussion groups or manipulation of materials, such as syringes.
Organization	The information should be in a predetermined organized format, moving from simple to complex, and based on previous knowledge.	Assess learning needs and determine the plan prior to beginning.
Environment	Should be conducive to learning, free of distractions, well lit, and private.	Prepare the environment prior to the teaching-learning experience.
Physical and Emotional Ability	The patient should be physically and emotionally able to receive the information.	Assess physical and emotional state prior to beginning.
Reinforcement	Positive reinforcement and encouragement should be provided. Negative reinforcement (punishment) should not be used.	Encourage and praise positive behaviors. Provide immediate feedback.

Figure 12-1. Principles of Learning.

brain to process and retain information. This domain includes sorting, storing, recalling, and applying information. The highest level of the cognitive domain encompasses problem solving and evaluating the problem solving process. The information is purely objective and can be expanded easily with new knowledge.

The second domain, called the **affective** domain, encompasses attitudes, values, and emotions. This domain has its basis in family norms, religious practice, culture, and personal lifestyle. The associated values are not *consciously* learned or evaluated, making this domain more difficult to work with. The patient, for example, may not be sure of what his values are, if he is asked to list them. Since values and beliefs are ingrained in the unconscious and difficult to change, ethical issues are involved in changing someone's values. Is it ethical to attempt to change someone's value system because it differs from the nurse's? Is the client wrong? Is the nurse right? An important factor involved in learning in this domain is to allow the patient to evaluate his own values and incorporate new learning within his own framework of being.

The third domain of learning is the **psychomotor** domain, which involves learning physical skills. Examples of these skills are preparing and injecting insulin, changing dressings, irrigating colostomies, administering eye drops, or any number of skills that nurses teach patients and their families.

Learning Throughout the Lifespan

Learning occurs in humans from birth until death. As humans grow and develop, their ability to grasp ideas from their environment changes, and all of the domains of learning are affected. Young children grow and develop in all of the domains of learning, while adults continue to refine the knowledge and skills that they already have acquired.

Children. Infants and young children absorb information from the world around them through their senses of sight, hearing, touch, taste, and smell. Infants, for example, learn to distinguish their mother's voice and face from other voices and faces and begin to distinguish between their mother and themselves. Early learning occurs in all of the domains, but in infants it is most obvious in the cognitive and the psychomotor domains. Babies learn that crying brings relief from hunger, discomfort, or boredom. They learn that smiling and cooing results in getting picked up and cuddled.

As the child grows, the world around him expands, but he is still very egocentric, believing that he is the center of everyone's attention. Young children's thinking is concrete and based on experience. They are incapable of abstraction and learn by manipulating objects in the environment. Since the attention span of young children is short they learn through playing. For the young child, the acquisi-

tion of language opens up many new possibilities in the child's intellectual life, allowing him to learn from the words of others and to ask questions.[16]

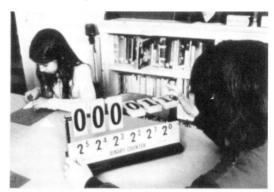

Figure 12-2. Young children learn through play.

The older child begins to learn values, acquires more knowledge, and increases his psychomotor skills. His attention span is longer, and he is able to learn from formal teaching experiences, as well as from play. Children between the ages of 7 and 11 have a basic understanding of their health state, and as they grow older and increase their knowledge base, the ability to understand more abstract ideas increases.

Adolescents. Important intellectual changes occur during adolescence. The knowledge base of adolescents has increased sufficiently for them to be able to understand concepts. The adolescent experiences an increased interest in abstract ideas and values, for example, the adolescent is able to think about abstract ideas such as truth, love, faith, liberty, and other concepts that cannot be seen or touched. Traditional values are questioned. Adolescents learn by seeing information, through questioning and reading, as well as by manipulating the environment. By using these methods of learning, they are able to understand relationships between ideas.

Adults. Adults have a great deal of basic knowledge and are able to think about abstract ideas. Values are well established and many psychomotor skills are highly refined. Adults are capable of learning information through reading, questioning, analyzing, and making decisions based on learning.

As individuals grow and develop, their ability to learn changes. As people experience life, they develop emotional, psychological, and intellectual strengths and weaknesses. These strengths and weaknesses affect an individual's ability to learn and are called facilitators and barriers to learning.

Barriers to Learning

Barriers to learning are things that get in the way of learning. They can come from within the patient (internal) or from the environment (external).

Internal factors are such things as present health or emotional states, previous experiences, and personal values that contribute to the way the patient thinks, acts, and behaves (See Figure 12-3). Nurses need to look at each one of these barriers to learning. Anxiety, an example of an internal barrier, is always present in the system to some degree, and can become debilitat-

ing if it occurs at high levels. High levels of anxiety do not permit satisfactory learning. If the client is worried about impending surgery or painful medical treatments, learning about home care might not be a priority.

Depression is another internal factor influencing learning. If the patient is depressed, he might not have the energy, motivation, or interest to learn.

Negative experiences with the health care system also can contribute to an individual patient's ability to learn. If a patient was hospitalized for a heart attack last year and a total diagnostic work-up proved to be inconclusive, he may refuse to learn about a diet, rest, medication, and exercise regime. This example also can demonstrate how denial can be a barrier to learning. If a patient denies that he has a serious illness, then he will not wish to learn about it. Previous negative experience with a disease process often can cause barriers to learning. A 40-year-old man, for example, whose father, uncles, or grandfather have had heart attacks and died in their 40s may be convinced that he too is going to die of a heart attack and may not be interested in learning about cardiac risk factors. This attitude of fatalism can be overcome, but it takes time and support from the staff and the family.

Educational level and intellectual ability both play an important part in the learning process. If the patient cannot understand what is being taught, it will not be meaningful to him and he cannot learn. These factors encompass young children, the uneducated, the culturally different, mentally disturbed, or learning disabled. Young children might not be developmentally ready to learn, or the material to be learned might be too complicated.

Readiness to learn is another potential barrier and has two components. The first component, emotional readiness, determines the patient's willingness to learn. The second component, experimental

Internal Barriers

anxiety
depression
denial of illness, crisis, or loss
negative experience with the health care system
previous negative experience with the disease
   process
educational and vocabulary level
lack of readiness to learn
pain
fever
inability to accept the sick role or over acceptance of the sick role
values and beliefs that are not congruent with the health care systems

Figure 12-3. Internal Barriers of Learning.

readiness, is determined by the patient's past experiences, skills, attitudes, and values.[17] The two components are closely related. If the patient with diabetes does not understand the purpose of insulin, he may not be motivated to learn about its administration. Furthermore, if the patient does not have the skill to administer insulin, he will be unable to prepare the injection correctly.

The client's present health state also can be a barrier to learning. If a patient is so ill that he cannot sit up or feed himself, he may not have the energy to learn about his condition and how to care for himself.

Inability to accept the sick role is another barrier that can affect a patient's ability to learn. For example, if a patient denies that he has a disease, he will not be interested in learning about it. If some patients overaccept the sick role, a maladaptive condition in which patients become preoccupied with their condition, they may not want to learn how to adapt or achieve a higher health state. For them, the gains of being ill are higher than the gains of being well. The attention that these patients receive has more value to them than does being well.

Finally, if the goal of the nurse is different from that of the client, learning may not take place. If attitudes, values, and beliefs conflict, the patient will block out what the nurse is teaching.

External barriers to learning include those factors that the patient may not be able to control, for example, the patient wants specific information from the doctor, but the doctor cannot be reached. (See Figure 12-4.)

Environment plays an important role in examining barriers to learning. The environment within which the teaching and learning take place needs to be controlled so that it is bright, free of noise, cool, and airy. It also should be structured so that privacy is assured if required.

Lack of family or group support can be

External Barriers

environment
time of teaching
the method of teaching
the level of the material presented
the nurse/teacher

Figure 12-4. External Barriers of Learning.

another external barrier to learning. For example, the hypertensive patient may not take his medication or cut his salt intake if the family is unwilling to assist him in these behaviors. Adolescents may be adverse to learning if they think the new behavior will not be accepted by the peer group.

The time of the teaching is an important consideration. After a rest period or first thing in the morning are usually the best times for teaching. Late in the day or any time the patient is tired would be a poor choice, since the patient may be too fatigued to concentrate.

Teaching methods need to be well-chosen in accordance with individual patient characteristics and needs. It would not be effective for example, to give a six-year-old child a book to read.

Certain characteristics and approaches by the nurse also can present learning barriers. The patient may not be motivated to learn if the nurse is distant, too busy, or judgmental. Failure to establish an effective nurse/patient relationship also can limit a patient's learning.

The nurse will be most successful as a teacher if she considers all of these learning barriers as possibilities when she assesses each client and plans for patient teaching.

Facilitators to Learning

Just as there are barriers to learning, there are facilitators to learning. A facilitator is something that helps. They are opposite from the barriers of learning, and can be viewed as internal and external as well. (See Figure 12-5.) Internal facilitators include positive experiences with the health care system, motivation and interest in the learning experience, a stable health state, and the ability to adapt to the sick role.

Internal Factors
Stable emotional and physical state
Positive experiences with the health care system in the past
Positive outcomes of previous altered health states
Desire or motivation to learn
Readiness to learn
Absence of fear, pain, fatigue
Ability to accept the sick role and to strive to attain a higher level of health

External Factors
Environment
Family support
Method of teaching
The nurse

Figure 12-5.   Internal and External Facilitators of Learning.

External facilitators include a pleasant environment conducive to learning, a supportive family, a teaching method that is based on the patient's learning needs, and a supportive nurse. Every effort should be made to break down barriers and to support facilitators.

TEACHING

Teaching can be described as activities presented by a teacher that help learners to absorb new material in a structured and sequential manner. The teacher controls the learning situation and introduces information that causes the learners to change their behaviors. Teaching, therefore, is an active process and a unique form of communication.

Health teaching is an important role for the professional nurse. Instructing patients to carry out their own care, administer their medications safely, and performing psychomotor skills, can make the difference between a healthy life and an un-healthy one, and in some cases may prevent severe complications or death.

Teaching is an art, and although some nurses are natural teachers, others are not. Everyone who engages in teaching must first learn the formalities of the teaching process. Like principles of learning, there are principles of teaching.

Teaching is a great deal more than simply the imparting of knowledge to another. Teaching a patient about a disease, for example, does not mean that the patient actually learned the material. Learning is the patient's option. Teaching offers the opportunity for learning. Teaching involves decreasing the threat of change, and it supports changing behaviors that facilitate positive adaptation.

There are many concepts that the nurse must consider before teaching. These concepts relate to the very nature of teaching,

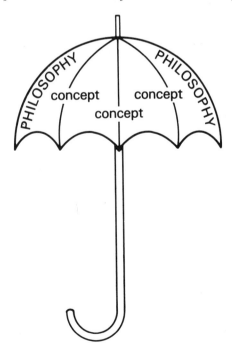

Figure 12-6.   Philosophy umbrella

and they are the framework on which to build. The broadest of these is philosophy. Philosophy is a belief about life, man, values, and ideals. Each of us has a philosophy of life, but most of us are not fully aware of it. Our philosophy is our overall outlook on life. It is like an umbrella composed of all the concepts we believe in. (See Figure 12-6.)

Reflect for a minute on your philosophy. (See Figure 12-7.) Is man good or bad? Is the environment passive or active? When someone fails to learn, is the teacher at fault or the learner? These are all questions that the nurse can answer when thinking about her philosophy.

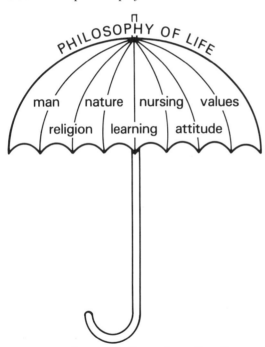

Figure 12-7.   Philosophy of Life Umbrella.

The next step is to compare the nurse's philosophy to the philosophy of the health care agency of which she is a part. The nurse will do well to inquire about the philosophy of any agency before accepting a job. Many agencies have a formal written philosophy that describes the goals of the agency and its view of the service offered

and reason for being. If philosophies are drastically different, nurses should question their ability to function adequately in that institution. In such a case, there is a high potential for conflict, and those nurses could be uncomfortable. If, on the other hand, the agency's and the individual nurse's philosophy are in agreement, the nurse will find the job much more agreeable. A nurse who does not believe in abortion, for example, would find it difficult to work on a unit that performed them.

Other factors arise when regarding philosophies. Redman states that, "Nurses face several questions of philosophy with regard to patient teaching. One such issue concerns how much and what information should be shared with the clients and how much independence clients should be allowed or should be required of them while participating in health care."[18] Other issues include: Who determines what is to be taught? How much should be taught? How much should the family participate in the learning? and Who should teach the actual material? These issues are all important. In many agencies, the physician decides what is taught and when. This can present a problem for the nurse, if the physician does not think that the patient is ready to know or should not know. The patient, on the other hand, is questioning every available person, trying to get more information. If the nurse provides the information, she may find herself in conflict with the physician. Another issue is how much should be taught. According to Redman, this issue can be resolved "when the patient's goals and the nurse's goals are congruent."[19] These goals can be determined mutually at the outset of the teaching process. This will provide both client and nurse with a set of goals to achieve.

A third issue, regarding family participation in the learning experience, should be established during the mutual goal setting period. If the patient wants the family to learn about the condition or the care, they should be included. If the patient is compromised by age, comprehension, or ability, the goal setting phase and teaching might be done exclusively with the family.

The final issue mentioned above, who should teach, is an important one. In many agencies the physician might do the teaching or delegate it to the nurse or another member of the health care team. For example, the dietitian teaches nutrition to a diabetic; an entrostomal therapist teaches colostomy care; the physical therapist teaches crutch walking and wheelchair transfer; occupational therapy might teach activities of daily living, and the nurse teaches footcare and insulin administration to diabetics.

The above discussion of philosophies regarding patient learning are important to examine, as they help determine the role of the nurse on the health care team. In many cases, there are not right or wrong answers, and many variables have to be considered.

A number of types of goals have been discussed, and a further description of the nature of goals will help clarify their importance. A **goal** can be defined as a statement of intent of outcome, and it is derived from needs. **Goals** are general statements and include short- and long-term goals. A goal is a general statement about a planned outcome. Both the nurse and the patient have goals. They may both wish for the patient to get well as soon as possible, but their means to the end may be quite different. It is important for the nurse to discuss goals with the patient and for the nurse and patient to negotiate mutual goals.[20] The patient and the nurse then strive to meet these goals together in order to reach an optimum health state for the patient.

Nurses must know if patients have achieved their goal, and this can be done by using objectives. **Objectives** are narrow statements about the outcomes derived from the goals (See Figure 12-8.). According to Mager, an objective "is an intent communicated by a statement describing a proposed change in a learner—a statement of what the learner is to be like when he has successfully completed a learning experience. It is a description of behavior (performance) we want the learner to be able to demonstrate."[21] In other words, they are **observable** changes in behavior.

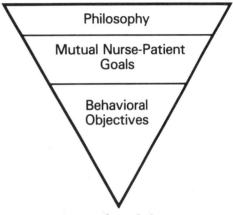

Figure 12-8. Goals and objectives can be derived from philosophy.

Objectives are stated in behavioral terms, and each goal may have several objectives. Objectives are structured in terms of several small steps as opposed to fewer large steps. They are more easily obtainable. Each objective, for example, can be seen as a step in the staircase to health. (See Figure 12-9.) Each objective is followed by an outcome criteria. The outcome criterion lists the behaviors and gives a reference to a period of time. This enables the nurse to evaluate the level of success of the teaching plan. Objectives also may reflect the philosophy of the patient, the nurse, and the health care institution (Figure 12-10), and can be united by the teaching-learning process. For example, the basic philosophy of the patient, the nurse, and the health care system is to restore the highest health state possible for the patient. Each has his own beliefs as to how that can be accomplished, and through ef-

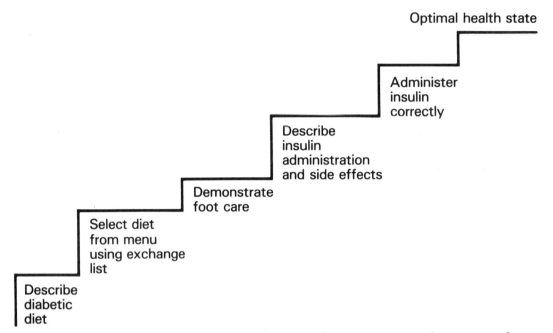

Figure 12-9. Behavioral objectives can be viewed as staircase reaching upward to a broad goal.

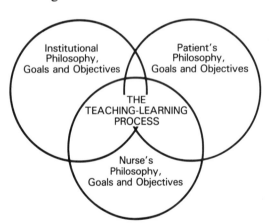

Figure 12-10. Congruent philosophies, goals, and objectives facilitate the teaching learning process.

fective teaching the philosophies can be blended to produce a successful outcome.

Once the nurse and the patient determine mutual goals, the nurse should prepare behavioral objectives and write them on the patient's care plan in terms of outcome criteria. If these objectives are lack-ing in clarity or definition, it will be impossible to evaluate the patient's learning. In addition to this, the patient can help evaluate his own progress as can other members of the health care team, if they are aware of the objectives and of the patient's progress.

Keep in mind that objectives and goals need to be attainable and realistic, and it is the joint responsibility of both patient and nurse to keep them so. When working with an obese patient who wants to lose weight, a realistic and obtainable objective might read: observes nutritional weight reduction diet and loses two pounds per week for four weeks. This objective adds another dimension to the ones discussed earlier, that of time. There is a demonstrated outcome, that of two pounds weight loss per week, that can be empirically measured or evaluated on a scale. Either the patient loses weight or he doesn't. At the end of the designated time, the objective could be reexamined to discover if it was reasonable and if the behavior was attained. In a case like this, where the behavior change (or goal attainment) may take a long period of time, a series of progressive objectives can be written for one goal. To use the same example, the broad goal might read: to attain normal weight as indicated by body build, height, and age. The time set objectives might be written as: patient loses 2 lbs/wk for 4 wks; 1 1/2 lbs/wk for 8 wks; 1 lb/wk for 8 wks; 1 lb/wk until ideal (or negotiated) weight is reached. Thus, a series of objectives are met until the goal is reached. The nurse, the patient, and other members of the health care team can evaluate the progress or lack of progress. In addition to this, the objectives are not overwhelming. The patient is able to cross each hurdle. If the objective had been written as: the patient will loose 100 lbs. in one year, it might defeat the patient before the first pound were lost. First, 100 lbs. is a great deal of weight to lose, and a year is a long time to be on a calorie restricted diet.

Another important factor to consider when writing patient objectives is that of setting priorities. Are certain things necessary to learn first for the patient's safety, or must some things be learned first so that they lay the foundation for future learning? If so, then the objectives should be written to comply with this effort.

When writing mutual nurse/patient objectives, it has been said that they must be written in behavioral terms. Let's examine what this means. Objectives should be written (on the chart or care plan) so that they can be observed readily by the nurse, thus enabling her to evaluate the patient's learning progress. Mager states that "there are many 'loaded' words, words open a wide range of interpretation."[22] Examples of these phrases include: to know, to fully understand, to have a basic knowledge, and to appreciate. What exactly do these statements mean? What does it mean to know something? How does the nurse "know" that the patient "knows." Objectives should be written so that they can be observed or measured. (See Figure 12-11.)

There are a variety of ways in which behavioral objectives can be written.

LIST OF SELECTED OBJECTIVE WORDS.

Weasel Words*	Clearly defined words**
know	describe
acquire knowledge	identify
fully understand	define
realize	compare
be familiar with	contrast
appreciate	list
value	state
feel	recall
	differentiate
	recite
	demonstrate
	write

*words open to interpretation
**words open to little interpretation

Figure 12-11. Behavioral objectives should be written so that they can be demonstrated by the patient.

A broad goal statement may proceed the step-by-step behavioral objectives. (See Figure 12-12(a).) Another way of writing behavioral objectives might be to list each objective without a broader goal. (See Figure 12-12(b).) As you can see from Figure 12-12(c), a time dimension has been added. Time, in the example, "at discharge" could mean days or weeks, and in a community setting, discharge could mean months or years. The ultimate goal of any series of mutually negotiated goals and objectives is the patient's adjustment to alterations in health state, with maximum adaptation of the patient and the family.

Each of the behavioral objectives in Figure 12-8 contains only one outcome. They were designed that way specifically for the purpose of evaluation. If the objective reads "prepares, administers, and lists the side effects of insulin," how could this be measured? Sometimes, yes, no? As you can

TYPES OF OBJECTIVES

Goal Directed Objectives

The patient will understand his diabetic diet. Related behavioral objectives. The patient:
- names all foods that are not to be eaten
- selects diabetic diet from the hospital menu
- describes the purpose of the diet
- describes the symptoms of insulin shock.

Behavioral Objectives

By discharge the patient will be able to:
- list all foods that are not to be eaten
- select diabetic diet from lists of foods using an exchange list
- describe the symptoms of insulin shock
- demonstrate proper foot care
- differentiate between his type of insulin and other types of insulin
- demonstrate correct insulin administration technique
- administer own insulin
- discuss insulin site rotation.

Time Reference Objective List

At the end of five days the patient will be able to:
- discuss administration of insulin
- list allowed foods
- describe foot care.

At the end of seven days the patient will be able to:
- demonstrate correct handling of syringe
- draw up prescribed amount of insulin
- observe the nurse administer insulin
- select balanced prescribed diet from menu
- compare and contrast insulin shock and diabetic coma

On discharge the patient will be able to:
- demonstrate correct syringe technique
- draw up prescribed insulin dose
- administer correctly and discuss site rotation
- prepare weekly menu using prescribed diet
- demonstrate foot care.

Figure 12-12.   Behavioral objectives can be written in a variety of ways.

see, a multiple objective could lead to problems.

No discussion on objectives would be complete without mentioning nursing objectives. Discussion to this point has revolved around mutual nurse/patient goals and objectives. These are the goals that the nurse and the patient discuss and agree are appropriate to the learning needs of patients. They are based on the assumption that the nurse can teach the patient, but only if the patient wants to learn. Nursing objectives appear on the patient's care plan, and they delineate what the nursing objectives are. To use the diabetic patient as an example again, a set of nursing objectives would outline what behaviors the nurse should demonstrate. For example, a nursing goal might be stated: prevent breakdown of tissue on the feet. Individual objectives associated with the goal would outline the various steps in meeting and evaluating this goal such as:

- wash the feet daily with mild soap and warm water
- inspect for reddened areas
- dry between each toe after washing
- examine the nails of the toes for integrity and condition
- apply lotion
- powder between the toes

These are behaviors of the nurse, and in most cases require the patient's cooperation, but do not necessarily involve his participation. Both nursing objectives and mutual nurse/patient objectives can be used simultaneously or individually, based on the nurse's individual assessment and evaluation of the situation.

The beginning nurse may experience difficulty in distinguishing between nurse/patient goals and nursing goals. A rule of thumb is to examine who is expected to perform the behavior. If it is the nurse, then it is a nursing goal. If it is the patient, then it is a mutual or patient goal. It takes practice and experience to be able to see the difference, and to write clear, concise, appropriate objectives.

It is also possible to arrange objectives in a hierarchy from simple to complex. This ordering of objectives evolved in the 1940s when psychologists and educators assessed a need for defining these behaviors and putting them into a common framework, so that all researchers and educators would use the same terms. This committee has become famous through educational publications and their work has been labeled as **Taxonomies of Educational Objectives.**

To further elaborate on the development of objectives, behaviors are divided into three domains: the cognitive, the affective, and the psychomotor. (See Figure 12-13.) The cognitive and psychomotor domains are arranged from simple to complex, and the affective domain from mild to increasing internalization.

TAXONOMIES OF OBJECTIVES

COGNITIVE DOMAIN*
  Knowledge
    defines terms
    identifies specific facts
    recalls information

  Comprehension
    translates information into own words
    identifies meanings of abbreviations and scientific terms
    summarizes information
    interprets information
    defines implications and consequences of actions

  Application
    applies facts to situations
    identifies steps in procedures

  Analysis
    distinguishes facts from hypotheses
    identifies relationships between ideas and facts

  Synthesis
    describes personal experiences, ideas, and feelings
    prepares plan of action using facts

  Evaluation
    evaluates behaviors using internal standards
    evaluates behaviors using external standards

AFFECTIVE DOMAIN**

  Receiving
    awareness
    willingness to receive information

  Responding
    responds with facts but has not internalized material
    responds with commitment
    responds with total commitment and is satisfied with the change

  Valuing
    accepts a value
    prefers a set of values

  Organization
    places values into a framework
    compares the relationships of values
    identifies prominent values in the framework

  Characterization by a value or value complex
    acts consistently according to value set
    contrasts values
    discusses a philosophy of life
    discusses a philosophy of health

PSYCHOMOTOR DOMAIN

  Perception
    observes skill
    identifies and describes skill
    recalls the skill

  Readiness
    states readiness to perform skills
    demonstrates the ability

  Response
    imitates the behavior of the skill
    performs skill independently

  Adaptation
    adapts the skill correctly to meet own needs
    performs the skill correctly without prior demonstration
    performs the skill correctly after a specified lapse of time

---

Figure 12-13.   Domains of learning are ordered from simple to complex.

*Adapted from Bloom, Benjamin S., Engelhart, Max D., Furst, Edward J., Hill, Walker H., Krathwohl, David R., **Taxonomy of Educational Objectives: The Classification of Educational Goals. Handbook I.** Cognitive Domain. New York: David McKay Co., Inc., 1957.

Adapted from Krathwohl, David R., Bloom, Benjamin, S., and Massia, Bertram B., **Taxonomy of Educational Objectives. The Classification of Educational Goals. Handbook II: Affective Domain. New York: David A. McKay Co., Inc., 1956.

We are concerned with the taxonomies of learning in order to analyze and plan what is to be taught and by what means it is to be taught. The nurse could use readings, facts, and printed information for the cognitive domain. For the affective domain she would use films, readings, discussion groups, role modeling, and various other techniques. The psychomotor domain could be best approached through manipulation of materials and practice. A further discussion of teaching methods will appear later in this chapter.

Ethics of Teaching

Of the three domains of learning, the affective domain is usually the most difficult with which to work. How does one change a patient's attitudes or values? An even more interesting question is should this be done? Since the affective domain is the "heart" of a patient, is it ethical to manipulate a patient? In addition to this, there are more practical issues, such as how does the nurse assess the affective domain? How does one write these objectives? How does one teach and evaluate learning?

Conley writes, "The hesitancy of teachers to use affective measures for evaluation of purposes stems partly from the inadequacy of appraisal techniques. Frequently, behaviors in the affective domain must be inferred from overt behaviors, which may or may not be valued. . . ."[23] Another factor that makes assessment of learning in this domain difficult is its very nature. This domain encompasses the value of privacy. Patients may be uncomfortable, embarrassed, or threatened with discussion of values, attitudes, and morals. They may become offended and not wish to pursue further nursing intervention, or they may simply refuse any nursing intervention in this area. Assessment in this area is also difficult because a patient may conform to the change while the nurse is observing and return to old behaviors when she is gone. This is not necessarily a devious maneuver, since patients perceive the teacher in several ways. They may simply conform momentarily because they are intimidated by authority. They may generally like the nurse and want to please her but have no real belief in the change, and they adapt their behavior in her presence and rapidly forget when she is gone. Finally, the affective domain requires that people examine their own philosophy and way of life in order to make changes. This is generally a slow procedure at best. It may take years to change a patient's attitudes and values. Conversely, some values can be changed rapidly with information. For example, the person who hasn't really valued his health might change after being told he will have a heart attack if he does not change his lifestyle. This person might immediately go on a diet, stop smoking, and institute an exercise program.

The role of the nurse in teaching values or assisting patients to change values is many faceted. First and most important, the nurse should examine her own values, which can get in the way when working with another's set of values. For example, the nurse who values cleanliness above all else may have difficulty in working with a person who does not. She may spend much time going over personal hygiene to no avail. The values of the nurse and the patient are quite different.

After the nurse has examined her own values, she can examine how she reacts to someone whose values are different. It is important to understand that judgmental attitudes are never helpful in a helping relationship. If, for example, the patient employs health practices that the nurse views as unusual or unhealthy, a values conflict is already taking place. For example, when a Mexican child becomes ill, the mother or grandmother may diagnose the child as having had the evil eye placed on him. One cure, according to them, is to place a raw egg under the child's bed. Nurses may view this as unusual or untidy and need to be aware of their own reactions to such behaviors.

A third thing to consider is the ethics of the situation. Is it ethical and in the patient's best interest to make a change?

The goals of teaching, in the affective domain, are the development of new sets of values that support healthful behaviors acceptable to the patient and his family.

Teaching in this domain is difficult. Once it has been established that learning is needed, the nurse can choose an appropriate teaching strategy. Conducting discussion groups is an excellent method for helping patients clarify their value systems. In groups with common problems, members learn from one another. They are accepted into the group easily and without judgment. Some examples of these groups include ostomy clubs, mastectomy groups, or Weight Watchers.

Involving the patient's family also can help to make changes in many instances. Another method of teaching in this domain includes active patient participation in the learning experience (such as role playing). Since changes in this domain take time for the patient to internalize, observed changes in behavior may be slow. This can be frustrating for nurses. Patience and the patient's freedom of choice should always be kept in mind. If the patient is slow to change, the nurse should focus on supporting identified strengths that will aid in positive adaptation.

Teaching through the Lifespan

Teaching strategies must be adapted for the level of the patient's understanding. This is particularly true when teaching children. The first step in this process is to assess the individual child's growth, development, and level of understanding. Infants and very young children are difficult to teach, because they have not yet acquired language. At this level, the nurse might just give tender loving care (TLC) to the child, and provide a safe and stimulating environment. Holding, rocking, smiling, talking, singing, and providing mobiles will be effective. This is also a Skinnerian type of conditioning. The child is conditioned, for example, not to be frightened. Health teaching of young children is generally focused on the child's mother or other care taker. Children as young as one year have been observed imitating behaviors of nurses and others on the health care team, and are able to learn through play.

Teaching of children usually focuses on play. Petrillo writes that, "Play is a natural phenomenon that leads to learning. . . ."[24] Concepts to be taught can be incorporated into games, puppet shows, coloring books, dolls, doll houses, doll hospitals, group play, arts and crafts, and many other methods. Teaching children is creative and fun. A plan should be used, however, to guide the teaching-learning process in order to present the material in an orderly fashion.

Slightly older children, from 1½ up, can be allowed to manipulate syringes, intravenous (IV) tubings, alcohol wipes, empty medicine bottles, and other equipment. They can be taught to put dressings on dolls, and give them "IVs" and "injections." Simple explanations of why the child will need to have these items should accompany the play. Art materials can be used as another media for teaching. A favorite with children is the butcher paper diagram, in which the nurse places the child on the paper and an outline of the child's body is traced. The nurse can then diagram the organ systems, make incisions, or put in an "intravenous". The child can also color the drawing or cut out colored body organ shapes to glue on it. While the nurse and child are engaged in this activity, the nurse can be teaching the child what to expect and how the organ subsystems relate to each other. Children two years and older are fascinated by this technique.

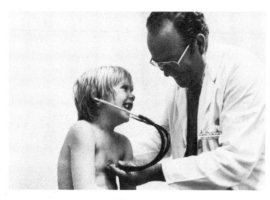

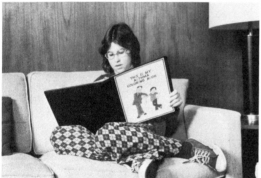

Figure 12-14. Teaching strategies must be adapted for the level of the patient's understanding.

Adequate time always should be provided for tours of the hospital, treatment rooms, operating rooms, and recovery rooms. Children who are going to experience painful treatments or surgery should always be taken on tours and permitted to ask questions.

Children, especially young children, need constant reinforcement and repetition. Parents should be encouraged to participate in these play learning experiences, because parental support increases the child's ability, and the parents can use these methods and reinforce the learning.

By adolescence, individuals are developing the ability to conceptualize and see relationships between things. Adolescents are able to understand more complex explanations, and their reading ability and vocabulary is considerably greater. They

are curious about what is going on and to the outcome of disease processes. Disfiguring diseases and conditions are very hard to deal with at this stage of life when peer group identity is so critical to development. Emotional support and role modeling is very important. Adult and child teaching strategies can be blended effectively to produce good teaching strategies for this age group.

Generally speaking, the adult patient has mastered reading, conceptualizing, perceiving relationships, and many other sophisticated behaviors that come with maturity and experience. Adults can be taught using a variety of teaching methods. The teaching methods can be used alone or in combination. (See Methods of Instruction and Educational Tools.) Some examples of these include: audiovisual materials, lectures, discussion, raising questions, and use of games. (See Figure 12-15.)

Occasionally, special consideration has to be given elderly patients. Because the aging process may reduce mental capacities, elderly people may have difficulty learning or remembering. They may not be able to understand the nature of the condition and the need for long-term medications in a chronic condition, such as diabetes, heart disease, or hypertension. Older people also may need more repetition of the material being taught. Other factors to be considered when teaching the elderly are alterations in vision and hearing. Teaching plans and educational tools might have to be adapted for the patient who can no longer see or hear as well as in the past.

Finally, keep in mind that all patients are under a great deal of stress when they are ill. All of their energy may be spent on worrying about the illness, impending surgery, or diagnostic tests that might be painful. These patients may not have much energy left to direct toward learning. They might be unable to focus on what the nurse is attempting to teach. For example, the patient who is going for coronary bypass surgery may not have the ability to learn about the heart-lung machine because of his great fear of the impending surgery, and his fear of the complex machine. This is not the case in all situations, however, so each individual should be assessed individually.

```
G B A C K L M E C T K A B S N U T R I T I O N C A I T N
L L L T O U E J H F S Y R I N G E A K W J H G F R N R L
O O U P L K P L U K Y L P A T D S D E O E J H G W S A Y
U O C C N P S R T A S V A N P O P R J P U S E F Y U H R
C D B D O N E P L U S J I P R S O G F L Y C U C U L J F
F S I E P S O S T O Q I N S F T L J U U T P T A I I T G
B U O A U O E F G G P D M F E W Y K T S K E E R E N R H
K G O N N N R G O G R D R G W Q U L Y W Z T I B R R I K
F A S T I N G B L O O D S U G A R E E I J T U O T E K L
T R K I N D K J G F T C F T F R I J C F T H Y H Y A L O
R I M M M M J K H R E C E C G E A R J G P I Q Y Q C H P
I N N A E D D D J E I E A A H U E J E H O R U D P T F W
N K I R S A C E T O N E O R Y X X K A K E S E R U I E E
K E V T P H L L I S S N V T E E J N N T T Y A V O R R
F O U R P L U S S G F E R R S U T T E E R F A T S N Y T
O I N S U L I N S I T E R O T A T I O N I E D E W A R D
U M A U M I N R E I N S U L I N E R E R N N O S U G A R
R N B M D Y I Y T N N O M I E R P T H R E E P L U S T D
P O C N P T O U J E X C H A N G E E U W W W E W E R G K
L E A H Y P O G L Y C E M I A A A W F A T I G U E T U R
```

CARBOHYDRATES	FATS
BLOOD SUGAR	SUGAR
FASTING BLOOD SUGAR	THIRST
ONE PLUS	EXERCISE
TWO PLUS	POLYURIA
THREE PLUS	INSULIN REACTION
FOUR PLUS	INSULIN
PROTEIN	INSULIN SITE ROTATION
ACETONE	NUTRITION
HYPOGLYCEMIA	SYRINGE
EXCHANGE	GLUCOSE
FATIGUE	FOOT CARE

Figure 12-15. Games can be an effective way of teaching terminology.

Methods of Instruction

Once goals and objectives have been mutually developed, specific methods of instruction are selected to meet the objectives. Methods of instruction are as important as writing the goals and objectives. Much teaching is done on a one-to-one basis with the patient, and is based upon interpersonal relationships. Some of this teaching comes about spontaneously during routine care when either the patient or the nurse questions the other. For example:

Patient: The doctor says that I have to take my insulin for the rest of my life. What will happen if I don't take it?

or

Nurse: Did the doctor tell you what will happen if you take too much or not enough insulin?

The quality of the nurse's interpersonal skills is very important in face-to-face teaching, as is her sensitivity to the patient's needs and wants. The nurse also should be aware of medical language and attempt to avoid this when teaching, since most patients do not know medical terms.

Other methods of teaching include such things as placing the patient in an identity group (Parents Without Partners, Al-Anon, AA) and use of audiovisual aids, self-study, or games.

The objectives generally determine what is to be taught and can determine the method to be used. Some types of information lend themselves best to one style of teaching, and some to others.

The one-to-one method of teaching requires the nurse to present the information, and the patient is an active participant in the learning experience. The nurse assesses the patient's learning throughout the experience. Factual information can be presented at a level that can be understood, and the patient can freely question the nurse.

Group discussion is another method of teaching. This method encourages patients to discuss their feelings and experiences. Patients learn from one another, and the nurse, as group leader, serves as a facilitator by clarifying when appropriate. This method is appropriate when members of the group have similar needs, such as a nurse-led diet and exercise group. While the discussion is going on, the nurse can interject information, clarify what has been said, add direction, and answer questions. Group discussion occasionally brings out some individual patient's erroneous thinking. Take for example, a group of hypertensive retirees enrolled in an exercise class. The class exercised for short periods (5 to 10 minutes), then rested, and then repeated the exercise. Discussion of diet and exercise occurred during the break. During one discussion period, Mrs. K said she was out of medication for her high blood pressure. Another member asked her the name of the drug that she was taking. Mrs. K gave the name and the other patient Mr. Z said "I'm not taking that but I am taking another medication for high blood pressure. You can have some of mine until you can get to the drug store." Everyone looked at Mr. Z who blushed and said, "I guess that I said something wrong?" The nurse then discussed the importance of taking one's own medicine and the dangers of taking someone else's. The impact of this learning experience was greater than lecture or other methods because they all had a chance to discuss the problem and learn from it. Discussion can be a very powerful learning experience if properly managed.

Chapter 24 provides further information on concepts of group dynamics and group teaching.

Lecture is another common form of teaching and probably the one most familiar to the student nurse. Lecture consists, basically, of a person presenting factual material to learners. Many hospitals have lectures for groups of patients about to share a similar experience, for example, classes presented to mothers-to-be on basic child care. This type of presentation does not require much interaction between the lecturer and the learner, but it can be effective when there is a need to present a number of facts to a large group of people.

Role playing, a more involving type of learning experience, is a teaching-learning technique where the patient consciously pretends to be someone else for a brief period of time. It is a type of play acting where the patient attempts to understand how the other person feels or reacts. This way of teaching tends to give the patient insight into a situation that he had not previously had. Role playing helps individuals to understand what another person is feeling and is a most effective teaching method in the affective domain.

Role modeling is another technique that assists in teaching in the affective domain. It provides teaching by example, and the nurse serves as the model to be copied. When the nurse is role modeling, she should always set a good example and be conscious that the patient is emulating her behavior. This technique works very well with children and adolescents, or with patients who are unfamiliar with the information or task. It is important to note that the nurse frequently acts as a role model whether she is aware of it or not. That is why personal behaviors such as hygiene, tone of voice, and various habits are important to pay attention to. Everyone looks to the nurse as a "model" whether she is consciously setting out to be one or not.

Demonstration and practice is a teaching technique for the psychomotor domain. The nurse demonstrates a procedure, such as insulin administration, and then allows the patient to manipulate the equipment, draw up the insulin, and inject an orange. Demonstrations may progress through several sessions until the patient is ready to administer the insulin to himself. Successive meetings might consist of the patient *returning the demonstration* from start to finish faultlessly. Demonstration as

a teaching technique is generally not good for large groups, because not everyone can observe, particularly if the demonstration requires small motions, such as drawing up insulin, or small areas, such as umbilical cord care of newborns. As with role modeling, the demonstrator must have perfect technique. In order for patients to learn the skill, they must practice with supervision, and it is important that the nurse ensure adequate time, space, and supplies for all members in the group.

Assessment of patient learning and progress is essential with technique learning. The patient must be provided with feedback about his progress and support when he is having difficulty performing the procedure.

Other ways of teaching include self-study, audiovisual aids, teaching machines, flip charts, and programmed instruction. Generally, these are used to **assist** the teacher and will be discussed in the section on educational tools.

Time, Space, Supplies, and Privacy

Teaching takes more time than one would expect, so nurses need to provide a block of time sufficient for the learning experience. The physical environment is another important factor to consider. Adequate space and chairs are necessary for a lecture or discussion. Well-lighted, well-ventilated areas in which to teach are also a priority. Supplies needed for demonstration, explanation, or clarification should be chosen carefully and assembled ahead of time. It is difficult to convey the idea of a syringe to someone who has never seen one. If return demonstration is a part of the plan, then enough supplies for each individual are also necessary. Finally, some things we may wish to teach might require privacy, for example, birth control information, or colostomy care. Drawing the curtain around a patient in a busy four-bed unit might not be adequate. Another place where no one will interrupt might be more appropriate. Sometimes in our cramped health care institutions, these places are hard to find and might mean the head nurse's office, the conference room, or some other place where privacy could be assured.

Educational Tools or Aids

Allowing patients to experience the same information through more than one method is an excellent way to repeat the same information. Recent research has demonstrated that certain individuals learn better through listening, while others learn best when they can see the material visually. Some learn best when combining listening and viewing, and still others learn from experience only. Very few people learn from only one route, so combinations of methods are a good idea. A mother-to-be, for example, can be given a pamphlet to read on bathing an infant, followed by a film, demonstration, and finally practice on a doll. This sequence provides the patient with several experiences, more or less sequential, ending with application. This example is known as a multimedia approach to teaching. In addition to stimulating more than one sense, it also provides information through a variety of methods.

Probably the most common educational aid available to the nurse is **printed material.** Materials such as pamphlets, booklets, printed cards, and specially prepared instructions are widely used to help meet the patient's objectives. Reading ability of the patient is a factor here. Is the patient able to read? Many people who cannot read are embarrassed and may not admit this problem. At what level does this patient read? Does the patient read English? If English is the patient's second language, does the patient prefer to read in his own language? Reading materials can be given to a patient to read before the more formal

teaching plan begins, followed by implementation of the teaching plan.

Another type of educational tools are **audiovisual (AV) aids.** The AVs are combinations of sound and sight, and occasionally touch and smell. They bring another dimension to the teaching plan. Some examples of AV aids include slide and tape presentations, speech and slide presentations, tape cassettes, photographs, slides, pictures, and workbooks. Models or replicas of body parts are sometimes used—in much the same way "Mrs. Chase" is used to teach student nurses. These methods should always be incorporated into an overall plan. It is not enough to turn on the patient's TV to a closed circuit program on infant care and expect that the patient will learn all of the material, so time for discussion and questions should be provided.

Programmed instruction (P.I.) manuals are another teaching aid. Programmed instruction is primarily a written guide. It begins with simple material, and becomes more complex as the reader progresses. It is designed so that the learner can move at his own pace. Each step is designed so that the learner masters it before he moves onto the next step. The nurse should always be available to provide additional information or answer questions when the patient is using P.I.

A newer device for patient teaching is the use of **games.** These can be devised by the nurse or the nurse and the patient together. The patient's participation in this activity engages him actively and helps him incorporate recently acquired educational material. Developing games depends upon the creativity of the designers. Again, they assist the patient in meeting learning objectives. Games are popular with adults as well as children and adolescents.

Coloring and workbooks are also teaching aids. These are especially good for children. Again, these are available from many agencies and in various languages.

Posters and attractively designed bulletin boards are also effective aids, especially when used in clinical waiting rooms and offices. For example, they may list cancer warning signs, signs and symptoms of disease conditions, chambers in the heart, diagram physical growth, or development from infancy through early childhood.

Flip charts can be used by the nurse when she is giving a talk to a group or to an individual patient. They also can be used alone by the patient before or after his contact with the more formal teaching presentation.

Most of these methods can be used in the hospital, the clinic, or the home. All of them can be used by an individual client or group of clients. Many can be used for adolescents as well as adults, but the level of the content and the speed of the presentation may be altered for understanding for younger patients and for patients whose reading comprehension is somewhat slower.

THE NURSING PROCESS AND THE TEACHING-LEARNING PROCESS

According to Yura and Walsh, "The nursing process can be applied in a variety of settings; it is flexible and adaptable, permitting the nurse to use judgment, and creativity in caring for the client in an organized, orderly, and systematic manner."[25] This definition of the nursing process fits nicely with the teaching process, since both are dynamic processes, and include assessment, planning, implementation, and evaluation. These processes can be integrated to provide realistic care.

Assessment

The first step in the nursing process is the assessment phase, in which the patient is observed and assessed by the nurse. The nurse identifies what the learner needs to know and specifies characteristics and behaviors of the patient. What the patient needs to know can be learned by questioning, listening, and observing behaviors. The patient can be asked to do a procedure such as a dressing change, a colostomy irrigation, or insulin administration, and the nurse observes the techniques and provides feedback. Many times this gives the nurse a clearer picture than if she asks the patient to describe the process. For example:

Miss Lorenzo, a third-year student nurse, went into Mr. Brown's room to administer his morning insulin injection. Mr. Brown asked if he might administer his own insulin, as he had been doing for eight years. After checking with her instructor, Miss Lorenzo allowed Mr. Brown to inject himself. Mr. Brown's technique was perfect until he injected himself. He carefully scrubbed his skin with alcohol wipes, then he injected himself intradermally, leaving a large wheal. He slapped the wheal on his thigh and it went flat. Miss Lorenzo questioned him as to why he did that. Mr. Brown said that a "bump" occurred every time he injected himself and slapping it made it go away.

The student nurse was able to identify specific areas where more teaching was needed. For example, where his insulin technique needed refining because he was injecting himself intradermally instead of subcutaneously. Ms. Lorenzo demonstrated the correct technique and gave an explanation. Mr. Brown never made that error again during his hospital stay.

Another factor to be assessed is potential learning, or anticipating learning needs. For example, a person who has diet controlled diabetes might be told that insulin administration might one day be necessary, and the nurse could give a brief overview and answer questions. Another example of an anticipatory learning need is that of a pregnant woman who needs to learn how to bathe and feed an infant.

Characteristics of the patient can be assessed by observation. One of these patient characteristics is readiness. Growth and development has impact on readiness to

PATIENT EDUCATION ASSESSMENT

Name _____ Age _____ Diagnosis _____ Date of Admission _____

Address _____ Phone _____ Date of interview _____

Marital status _____ Role in Family _____ Children _____

House _____ Apt. _____ Stairs to entrance _____ Stairs to bedroom _____

Occupation _____ Education level _____ English reading ability _____

Cultural orientation _____ Language spoken _____

Chief Complaint _____ Anxious _____ Depressed _____

Perception of Condition _____

How long has condition been present _____

What has physician told patient re: physical condition _____

What have other's told patient _____

What causes symptoms _____

What prevents symptoms _____

Questions about condition _____

_____

Compliance with previous health regimes _____

Past experience with disease and with health care _____

Ability to learn _____ Readiness to learn _____

Current health state _____

Family response to illness _____

Family member's interest and ability to learn _____

Physical limitations—Fever _____ Pain _____ Medications _____ Vision _____ Hearing _____

Figure 12-16. The Patient Education Assessment Tool

learn. A young child with diabetes, for example, just does not have the cognitive ability to understand the chronicity of the condition or the physical ability to administer insulin himself.

Patients who are ready to learn will ask questions, observe the nurse when she is caring for him, and ask for literature. For example, the patient who has just had a colostomy might first observe the nurse irrigate and change the colostomy bag, and then ask to assist with the procedure the next time.

Patients who are not ready to learn about their condition will not ask direct questions and will not make much effort to participate in the care. A patient with a colostomy might avert his eyes when the nurse is changing the colostomy bag. Patients might also become restless, anxious, or depressed when related topics are raised by the nurse or refuse to discuss them. Frequently, people who are not ready to learn are depressed or employing defense mechanisms such as denial. Others have maladaptively accepted the sick role in order to receive secondary gains, such as the diabetic man who says, "My wife will take care of me. Teach her about the diet, since she does the cooking anyway. I can't inject myself. She will do it for me. She likes to take care of me."

Another characteristic of **motivation** is wanting to learn. Motivation to learn is greatest when the patient is ready to learn. This type of motivation is self-generated and called **internal motivation.** The learner usually learns more and retains it longer.

External motivation comes from without and is usually created by the teacher. Rewards and praise are useful in fostering this type of motivation. A mother who is toilet training her toddler might reward him everytime he uses the bathroom. Skinner found that punishment or threats did not do much to motivate individuals to learn, because they tend to generate a high level of anxiety. If the nurse is able to determine the patient's internal motivation, she may be able to increase it by helping the learner see relationships between things. The patient who has had a heart attack wants to get well so that he can go home and is, therefore, motivated to learn about his medications and exercise.

If there appears to be major learning barriers or significant problems related to any part of the teaching-learning process, it may be appropriate to state these as nursing diagnoses. Examples of such nursing diagnoses are as follows:

- potential alteration in ability to learn due to cultural/language barriers
- non-compliance with teaching plan due to family pressure
- inability to learn side effects of medications due to fear.

Planning

Once the nurse has carefully assessed the patient's educational needs, she begins the second phase of the nursing process, *planning.* In the planning phase, what to teach, how to teach, who will teach, where to teach, and when to teach are addressed. These all can be incorporated into a broad teaching plan (Figure 12-17) and directed by goals and objectives.

What to teach is based on the nurse's assessment of the patient knowledge base and condition. Teaching-learning relies on the health state and on the patient characteristics of readiness and motivation. What to teach can be determined by what the patient wants to learn, and relates to readiness to learn. For example, the colostomy patient may want to learn what a colostomy looks like and how it works, but not how to irrigate it himself.

How to teach is the next decision that the nurse must make. The method chosen should reflect both what is to be taught and the patient characteristics. Methods chosen should be the ones that involve the patient the most, that is, the ones that stimulate his interest. The domain in which the learning is to occur also should be considered when choosing a method, because of the different methods used in each domain.

Who will teach the patient is another consideration. Generally, the nurse and others on the health team teach the patient. A teaching plan for a diabetic patient might involve the physician, the nurse, and the dietitian. The nurse can serve as the link between all of the departments by reinforcing what the patient has learned.

In addition to the patient, who in the family needs to be taught about the patient's condition and care? This can be determined by assessing cultural and developmental aspects, and cognitive development. Does the patient's culture allow health teaching? Can the mother make decisions about followup care, and can she implement the teaching? Developmentally, is the individual old enough to learn the material? Do the parents or caretakers

Patient's Name _____ Age _____ Culture _____ Language _____ Address _____ Phone _____

Diagnosis _____ Others to be taught (who) _____ Address _____ Phone _____

Goals _____

Objectives _____

Objective	Content to be taught (what)	Teaching method (how)	Health Care Provider Dept. (name) (who)	Time Date (when)	Location (where)	Evaluation Method	Comments and Observations

Figure 12-17.   An example of a patient teaching plan.

need to be included in the teaching plan? Does the patient understand? Can he read? Does he accept the sick role? All of these questions need to be considered when developing a teaching plan.

Where to teach is another issue and fairly easy to answer. Location of teaching depends on the method to be used, the patient's condition, and the patient's location. If a film, lecture, or group discussion is to be used, then it is important to secure a large enough room to accommodate the group. This usually takes advance planning, because space is often at a premium in today's health care facilities. If flip charts or programmed instruction are to be used, then the bedside or the home is as appropriate as the hospital. If filmstrips are to be used, the bedside or home can be used as well, but generally involves reserving a portable projector. When one-to-one teaching is done, adequate time and privacy are required, and that involves preplanning. In many instances, pulling the curtains around the patient is not enough; therefore, arranging to take the patient out of the room must be considered.

The best time for teaching is when the patient is free of fatigue, fever, and pain, is ready to learn, and is motivated to get well. By careful assessment, planning, and implementation, these factors can be controlled, to an extent, when both the nurse and the patient have a block of time to devote to the activity.

For major teaching needs, a specific teaching plan should be written to provide an organized structure of the who, what, where, and how of teaching. (see Figure 12-17.) The plan is written and is placed on the patient's Kardex. A plan provides for a consistent approach for the nurse, and it provides structure. When patient teaching is not the highest priority or only involves a few simple points, the teaching objective is listed on the regular care plan, and a separate teaching plan may not be necessary.

Implementation

Once a plan has been written, the next phase of the process is to implement the plan. During the implementation process, the person teaching needs to draw from her knowledge of the theories of learning and from teaching principles. While teaching, the nurse should allow the learner to proceed at his own pace, because not all people learn at the same rate. Some individuals need a great deal of repetition, while others can grasp difficult concepts at once. The duration of the teaching experience should be kept to a minimum, as attention spans can be short when people are anxious or in pain, but should be long enough to present the material.

Other steps in implementation should include giving the patient advance knowledge of the content of the teaching plan. This can be done with a written outline or by saying what you are going to include. Charting for the teaching plan should be done so that others know what has been taught, and providing feedback to the patient is helpful so that he knows the strengths and weaknesses of his knowledge base. It allows him to know what he knows and what he doesn't know.

Evaluation

Feedback brings us to the final step in the nursing process, **evaluation.** Evaluation is a form of assessing what the patient has learned, and how his behavior has changed as a result of nursing intervention. Evaluation is a crucial step in the process, because it allows the nurse to see if her plan is effective and where reassessment is necessary.[26]

Very specific criteria are needed in order to determine if the patient has met the goals and objectives. The major purpose of goals and objectives serves to list observable items that are expressed as outcome criteria. Did the patient meet those objectives and outcome criteria? If he did, he has learned the material, and modified his behavior accordingly. If not, then the situation needs to be reassessed, the nursing plan rewritten, and the new plan needs to be implemented and reevaluated.

Evaluation also serves to redirect or refocus nursing actions. If the patient has learned some of the material, the nurse can go back to the assessment phase and begin the process again.

There are a variety of ways to evaluate learning. The one that we are most familiar with is the **test**. A test can be written (essay, short answer, multiple choice) or oral. We also can observe the behaviors that the patient has learned. This is especially true when evaluating psychomotor skills. One way is to use check lists that test the necessary behaviors. The patient gets a score that is compared with a predetermined acceptable pass or fail rate.

Evaluation is a continuous process. Because someone can repeat a list today does not mean that he will be able to do it tomorrow or in a week, so we must constantly and consistently monitor the patient's learning. By using a formal teaching plan and proceeding through the evaluation phase, the nurse refocuses her nursing interventions and the patient's learning.

SUMMARY

Teaching is a primary role of the nurse and has been recognized as such for over a hundred years. The nurse's role in teaching is to assist patients to get well and to stay well.

In order to comprehend the teaching-learning process, nurses need to know how and why people learn. Many leaders from the fields of philosophy, education, and psychology have developed theories relating to this. By knowing the writing of several theorists, the nurse can determine her own theory of teaching and develop specif-

ic teaching methods based on it.

There are three domains of learning. These are the cognitive, the affective, and the psychomotor domains. The cognitive domain refers to sorting and storing information in the brain for future use. The affective domain encompasses attitudes, values, and emotions. Culture, religion, and beliefs about life belong to this domain. Ethical issues are raised when one attempts to change another person's value system. The psychomotor domain involves the learning of skills.

Learning ability and learning needs change throughout life. Learning needs are different at all levels of development.

Many factors influence the learning process, and these can be grouped into barriers and facilitators. Barriers impede learning and include previous negative educational experiences, poor psychological and physical state, values, family support systems (that are either maladaptive, nonexistent, or different from the nurse's), poor past experiences with the health care system, and an environment not conducive to learning. Facilitators to learning enhance the ability to learn and include adequate education and positive experiences with the health care system, adaptive psychological and physical states, strong family support, congruent values, and an environment conducive to learning. Both facilitators and barriers to learning need to be assessed by the nurse in order to formulate a comprehensive teaching plan.

Most nurses must learn how to teach their patients. Teaching is an art, and before nurses can begin to teach, must reflect on their philosophy of man, the role that environment plays in the learning situation, who fails when the patient does not learn, and what is the best method of teaching. Once this has been accomplished, the nurse and others on the health care team determine what is to be taught and who will teach it. Realistic mutual goals and objectives to guide and direct the teaching plan are written in behavioral terms with the expected outcome of the teaching experience stated so that changes in behavior that indicate learning can be observed by the nurse. Teaching methods and content vary depending on the age of the person being taught. Simple explanations are best for children. Explanations should increase in complexity as the age of the person increases.

Methods of teaching also vary and are determined from the objectives. Methods used also depend upon location of the teaching, the type of recipient (individual or group), the resources available, and the type of material to be presented (facts, values, or skills).

In the role as teacher, the nurse uses a variety of teaching aids, including films, reading material, filmstrips, and programmed instruction. These are very valuable, in that they add another dimension to the patient's learning experience.

The nursing process can be used as a model for patient teaching. Learning needs and personal characteristics of the patient are assessed, the material and method planned, a teaching plan written, the plan implemented, and then evaluated from the objectives on the teaching plan.

It is through careful assessment and use of the teaching process that the nurse can be an effective change agent and help patients attain their highest levels of wellness.

STUDY QUESTIONS

1. Why is it important to know learning theory?

2. What are the three domains of learning? Give an example of each.

3. Devise a teaching plan for a diabetic child. Compare this plan to an adult teaching plan.

4. List several barriers to learning. Give examples of how nursing actions can change them.

5. Write three behavioral objectives for an obese patient with heart disease.

6. List four teaching methods and give an example of what could be taught by each method.

7. Why is using more than one teaching method beneficial to patient learning?

8. Give examples of teaching aids. How could they be used in patient teaching?

9. What is a teaching plan? Why is it necessary?

REFERENCES

1. American Nurses' Association. **Standards of Nursing Practice.** (Kansas City: The American Nurses Association) 1973.
2. American Hospital Association. **A Patient's Bill of Rights** (Chicago: The American Hospital Association). 1972.
3. E. Lee and J. L. Garvey. "How is Inpatient Education Being Managed?" **Hospitals,** 51(1977), p.75–82.
4. Barbara Klug Redman. **The Process of Patient Teaching.** 3rd Ed. (St. Louis: The C. V. Mosby Co., 1976) p.9.
5. P. Jones and W. Oertel. "Developing Patient Teaching Objectives and Techniques: A Self-Instructional Program." **Nurse Educator,** 2 (1977).
6. Aristotle. "The Golden Mean," in **Classics in Education.** Baskin, W. (Ed) (New York: Philosophical Library Inc.) 1966.

7. Virginia C. Conley. **Curriculum and Instruction in Nursing**. (Boston: Little, Brown and Company, 1973). p.191.
8. C. H. Patterson. **Foundations for a Theory of Instruction and Educational Psychology**. (New York: Harper & Row, Publishers, 1977) p.188.
9. Patterson. **Theory of Instruction**, p.189–190.
10. Conley. **Curriculum and Instruction**, p.194–196.
11. B. J. Skinner. "The Science of Learning and the Art of Teaching." **Harvard Educational Review, 24**(1954), p.86–97.
12. J. S. Bruner. "Notes on a Theory of Instruction," in P. E. Johnson (Ed) **Learning: Theory and Practice** (New York: Thomas Y. Crowell Company, 1971) p.339–363.
13. Robert M. Gagné. **The Conditions of Learning**. (3rd Ed) (New York: Holt, Rinehart, and Winston, 1977).
14. Benjamin S. Bloom et al. **Taxonomy of Educational Objectives: the Classification of Educational Goals. Handbook I. Cognitive Domain**. (New York: David McKay, Company, Inc. 1959).
15. David R. Krathwohl, Benjamin S. Bloom, and Bertram B. Masia. **Taxonomy of Educational Objectives. The Classification of Educational Goals. Handbook II: Affective Domain**. (New York: David McKay Company, Inc. 1956).
16. William D. Rohwer, Jr., Paul R. Ammon, and Phebe Cramer. **Understanding Intellectual Development**. (Hinsdale, Illinois: The Dryden Press, 1974) p.2.
17. Redman. **Patient Teaching**. p.59.
18. Redman. **Patient Teaching**. p.59.
19. Redman. **Patient Teaching**. p.59.
20. Baccalaureate Curriculum Subcommittee. **CUA—Systems Adaptation Model**. (Washington, D.C.: The School of Nursing, Catholic University of America, 1978). Unpublished.
21. Robert F. Mager. **Preparing Instructional Objectives**. (Belmont, Ca: Lear, Siegler, Inc., 1962) p.3.
22. Mager. **Instructional Objectives**. p.11.
23. Conley. **Curriculum and Instruction**. p.224.
24. Madeline Petrillo and Sergay Sanger. **Emotional Care of Hospitalized Children. An Environmental Approach**. 2nd Ed. (Philadelphia: J. B. Lippincott, 1980). p.159.
25. Voncile M. Smith and Thelma A. Bass. **Communication for Health Professionals**. (Phila: The J. B. Lippincott Co. 1979). p.111.
26. Helen Yura and Mary Walsh. **The Nursing Process**. 3rd Ed. (New York: Appleton-Century-Crofts, 1978). p.158.

ANNOTATED BIBLIOGRAPHY

Cohen NH: **Three Steps to Better Patient Teaching.** Nurs 80 72–74;1980. This article discusses the need for accurate assessment of the patient's learning needs, resources available, and the content to be taught. It also includes a brief assessment tool of patient learning needs.

Cosper B: **How Well Do Patients Understand Hospital Jargon?** Am J Nurs 77:1932–1934;1977. This brief research study describes how patients can be overwhelmed by medical language and offers some advice to avoid pitfalls.

Kratzer JB: **What Does Your Patient Need to Know?** Nurs 77 7:82–84; 1977. This article discusses use of a teaching plan to direct teaching and provides an example of a patient teaching plan.

Haferkorn V: **Assessing Individual Learning Needs as a Basis for Patient Teaching.** Nurs Clin North Am 199–209; 1971. Use of the nursing process for teaching is the crux of this article, which provides an excellent assessment tool.

Jones P, Oertel W: **Developing Patient Teaching Objectives and Techniques: A Self-Instructional Program.** Nurs Educator 2; 1977. This programmed instruction stresses the importance of writing learning objectives to direct teaching. It provides space for the reader to write objectives and provides answers to help clarify problems.

Murray R, Zentner J: **Guideline for More Effective Health Teaching.** Nurs 76 6:44–53; 1976. This excellent article provides a down-to-earth format for effective teaching.

Smith D: **Writing Objectives as a Nursing Practice Skill.** Am J Nurs 71:319–320;1971. This classic article concisely discusses writing objectives that can be measured in terms of changes in patient behaviors.

13

Change Theory

Janet-Beth Flynn

CHAPTER OUTLINE

OBJECTIVES

Upon completion of this chapter, the reader should be able to:

- Define change
- Identify the three stages in the change process described by Lewin
- Compare and contrast barriers and facilitators of change
- Discuss the role of the nurse as a change agent.

GLOSSARY

Active change—change that is planned and directed.

Barriers—obstacles that block change.

Change—an alteration in behavior.

Change agent—a person who effects change through intentional intervention.

Change theory—a framework for organizing change.

Covert change—change that occurs without an individual's knowledge.

Evolutionary change—a slow change over time.

Facilitators—enhancers that support change.

Overt change—change that occurs within a person's awareness.

Passive change—unplanned change that occurs as time passes.

Planned change—a change that is approached systematically.

Revolutionary change—a rapid and drastic change.

Targets for change—individuals, families, groups, or subsystems within the community who have health behaviors that are not good practice.

INTRODUCTION

Throughout life, man grows, develops, and adapts. This process is known as **change.** Change is a natural part of our lives and is necessary to maintain personal equilibrium, which occurs in response to an upset in previous behavior patterns. Change occurs daily on all levels—from the cellular level, organ level, organ system, patient system—to the more complex family, social system, and environmental systems. Change, a dynamic process, can be subtle and continuous, like growth and development, and occur without noticeable changes in behavior. Or change can be cataclysmic, occurring overnight. Without the ability to change, man would be unable to adapt to change.

Teaching a patient about a disease process or bodily change provides the patient with an opportunity to change. Learning, by its definition, indicates an observable change of behavior.

In a role as teacher, nurses assume the role of **change agent.** A change agent is a person who affects the change process through intentional intervention. In this role, the nurse initiates planned change. **Planned change** is change that is not accidental, but is systematically assessed and carefully implemented. Planned change has goals and objectives to guide it.

Welch states, "The ability to identify and carry out planned changes is an integral part of the role of the professional nurse."[1] In order for nurses to engage in the process of change, they must have the knowledge base and the skills necessary to bring about change. According to Olson, nurses should be guided by a framework for effecting the change process.[2]

One framework for planned change was formulated by Kurt Lewin[3] and is known as change theory. **Change theory** describes the process of change and identifies six components of change. The first is recognition of the area where the change is needed. The second component involves a careful assessment of the situation in order to learn what is operating to maintain a status quo (barriers) and what is operating to change the situation (facilitators). A third component is identification of the methods to be used in order to produce change, and a fourth is the planning of the change. A fifth involves what the person's culture identifies as a method of change, and the final component is the process of change itself.

These six components cause three distinct stages in the change process—the stage of unfreezing, the stage of moving, and the stage of refreezing. In the unfreezing phase of the change, the discovery that change is needed is made, and the individual is motivated to change. The second stage, moving, is the change itself. The third stage is that of refreezing, in which the new changes are incorporated into the person's behavior and are stabilized.

Lewin advanced another theory about change that includes the idea that opposing forces facilitate the change process or impede it. It is important to identify these forces in order to activate the process of change.

Since the change process is dynamic, it is important to keep in mind that none of the stages or steps in the change process are rigid. There will be flow between the steps and there is no way to determine how much time will be spent in each step. The change process may move quickly through some steps, only to stop in another phase. Nurses must use all of their skills to keep the process moving to a positive outcome.

The target for change can be an individual, a family, a group, or a subsystem of the community with real or potential health problems.

Change is an important concept for nurses to understand so that they can serve as change agents when working with patients, families, or groups. In identifying the steps in the process of change, the nurse can incorporate them within the four steps of the nursing process.

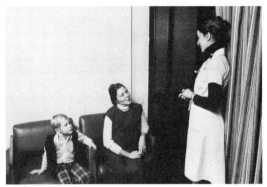

Figure 13-1. In the role of change agent, the nurse works with individuals, families, and groups.

TYPES OF CHANGE

There are several types of change with which the nurse comes into contact. **Evolutionary change** is characterized by gradual change. Examples of this type of change might include becoming parents or gradually becoming crippled due to rheumatoid arthritis. This process is slow and does not require rapid adaptation or shift in personal goals. Because it is gradual and gives the person an opportunity to adapt, it is a less threatening form of change.

Another form of change is **revolutionary change,** which is more rapid and drastic and may upset the equilibrium of the individual. There is a need here to alter life goals and perhaps even redesign patterns of behavior in order to cope and successfully adapt. Individuals experiencing this type of change generally have little or no warning or time to prepare. This type of change is very threatening and causes people to use high levels of energy. Defense mechanisms are often necessary to cope, and the result may be a crisis state. Some examples of revolutionary change include: loss of a limb, loss of a loved one, loss of vision (see Chapter 22), heart attack, stroke, and accidents.

Covert change is change that is constant and often occurs without the person being aware of it. Aculturation is a good example of covert change. **Overt change** is within the person's awareness. This type of change is generally revolutionary, and individuals may react with feelings of anxiety and apprehension. These are related to the individual's feeling of autonomy, since it may involve an involuntary change in behavior without regard for his feelings, needs, and desires.

Passive change occurs with the passage of time. It is like evolutionary change but generally is not planned; it just happens. **Active change,** on the other hand, is planned, and goal directed.

Facilitators of Change

Facilitators of change are things that increase the chance of change and enhance it. Facilitators of change are much like facilitators to learning and depend on a combination of the following behaviors on the part of the patient:

- Desire for change on the part of the patient
- Motivation to change behavior patterns
- Positive past experience with change
- Change not perceived as a threat
- Trust in the nurse as a change agent
- Clear communication systems with the nurse and others on the health care team
- Goals that are congruent with the health care system's goals
- Ability to compromise in order to attain the above goals and to accept change
- Family support and identity group support and acceptance
- Ability to use the health care system and other resources available

- Dedication to the change.

Facilitators are extremely useful tools to use when implementing planned change. They should be carefully assessed and incorporated into the change process.

Barriers to Change

Barriers to change are factors that block effective change and can increase an individual's resistance to change. Barriers to change can be adaptive at times, and should be carefully assessed. For example, it can be important for patients to deny health state changes for short periods of time. Barriers can lead to poor decision-making and problem solving skills in the patient's repertoire of behavior. A clear assessment of these behaviors can lead the nurse to methods of correcting them. Barriers to change include:

- Desire to maintain the status quo
- Satisfaction with things as they are
- Threat of the change
- Overacceptance of the sick role
- Lack of motivation for change
- Perception of change as a threat to the self
- Perception of change as a threat to the family or group
- Negative past experiences with change
- Lack of trust in the health care system
- Poor communication skills
- Goals that are not congruent with those of the health care system or the nurse
- Unrealistic goals
- Traditions, attitudes, values, and culture that are not congruent with the health care system
- Inability to compromise
- Lack of family support for the change

- Lack of cultural group support for the change
- Focusing on one point of the situation instead of seeing the whole picture
- Lack of understanding of what is needed in order to change
- Lack of ability to use health care resources
- Lack of dedication to the change
- Fear of failure
- Expense of the change.

THE NURSING PROCESS

Nurses act as change agents in almost all interactions with patients. The nurse's fundamental role is to recognize that a change is occurring or not occurring. It is the nurse's responsibility to assess and gather data on barriers and facilitators and plan the methods of change. Change should be planned in a nonjudgmental way, taking the patient's needs, wants, and values into consideration. Sensitivity to how much and what can be changed and not changed is a valuable asset to any nurse.

Assessment

The initial assessment will provide the data needed to determine what changes are necessary for the patient to adapt. In order to do this, the nurse must establish a trusting nurse/patient relationship based on a system of open communication. The nurse needs to assess her own abilities and values. Many times, a proposed change might be unrealistic for the patient. For example, a patient who has smoked two packs of cigarettes a day for 30 years may be unwilling to stop smoking completely. The nurse should realize that she wants the patient to stop smoking and establish a workable plan for the patient such as decreasing the number of cigarettes smoked

until the desired number is reached.

Many times a patient's beliefs and behaviors cannot be changed, for example, a religous belief about not receiving blood transfusions or taking certain medications. Trying to change behaviors that cannot be changed is frustrating for both the patient and the nurse, and may destroy the nurse/patient relationship. Sometimes one change in a patient's system leads to another. Occasionally behavior assessed as unchangeable may begin to change as a

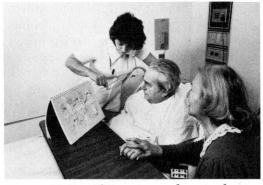

Figure 13-2.   The nurse works as a change agent in many nurse/patient interactions.

result. Change is viewed by many as a threat, but by making a small unthreatening change, other changes may follow.

The nurse also should determine the ethical issues involved in the change process. Does the nurse believe that the change is in the patient's best interest? Is she committed to assist the patient change his behavior? (For a discussion of ethics see Chapter 12).

The health state of the patient must be assessed. In order to change his behavior, the patient must be physically able to commit himself to the change.

Barriers and facilitators to change need to be carefully assessed and incorporated into the health care plan. Change cannot be instituted or supported without knowledge of these aspects of the patient's situation. It is important to assess facilitators of change, so that they can be supported and built upon. It is equally important to assess barriers to change, so that they can be modified or eliminated, or at least identified.

Most problems have more than one cause, therefore as many factors as possible should be assessed. For example, Mr. J.B., a 56-year-old man with congestive heart disease, and chronic bronchitis, had numerous problems. He was intellectually slow and could not read. His income was well below the poverty level because he was disabled, and it was difficult for him to work to supplement his disability income. He lived in one room on the first floor of an unairconditioned building and served as the doorman. He kept his room spotlessly clean and prided himself on his ability to cook on his one burner electric stove. He washed his dishes in a pan of water carried from the bathroom down the hall. He rotated shifts, and on his off hours, he washed and waxed cars at the corner gas station for extra money. In the summer, all of his activity aggravated his symptoms, causing him to be hospitalized repeatedly. He did not want to be sick and took all of his medicines faithfully. The following facilitators were assessed: a desire for change, motivation, trust in the nurse; clear communication; ability to compromise; ability to use the health care system (but in a limited way); and dedication to a change. The barriers included: desire for status quo; unrealistic goals, habits, values, and culture; lack of family and group support; focusing on one part of the problem; and lack of understanding of the need for change.

The nurse assessed areas for change that were then discussed with Mr. B. and established a mutual nurse/patient relationship. This initiated the unfreezing phase. The type of change was active and overt. On the next visit, one week later, Mr. B. had a fan, which a neighbor had given him. He was working the day shift but he was still waxing cars, because he needed the money. Fi-

nally, a compromise was reached. Mr. B. would rest with the fan on during the day, between calls at the door. He would continue with his medications, and he would wax the cars in the early evening when it got cooler. In this way, his old behaviors could be maintained but slightly altered, and the patient continued to trust the nurse. The nurse was able to alter her plan to enable Mr. B. to continue what he was doing in a more healthful way.

The degree to which the nurse initiates change depends upon the patient's present state of wellness and adaptation, his understanding of his disease and the change process, his ability and desire to change, the resources available, and the nurse's knowledge and ability to implement planned change. At the conclusion of the assessment phase of the nursing process, the nursing diagnoses are formulated. Examples of nursing diagnoses regarding change might include:

- barriers to change related to cultural expectations
- facilitators to change related to desire to get well.

Planning

Planned change needs to be directed by written goals and objectives that identify how the change will occur. Objectives need to be written and stated in terms of observable behavior. They should state a reasonable amount of time for the change to occur. Objectives should be discussed and agreement should be reached by the nurse and the patient.

Strategies for change must include the person and his family, friends, or group. Level of growth and development and level of knowledge are two other factors to keep in mind when planning change. Motivation and the patient's physical ability also need to be considered when planning change, too. All of these factors must be included in the change plan if it is to succeed.

In the example of Mr. B., the appropriate strategies were incorporated in the plan. He did not have close family ties, but he did have neighbors who provided emotional support and aid. Also, since he could not read, alternative methods had to be planned for him in order for him to keep clinic appointments and take medications.

At this stage, the problems needing change have been identified and the methods for change selected. This is the beginning of the "moving" stage described by Lewin.

Implementation

Once the change has been planned, the next step is to implement the plan. Lewin's stage of moving continues throughout the implementation phase of the nursing process. Frequent feedback and open lines of communication between the patient and nurse are essential. Depending on the type of change involved, implementation may be short and relatively easy to accomplish or painfully slow and difficult. As in the latter case, a great deal of patience on the part of the nurse and client is often necessary and emotional support given by the nurse can make the difference between success and failure. At the conclusion of the implementation phase, the patient's new behaviors should be stabilized and refrozen.

Evaluation

"Evaluation involves measuring behavior and interpreting the results in terms of desired behavior change."[4] Evaluation is always considered in terms of how the patient met the written objectives in the care plan. If the patient met the objectives, further changes in behavior may not be needed. If the patient did not meet the objec-

tives, a reassessment of the situation is needed, followed by plan revision and implementation.

The change process enables the nurse to help individuls or groups to change and therefore to adapt positively.

Olsen writes that:

> inaction and frustration are inevitable during the change. In order to meet the realities of the situation, persistence and flexibility are essential attributes for the nurse change agent. She must be realistic about what she can accomplish. Persistence is essential, for if the identified change fails, she must try again.[5]

Planned change is an integral part of the nurse's role. The ability to assess the need for change is essential for promoting positive adaptation.

SUMMARY

Change is a natural part of our lives, and it is necessary for humans to adapt in a dynamic environment. The nurse, in her role as a change agent, is able to bring about planned change by careful use of the nursing process.

In order for nurses to implement planned change, they should be guided by a theoretical framework for the change process. One framework formulated by Lewin divides the change process into three distinct stages: the unfreezing stage, the moving stage, and the refreezing stage. Lewin also proposes that there are opposing forces at work that facilitate or impede the process of change.

The target of a planned change can be an individual, a family, a group, or a subsystem of the community. The change target may have real or potential problems.

Change can occur in several ways. Evolutionary change is change that evolves slowly and allows adaptation. Revolutionary change is rapid, drastic, and does not allow for adaptation. Covert change occurs without the individual's awareness of the change, and overt change occurs within an individual's awareness. Change also can be passive or active.

Many things affect change. Things that increase the chance of change are called facilitators, and things that slow or impede change are called barriers.

Most problems with which the nurse comes into contact have more than one cause, so by careful use of the nursing process, the nurse can act as an agent of planned change.

STUDY QUESTIONS

1. How has your life changed since entering school?

2. Identify some barriers to change in your life.

3. Identify some facilitators of change in your present life.

4. How could you act as a change agent on your campus or community?

REFERENCES

1. L. B. Welch. "Planned Change in Nursing: The Theory." **The Nursing Clinics of North America, 14** (1979), 307–321.
2. E. M. Olson. "Strategies and Techniques for the Nurse Change Agent." **The Nursing Clinics of North America, 14** (1979), 323–336.
3. K. Lewin. "Quasi-Stationary Social Equalibria and the Problem of Permanent Change." W. G. Bennes, K. D. Benne, and R. Chain (eds.). **The Planning of Change** (New York: Holt, Rinehart, and Winston, 1962).
4. Barbara K. Redman. **The Process of Patient Teaching in Nursing.** 3rd ed. (St. Louis: The C. V. Mosby Co., 1976), p.183.
5. Olson. "Strategies and Techniques". **Nursing Clinics.** p.324.

ANNOTATED BIBLIOGRAPHY

Dean LP: **The Change from Functional to Primary Nursing.** Nurs Clin North Am 14:2:357–364; June 1979. This article discusses use of an outside consultant to make changes on an established dialysis unit.

Olson EM: **Strategies and Techniques for the Nurse Change Agent.** Nurs Clin North Am 14:2:323–336; June 1979. This article discusses the role of the change agent and suggests potential strategies for implementing the change process. Three frameworks for change are presented.

Reynolds BC: **The Nurse as a Change Agent.** Occup Health Nurs 28:19–21;1980. This brief article discusses the concept of change and the nurse's role as a change agent.

Welch LB: **Planned Change in Nursing: The Theory.** Nurs Clin North AM 14:2:307–321;June 1979. This article describes the process of change and discusses a variety of change theories.

Section 3

Concepts Related to the Care of Individuals

This section discusses selected concepts as related to individuals. They are broad in scope and were selected because they are concepts that affect a great many patients of all ages, in any health care setting. In most instances nurses relate to these concepts every day and their nursing practice can be greatly enhanced by the understanding of basic principles and applications of each.

Chapters in this section begin with the theoretical discussion of how individuals develop into persons and how they develop concepts of themselves as individuals.

Subsequent chapters in this section introduce the reader to other concepts that may have an impact on the lives of patients and in some instances, the lives of other family members.

The chapters included in this section build on the concepts introduced in the previous sections. Each of these chapters reviews the theoretical basis for the concept and then discusses the relevance of the concept to nursing. A nursing approach is used throughout these chapters, with patient examples, when appropriate.

14

Theories of Personhood

Mary Ann Schroeder

CHAPTER OUTLINE

OBJECTIVES

After completion of this chapter, the reader will be able to:

- List the different theories regarding personality.
- Compare and contrast each of the major theories.
- Describe the role that events in history, philosophy, science, and changes in society have had on the development of the individual.
- Describe the ongoing process of personhood throughout the life of the individual.
- Discuss the application of two theories of personality to each component of the nursing process.

GLOSSARY

Accommodation—part of the mediating process that seeks to change input.

Anxiety—feeling that can range from extreme discomfort to being ill at ease.

Avoidance—mechanism or process in which situations are seen as undesirable, and the person withdraws or moves away from the situation.

Complexes—set of associated ideas or feelings that motivates certain ways of interacting.

Congruence—state of harmony or consistency between what is said and what is meant.

Conscious—state of mind wherein readily available awareness or information exists.

Drives—underlying forces that propel a person toward a course of action; the source of dynamics of thinking, feeling, and behaving.

Ego—mediator between the id and superego; the part of the mind that has contact with reality.

Extroversion—the interest of the individual is directed outward, such as in seeking satisfaction in external ways.

Id—animal instincts, innate desires.

Introversion—the individual seeks satisfaction from his inner life, and his interest is directed inward.

Narcissism—self-love.

Self-disclosure—technique in which people share honest thoughts and feelings.

Stimulus-response—the stimulus is something that triggers a reaction; the response is that reaction.

Superego—the conscious; the way society has instructed the individual to behave.

Unconscious—state of mind when material is or has been pushed out of awareness.

INTRODUCTION

Personality and the more comprehensive concept of personhood involve the study and integration of numerous characteristics and theories. Over the years, people have been interested in such things as why people behave as they do, whether individuals can be described in terms of characteristic traits, what the relationships are between growth, development, and personality, and how we can predict the outcomes of various kinds of personality behaviors.

Theories and ideas that shed light on these kinds of questions are of great value to professional nurses. Because of the nature of the nursing process and the fact that nurses work most frequently on a one-to-one basis with people, they rely heavily on individual assessment skills and effective communication. Without a basic working knowledge of the processes of personality development and the relationship between personality and behavior, there is a great danger for faulty assessments to be made and communication to be ineffective. Appropriate planning for nursing care also can be highly dependent on personality factors.

This chapter presents material about personality theories from the social sciences, primarily psychology, and other closely allied fields. It is important to note that these theories, ideas, and concepts tend to overlap. A primary reason for this is that later theories are based, to a great extent, on earlier ones. Also, in the general literature, there are varying opinions about the relative importance and validity of selected theories.

This chapter provides basic definitions and descriptions of selected major theories of personality and personhood, and gives specific examples on how the associated concepts can be applied to nursing actions. An additional aim of this chapter is to stimulate further interest in those ideas or concepts that seem particularly useful to the reader working with patients in the clinical setting. Each subject area can be explored in greater detail, as there has been much work and research done on all of these theories. Besides gaining a better understanding of the people nurses care for, a knowledge base of personhood can foster a greater understanding of the self and the dynamics of interpersonal relationships; both are important aspects in the preparation of professional nurses.

PERSONALITY

There are many theories regarding personality and, consequently, personality has been defined in many different ways. The dictionary states that personality is the quality of being a person rather than an abstraction, thing, or lower being. Personality is not an isolated state but involves the relationship of the individual to the society. This relationship is influenced by a complex set of characteristics (such as traits, habits, attitudes, and patterns) that, in some manner, distinguishes a particular individual from others.

Allport, in a definition that is almost half a century old yet seems fresh and up-to-date, states that "personality is the dynamic organization within the individual of those psychophysical systems that determine his unique adjustments to his en-

vironment."[1] There are several key thoughts in Allport's definition that seem especially relevant to understanding most theories of personality. The first idea is the use of the word dynamic, which indicates change and movement. Dynamic also means energy. It is the opposite of static, to stand still or not to move forward. Static is passive, while dynamic denotes action. Another concept important to Allport's definition is the word organization. Organization conveys a feeling of putting in order to make up a whole. It also means a method or model on which to look totally or as a complete overview. Organization, in this sense, is the opposite of being haphazard. The concept of systems, as expressed by Allport, connotes homeostasis and equilibrium. The various systems' balance or lack of balance is related. If there are problems in a system, the whole organism is influenced. The term unique, also part of Allport's definition, emphasizes that personality is primarily a product of an individual experience, rather than the perspective of society collectively. Finally, the word adjustment involves adaptation, development, and movement toward change. It indicates an attempt by the individual to bring things into harmony by altering positions for a more satisfactory condition.

Personality is the sum of the parts of an individual, plus an evolving pattern of relating to the world. It is an ongoing adjustment that is influenced by the society, the person's past, present, and aspirations for the future. It is a way to describe the essence of a person.

PERSONHOOD

How does the concept of personhood differ from that of personality? Once again, turning to the dictionary there are six distinct meanings of the word personality. But the term personhood is not specifically cited. Therefore, to define personhood, we must break up the word. You already have some idea of what a person is. So it is the suffix "hood" that needs further explanation. According to Webster, hood means "an instance of specific state, condition, quality, rank, character. . . ."

A theory of personhood is mingled with the philosophy of the nature of human beings. It is important to note that the spirit of the time and the view of life truly influences how the essence of the nature of a person is defined. For instance, in societies that believe people are basically good, an individual's worth is viewed quite differently than in a culture where persons are seen as inherently evil and sinful. So, too, if the major belief of society is that people have free will to choose their fate, then an individual is seen differently from individuals who reside in a culture that sees human beings as being predestined. Whatever is the predominate belief system is reflected in how the nature of humanity is defined. Most likely there will be a great correlation between a definition of the nature of human beings and the view of the person.

The current use of the term personhood conveys a spirit of dignity. People are felt to have worth. To support this position, think about what terms are linked to the suffix "hood"—knighthood, motherhood, priesthood, and maidenhood all express a rather noble view of the state of being a knight, priest, mother, or maiden.

If individuals are thought to be worthy of respect, then it follows that their desires and wishes should be considered. One modern nursing theory that capitalizes on dignity is the theory of self-care as advocated by Orem.[2] A basic tenet of self-care is that people should have control over their own health. This means a nontraditional role for health care professionals. It emphasizes that goals should be mutually agreed upon, and that planning is jointly considered. People with health needs come to health care providers, and together they negotiate care plans and health strategies.

When people indicate needs, these must not be discounted, but rather, should be fully explored.

Personhood is a positive view of individuals, as people worthy of respect and dignity. The person is seen as having strengths and positive attributes that influence decisions about courses of action.

BENEFITS OF LEARNING ABOUT THEORIES OF PERSONHOOD

Why should nurses learn about various theories of personality and personhood? Nursing is a practice discipline that bases its actions on a body of knowledge. The body of knowledge regarding individuals and how they relate to others is especially important in the areas of mental health, community health, rehabilitation, and normal growth and development. It follows that if these theories are important in health and wellness, they are also important in attempting to understand disease, illness, and psychopathology. This chapter presents a multitude of theories. These theories can help to provide a better understanding of the dynamics of human behavior. They give clues to why individuals in given situations behave in a specific manner.

Along with understanding the whys of human behavior, personality theories also afford understanding about how individuals think and feel about their existence. Theories can help the nurse choose a certain course of action rather than another, based on the patient's developmental stage. Knowledge of stages of growth and maturity give the nurse a basis for anticipating future needs that a patient may have, as well as awareness that certain problems may occur at a given stage. Theories also provide an ideal of what the person might strive for in life goals.

One other point is that new theories are

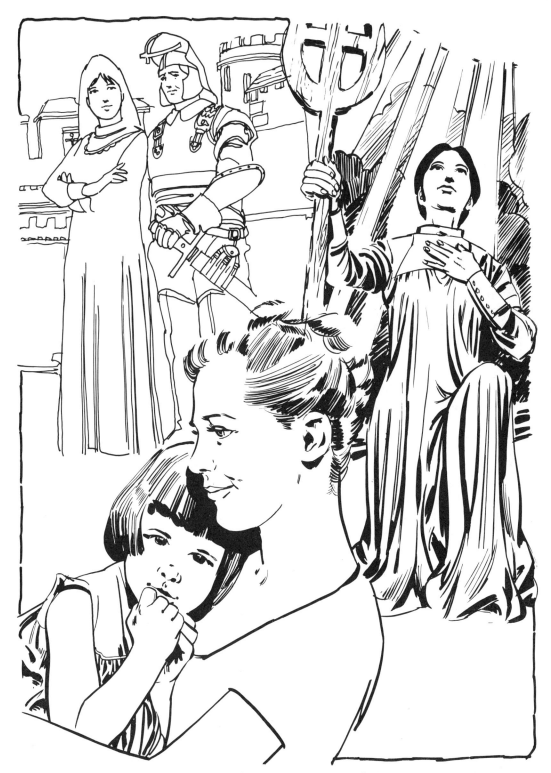

Figure 14-1.   The Term Personhood Conveys a Spirit of Dignity.

being generated continually as practitioners, theorists, and philosophers attempt to organize what they have observed in a logical fashion. A theory can provide a framework in which to conduct nursing practice.

SELECTED THEORIES OF PERSONHOOD

Theories regarding personality began early in the history of civilization. The theories were an attempt to make sense of or explain observations. Hall suggests that the early theories were generated as offspring of philosophy, and that philosophers such as Plato, Aristotle, Kierkegaard, and Locke had their own ideas of what constituted personhood.[3] According to Allport, from 400 B.C. to the 1600s, the unit of analysis for the majority of scientific material in all branches of inquiry was the Humors Theory.[4] This theory categorized all phenomena according to the elements of earth, air, fire, and water. The elements then were subdivided into specific parts.

For example, if a person demonstrated a predominant mood of sadness or melancholy, it was thought that that person was under the control of "blue bile," one of the established humors. Allport goes on to state that this theory was not seriously challenged until Darwin's work, when a theory of instincts and drives emerged. Hall further traces the development of scientific thinking as becoming more involved with the experimental method, which Pavlov perfected. This experimental method related to personality, because ideas of motivation and situational variables came forth. At this time, case studies of individuals also enhanced the knowledge bases.

Some theories were born, disproved, and discarded. For instance, some theories, even though they sounded reasonable, did not stand up to scientific scrutiny. Specifically during the 1940s and 1950s, William Sheldon's theory of somatotyping was very popular in attempting to explain personality makeup, based on a person's body type. Categories included the endomorph (short, fat build), the ectomorph (tall, thin physique), and mesomorph (muscular, well proportioned). Specific personality traits such as orderliness, self-sufficiency, and cooperativeness then were postulated as being associated with each body type.[5]

The four categories presented here for consideration—psychoanalytic, interpersonal, existential-humanistic, and learning—are still considered as either valid or potentially useful. In other words, even though these theories originated in the early half of the century, there are still people who find them useful in analyzing and explaining human behavior.

Psychoanalytic Theory

Psychoanalytic theory had its beginning in the work of Sigmund Freud, an Austrian neurologist, who produced much of his work in the early decades of the 20th century. Freud based his theory on his clinical practice. He worked with people suffering from mental disorders and published many papers about his theory. He also founded the Vienna Psychoanalytic Society, which was an important force in developing this theory.[6] Many clinicians and theorists joined Freud both physically and intellectually. Another school of thought, the neo-Freudians, broke off from the Vienna Society, acknowledging that the early work done by Freud had influenced their thinking. Even today, both Freudian and neo-Freudian analysis are used in treatment.

Basic to psychoanalytic theory are the concepts of the **conscious** and **unconscious**. Consciousness is the state of the mind wherein readily available awareness of information exists. Unconsciousness is the state in which material has been pushed out of the sphere of awareness. Generally, conscious material is not anxiety provoking, while unconscious material is emotionally charged and more likely to provoke anxiety. For this reason, it often is hidden from conscious awareness in order for the individual to be comfortable. Much has been written about the mental mechanisms that operate to help push material into the unconscious. These mechanisms, such as suppression, repression, sublimation, denial, rationalization, and numerous others, are discussed thoroughly in Chapter 20. The purpose of all these mechanisms is to reduce the discomfort of the individual.

Other concepts identified by Freud were the parts of the mind, in his structural theory. The mind is made of the **id, ego,** and **superego.**

Generally, the superego is considered the structure concerned with incorporation of parental and societal attitudes of right and wrong. It represents the values of the individual developed through the growing up process. The superego is the source of guilt feelings.

The ego has two major functions. It mediates between the id and the superego, and is the part of the mind in contact with reality. The id is involved with wants and desires. The superego is the person's conscience. The ego seeks to bring the id and superego into balance. It resolves conflict through compromise.

Bruno Bettleheim, in a more recent article, redefined these terms slightly differently than do most textbooks.[7] Bettleheim contends that the original translations of Freud from the German to English distorted Freud's true meaning. Bettleheim states that the best definition of id is that part of the personality that means "it," as in a force, such as "the it" that made the person do a certain action. The "it" is something in the individual, and the person does not know what, that pulls in a certain

direction. Bettleheim goes on to state that the ego is the "I," or the conscious, rational part of the person. He indicates that it is the ego in operation when a person says "I am trying to understand why I did this." The third concept is the superego, which literally means "overself." This part of the mind is created by the person as a response to inner needs and external pressure that, Bettleheim feels, have been internalized. In the successfully adjusted person, according to the psychoanalytic school, the I, it, and over-I are in balance, and the person is in control of his "self."

Stages of development are also important concepts from Freud's theory. The psychosexual stages of development are the oral, anal, oedipal, and genital. These are the four stages through which the normal individual passes. According to this school of thought, the stages become important if a person fixates at or regresses to an earlier stage. This aspect of the theory has given rise to a jargon of descriptive phrases that can be heard about patients. For example, it is not uncommon to hear someone described as an "anal personality." The anal personality frequently demonstrates traits of excessive cleanliness or frugality. For example, people who are perfectionists about housekeeping are sometimes called anal personalities. The stage of anal development is marked by the task of toilet training, which involves attempts by the parent to get the child to control bladder and bowels. This task involves learning to eliminate feces and urine in an appropriate place and generally pleases significant others. The individual, according to psychoanalytic theory, becomes aware of the power he has to make another individual either happy or frustrated by the control of bodily functions. This stage is seen when the individual becomes an active force in relationships, in contrast to the earlier oral stage, in which the individual has a much more passive role. The issue of control becomes important. The psychoanalytic theory frequently uses the premise that either the function or symptoms related to the function can be and frequently are symbolic rather than actual. For instance, the symptoms manifested in the anal personality are symbolic of the functions involved in toilet training, such as giving, withholding, cleaning, and disposing.

Carl Jung, a contemporary of Freud and a proponent of the psychoanalytic theory, focused on the two major orientations of personality—**extroversion** and **introversion.**[8] Extroversion is apparent when the interest of the individual is directed outward. The extrovert seeks satisfaction in external ways. Introversion is the opposite. Introverts seek satisfaction from their own inner life, and their interest is directed inward, rather than toward people and things. Rarely, if ever, is an individual totally one or the other. Another concept that Jung identified was **complexes.** Complexes were seen as energy systems. The person has a recurring idea that frequently drains energy from the conscious personality. Examples are superiority, inferiority, mother, or father complexes. These complexes have corresponding patterns of behavior that indicate the person's inner feelings about themselves.

Adler was another Austrian physician involved in the Freudian school. He was the first to break away from the Vienna Psychoanalytic Society, and went on to found his own analytic group.[9] **Holism** was one of Adler's major concepts. The idea of holism is that human beings must be viewed as a unit, not just a collection of parts. Adler was particularly interested in the instincts—basic motivating forces—that play a role in the decisions individuals make. He was especially intrigued when instincts seemed to be in opposition.

Two other concepts derived from psychoanalytic literature are **drives** and **narcissism.** Drives are the underlying forces that propel a person toward a course of action. Initially, the drives indentified by

Freud were seen quite specifically as either destructive or sexual drives. But drives can be seen as the source of dynamic thinking, feeling, and behaving.

Narcissism can best be described as self-love. Currently the concept is seen rather negatively, as someone who is self-centered and generally nonresponsive to the needs of others. Narcissism, however, is normal and expected at certain stages of life, especially in childhood. The baby, for example, is self-centered. Only when this concept is predominant in adult life is it pathological.

Many concepts have been identified by people associated with the psychoanalytic school of thought. Some of these concepts are no longer in vogue, while others have laid the groundwork for subsequent theories. The psychoanalytic theory was one of the earliest of the currently used models for understanding the nature of personhood. The people who advocated this method wrote extensively. The literature is rich with clinical examples. Perhaps the greatest contribution of this theory was that it was an organized effort at defining what motivated people.

Interpersonal Theory

Interpersonal theory was, to a large extent, based on the earlier works of the psychoanalytic school of thought. The major difference was in its focus. The psychoanalytic theory's thrust was on the intrapsychic life (the internal drives, strivings, and conflicts) of the individual. The focus of the interpersonal theory was that human beings, although certainly affected by the intrapsychic life, are mainly influenced by what happens in their relationships with others. This involves the ideas advanced by George H. Mead[10] and Eric Berne,[11] that people not only reflect their own perceptions of their worth, but also are products of how others view them.

Relationships with others mold an individual's personality, thought, feeling, and behavior. For example, if a mother sees her son as naughty, most likely that is the way the child will act. Who is to say whether the acting or the perception of naughtiness came first?

Harry Stack Sullivan, an early proponent of this school of thought, defined developmental tasks not very dissimilar from the psychosexual ones of the psychoanalytic school. The central focus of the interpersonal tasks was on the reciprocal nature of need expression and satisfaction.[12] Sullivan felt that infancy was a time when the individual learns the basic cultural patterns. As the child masters language, the finer but equally important points—cooperation and socialization—emerge. Sullivan emphasized that by adolescence, either a "well-behaved" citizen had developed, or the child had basic problems in his interpersonal relationships. These problems yielded a great deal of discomfort and dissatisfaction to both the individual and those who interacted with the individual.

Clarity of communication was seen by several theorists (including Berne and Virginia Satir) as one major objective in personality development. (For a more detailed explanation of this aspect, see Chapter 11.)

Carl Rogers, basically an existential-humanistic psychologist, but eclectic, identified the concept of **congruence,** especially in communication, as one of the laws of interpersonal theory.[13] Congruence is seen as the state of harmony between what is said and what is meant. In other words, what a person conveys is what he means. For example, if a person declares "I am happy," and yet his facial expression appears depressed and he demonstrates otherwise, one would say that there is incongruence—lack of harmony between words and expressions. Rogers speculated that the greater the congruence of experience and awareness to communication, the more mutually satisfying would be the resulting interpersonal experience. For in-

stance, the child learns the mother means business when she says "no" or learns that when the mother says "no" it may or may not mean no. Mixed messages with a lack of clarity lead to uncertainty. What is meant is open to speculation, as in the old song, "her lips say no, no; but there's yes, yes in her eyes." The implication of lack of congruence in personality development is that the child grows secure or insecure in message transmission. Clarity of communication promotes trust of others. If one cannot be certain what is being said, then he becomes wary or lacks trust.

Another variation on the theory of interpersonal relationships is that of the transactional model, developed by Berne to explain and explore interactions.[14] Berne looked at the inner individual quite like Freud had done in terms of the structure of the mind. But instead of calling these parts the id, ego, and superego, Berne called these aspects the child, the parent, and the adult. According to Berne, the child, which was analogous to the id, was seen as the part of the personality concerned with gratification of needs. Berne saw the child as rather short-sighted, primarily considering the now rather than looking to the future. The parent was in conflict with the child. The parent had incorporated the values of the society and reflected what is held in esteem by others. The adult, similar to Freud's ego, had as a major function the mediation between the child and parent, as well as helping the individual adjust to reality.

Berne focused on how the individual functioned in society or in interpersonal situations. One major difference between the Freudian orientation and Berne's is that Freud specialized in using his framework to analyze psychopathology, such as his work on neurosis. Berne, however, chose to explore his theory of personality development with a backdrop of social situations. These social situations were called games by Berne. In games, people took roles in acting out scripts. For example, many overweight people respond differently to refusing food than do thin people. The overweight individual may feel a need to explain why they aren't eating; the thin person says merely "no, thank you."

One major concept underlying interpersonal theory is that of **anxiety**. Anxiety can range from extreme discomfort to simply feeling ill at ease. The interpersonal theorist speculated that behavior is motivated by attempting to reduce anxiety, especially that which occurs because of difficulties in interpersonal interactions. Anxiety can be manifested by physical symptoms, such as sweaty palms or a fast pulse. It is an unpleasant, painful state. A little anxiety, say for instance about a forthcoming exam, causes the individual to spring into action, which is a positive aspect of anxiety. Huge amounts of anxiety, however, immobilize the individual and prevent him from functioning. You have heard of people so overwhelmed with anxiety that they cannot speak. It does not matter what the cause of the anxiety is—a threat is real or perceived. The basic task of people is to learn effective methods to handle anxiety so that life becomes more pleasurable.

Existential-Humanistic Theory

Ideas of existential philosophers, such as Martin Heidegger and Rollo May, merged with the efforts of humanistic psychologists, including Carl Rogers and Sidney Jourard. Existential-humanistic theory is quite different from either the psychoanalytic or interpersonal but they overlap. The major thrust of this theory is the holistic nature of human existence. Basic to all existential and humanistic theories is the belief that all human beings have potential for growth, and that it is up to the individual to decide and determine his fate. The goal of development is to achieve or move closer to potential, by means of "becoming." "Becoming" is a process rather than an outcome. The process consists of the individual attempting to liberate himself from the external world's view, and gaining insight into his own nature. There is an emphasis on freedom to choose and the responsibility of the individual to achieve his goals.

Inherent in this theory is the aim to help people live more authentically. To live authentically means to stop misrepresenting oneself to others. One concept important in becoming more authentic is **self-disclosure**. Self-disclosure is a technique in which people share honest thoughts and feelings rather than "shoulds," "musts," and "oughts."[15] Jourard maintained that the greater the level of human potential reached, the higher the level of wellness. Jourard also stated the corollary—the more unauthentic the person, the greater the disorganization, and therefore, a lower resistance to stress and illness would result.[16]

Rogers focused on such tasks as the dropping of facades, discovery of unknown elements in oneself, freeing oneself in the discovery process, and gaining trust and confidence in one's perception, especially in regard to choices and decisions.[17] Both Jourard and Rogers acknowledge the unending nature of the process of "becoming."

Abraham Maslow, focusing on motivational aspects of becoming a whole healthy person, brought forth a paradigm on the hierarchy of needs.[18] This hierarchy established an integrated, organized approach to consider human existence as related to needs. Maslow identified five broad categories of needs, starting with the basic ones of physiology and safety, and then moving to more sophisticated and advanced needs of belonging, esteem, and self-actualization.

The concepts inherent in the physiological needs were those of homeostasis and appetites. Examples of physiological needs are those for water, minerals, oxygen, food, an acid-base balance, and appropriate temperature. The need for safety brought concepts such as security, stability, protection, dependence, freedom from fear, anxiety, and chaos, and a need for structure, order, law, and limits. The need of belonging included concepts of love, affection, friendship, and affiliation. The esteem need involved attempts at self-respect, self-confidence, worth, and feelings of adequacy, prestige, appreciation, dignity, and having some status in the world. The most sophisticated of Maslow's hierarchy was the need for self-actualization, which included the individual seeking self-fulfillment and achievement of potential. Maslow contended that until the basic needs were satisfied to some extent, more mature needs could not emerge. As an example, it is difficult for a nurse to try to teach a patient how to give insulin while the patient is worried about being in a diabetic coma. First the nurse must deal with the needs presented by the patient, in this case the fear.

Another existential-humanistic theorist was Erik Erikson.[19] Erikson, who began his career as a psychoanalytic thinker, devised a framework wherein the level of functioning was assessed by considering the tasks of the lifecycle. (For a detailed identification of the tasks that Erikson delineated, see Chapter 13).

Erikson felt that these tasks showed the conflicts, possible crises, and critical steps in becoming a highly functioning adult. Erikson, as did the other theroists of this school, acknowledged that time was important in movement toward growth. But time alone was not the most important variable, as someone could be old in actual number of years, but quite immature in terms of growth toward potential. As an example, one of the tasks Erikson wrote of was initiative in contrast to guilt. Imagine a person who, although 50 years old, is mainly motivated to action by guilt rather than because he wants to do something.

This frequently underlies behavior of people who say "I should" or "I ought," rather than "I want to."

Erikson saw growth as somewhat painful. He felt that childhood was the time when the society systematically trained the individual to become a productive member.

Erich Fromm, another existential-humanistic theorist, took a slightly different point of view. He first analyzed the society, and then decided what tasks of "social character" are developed. Fromm also stated that different classes in the same society will enforce or reinforce certain ideals based on what is or is not acceptable to certain groups.[20] Fromm thought that social character harnesses human energy primarily to meet the needs, economic or social, of a given system. This would affect what virtues are seen as important, depending on the developmental plan of the society. For instance, in a hunting and gathering society, traits such as artistic creativity or being articulate might be held in low esteem, while in a highly industrial society these same traits might be considered very worthwhile and rewarded with fame or money. Subgroups of society may have different values from the majority. Teenagers may place a high value on a certain hair style, while their parents view it with less esteem. Fromm extended thinking about "becoming" as a societal and individual process.

The existential-humanistic scholars acknowledged needs, including individual and societal. They also speculated that people could go beyond basic needs and identified ideals. They offered explanations as to why people could become martyrs, giving up their lives, for an ideal. The theories of the existential-humanistic individuals paid heed to the society, but advanced a position that individuals could be more mature than the culture in which they existed.

Learning Theory

This theory regarded personality development as a learning process, with learned responses as a major factor in dictating how a person reacts in specific situations. At one time this theory was considered to be antihumanistic and concerned mainly with putting human beings and the motivating forces of human behavior in the category of animals. But presently this theory is seen less negatively.

Much of the early work on which some aspects of this theory are based comes from the experimental method of study. The experimental method frequently studied laboratory animals to understand certain elements of the learning process.

B.F. Skinner's work looked at behavior in terms of the **stimulus-response** (S-R) interaction.[21] The stimulus is something that triggers a reaction. The response is the reaction. For example, a stimulus might be a brightly colored baby rattle; the response would be the baby reaching for the rattle. Another example is a hypodermic needle being the stimulus in a pediatrician's office. The response on the part of a 5-year-old child is crying. The S-R is a process. Skinner, expanding on the early work of Pavlov, added to the body of knowledge about how organisms learn. Using observation and carefully controlled studies, Skinner articulated relationships between two sets of variables. The variable of the stimulus was not merely a one-stimulus, such as an electric shock device or a push-bar that gave out grain, but generally a class of variables that contained many things—the environment. The other variable, the response, was seen as a behavioral response that could and frequently did contain complex patterns of behavior. In addition to the concepts of stimulus and response, the terms **avoidance** and **approach** are used. Avoidance is the mechanism or process in which situations are seen as undesirable, and the person withdraws or moves away from the situation. Approach is the process of coming closer to or engaging in the activity.

The behaviorists were just one branch of learning theory scientists. Many others advocated learning as a theoretical framework for understanding personality. Piaget, working during the mid-portion of the 20th century in Geneva, Switzerland, speculated that within the cognitive functions of the individual, a process took place that enabled an individual to adapt to new situations.[22] This process involved the person organizing past experiences and applying them to the present. Piaget's efforts were concentrated with the structure, the "hows" of learning, rather than looking at the content, or the "whats" of learning. Much of Piaget's work was done by observation of children. His method was to clinically observe the child, formulate a hypothesis, and then test the hypothesis by slightly altering the child's surroundings. Piaget identified that a complex process, involving assessment of the stimulus, takes place within the individual. The present stimulus is viewed not merely on the perception of the current stimulus, but also on knowledge gained by the individual through previous situations.

According to Piaget the biological make-up of the child was not discounted, but the focus of his work was based on the ongoing interactions with the environment. Concepts important in Piaget's theory were **assimilation** and **accommodation.** Assimilation is the aspect of the mediating process where incoming sensory data interacts with that which has already gone on within the brain. It is a type of incorporating process. Accommodation is that other part of the mediating process that seeks to change the input. The goal of both these functions is to promote a general state of stability in the person. They both lead toward individual gain (or regain) of equilibrium. Piaget speculated that there is a better level of functioning if the person is in balance.

Piaget felt that language was the vehicle by which thought was socialized and rendered logical to the individual. People, by understanding structure and action, could transfer this understanding in the application of new knowledge. It should be noted that Piaget, like Erikson and Maslow, is frequently identified as a growth and development theorist.

One other aspect of learning theory work was done by Kurt Lewin on perceptional theory.[23] Lewin focused on how the individual perceives stimuli. One cannot examine stimulus apart from the environment. In other words, in order to understand one part of a situation, one must understand the broader field. One cannot look at a tree, for example, without realizing that the tree is just a part of the forest.

People, according to the learning theorists, think and act the way they do because, to a great extent, they have learned that they should do so. This theory does not negate the other theories, but adds another dimension to an understanding of the nature of personhood.

THE NURSING PROCESS

In carrying out the nursing process, the nurse uses her knowledge of many different theories and concepts as she collects data, analyzes it, and plans care. The contributions of personality theorists may assist in the assessment phase, in planning and implementation, or in evaluation. Nurses who work in psychiatry or with clients who have significant personality or behavioral difficulties may base their entire practice on one or more theories of personality. Some of the concepts identified in this chapter might be used solely to better understand the motivation of individuals or to decide on interventions to help the patient adjust to illness or choose a more healthy lifestyle. Some concepts may seem more useful than others. Your use of this knowledge also will depend on the area of professional practice you are engaged in, how much experience you have had, and what your role is.

The following discussions on each of the phases of the nursing process will show, by example, how several of these theories can be clinically applied to nursing.

Assessment

How might the nurse use the concept of unconscious from the psychoanalytic theory in the assessment phase of the nursing process? It is not suggested that the nurse, unless quite sophisticated in both theory and practice, seek to undercover unconscious material. Unconscious material is hidden precisely because it is painful to the person.

Assume that a patient who has been diagnosed as hypertensive is given a prescription for medication that will lower the blood pressure. While the nurse is visiting the home, giving prenatal instruction to the hypertensive patient's wife, the nurse discovers that the patient never had the prescription filled. Obviously, the patient is not taking the medicine. The nurse should suspect that this noncompliance with the medical regimen is not merely a case of the patient "not wanting" to take pills.

What might be the reason the patient is not taking his blood pressure medicine? The nurse begins by asking questions. "Why" questions are difficult to answer. Many times patients respond with "I don't know," and frequently they really do not recognize what motivates them to engage or to not engage in certain activities. One hidden reason for noncompliance might involve that patient's perception that he feels he is not a "good provider," and therefore, his taking money to purchase the medicine might deprive his family. The nurse does not introduce this suspicion, but considers it as a possibility in speaking with the patient. The goal is not to get the patient to acknowledge unconscious thoughts, but merely to help the nurse better understand the dynamics of the situation. In this case, the plan of the nurse might be to help the patient identify the value of taking medicine. There should be reinforcement that medicine is important for several reasons. One reason might be that if the blood pressure is controlled, the patient will be in better health to enjoy the baby and be better able to provide for his family.

Planning

Another example of theoretical application would be to consider the concept of anxiety for planning patient care. Imagine the nurse trying to help plan care for a bedridden, arthritic patient. Arthritis is a chronic condition that affects the patient's joints, and frequently involves pain on movement.

In planning care, the nurse needs to consider patients' and their families' feelings and fears. For instance, in planning for the arthritic person, the nurse is attempting to enlist the aid of a patient's elderly sister to do frequent turnings to prevent bedsores from forming. After a great deal of discussion, the nurse recognizes that the sister seems reluctant to do the turning for two reasons. She feels she might hurt the patient, and she fears that by moving the patient she might injure her own back. The nurse could use a straightforward approach to try to alleviate the anxiety. To deal with her fear about herself, the nurse might say, "I will teach you how to do it, and make certain that you are not putting yourself in danger of injury. I will make sure that you can do it correctly before you do it on your own." By providing an example, supervision, and suggestions, the nurse can help the sister reduce her anxiety. In regard to the expression about hurting the patient, the nurse might say, "You may hurt your sister a bit, but it is far

better for her to experience a bit of discomfort during turning than to suffer bedsores." Anxiety frequently can be diminished by confronting the issues that make the person anxious. When anxiety is reduced, the person is able to help in planning care.

Implementation

Intervention or implementation might be considered in using the concept of stimulus-response from the learning theory. One example of using this concept might be in working with a mother who is trying to help her mentally retarded child stop biting his nails. The nurse would help the mother identify what situations (stimulus) seem to cause the child to chew on his nails (response). The mother then would be aware of those times that are especially stressful for the child. Together, the nurse and the mother might consider ways to see that the stimulus is diminished so that the response does not take place. This might be done by the mother offering a diversion, such as game playing at the stressful time, or maybe just holding the child, in order that the response, the nail biting, does not happen.

Evaluation

Evaluation, which measures the effectiveness of nursing practice, including assessment, planning, and intervention, might be influenced by some of the concepts of needs theory, which is one aspect of existential-humanistic theory. One example might be to use Maslow's concept of self-actualization to determine the effectiveness of group therapy. Many psychiatric patients have problems with interpersonal relationships because they view their own self-worth unrealistically. In other words, because of their low self-esteem, their interactions with others may be disturbed. Treatment in psychiatric settings frequently is multifaceted, and group therapy is one common treatment mode.

One goal of a therapy group might be to increase self-esteem. In order to measure self-esteem, one would have to decide on behavioral aspects that could be noted and would be linked to self-esteem. The measure could be the frequency with which patients in a group speak disparagingly about themselves. It is assumed that as patients' self-esteem increases, the negative comments they make about themselves will decrease. The measure is behavioral change, which the nurse thinks is related to an affective change.

CONCLUSION

One of the major concepts that has been identified and appears in all these theories, is that of growth—the possibility of change. Growth is viewed as a positive movement toward a higher level of functioning and a more healthy way of relating to the world and those in the world. In terms of personhood, growth is a movement toward a greater feeling of worth and dignity and an increasingly positive view of oneself as a unique individual. No matter how seemingly disabled or distraught a patient appears, the nurse can help the patient becomes less so by capitalizing on his potential for personal and emotional growth.

The nurse might help patients grow in many situations. One opportunity may be leading a group of aged individuals with a focus on adjusting to moving into a retirement home. Giving parenting classes may help parents grow in their skills and self-confidence. Still another situation where a nurse can help patients grow is in health teaching in a junior high school. If the nurse works in a crisis intervention setting, growth may take place by helping the patient learn from one situation to another.

One other important consideration is the nurse's own potential for growth. Within each of us, there exists a quality of striving, which involves doing better or becoming more mature. Growth includes being aware of our strengths and limitations. In order to grow, we must seek to capitalize on our strengths and work on our limitations. It is a constant process, but one with great rewards.

SUMMARY

This chapter presents several concepts that have emerged from various theories of personhood. The goal has been to identify concepts that are fundamental to the mental health, growth, and development aspects of people. The chapter gives a few examples of how the nurse might apply some of these concepts to nursing practice.

Personhood, as a state of being, depends on many things. Some of the factors that influence it are age, maturation, heredity, culture, state of health, and beliefs. These theories can improve our understanding of people. The more we understand about people, the more likely we are to be able to help them and care for them.

Nursing involves gaining knowledge in order to apply that knowledge to more fully serve others. Gaining an understanding of personhood is basic to treating people with respect and dignity. In your own nursing practice, you should try to apply some of the concepts discussed to help you address the needs of your patients.

STUDY QUESTIONS

1. Go to a playground and observe children. Are some introverted and others extroverted? How can you tell? List the behaviors.

2. Do you have a bad habit—maybe smoking, or handing in school work late, or not hanging up your clothes? Make an effort for a week to try and break that

habit. Notice how "breaking the habit" influences your feelings and thoughts. Keep a diary of what you think and feel about not following your usual behavior.

3. Try telling a friend a story. Say all the "right" words, but attempt "wrong" behavior (nonverbal clues). For instance, tell about a funny movie, but appear to be on the verge of tears. Does your friend notice? What does your friend say nonverbally? What does he say in words? Does the lack of congruence influence whether or not your friend thinks the movie is funny?

4. Keep a log for a week of when you feel anxious or uncomfortable. Try to determine the origin of these feelings. What do you do to become more comfortable? Does it work? If not, why not?

5. In what ways have you grown since you entered nursing?

REFERENCES

1. Allport G: "What units shall we employ?" In the **Assessment of Human Motivates.** Rinehart, New York, p.48, 1958.
2. Orem D: **Nursing: Concepts of Practice,** 2nd ed. McGraw-Hill, New York, 1980.
3. Hall C, Lindzey G: **Theories of Personality,** 2nd ed. John Wiley and Sons, Inc., New York, 1957.
4. Allport: **Assessment of Human Motivates,** p.48.
5. Hall: **Theories of Personality,** 1957.
6. Freud S: **The Basic Writings of Sigmund Freud.** Modern Library, New York, 1938.
7. Bettelheim B: **Reflections (Freud),** The New Yorker. pp.52–93, March 1982.
8. Jung C: The symbols of the self. **In** the **Collected Works** Pantheon, New York, 1960.
9. Alder, A: **Individual Psychology.** Clark University Press, Worcester, Mass., 1930.
10. Mead, G: **Mind, Self and Society.** University of Chicago Press, Chicago, 1934.
11. Berne, E: **Games People Play.** Grove Press, New York, 1964.
12. Sullivan, H: **The Interpersonal Theory of Psychiatry.** W.W. Norton and Company, Inc., New York, 1953.
13. Rogers, C: **On Becoming a Person.** Houghton Mifflin, Boston, 1961.
14. Berne: **Games People Play,** 1964.
15. Jourard, S: **Self-Disclosure an Experimental Analysis of the Transparent Self.** Wiley-Interscience, New York 1971.
16. **Ibid**
17. Rogers, C: **On Becoming a Person.**
18. Maslow, A: **Motivation and Personality.** 2nd ed., Harper and Row, New York, 1970.
19. Erikson, E: **Childhood and Society.** 2nd ed., W.W. Norton, New York, 1963.
20. Fromm, E: Character and the Social Process **In Appendix to Escape from Freedom.** Rinehart, New York, 1941.
21. Skinner, B.F.: **The Behavior of Organisms: An Experimental Analysis.** D. Appleton Century, New York, 1938.
22. Phillips, J: **The Origin, of Intellect Piaget's Theory.** W.H. Freeman and Co., San Francisco, 1969.
23. Lewin, K: **A Dynamic Theory of Personality; Selected Papers.** McGraw-Hill, New York, 1935.

ANNOTATED BIBLIOGRAPHY

Fromm E: **The Art of Loving.** New York, Harper and Row, 1956. (Available in paperback) This classic book presents Fromm's ideas about the nature of love in terms of personality development. It is an excellent resource for assisting in self-development. Fromm emphasizes the importance of ongoing self-responsibility for reaching one's potential in life, particularly one's highest capacity for love relationships. It supports Fromm's personality theory.

Hymovich D, and Chamberlain R: **Child and Family Development: Implications for Health, Primary Health Care.** New York, McGraw-Hill, 1980. This is a family oriented textbook that presents growth, development, and personality theories as they relate to nursing and health care. It is comprehensive and includes a section on theoretical frameworks.

Mussen P, Conger J, and Kagan J: **Child Development and Personality,** 4th ed. New York, Harper and Row, 1964. This is a comprehensive, basic textbook on general growth and development with an emphasis on personality development through adolescence. It presents an excellent overview of all the possible factors that contribute to personality makeup.

Satir V: **Peoplemaking.** Palo Alto, Science and Behavior Books, Inc., 1972. This is primarily a book about the family process and parenting, but it gives tremendous insight into the complexities of personality development. It does not present personality theory per se, but gives practical information and interesting viewpoints on interpersonal relationships within the family setting.

15

Self-concept

Linda Manglass Shapiro

CHAPTER OUTLINE

OBJECTIVES

At the completion of this chapter, the reader will be able to:

- Identify self-concept as one way in which man adapts to bio-psycho-social influences
- State a definition of self-concept congruent with theories of self-concept development
- Identify components of self-concept using an adaptation approach/model
- Identify factors useful in assessing self-concept in clients
- Describe nursing intervention strategies effective in the development of an adaptive self-concept and in promoting positive responses to influences on self-concept.

GLOSSARY

Body image—an individual's concept of the shape, size, and appearance of his body and its parts.

Looking Glass Self—a person's view of self resulting from his perception of others' responses to him.

Self-actualization—a term coined by Abraham Maslow referring to a level of development; making full use of one's talents and potentials.

Self-concept—an individual's self-definition; the composite of beliefs and feelings one holds about self.

Self-esteem—evaluative attitudes toward self.

INTRODUCTION

Understanding of self-concept is important in nursing because an individual's self-concept affects and is affected by his health and any deviation from health. How an individual functions in a given situation is dependent on how he perceives himself and how he perceives the situation. The self-concept is the point of orientation for all behavior.

Nurses are very concerned with individuals' physical, psychological, and social behaviors. Understanding the relationship between these and the self-concept will aid the nurse in promoting behaviors that are positive and adaptive.

Any time there is a change in an individual's state of wellness or illness, he must adapt as a total person. How well he is able to adapt, in part, depends on how he views himself. This view of self is the self-concept.

Using a framework for assessing the client's self-concept enables the nurse to predict problems the person may have in adapting and promotes adaptation through identification and use of client strengths.

DEFINITIONS AND THEORY DEVELOPMENT

Self-concept is a composite of beliefs and feelings one holds about oneself. Self-concept is formed partly from perceptions or reflected appraisals of significant others, partly from environmental influences, and partly from inner resources. Self-concept is constantly evolving and directs one's behavior.[1]

This eclectic definition of self-concept is a composite of the major schools of thought regarding self-concept and reflects the what, how, and why of self-concept development.

THEORISTS

The term "reflected appraisals" and "significant others" are concepts originated by Harry Stack Sullivan,[2] one of several social interaction theorists who wrote about self-concept development. He used the term "reflected appraisals" to refer to the inferences we get about ourselves as a result of ways we are treated and judged by significant others. "Significant others" are those people who provide rewards and punishments; most commonly, parents, spouses, helpmates, and best friends.

Another theory of self-concept development based on social interaction theory is the "Looking Glass Self" by Charles Horton Coolie.[3] This is seeing oneself through the eyes of others. An individual imagines how he is perceived by another person, how the other person appraises him, and then makes a value judgment about that appraisal (i.e., he is proud of his perception or ashamed of it).

Both of these theories are based on the belief that interaction with others in a social world determines an individual's concept of self.

Perceptual psychology discusses self-concept in terms of individual perceptions. How a person behaves is determined largely by how he views himself. This self, referred to as his **perceived self,** is the point of reference for everything he does. These concepts are the core of personality.[4] Raimy said of self-concept that it is more or less an organized perceptual object resulting from present and past observations. It is what a person believes about himself. The self-concept is a map that each person consults in order to understand himself, especially during moments of crisis or choice.[5] The self-concept is the self at all times and in all situations, and once established, has a high degree of stability.[6]

SELF-CONCEPT DEVELOPMENT

It is thought that an individual's concept of self actually begins at or soon after birth. This process begins in its earliest phases when the infant begins differentiation of self from others. The infant's first differentiations are tactile, and the sense of who and what he is comes with exploration of his own body and his discovery that he is separate from the surroundings. As the child matures, this process becomes less difficult and is greatly accelerated by the development of language. Initially, communication occurs on a nonverbal level with mother (or significant person). This nonverbal communication is the response the infant receives. Language, particularly the use of his own name, aids the child's clarification of self-concept. Using the child's own name helps him to identify himself and see himself as unique and special. The use of nonverbal language also allows approval and disapproval, affection and rejection. At this time, for example, it is particularly important for the difference between "bad boy" and "bad behavior" to be made clear.

Significant research by Stanley Coopersmith, has been done on development of self-concept in school age boys. The results of his research, published in 1967, provided valuable information regarding the effect of the family on self-concept development.[7]

> "No experience in the development of a child's concept of self is quite so important or far reaching as his earliest experiences in his family. It is the family which introduces a child to life which provides him with his earliest and most permanent self definitions. Here it is that he first discovers those basic concepts of life which will guide his behavior for the rest of his life."[8]

It is necessary, therefore, to understand what contributes to positive self-concept

development and what does not.

Coopersmith used the term self-esteem to refer to evaluative attitudes toward self—the individual's perception of his worth. He looked at many different areas in the family life of school age boys in order to determine what kinds of parental characteristics and influencing familial factors had an effect on the feelings the boys developed about themselves and their resulting behavior. Some of the areas he studied and drew conclusions from are as follows:

- He found no clear or definite pattern of relationships between social class and positive or negative levels of self-esteem.

- He found no difference between religious classes—Jewish, Protestant, or Catholic.

- The prestige of the father's work had no bearing on levels of self-esteem. It was found that regular employment enhanced self-esteem, and that there was an exception with the children of police and members of the armed forces, who demonstrated lower levels of self-esteem.

- Whether or not the mother was employed made no difference in levels of self-esteem.

- Family size was unimportant, except that self-esteem was found to be higher in first-borns and only children.

General characteristics of family life that were shown to contribute to the development of positive self-esteem were acceptance by parents, clearly defined and enforced limits, and respect for individual action that exists within those limits.

Coopersmith summarized characteristics of children identified with low self-esteem and those with high self-esteem (see Figure 15-1). These factors are important in the process of assessing levels of self-esteem in clients.

Low self-esteem	High self-esteem
isolation	maintains fairly constant image of self as a person
inability to give or receive love	capable of active expression
decreased interactions	can move realistically toward goals
decreased socialization	
fears and self-doubts	

Figure 15-1. Characteristics of Low and High Self-Esteem.

As in any research study, Coopersmith reviewed the literature on self-concept and theoretical aspects of the development of self-concept. He found many of the same ideas in the existing writings. He summarized four factors inherent in any self-concept theory.

- The amount of respectful, accepting, and concerned treatment a person receives from significant others.
- The individual's history of successes.
- The person's experiences are interpreted and modified in accordance with aspirations and values (what is perceived as important).
- The individual's manner of responding to devaluation.

Callista Roy, in her adaptation model, presents a similar summarization of stimuli affecting the individual's self-concept:[9]

- The individual's previous perceptions of feedback about self from significant others.
- The individual's previous maturational and situational crises and how he has rearranged his self-concept in response to the crises.
- The person's self-expectations and experiences with success and failure.
- Any experiences, such as interpersonal ones, that generate in the individual positive feelings and a sense of value or worth, or conversely, negative feelings.

- The individual's physiological integrity.

THE NURSING PROCESS

Potential nursing problems related to self-concept are many and varied. The adaptation approach to nursing provides a useful framework for understanding self-concept and its relationship to individuals' behavior in health and illness.

Just as man adapts physiologically to his environment (i.e., an increase in temperature causes sweating, which results in cooling), he also adapts through self-concept. Roy calls this the self-concept mode of adaptation.[10]

Individuals with positive self-concepts function effectively because they view themselves and their worlds positively. Negative self-concepts are associated with problems in many areas. For example, research has shown that patients with negative self-concepts believe their illnesses have a greater negative effect on their lives, have less hope and optimism about the future, and are more anxious about their illnesses.[11]

To understand and use the self-concept mode more easily, it is broken into components. These components are parts of the self that contribute to the overall concept of self that a person holds. The components provide a framework for assessing the individual's self-concept. The following definitions with discussions on each mode and

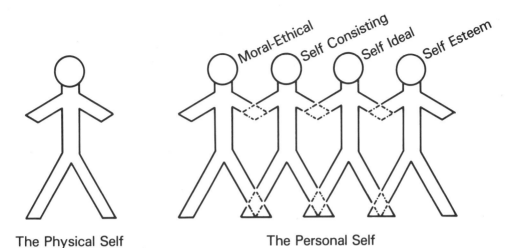

The Physical Self   The Personal Self

Figure 15-2.   The Components of the Self.

component are adapted from Roy. There are two basic components: physical self and personal self. The personal self is further divided into moral-ethical self, self-consistency, self-ideal/self-expectancy, and self-esteem.

Assessment

Behaviors to look and listen for, in assessing self-concept, that indicate adaptation include general physical appearance reflecting a "cared for" look, appropriate height/weight proportions, good posture and gait, comfortable (for nurse and client) degree of eye contact, an energy level that reflects participation and enjoyment of a reasonable number and variety of activities, an accurate view of reality, emotions within a range of normal, consistent verbal and nonverbal behavior, an ability to establish and maintain mutually satisfying interpersonal relationships, an ability to problem solve and make decisions, task achievement appropriate to developmental level, appetite and sleep patterns within normal limits, use of adaptive defense mechanisms, and what a person says about himself.

Behaviors that may indicate less than positive adaptation are discussed next un-

der problems commonly encountered in each component.

Physical self refers to the person's appraisal of his physical being; his image of

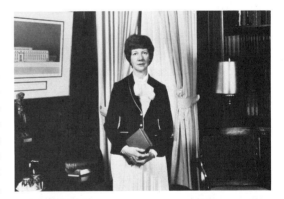

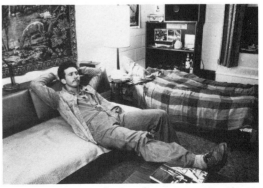

Figure 15-3.   Physical appearance is an indicator of self-esteem.

himself physically. It includes physical attributes, functioning, sexuality, wellness-illness state, and appearance. The physical self is commonly known as **body image.** As with self-concept generally, a person's mental image of his body (his concept of physical self, or body image) may not correspond to his actual body structure. In other words, he may not see himself as others see him.

Problems encountered in nursing related to physical self often are caused by loss—real, imagined, or symbolic. Loss is defined as a situation, either actual or potential, in which a valued object is rendered inaccessible to an individual or is altered in such a way that it no longer has qualities that render it valuable. The object, in its broadest sense, includes people, possessions, an individual's job, status, home, ideals, and parts and processes of the body.[12] (See Chapter 22 for a more thorough discussion of this important concept.)

Changes in physical body structure (e.g., amputation or mastectomy) commonly precipitate feelings of loss. Changes in physical functioning, loss of strength, central nervous system diseases, the aging process, pregnancy, a colostomy, obesity, and disfiguring surgery are losses that frequently are encountered in nursing situations.

The nurse can tell a great deal about how an individual feels about himself by looking at him and listening to what he has to say about his body and appearance. Areas to observe and listen for in assessing physical self include appearance, height/weight proportions, posture and gait, eye contact, and references made to body image. Individuals who feel good about themselves tend to take care of themselves and look like they care about themselves. If an individual is unkempt, unable to make eye contact, and walks slumped over, for instance, it may be an indication that he doesn't think very much of himself.

Physical changes, such as those described previously, always demand adaptation, and the individual will experience concerns and possibly anxieties as a result of the changes. How well he is able to adjust will be determined by numerous factors, such as previous perceptions of self, feedback from others including the nurse, suddenness and severity of change, and previous experiences.

Personal Self. The first component of personal self is the **moral-ethical self,** which refers to the aspect of self that functions as observer, standard setter, dreamer, comparer, and most importantly, evaluator of who this person says he is. Moral-ethical self judges desirability and undesirability of self-perceptions. Judgments a person makes about himself influence the value or esteem he feels about himself.

Since moral-ethical self has a great deal to do with values an individual holds, problems in moral-ethical self commonly take the form of guilt. Areas to observe and listen for in assessing guilt include disparaging remarks about self, depression, apologies, self-blaming statements, blushing, and stammering.

Self-consistency refers to a person's striving to maintain a consistent self-organization, and thus avoid disequilibrium. People have a need to maintain a consistent or stable self-image; so, for example, a person who achieves a weight loss may still have an image of self as heavy. Only through consistent, repeated experiences of "thin" can this person change his concept of self from heavy to thin.

Problems in self-consistency produce anxiety. Anything that threatens who or what that person believes himself to be will result in anxiety. Problems in the self-consistency component of self-concept reflected as anxiety are encountered daily in all areas of nursing. Hospitalization alone is a threatening, anxiety provoking experience. Addressing problems of anxiety in clients should be a part of every client's care plan. (See Chapter 21 for assessment factors and intervention strategies.)

Self-idea/self-expectancy is the aspect of the self that relates to what the person expects himself to be and do. It is also the ideal of what he wants to become. These concepts guide his behavior toward achieving identified goals.

Problems in achieving ideals and expectations often result in powerlessness. Feelings of powerlessness may be seen as a decrease in motivation and energy, depression, anger, passivity, or apathy. Illness and hospitalization may result in feelings of powerlessness, and nurses can intervene by assuring that clients are given as much control over their experiences as possible. Control is enhanced by offering choices, giving information, and allowing time for questions and discussions.

Self-esteem refers to an individual's perception of his worth and is integral to each component of self-concept. For example:

- physical self-capacity and control of bodily functions affect feelings of self-worth;
- moral-ethical self—judgments about self affect esteem;
- self-consistency—it is only when a person has a consistent concept of self that he is able to place value on that self;
- fulfilling self-ideal and expectancies directly influence levels of self-esteem.

This framework is one that can be used to organize data in assessing areas of self-concept that may be causes of concern or problems.

At the conclusion of the assessment phase, nursing diagnoses can be formulated from the data gathered. Some sample nursing diagnoses include:

- Alteration in self-concept due to loss
- Alteration in body image due to amputation
- Alteration in body image due to pregnancy.

Planning

In the planning phase of the nursing process goals and outcome criteria are established. Identifying precisely what the nurse is trying to achieve helps organize and direct nursing interventions. The plan should be in writing and placed either on the client's chart or on the Kardex.

Using the nursing diagnosis stated above examples of goals might be:

- The patient will be able to look at his amputation site within seven days and clean and care for site by discharge
- The client will state three positive aspects of self.

In establishing goals to address problems in self-concept, keep in mind realistic time parameters. It is unlikely you will be able to raise a client's self-esteem and improve his body image during a short hospital stay, for example.

Implementation

The importance of helping individuals develop and maintain positive feelings about themselves cannot be over-emphasized. Individuals function in any given situation according to how they perceive themselves and how they perceive the situation in which they are involved. The nurse's role in assisting clients to feel valuable and worthwhile and view themselves with confidence is paramount in the overall goal of working with clients to achieve maximum levels of adaptive functioning.

This is not an easy task. One characteristic of the self is stability. The self represents our fundamental frame of reference, our anchor to reality. Even an unsatisfactory self-organization is likely to prove highly stable and resistant to change.[13] You know, for instance, how difficult it is to change a friend's view of himself if he doesn't like himself much. He may be pleased by the praise, but continues to act in the same manner. Because of this characteristic stability, you can't "change" an individual's self-concept. That is not a goal. What you can influence is the individual's perception of the situation. How does this happen?

A change in the view of self occurs upon repetition of experiences of adequacy and with much praise and encouragement. For example, a student who believes he is dumb will not change that view of self with one high grade. It will require many high grades. A client who feels unattractive and unlovable as a result of a physical alteration will only begin to be able to change that view of self with many positive interpersonal interactions and experiences.

Nurses are in unique and powerful positions with clients in influencing how they view themselves and the situations in which they find themselves. They often become, at least temporarily, a "significant other" to the client. For example, it is the nurse who usually works first and most closely with the client following surgery. How the nurse behaves with the client following her mastectomy, what kind of information she gives her, and how she treats her will have an impact on how the client incorporates this new aspect of self into her self-concept. If she is accepted, esteemed, and valued by the nurse, she will be more likely to accept, value, and esteem herself and incorporate her new self-image in a positive, adaptive manner. This relationship between nurse and client is the primary tool of the nurse in intervening with clients experiencing problems related to self-concept.

Another important aspect of planning intervention strategies for clients is recognizing the client's strengths and looking for ways to focus on those strengths consistently and continuously. Focusing on strengths helps clients feel more confident and positive. If they can recognize worthwhile, positive qualities of self, then they will feel better able to cope with whatever situation comes along.

Evaluation

Evaluating your client's progress is necessary to determine whether your interventions are working. You are looking for the client to be able to view his situation in a different way that allows him to behave in a more positive, adaptive manner. You will know your interventions are working if and when the client begins to talk about himself in an accepting, positive way and with realistic confidence in his abilities. The client's ability to interact with others and to identify with them is another area to evaluate. Remember that change takes time. Adapting to changes that occur in states of wellness and illness and that affect self-concept are difficult and challenging for both client and nurse.

SUMMARY

This chapter has introduced self-concept as an integral component of the total person. Self-concept influences and is influenced by an individual's state of wellness and illness and is, therefore, important for nurses to consider in providing total care to clients.

Social interaction theory and perceptual psychology were presented as two theories of self-concept development. Research was included on self-concept development in children, which is also useful in assessment of self-concept.

Adaptation, as a framework, offers one approach to examining the self-concept of an individual. This approach allows for the steps of the nursing process to be carried out in assessing self-concept, planning and implementing nursing approaches, and evaluating the effectiveness of those nursing interventions.

STUDY QUESTIONS

1. List ten of your own strengths.

2. What is self-concept?

3. Relate two theories of self-concept development.

4. How does self-concept relate to self-esteem? body image? self-actualization?

5. Why is self-concept important in nursing?

6. What nursing strategies do you use to assess self-concept?

7. Indicate characteristics of positive self-concept and characteristics reflective of low self-concept.

8. Describe interventions appropriate in developing and promoting an adaptive self-concept.

REFERENCES

1. Callista Roy, **Introduction to Nursing: An Adaptation Model.** (N.J.: Prentice-Hall, Inc., 1976), p.174.
2. Harry Stack Sullivan, **The Interpersonal Theory of Psychiatry.** (N.Y.: W.W. Norton and Co., Inc., 1953), pp.49–61, 158–171.
3. S. Epstein, "The Self Concept Revisited or a Theory of a Theory," **American Psychologist,** 28, (May 1973), pp.404–416.
4. Arthus Combs, Anne Richards and Fred Richards, **Perceptual Psychology.** (N.Y.: Harper and Row Publications, 1976), p.154.
5. V. Raimey, **The Self as a Factor in Counseling and Personality Organization.** Doctoral dissertation, Ohio State University, 1943. (Columbus, Ohio State University Libraries, 1971).
6. Combs and Richards, **Perceptual Psychology,** p.160.
7. Stanley Coopersmith, **Antecedents of Self-Esteem.** (San Francisco: W.H. Freeman and Co., 1967).
8. Arthur Combs and Donald Snygg, **Individual Behavior: A Perceptual Approach.** (N.Y.: Harper and Row Publications, pp.134–135.
9. Roy, **Introduction to Nursing,** p.190.
10. Roy, **Introduction to Nursing,** p.171.
11. J. Schwab, R. Clemmons and L. Morder, "The Self Concept: Psychosomatic Implications," **Psychomatics,** 7 (January–February, 1966), pp.1–5.
12. Roy, **Introduction to Nursing,** pp.193–194.
13. P. Lecky, **Self Consistency. A Theory of Personality,** ed. interpreted F.C. Thorne (Hamden, CT: Shoe String, 1961), p.162.

ANNOTATED BIBLIOGRAPHY

Chrzanowski G: **The Genesis and Nature of Self Esteem.** Am J. Psychother 35:38–46; January 1981. This article discusses self-esteem as a foundation for understanding human behavior and in the psychotherapeutic situation.

Gruendemann B: **The Impact of Surgery on Body Image.** Nurs Clin North Am 10:635: 1975. Discusses the impact of surgery on the individual's concept of self. Includes assessing, planning, and intervention.

Jourard S: **The Transparent Self.** New York, Littan Educational Publishing Co., 1971. The concept of self-disclosure and its implications for the nurse/client relationship is discussed.

Maslow A: **Toward a Psychology of Being.** Princeton, D. VanNostrand Co., 1962. Presents a theory of functioning based on needs including self-esteem. It is particularly noted for the concept of self-actualization.

Money J, Ehrhardt A: **Man and Woman, Boy and Girl.** Baltimore, Johns Hopkins University Press, 1972. Presents the results of the author's research on the development of sexual identity and sex-typed behavior.

Norris C: **The Professional Nurse and Body Image.** In Carlson C (ed): Behavioral Concepts and Nursing Interventions, Philadelphia, J.B. Lippincott Co., 1970. Identifies problems related to physical self and discusses factors that influence the degree of threat to one's body image.

Otto HA: **The Human Potentialities of Nurses and Patients.** Nurs Outlook August 1965. This widely read and cited article discusses some of the findings of a human potentialities research project. Interesting and enlightening findings.

Satir V: **Peoplemaking.** Palo Alto, Science and Behavior Books, Inc., 1972. Highly readable, practical book that addresses the importance of self-concept in family relations.

16

Human Sexuality

Carol N. Knowlton

CHAPTER OUTLINE

OBJECTIVES

At the completion of this chapter, the reader will be able to:

- Describe human sexuality as a function of the total personality.
- Differentiate between sex and sexuality.
- Describe the influence of family and society on the child's psycho-sexual development.
- Define gender identity, sex role, and sexual orientation.
- Describe potential threats to an individual's sexual integrity.
- Identify the effect of one's own feelings and value system on patient care.
- List some sexually related behaviors that may occur in the hospital setting.
- Use a brief sexual assessment guide.
- Describe nursing attitudes and interventions related to sexual health that will help the patient maintain a positive sense of self.

GLOSSARY

Biological sex—anatomical and physiological "givens"—the sex organs, hormones, nerves, and brain centers.

Bisexual—a person sexually attracted to both males and females.

Celibacy—abstention from sexual intercourse.

Chromosomes—the genetic material in the nucleus of every cell of the body.

Gender identity—the inner persistent conviction that one is male or female.

Gender role—behavior that conveys to others that an individual is either male or female.

Genital(s)—pertaining to the sex organs in the pelvic region; customarily refers to the penis, the testes, and the scrotum in the male; the vulva and the vagina in the female.

Gonad—ovary or testicle.

Heterosexual—person with a sexual preference for partners of the opposite sex.

Homosexual—person with a sexual preference for partners of the same sex.

Hormone—chemical substance secreted by the endocrine system in the blood stream to be carried directly to the tissue on which it acts.

Masturbation—self-stimulation of the sexual organs resulting in orgasm.

Ovaries—paired structures located on each side of the uterus that contain and release eggs. Female gonads.

Secondary sex characteristics—those body characteristics that develop during puberty that distinguish the sexes.

Sex—gender—male or female; sexual behavior; sexual anatomy; sexual intercourse.

Sex identity—see gender identity.

Sex role—see gender role.

Sexual differentiation—the process that begins at the moment of conception to create a normal male or female.

Sexual integrity—a comfortable secure gender identity and sexual orientation; experiencing an increasingly satisfying sexual life, free of sexual dysfunction.

Sexual orientation—preference for sexual partner.

Sexuality—a pervasive life force that includes a person's total feelings, attitudes, behavior, and beliefs that relate to being a male or female.

Testes—paired male reproductive glands contained in the scrotum; the male gonads.

Transsexual—a rare condition in which there is a persistent sense of discomfort about one's anatomical sex and the desire to change one's sexual anatomy and live as a member of the opposite sex.

INTRODUCTION

Sexuality is a complex, unique, and human characteristic that pervades the whole of an individual's life. No other biological function is so personal and emotionally charged and yet so subject to legal and ethical regulation. The term **sexuality** is a broad concept and it includes more than just biological sex. Sexuality encompasses the biological, psychological, social, cultural, and ethical aspects of sexual behavior. It designates the totality of being, one's experience of maleness or femaleness, and the way one expresses these attributes.

In contrast, the word **sex** generally connotes genital sex, physical sex, or the sex act; thus, sex has a much narrower meaning than sexuality. Sexuality is a broad, integrating concept, synthesizing the varied aspects of an individual's expression of self, and in many ways refers to what a person is. It does not exist only in the young and attractive or only between partners. It is a deep and pervasive aspect of the total human personality and of the total self from birth to death. It is observable in everyday life in endless variations conveyed by the way one dresses, moves, speaks, and relates to other human beings. Sexuality includes the need for attachment, sensuality, tenderness, intimacy, caring, and procreation. Attitudes towards relationships with people the same and opposite sex, toward touching and being touched are also integral parts of sexuality.

As a significant concern throughout life, sexuality has the potential to enhance the quality of life, foster personal growth, and contribute to human fulfillment. Today, sexuality is seen as an important aspect of health for people of all ages.

Professional interest in sexuality as an integral part of human behavior has increased greatly in the past 20 years. Tremendous changes in openness about sexuality followed the publication in 1948 of Alfred Kinsey's first research in sexual behavior.[1] As a result sexual concerns are readily discussed today by both individuals and health professionals, and there has been a definite relaxation of societal norms pertaining to sexuality. Openness and candor about sexuality seem to be the norms of the 1970s and 1980s, in contrast to a taboo about discussion of sexuality in previous decades. In addition, a larger knowledge base now exists in the area of human sexuality. Sex research is a legitimate area of scientific inquiry for researchers in fields such as biology, anthropology, sociology, psychology, nursing, and medicine. The basic facts about sexual functioning are now known, and the body of knowledge about human sexuality is continuing to grow at a rapid rate. Because of the marked expansion in knowledge and the increased availability of information on sexuality, our society has become more informed in sexual matters. Yet for many, sex myths still prevail or persist.

Myths, or beliefs with no foundations in truth, are by no means held only by the uneducated and unsophisticated. Health care professionals, such as nurses and physicians, can have a variety of misconceptions about sexuality. A few of the more common sexual myths and fallacies are listed in Figure 16-1.

This increase in professional interest and knowledge in human sexuality has extended to the nursing profession as well. Prior to 1970, there were relatively few sexuality related articles in the nursing literature. In 1976, 118 articles dealing with sexuality appeared in nursing journals, and in 1978, over 200 such articles were published. The first nursing text dealing exclusively with sexuality was published in 1974.[2] At least a half dozen nursing texts on sexuality have since been published. Since health care professionals are often the primary source of information for people with sexual concerns, it is essential that nurses be prepared and willing to manage

COMMON SEXUAL MYTHS

1. Old people do not want or need sexual intimacy.

2. Blacks have a greater sex drive than whites.

3. A large penis is of great importance to a woman's sexual gratification.

4. Menopause or hysterectomy terminates a woman's sex life.

5. Homosexuals are usually identifiable by their appearance.

6. Sexual intercourse should be avoided during pregnancy.

7. Alcohol is a sexual stimulant.

8. Emotional instability is caused by masturbation.

9. A couple must have simultaneous orgasms for conception to occur.

10. There is an absolutely "safe" period for sexual intercourse during which coitus cannot cause impregnation.

All of the above statements are false.

Figure 16-1. Sexual Myths.

sexually related health problems. Human sexuality content in nursing programs generally provides factual information about sexuality, modifies attitudes that block understanding of sexuality, and develops skills for assessment and management of sexually related concerns.

To comprehend how each person becomes the particular sexual being he is, certain fundamental principles must be understood. One's sexuality and sexual behavior result from the interplay of many influencing factors—a combination of inherited biological and physiological capabilities influenced by cultural factors—transmitted through the family and society. Human sexual feelings develop throughout the entire lifecycle. One's sexual feelings, attitudes, and behavior are primarily learned, and the earliest sexual attachments are to one's parents.[3] Infantile sexuality begins as the baby learns to enjoy the sexual pleasure of his own body and

that of his mother's. The physical and psychological closeness between parent and child that develops through holding, touching, and cuddling is essential to the child's development of a belief that he is worthwhile and lovable. These early influences affect later behavior and attitudes in the area of sexuality. No aspect of human sexual expression can be fully understood without knowing how it is developed. The family's attitudes, feelings, and values about sexuality are influenced by the surrounding society and culture. Each society and culture determines what is sexual and what is not; what behavior is appropriate or acceptable and what is not. Each society and culture governs in what way each generation will learn the behavior of sex.

A sexual practice that is advocated in one society may be forbidden in another. For instance, sexual activity before marriage is encouraged by some societies and condemned by others. Premarital coitus is permitted by nearly half of the societies of which there is a record of sexual customs.[4] There are no predetermined, universally accepted sexual values or norms; in fact, it is virtually impossible to achieve consensus about sexual values. Each person assimilates family and societal norms and develops his own religious belief system regarding the purpose of sex.

The concept of sexuality refers to the totality of being a person. It includes all those aspects of the human being that relate specifically to being a boy or girl, woman or man, and is an entity subject to life-long dynamic change. Sexuality reflects our human character, not solely our genital nature. As a function of the total personality it is concerned with the biological, psychological, sociological, spiritual, and cultural variables of life which, by their effects on personality development and interpersonal relations, can in turn affect social structure.

Sex Information and Education Council of the U.S., Inc. (SIECUS). "The SIECUS/Upsala Principles Basic to Education for Sexuality." **SIECUS Report**, 1980, 8(3), 8.

Figure 16-2.· SIECUS Definition of Sexuality.

COMPONENTS OF SEXUALITY

To understand sexuality, the interrelated components constituting the totality of the sexual self must be described. These components are **biological sexuality, gender identity, sex role** or **gender role**, and **sexual orientation.**

Biological sexuality refers to the chromosomes, hormones, and primary and secondary sex characteristics that distinguish male from female. Before birth, in the prenatal period, sexual development is controlled mainly by biological forces. Normal sexual development or differentiation begins at the moment of conception. The chromosome pattern from each parent determines whether the gonads will be ovaries or testes. Subsequent genital development of specific physical differences depends on hormones derived from the fetus and the mother. Growth of the testes begins about the sixth week of life after conception. For male sexual differentiation to occur, certain hormones (H-Y antigen and testosterone) must be present in adequate amounts at the right time of development.

Female sexual differentiation does not require hormonal stimulation. The ovaries develop by the twelfth week after conception. Prenatal sex differentiation in both sexes involves the genital, the internal reproductive structures, and probably the brain.[5]

Current research is exploring the effects of fetal hormones on the brain. Some of this research theorizes that the brain is a bi-potential structure; that is, it has the potential to differentiate differently in males under the influence of testosterone. (For a detailed description of the differentiation processes, see the annotated bibliography for suggested readings.)

At puberty there are further physiological changes, as the secondary sex characteristics appear in response to increased hormone levels. Thus, the biological aspects of being male or female are determined by chromosomes, hormones, and internal and external sexual anatomy.

From the moment of birth, biological sex development is influenced by psychosocial factors. When a baby is born, it is declared to be either a boy or a girl. This **gender assignment** based on anatomy will greatly influence how the child is to be reared, because society prescribes different treatment for boys and girls.

Research has indicated that caretakers of babies, particularly parents, treat infant boys and girls differently. For example, during the first six months of life, boys receive more physical contact (being touched, held, nursed) and less nonphysical contact (being looked at and talked to) than girls. Girls are treated as though they were more fragile than boys.[6] The infant and older baby is receptive to and influenced by the input triggered by adult reactions to the baby's sexual anatomy.

As a result of these inputs, each child will develop a **gender identity,** an internal sense of sexual self. Gender identity is a persistent conviction that one is either male or female, an awareness of one's masculinity or femininity. It encompasses much more than genital functioning. The child's gender identity, usually corresponding with his or her genetic makeup and anatomical sex, will be solidified between the ages of 18 months and three years. Positive solid feelings about self are important foundation for the development of future healthy sexuality.*

Gender role or **sex role** is an external or outward expression of one's maleness or femaleness and is a learned behavior. Every society ascribes different roles to

---

*Transsexualism** is a disorder of gender identity. An anatomically normal person believes he or she is a member of the opposite sex and sometimes seeks sex-change surgery to alter his/her genitalia to conform with his/her identity. Currently there is disagreement whether surgery is the optimal treatment for this disorder.

males and females. For example, in American society, boys are often expected to be tough and action-oriented, while girls are expected to be domestic, quieter and refined. Gender roles permeate all human interactions. They affect how one perceives the other person, they allow one to know

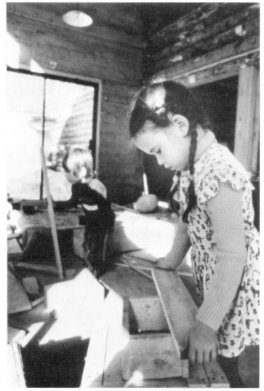

Figure 6-3.   In the past, girls were treated as though they are more fragile than boys.

how to act, and what to expect from other people. Fulfilling gender role expectations can give a feeling of success and competence. Gender roles are probably learned in a variety of ways through the social and psychological mechanisms of **reinforcement, role modeling,** and **socialization.**

From the moment of birth when the infant is identified as a boy or a girl, **reinforcement** is given, by the parents or care givers, to behaviors that society sees as masculine or feminine traits. Through praise or discouragement, parents reinforce girls for what they believe to be feminine behaviors and discourage them from masculine behaviors. Likewise, parents and teachers give positive reinforcement to boys for masculine behaviors and negative reinforcement for feminine behaviors. In American society, it is much more acceptable for a girl to exhibit behaviors that are seen as masculine than is the reverse. Boys are strongly prohibited from exhibiting what are viewed as feminine behaviors.

A second way that children learn gender role behaviors is through imitation or **role modeling.** Children choose the same sex parent as a role model and use these models to form their own behavior.

The third way a child learns role behaviors is through **socialization.** The child observes what goes on about him and then tries to fit his behavior into the norm for the social group. Socialization begins with the parents or care givers, then extends to toys, clothes, television, books and a whole myriad of sources in society. In American society, the overlap between male and female role behaviors has greatly increased in the past 10 years. Many previously considered male role behaviors are being assumed by women, such as head of family, assertiveness, and competitiveness.

In addition, contrary to older views that looked at masculinity and femininity as mutually exclusive opposites, it is now evident that masculine and feminine traits coexist in many people. Males and females are far more similar than different.[7]

Throughout the lifecycle, various components of biological sexual function develop. For example, in infancy and childhood, the sexual reflexes for males and females are all present except for the ability of the male to ejaculate.[8] At puberty, with the increases in sex hormone levels and concomitant development of secondary sex characteristics, sexual orientation comes into full force. The term **sexual orientation** is used to describe an individual's preference for one or several means of expression of sexual thoughts and feelings. Sexual behavior, like all human behavior, is varied, complex, and defies simple classification. Sexual feelings are most commonly expressed in a **heterosexual** relationship between males and females. In most societies, heterosexual behavior is the preferred pattern. Alternate forms of sexual expression include **homosexual** relationships, where sexual satisfaction is obtained in a relationship in which partners are of the same sex. **Bisexuals** choose both the same and opposite sexed partners at various points in time. Some persons may choose to be **celibate,** abstaining from sexual intimacy and intercourse as a temporary or lifelong pattern. For some, solitary sexual behavior, such as **masturbation,** will be a source of sexual gratification. The factors determining sexual orientation are incompletely understood but include some combination of genetics, hormones, and environment. One's sexual orientation is probably established by the age of five to seven years, but is thought to be a dynamic, lifelong process of growth.[9]

Homosexuality, or sexual attraction to the same sex, requires special mention. Within the context of both male and female homosexuality, it is a prevalent, controversial, and poorly understood form of sexual orientation. Attitudes towards homosexuality range from acceptance to condemnation. The causes of homosexuality may include genetic factors, hormonal imbalance, and faulty child-parent relations. There is no firm research evidence for any of these, possibly because there may be different types of homosexuality, each of which originates in a different way.[10] Some persons enter a homosexual relationship because they are strongly attracted to someone of the same sex. Others may enter a homosexual relationship because heterosexual partners are unavailable, out of loneliness or rebellion. Transitory homosexual experiences during adolescence are not uncommon. (See the annotated bibliography for additional references on homosexuality.)

HUMAN SEXUAL RESPONSE

The human sexual response represents an integration of physiological responses with thoughts and feelings within an interpersonal relationship. Masters' and Johnson's[11] work in the area of human sexual response greatly contributed to understanding of the physiological aspects of sexual expression.

Sexual arousal is very individual and can occur in response to a wide variety of stimuli including touch, visual input, and fantasy. Masters and Johnson identified four basic phases of sexual response experienced by both men and women: excitement, plateau, orgasm, and resolution. The **excitement** phase begins with responses to sexual stimulation and is characterized primarily by vasocongestion of the genitals and breasts, vaginal lubrication, and erection of the penis.

The **plateau** is characterized by the maintenance of sexual arousal and the building of excitement toward orgasm.

The **orgasmic** phase is a highly pleasurable reflex characterized by muscle

---

Sex is a part of sexuality; a part of total personality.

All people are sexual from birth to death.

All people have the right to facts about sex and sexuality.

Sexual behavior will vary greatly from one person to another and in the same person over time. A wide range of sexual behavior is normal.

Because sex is a natural function, guilt need not be associated with sexual thoughts and feelings. Sexual feelings and fantasies are normal. All people experience them.

Health professionals can help clients deal with sexual concerns if the professionals are comfortable with their own feelings and values about sexuality.

Figure 16-4.   Basic Assumptions About Sexuality.

spasms and accompanied by ejaculation in the male.

The **resolution** phase is characterized by a gradual return to the preexcitement phase. A **refractory** period in males occurs immediately after orgasm during which ejaculation is impossible, but women have the capacity to be multiorgasmic.

THE NURSING PROCESS

As a basic human need, sexuality is one of the essential dimensions of holistic health care. Nurses are recognizing sexual integrity as an integral part of a client's health and well-being as well as recognizing the impact of illness on sexual functioning. Nurses encounter many clients whose sexuality is threatened by disease, trauma, surgical intervention, situational or maturational crises, or psychological problems. The resulting alterations in self-concept, changes in body image, and inability to meet role expectations are significant areas of concern.

Many nurses believe they have a responsibility for promoting sexual health in their professional practice. To be effective in helping people with sexual concerns, nurses must:

1. confront feelings, values, and attitudes of sexuality in themselves and in those differing in sexual orientation and practices;

2. develop a sound and comprehensive body of knowledge about sexuality; and

3. develop assessment, intervention, and communication skills in all aspects of health.[12]

Much personal and professional effort is necessary to develop these skills. However, it is appropriate for the beginning nurse to begin to develop sophistication in each of these areas.

A clinician who has achieved a healthy attitude toward his own sexuality can deal most effectively with the client's sexuality. Sexuality is an area to which many people attach strong emotions, religious ideas, and rigid opinions. Sexual attitudes, values, and behaviors that are acceptable to one person may be repulsive to another. There is no consensus about sexual values in our society. The nurse must be able to clarify and acknowledge her own feelings, attitudes, and opinions about sexual issues as well as developing a value free attitude toward sexual practices. In identifying the effect of her attitudes and values on her nursing practice, she does not have to give up her own moral standards. Her goal is to develop an atmosphere of acceptance and respect for the rights of individuals to self-determination.

For instance, attitudes of nurses and medical staff toward homosexuals or transsexuals may be negative (e.g., the focus of jokes). Negative staff feelings may compromise the health care they offer these individuals. These patients are often struggling for acceptance as persons and deserve to be treated with the same dignity and respect as heterosexual individuals.

Assessment of one's own attitudes is a time consuming but invaluable process. One can begin by listing topics related to sexuality (such as male and female anatomy, intercourse, masturbation, homosexuality) and then record how one feels about each topic. Discussing feelings about sexuality in small groups guided by an experienced professional can contribute not only to clearer identification of feelings, but increased comfort in discussing emotionally laden topics. Courses in human sexuality often focus on desensitization to sexual topics. In helping people with sexual concerns and questions, the single most important factor is the ease and comfort of the professional in discussing sensitive and value laden topics.

Sexuality and Illness

There is increasingly widespread recognition that there is a reciprocal relationship between most medical illnesses and an individual's sexual functioning. Illness may cause changes in one's self-concept, role, sense of self as a man or woman, as well as physical ability to function. It is known that over 50 chronic illnesses and surgical conditions adversely affect sexuality,[13] and that their medication, plus the depression, stress, and fatigue that are often a part of chronic illness also can affect sexual functioning.[14] For instance, diabetes has a potentially destructive effect on sexual function. Some prostatectomy procedures destroy or interfere with normal sexual response. Many medications used to treat hypertension interfere with sexual function.

Transient disinterest or lack of desire in sexual activity occurs in most persons when they are preoccupied with the symptoms of illness. Sexual problems often disappear when the illness improves. The fear that sexual behavior may cause or aggravate existing physical illness is common in patients. For example, although a myocardial infarct has no direct effect on sexual response, many male post-myocardial infarction (MI) clients are unable to achieve an erection. The client fears that sexual activity will cause another attack or that sex will be "weakening." Fear may last long after recovery—and this fear may be experienced by both partners.

Effects of Hospitalization

Hogan states that admission to the hospital, physical exams, and diagnostic procedures may be more disturbing to the individual's sexual integrity than the disease itself. Hospitalized individuals are separated from significant others and stripped of their identity by removal of accustomed clothing, jewelry, and personal possessions.[15] Assessments and treatments such as rectal temperatures and pelvic exams may be perceived as intrusive. Questions focus on areas that have been considered private and that may be embarrassing to discuss. Invasion of one's privacy and violation of one's territory might surely be viewed as threats to one's sexual integrity. For instance, women often have feelings about a pelvic examination such as fear of the procedure, embarrassment, concerns about normalcy. Nurses can be a positive influence here. They can use knowledge and sensitivity to create an atmosphere of caring and consideration. Explaining the procedure, providing verbal support, and answering questions can contribute to maintaining the patient's sense of self.

Patients react to illness and hospitalization in various ways—some with **overt sexual behavior.** Sexual behavior within the hospital setting may be the expression of a variety of needs, such as the need to reaffirm one's sexual identity, to express sexual feelings, to affirm one's ability to function sexually, or to control the situation.

Most patients will conduct sexual behavior privately, but there are times when staff members are confronted with a patient's sexual behavior. This may be embarrassing and anxiety-producing for nurses. Health care professionals sometimes respond by ignoring the behavior, humiliating the patient, punishing the patient, becoming angry, or avoiding further contact with the patient. Instead, the nurses need to look at the meaning of the patient's behavior as a basis for choosing the response most therapeutic for the patient. The way nurses respond will be dependent on their knowledge of sexuality and comfort with sexual issues. They may see the patient as asexual, or not having sexual needs because of age or illness. They may see the patient as not having a right or need to express his sexuality. For instance, it is sometimes assumed that sexuality is not a concern for older people, especially in nursing home settings. For an older person to exhibit interest in sex is often considered perverse or pathological. Interest in sex, despite age or illness, is a component of health throughout the lifecycle and is a positive, vitalizing force.

In providing care, nurses have the responsibility to help the individual maintain a positive sense of self and sexual integrity within the limits of the patient's particular capacity. Nurses can accomplish these objectives by avoiding practices that contribute to shame, by helping to ameliorate guilt related to sexuality, and by providing privacy.

Overt Sexual Behaviors

There are several overt sexual behaviors that commonly occur in health care settings. **Erections** often occur spontaneously in men and are not under conscious control. An erection occurs when arterial blood rushes into the body of the penis. Erections are of two types—psychogenic and reflexogenic. Psychogenic erections can be triggered by fantasies, thoughts, and memories. Reflexogenic erections are stimulated by tactile stimulation of the penis or genital area or by a full bladder. By giving the patient a few minutes warning before any procedure involving exposure of the genital area, the nurse can usually avoid confronting erections. The nurse can respond to the presence of an erection by ignoring it or by acknowledging the patient's sexuality by saying, "It looks like it's frustrating to be in the hospital!"

Masturbation or self-stimulation is a normal part of sexual maturation and behavior. It can be a healthy outlet for sexual drives, an alternate method for experiencing sexual release. Masturbation is especially significant for the hospitalized individual who does not have access to a sexual partner. It can also serve to reduce anxiety. It is the responsibility of health care personnel to provide privacy for patients. Allowing predictable times during which they can enjoy solitude, drawing curtains, closing doors, knocking on doors before entering show respect for the patient and contribute to privacy.

Masturbation can also be used in a dysfunctional way if it is conducted publicly without respect for the rights of others. The possible meanings of this type of behavior are to draw attention, to express hostility, or to embarrass the staff. If the nurse encounters this type of behavior, she should confront the behavior and request that the patient seek privacy for masturbation.

Certainly, the need for **sexual interaction** is normal, and the hospital setting is not conducive to intimacy. The nurse needs to be sensitive to patients' sexual needs, help them gain privacy, yet ensure that the rights of other patients are protected. If the nurse encounters a patient and partner engaging in sex, her response might be, "Pardon me, I didn't realize you had company. I'll close the door."

Seductive or sexual acting-out, such as sexual overtures, compliments, sexual jokes, exhibiting one's genitals, provacative suggestions, attempts to touch the nurse and bragging about sexual capabilities may be directed at the nurse. Both male and female nurses may become objects of seductive behavior by patients of the opposite sex. Again, the nurse must kindly but firmly set limits on the behavior. Reject the behavior, but not the person. Sometimes a sense of humor is helpful. The nurse must attempt to understand the meaning of the behavior as an expression of an underlying need. The patient may doubt his attractiveness and consider the nurse a safe person on whom he can test his desirability. It is possible that the nurse may have been provocative or have given mixed messages about her own needs. Nurses are sexual people, too, but they must make their role clear without reacting negatively to the patient or humiliating him.

Promoting sexual integrity for the patient is a complex task, especially for the beginning nurse. By discussing experiences one has had with patients who were sexually acting out, one can master feelings and understand the needs underlying the patient's behavior. In this way, the nurse can devise more effective strategies for future interactions with patients.

Skills in assessing, interviewing, teaching, and counseling are needed if the nurse is to become able to promote sexual health. Nurses must become sensitive in recognizing sexual concerns and problems in clients. Establishing a therapeutic atmosphere is a first step.

Despite increasing openness in American society about sexual matters, a patient will seldom initiate discussion of a sexual concern. He may not wish to reveal his ignorance, feel guilty about having a problem, be uncertain how to state the concern, or fear being viewed by the staff as overinterested in sex. Sexuality is an area of self that needs to be treated with discretion, but the secrecy and taboos related to sexuality have often led to shame and guilt. Health care professionals, through their own openness, help to change this atmosphere. It is the nurse's responsibility to provide a climate in which the patient feels comfortable expressing sexual concern. The nurse needs to give the patient permission to discuss such concerns. This can be done indirectly in several ways. The nurse can bring up the topic of sex by saying, "Many patients with your condition note changes in their sexual feelings. How about you?" Or the nurse can give reading material that includes information on sexual activity to the patient. When the patient has read the material, the nurse can discuss questions and concerns related to the patient's situation. Once the nurse has sanctioned the topic of sexuality, the patient will be much more likely to express sexual concerns. The nurse can assess whether the patient has correct information or misconceptions about sexuality and especially about the effects of his illness on sexual function. She can listen for nonverbal cues of sexual problems. For example, telling sexual jokes, bragging about sexual prowess, or exhibiting one's genitals may be clues about underlying concerns the patient may have.

Sexual Dysfunctions

Sexual dysfunctions are conditions in which the ordinary physical responses of sexual function are impaired. Women can experience problems in getting aroused and maintaining arousal as well as having difficulty in reaching orgasm. Men can have difficulty getting or maintaining an erection, ejaculating too quickly, or difficulty in ejaculating. Sexual dysfunctions most often have psychological or relational causes (such as fear of failure or marital conflict), but about 10 to 20 percent have an organic cause such as diabetes, neurological disease, alcohol, or prescription medications.[16] When confronted with a client's expressed anxieties and concerns, the nurse can gather data as the basis of a referral to a sex counselor or therapist. Because of the possibility of an organic cause of the dysfunction, it is imperative that the client have a thorough medical evaluation.

Assessment

Assessment of patients' sexual health can be ascertained as early as admission to the hospital. The scope of sexual assessment will be dictated by the professional's preparation and experience as well as by the patient's health situation. Sexual health assessment is a legitimate concern of the health professional and is the first step for the health care team in meeting its responsibilities for maintaining the patient's sexual integrity.

Sexual health assessment requires greater skill than any other interview. If the nurse is ill at ease, this discomfort will be conveyed to the client. A sexual health assessment should be part of every routine history. Including a sex history early in the nurse/client relationship communicates to the client the nurse's appreciation of the importance of sexual health and her comfort in discussing these health needs. Whether or not the initial assessment elicits problem areas is insignificant. Perhaps none exists, or perhaps it will take time for the client to develop sufficient comfort and trust to confide a longstanding problem. When a problem does arise, the client will seek out the nurse as someone in whom to confide.

Several strategies can be used to facilitate obtaining a sexual health assessment:

- Provide privacy while conducting the assessment; ensure confidentiality.

- Prepare client for the assessment with an introductory statement by briefly explaining the purpose of the interview. "To plan care for your health needs, I am going to ask you for information. You may find some of the questions personal, but these are issues about which patients often have questions or concerns."

- Ask questions in an open ended manner that helps the client to explain their situation rather than merely answer "yes" or "no." "Many people, after an operation (illness, accident) like yours, have concerns about their sexuality. What are your concerns?"

- Allow the client to refuse to answer. "You seem reluctant (anxious, embarrassed) about answering that question. Would you prefer I bring it up later?"

- Give the client a chance to ask questions. "What questions about sexual health would you like answered?"

Woods suggests three broad questions that can be asked to assess the effect or potential effect of illness or hospitalization on self as a sexual being, and on the individual's ability to function sexually:

- "What about your illness (surgery, accident, pregnancy), has it interfered with your being a (mother, wife, father, husband)?"

- "Has anything (for example, heart attack) changed the way you feel about yourself as a man (woman)?"

- "What about your illness (surgery, accident, pregnancy), has it changed your ability to function sexually?"[17]

By including questions related to sexuality

Variables Affecting Nurse's Ability to Deal Effectively with Patient's Sexual Concerns	Responsibilities of Health Care Team for Maintaining Sexual Integrity of the Patient	Desired Patient Outcomes
Comfort level in discussing sexual concerns.	Anticipating potential sexual problems.	Client feels free to verbalize sexual concerns.
Knowledge level about concepts related to sexuality.	Preventing problems from developing.	Client understands effect of illness on sexual behavior.
Awareness of own sexual value system.	Validating normalcy.	Client maintains a positive sense of self.
Ability to perceive the underlying meaning and needs expressed by the patient's behavior.	Offering early treatment for problems that develop.	Client functions sexually to the limits of his particular capacity.
Interpersonal skills, such as communication, interviewing, and teaching techniques.	Seeking consultation or offering referral for problems beyond the expertise of the health care team.	

Figure 16-5.   Nursing Variables Fostering Client Sexual Integrity.

ASSESSMENT Data	NURSING DIAGNOSIS Problem and its probable cause	GOAL	PLAN AND INTERVENTION	OUTCOME CRITERIA Evaluation
Parental fear that sex education in the schools will cause promiscuity in their teen-age children	Fear secondary to lack of information	Client feels free to verbalize sexual concerns and values Client has accurate information	Provide opportunity for discussion of concerns about sex education Involve parents in planning of sex education program Validate normalcy of adolescents' interest in sexuality	Parents understand that increased knowledge of sexuality does not cause promiscuity Parents feel free to verbalize additional concerns about sexuality
Belief that hysterectomy (removal of the uterus) will cause loss of sexual desire	Sexual misinformation secondary to lack of information	Client understanding of effect of hysterectomy on sexual desire Prevent sexual problems from developing	Anticipatory guidance: Provide accurate information preoperatively Offer reading materials on hysterectomy Give permission to discuss sexual concerns	Client understands that hysterectomy will have no effect on sexual desire Client aware of source of accurate information on sexuality

Figure 16-6. Nursing Care Plans

on the health history, the nurse conveys the message that sexuality is a matter of legitimate concern and that sexuality is a topic she is comfortable discussing. It also provides an opportunity to provide education and to dispel myths and misinformation. Nursing diagnoses are formulated at the end of the assessment phase of the nursing process. Examples of these can be found in Figure 16-6.

Implementation

Education and counseling are the prime interventions that promote sexual integrity. The assessment process is, by its nature, a positive force toward health and can be considered to have the effect of an **intervention.** The nurse's comfort level in discussing sexual matters will encourage and facilitate clients' discussion of their own sexual problems and concerns, and this openness will contribute to self-understanding and enhancement of sexual integrity.

Secondly, clients frequently approach professionals to find out if what they are experiencing is acceptable or normal. By validating the normalcy of a particular practice, the nurse is contributing to problem prevention. Providing anticipatory guidance is another intervention useful in promoting sexual health. This involves providing the client with information about what to expect. For example, the nurse can provide a middle-aged woman with information about predictable physiological and emotional changes related to menopause or reassure a hospitalized patient that loss of interest in sex after surgery is a normal but transient feeling.

Evaluation

Evaluation completes the nursing process. The nurse establishes whether or not her interventions have been successful. In conclusion, according to her knowledge base, the nurse can provide accurate infor-

mation and dispel myths and misconceptions. As a member of the health care team, she can anticipate potential sexual problems and, through education and counseling, prevent some problems from developing. The nurse needs to have referral sources for interventions beyond her ability. As with any skill, practice is needed for proficiency in sexual history taking, education, and counseling.

SUMMARY

Sexuality is a function of the total personality. It is a lifelong process that has many variations.

The concept of sexuality, a function of the total personality, is concerned with the biological, psychological, sociological, spiritual, and cultural aspects of life. The interrelated components constituting the totality of the sexual self are biological sexuality, gender identity, sex role, sexual orientation, and sexual response.

Sexual behavior is varied; each person has a right to his own values and beliefs about sexuality.

Sexuality is an essential dimension of health care, and nurses have a role in promoting sexual integrity in their clients. By becoming comfortable with their own feelings and values about sexuality, health professionals can more effectively help clients deal with sexual concerns. A sound and comprehensive body of knowledge about sexuality is essential for the care giver.

The nurse's ability to use the nursing process effectively in caring for patients with sexual concerns will depend on her preparation, level of self-awareness, and ability to communicate effectively through listening, eliciting feelings, acceptance, and problem solving. Mastery of these interpersonal skills will enable the nurse to create a comfortable atmosphere in which the patient can express concerns.

In providing care, nurses have the responsibility to help the individual maintain a positive sense of self and sexual integrity within the limits of the patients capacity.

STUDY QUESTIONS

1. What is the role of the family in determining the child's sexual identity and sex role?

2. Who was your most important role model when you were a child? When you were a teenager?

3. Differentiate between sex, sexuality, sexual identity, and sexual orientation.

4. For you, what is the meaning of touching? of companionship? of intimacy?

5. What is the relationship between human sexuality and nursing?

6. Whose responsibility is it to talk with patients about sexual concerns?

7. What are some of the reasons health professionals are reluctant to talk with patients about sexuality?

8. What are some nonverbal cues of sexually related problems a patient may express?

REFERENCES

1. Alfred Kinsey, Wardell Pomeroy, Clyde Martin, and Paul Gebhard, **Sexual Behavior in the Human Male.** (Philadelphia: Saunders, 1948).
2. Nancy F. Woods, **Human Sexuality in Health and Illness.** (St. Louis: C.V. Mosby, 1974).
3. Warren Gadpaille, **The Cycles of Sex.** (New York: Charles Scribner's Sons, 1975), p.3.
4. Frank A. Beach, ed. **Human Sexuality in Four Perspectives.** (Baltimore: The Johns Hopkins University Press, 1977), pp.115–163.
5. William Masters, Virginia Johnson, and Robert Kolodny. **Human Sexuality,** (Boston: Little Brown, 1982), pp.152–155.
6. Eleanor Maccoby and Carol Jacklin, **The Psychology of Sex Differences.** (Stanford, CA: Stanford University Press, 1974), p.309.
7. Masters, Johnson, and Kolodny, p.224.
8. Masters, Johnson, and Kolodny, pp.152–173.
9. Robert C. Francouer, **Becoming a Sexual Person.** (New York: John Wiley and Sons, 1982), pp.512–513.
10. Masters, Johnson, and Kolodny, pp.315–339.
11. William Masters and Virginia Johnson, **Human Sexual Response.** (Boston: Little Brown, 1966).
12. Fern H. Mims and Melinda Swenson, **Sexuality: A Nursing Perspective.** (New York: McGraw-Hill Book Co., 1980), p.4.
13. Helen S. Kaplan, **The New Sex Therapy.** (New York: Bruner/Mazel, 1975), pp.75–103.
14. Gadpaille, pp.427–433.
15. Rosemary Hogan, **Human Sexuality, A Nursing Perspective.** (New York: Appleton-Century-Crofts, 1980), p.297.
16. Masters, Johnson, and Kolodny, pp.399–404.
17. Nancy F. Woods, **Human Sexuality in Health and Illness,** 2nd ed. (St. Louis: C.V. Mosby Co., 1979), pp.79.

ANNOTATED BIBLIOGRAPHY

Beach F (ed): **Human Sexuality in Four Perspectives.** Baltimore, The Johns Hopkins University Press, 1977. An outstanding discussion of cultural variance in sexual matters.

Boston Women's Health Collective: **Women, Our Bodies, Our Selves.** New York, Simon and Schuster, 1979. A book by and for women about how women feel about their sexuality.

Francoeur RT: **Becoming a Sexual Person.** New York, John Wiley and Sons, 1982. A comprehensive textbook on human sexuality with a strong emphasis on self-health, cultural influences, and values. Extensive information on gender differentiation, contraception, sexually transmitted disease, and the quest for intimacy.

Gadpaille W: **The Cycles of Sex.** New York, Charles Scribner's and Sons, 1975. Detailed portrayal of each of the developmental phases of normal psycho-sexual development.

Hogan R: **Human Sexuality, A Nursing Perspective.** New York, Appleton-Century-Crofts, 1980. Coverage of biological, psychological, and sociocultural aspects of sexuality in health and illness with emphasis on the nurse's role in promoting and maintaining sexual health. Good chapters on effects of illness/hospitalization on sexuality, and sexual problems throughout the life cycle.

Kaplan HS: **The New Sex Therapy.** New York, Brunner/Mazel, 1975. A detailed handbook on sex therapy.

Kinsey AC, Pomeroy WB, Martin CE, Gebhard PH: **Sexual Behavior in the Human Male.** Philadelphia, Saunders, 1948. A classic statistical survey of the varieties of male sexual behavior.

Maccoby E, Jacklin C: **The Psychology of Sex Differences.** Stanford, Stanford University Press, 1974. The definitive work on this topic. Tough reading, but exhaustive in coverage.

Masters WH, Johnson VE: **Human Sexual Response.** Boston, Little, Brown and Co.,

1966. A classic work on this topic. Difficult reading.

Masters, WH, Johnson VE, Kolodny RC: **Human Sexuality.** Boston, Little, Brown and Co., 1982. Comprehensive coverage of the field of human sexuality written in an interesting and lively manner. Striking art work. Especially good coverage of gender identity, sex roles, homosexuality, bisexuality, fantasy, sexual assault, and contraception.

Mims FH, Swenson M: **Sexuality: A Nursing Perspective.** New York, McGraw-Hill Book Co., 1980. An excellent, concise text on promotion of sexual health with focus on prevention and health maintenance and care of individuals with acute, chronic, or terminal illnessess affecting sexual health. Especially good chapters on drugs affecting sexuality, sexuality and dying, and taking a sexual history.

Morison E, Price M. **Values in Sexuality.** New York, Hart Publishing Co., Inc., 1974. A collection of group exercises, games, and role playing suggestions useful in values clarification and in increasing the comfort level in discussing sexuality.

Moses AE, Hawkins R: **Counseling Gay Men and Women.** St. Louis, C.V. Mosby Co., 1982. Coverage of many of the aspects of being homosexual in American culture with specific information on counseling approaches.

Woods NF: **Human Sexuality in Health and Illness,** 2nd ed. St. Louis, C.V. Mosby Co., 1979. An excellent text with emphasis on sexual health, health care, and clinical aspects of human sexuality. Good chapters on assessment of sexual health, roles for professional nurses in sexual health care delivery, fertility and infertility, and sexual assault.

17

Pain

Marion R. Johnson
Joann M. Eland

CHAPTER OUTLINE

OBJECTIVES

After reading this chapter, the reader will be able to:

- Discuss the concept of pain and relate it to the gate-control theory of pain.
- Describe differences in types of pain: acute, chronic, and progressive.
- Identify variables that may alter the perception of and response to pain.
- Describe physiological and psychological responses to pain and relate them to types of pain.
- Apply pain assessment techniques to a patient situation.
- Discuss factors to be considered in selecting a nursing intervention for the patient experiencing pain.
- Describe a process that may be used in relaxation and in distraction of patients who are experiencing pain.
- Identify how various types of analgesics may be used most effectively in pain control.
- Discuss the use of placebos in pain control.
- Identify behavioral outcomes that may be used to evaluate pain control.

GLOSSARY

Analgesic—medication used for the purpose of pain relief.

Pain reaction—multiplicity of events or responses set up by a pain sensation.

Pain sensation—recognition of perception of pain.

Pain threshold—the lowest stimulus value at which pain sensation is reported.

Placebo—an inactive substance used as an analgesic reaction.

INTRODUCTION

Pain is a symptom commonly encountered in individuals seeking health care, and it is, therefore, an important concept for nursing. The person with pain may be encountered in any clinical area and in any health care setting. Nurses are often responsible for pain assessment and alleviation on a continuous basis. Because of the frequency with which the nurse encounters persons with pain, it is necessary to develop skills to assist the person experiencing pain.

What is pain? A warning, a sensation, a perception? Despite intensive study and research during the last decades, a concrete definition of pain, acceptable to all disciplines, has not been formulated. Richard Sternbach has defined pain as an "abstract concept which refers to (1) a personal, private sensation of hurt; (2) a harmful stimulus which signals current or

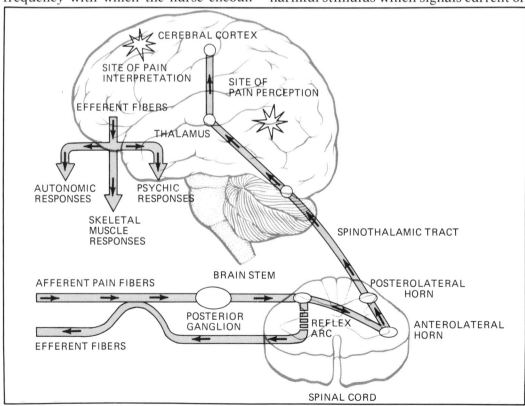

Figure 17-1. Specificity Theory of Pain

impending tissue damage; (3) a pattern of responses which operate to protect the organism from harm."[1] Although this definition separates components of pain for the purpose of clarification and research, it must be recognized that these components overlap or occur simultaneously in the pain experience. Margo McCaffery's definition of pain is perhaps the most useful to the practicing nurse; she defines pain as "whatever the person says it is, existing whenever he says it does."[2] This definition of pain requires nurses to approach the pain experience from the perspective of the suffering individual.

PAIN THEORIES

Many theories regarding the actual pain mechanism have been proposed. Three of the more popular are the specificity, pattern, and gate-control theories. The **specificity theory** is perhaps the most traditional of the three (See Figure 17-1). It proposes that there is a specific pain modality that can be stimulated only by pain and perceived as pain. The impulses are picked up by undifferentiated free nerve endings and carried by peripheral nerves to the spinal cord and then transmitted to the pain center in the thalamus. Those opposing this

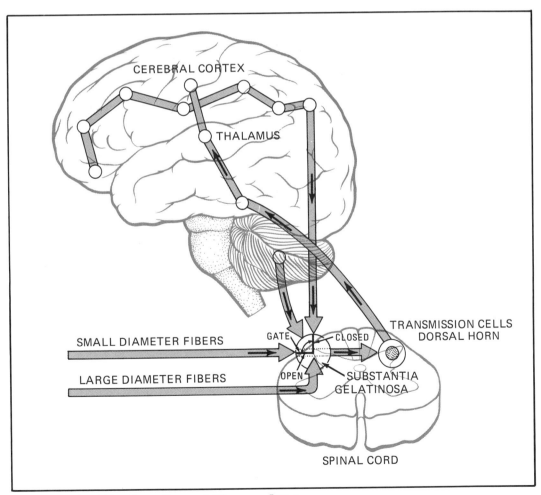

Figure 17-2.   The Gate-Control Theory of Pain

theory have taken issue with its failure to explain why the same stimulus presented to two different people is not always felt as pain.[3]

Pattern theory evolved from specificity theory and includes several slightly different theories. All of the pattern theories agree that the patterning of nerve impulses generated by the receptors forms the basis of a code that provides the information that there is pain.[4]

In 1965, Melzack and Wall proposed what is now the most commonly accepted theory of the pain mechanism, the gate-control theory.[5] The **gate-control theory** suggests that there is a gating mechanism (See Figure 17-2) in the dorsal horn of the spinal cord that can increase or decrease the flow of nerve impulses from peripheral fibers to the central nervous system. This gating mechanism is influenced by the activities of the larger-diameter A-Beta, smaller-diameter A-Delta and C fibers, and by descending influences from the brain. The small-diameter afferent fibers (A-Delta and C) conduct excitatory pain signals. Stimulation of the large-diameter cutaneous afferent fibers (A-Beta) inhibits the transmission of pain impulses. Both the small- and large-diameter fibers terminate in the dorsal horn of the spinal cord in an area known as the substantia gelatinosa (the gate and T-cell). The spinal gating mechanism also is influenced by nerve impulses that descend from the brain.

A specialized system of large diameter fibers rapidly conducts impulses directly to the brain, activating selective cognitive processes that can influence the gating mechanisms by the descending fibers. This specialized system explains how an individual's past and present experiences influence current pain responses. The T-cell within the substantia gelatinosa acts as a calculator to sum information from the small fibers, the large fibers (A-Beta), and the descending fibers. When the excitatory input from the small fibers outnumbers input from the inhibitory (A-Beta) and descending fibers, the T-cell "opens" the gate and allows information about pain to be transmitted to the brain. These messages are transmitted via the *neospinothalmic system* and the *paramedial ascending system*. (For further information consult a physiology text.)

The paramedial ascending fibers and neospinothalmic system enter the thalamus, which is a major relay system. Within the context of pain, its function can be compared to a major telephone switchboard where thousands of messages are routed to specific destinations. Messages from paramedial ascending fibers are routed to reticular and limbic structures and then processed by the cerebrum. The reticular and limbic structures produce the *unpleasant affective quality* associated with pain, activate the stress response, and motivate the organism to stop pain. Sensory discriminatory messages are routed directly to the cerebrum. The cerebrum and thalamus together are called the *central control* center by Melzack and Wall.

Central control processes information from three sources: sensory discrimination information; motivational affective information, the body's fight or flight response; and cognitive information including such things as past experiences and response alternatives.[6]

Each person has cataloged, in central control, a variety of previous experiences involving pain as well as a number of intervening variables in the pain response, such as age, sex, socioeconomic status, race, and ethnic group expectations. Because pain stimuli are processed within each individual's own context, a wide variety of pain responses is seen.

THE NATURE AND TYPES OF PAIN

Although agreement on definitions and theories of pain is not presently available in the literature, some attributes of the pain experience are more consistently described than others. Pain **threshold** identifies the lowest stimulus value at which the sensation of pain is reported, while pain **tolerance** identifies the maximum level of sensory stimulus one is willing to tolerate.[7] The difference between pain threshold and pain tolerance may be referred to as the **sensitivity range.**[8] Research has shown the pain threshold to be relatively constant, providing the central nervous system is intact, while significant variations occur in pain tolerance. Pain threshold depends on physiological factors, whereas pain tolerance depends on psychological and social factors.[9] It is also important to note that pain tolerance may vary in the same individual in differing circumstances. For example, an individual may be less aware of, or more willing to tolerate muscle spasm while involved in competitive sports than while recovering from an appendectomy. Studies of pain tolerance have significance to the nurse, since efforts to alter the pain experience will often be directed at altering the pain tolerance level rather than the pain threshold level.

Researchers usually distinguish between the pain sensation and pain reaction. **Sensation** is the recognition or perception of pain and could be equated with the pain threshold. **Reaction** is the events or responses set up by the original sensation. This term may be used to include only the mental processing. The typical pain response seems designed to protect the individual from further harm and may consist of automatic behaviors and responses learned as methods of coping with pain. The pain response will be affected by:

- the integrity of the central nervous system
- the level of consciousness
- previous experience with pain
- learned coping mechanisms

- attention and distraction
- fatigue
- emotions.[10]

The pain sensation cannot be observed but must be reported by the subject; the reaction will be observable as the behaviors elicited by the pain stimulation. Both sensation and reaction are evaluated during a clinical assessment of pain.

A very simplified example of the components in a common pain experience may clarify the concepts. Slamming one's finger in a door causes two distinct sensations in most individuals—a sharp, quick pain followed by a throbbing or dull ache. This is the basic sensory component and will be quite consistent with most people. What the individual does—his verbal expression of pain as well as motor behaviors, such as squeezing the finger—can be considered indicative of the reaction component. Even with such a simple pain, we might observe different verbal motor responses; this helps us appreciate the variety of responses that can occur with more complex pain experiences. What the individual feels and the degree of hurt experienced is the personal, subjective aspect of pain that can be shared only through verbal communication and only imperfectly, because of the constraints imposed by language.

Pain is often labeled as psychogenic or organic, depending on whether a physiological cause for the pain can be determined. There is a tendency to treat organic pain as "real" pain and psychogenic pain as "imaginary" pain; this dichotomy carries the implication that suffering does not occur without demonstrable pathology. A more accurate and fruitful approach is to view pain as a continuum in which physiological and psychological factors play greater or lesser roles depending on whether the pain is triggered by a mental or physical stimulus. Psychological factors may cause pain or augment its severity. Three psychological mechanisms that may precipitate or increase pain are:

- the occurrence of pain as a hallucination in conjunction with schizophrenia or endogenous depression
- pain due to muscle tension, vascular distention, or other physical changes caused by psychological factors
- pain associated with conversion hysteria.[11]

Anxiety may intensify pain, and anxiety may need to be controlled if pain relief is to be obtained. Determining the degree to which psychological factors are important is a necessary requisite for determining the method of treatment that will prove most successful.

The type of tissue or organ that is the source of pain may determine aspects of the sensory characteristics of pain. Three distinctive sources of pain are cutaneous, deep somatic, and visceral. **Cutaneous or superficial pain** generally is well localized and may occur along dermal segments. **Deep somatic pain** may be more diffuse, may be felt as three-dimensional, and may be referred to other deep tissues. **Visceral pain** tends to be diffuse but may localize if pain continues. It may be accompanied by symptoms of autonomic stimulation and by pain and tenderness referred to the body surface in locations adjacent to or removed from the affected organ. The quality and chronology of the pain also may be determined to some extent by the source of the pain. Characteristics of pain that may be related to the pain source can be identified.

Pain of neurological origin is not well understood, and acceptable models for

Source	Location	Intensity	Quality	Associated Factors
Superficial	Surface; well localized	Correlates with intensity of the stimulus; sharp, cutting, boring	Described in terms of familiar surface injuries; sharp, cutting	May be intensified by contact; may protect area
Somatic	Deep; poorly localized. May radiate or be segmental; may be referred to body surface	May be mild to severe; correlates with stimulus. May be increased by muscle spasm	Vague, aching, boring, pounding, sharp, or cutting	Intensified by movement; may move awkwardly to prevent pain
Visceral	Deep; poorly localized. May radiate or be referred	Varies; may be mild to severe. Intensity may not remain stable	Gripping, cramping, aching, burning, stabbing. May be vague; an ache or soreness	May be intensified by motor activity or by compression of involved organ. May have found factors that relieve pain
Neurogenic	Follows neural distribution; may be on surface or deep; may radiate	Usually intense; does not necessarily correlate with stimulus	May be combination of painful sensations; difficult to describe. Burning, stinging, stabbing	Provoked by minor stimulation; guarding and protection of area is prominent

Adapted from Engel GG: Pain in MacBryde CM, Backlow RS (eds): *Signs and Symptoms* Philadelphia J.B. Lippincott Company; 1970

Figure 17-3.   Characteristics in Relation to Pain Source.

such pain are not available. The term **central pain** traditionally has been used to describe pain arising from the brain and spinal cord; however, it more recently has been enlarged by some authors, to include pain arising from within the central nervous system, regardless of the location. Central pain may be described as episodic or constant.[12] Central pain is usually experienced as intense pain and may be accompanied by a variety of sensations, such as cold, burning, itching, and tingling. Phantom limb pain is an example of central pain, which may be constant or cyclic in nature. It is frequently described as twisting, cramping, or shooting, and occurs in the vicinity of an absent body part.[13] Melzack identifies four characteristics of phantom pain that also might be used to describe central pain.[14] These are: pain endures after healing and may persist for years, pain may be caused by the stimulation of trigger zones, phantom pain is more common in cases where pain existed prior

to amputation, and pain may be decreased or abolished by changes in somatic input.

The nature of pain cannot be adequately described without considering a model of pain as related to pain chronology and duration. A model helpful in describing acute and chronic pain differentiates chronic pain as progressive or long-term. **Progressive pain** is frequently found in pathological conditions that progress over time and ultimately end in the patient's death. Long-term pain occurs in pathological conditions that may remain stable or progress but are not of themselves terminal. Long-term pain also may occur when no known pathological cause can be identified, for example, some cases of low back pain. The model relied on most frequently in health-care settings is that of **acute pain,** and certainly many of the pain experiences encountered in a hospital setting fall into this category—incisional pain, renal colic, labor pains. Individuals experiencing chronic pain are not immune from hospitaliza-

FACTORS	TYPE OF PAIN		
	ACUTE	*CHRONIC*	*PROGRESSIVE*
Duration	Minutes--->Weeks.	Weeks--->Lifetime.	Until death, remissions may occur.
Cause and treatment	Known and treatable.	May be unknown or untreatable or both.	Usually known but may be difficult to treat.
Intensity	Moderate--->Severe.	Low--->Moderate Severe episodes may occur.	Low--->Moderate Severe episodes may occur.
Function	Warning.	No useful function.	May warn of change.
Related emotional component	Anxiety.	Depression.	May vary.
Interference with activities	Temporary.	Indefinite.	Varies with remissions.
Social acceptance of pain behaviors	Acceptable, no stigma.	Not acceptable, stigma attached.	Acceptable.
Adaptation	No change, temporary.	May lead to decreased self-esteem. Requires behavior modification.	May be associated with fear of greater pain. Requires some behavior modification.

Figure 17-4. Pain Model Relating Characteristics to Duration.

tion, and the characteristics that differentiate acute and chronic pain must be recognized.

Physiological signs that result from autonomic stimulation in acute pain do not occur with chronic pain. The body cannot sustain changes in blood pressure, pulse, and other physical symptoms that may occur with acute pain over prolonged periods without resulting in physical harm to the body. Thus, physical symptoms are absent or sharply modified in chronic pain. Many persons also adapt to chronic pain by eliminating behaviors normally associated with pain. One of the goals of a pain treatment center may be to decrease pain behaviors while increasing participation in daily activities. Individuals may learn coping mechanisms that allow them to increase their control over pain behaviors. These mechanisms may vary from increased activity as a method of distraction to sustained periods of quiet and meditation. An awareness of the potential differences in expression of acute and chronic pain is of importance to the nurse in assessing and evaluating pain; it emphasizes the need to rely upon the individual's report of pain.

Chronic pain may wear many faces, but whatever else, it becomes a constant companion, to be controlled if possible, but always to be lived with. It imposes stress on the individual and can become the most debilitating and potentially destructive force in a person's life. Mental and physical resources of the individual may be drained as energy is focused on the pain. In his classical description of the world of the patient in chronic pain, Le Shan compares chronic pain with a nightmare.[15] Terrible things are occurring to the individual with the possibility of worse to come, there is a lack of control in what the individual can do to provide relief, and there is no time limit—no known end to the nightmare. Chronic pain becomes a state of existence and, perhaps most tragic, this suffering no longer serves a useful purpose in warning the individual of potential harm. Chronic pain may, however, serve to enforce rest as an aid to healing.[16]

Fordyce suggests that a component of learned behavior may exist in chronic pain.[17] Reinforcement of pain behaviors may occur when the health care worker provides attention only when pain is experienced and withdraws this attention when the person is comfortable. If this theory proves to be correct, we may unwittingly increase the learning of pain behaviors by activities such as medicating on an as needed (p.r.n.) basis for severe pain and increasing activity until painful.

INTERVENING VARIABLES

Age becomes a factor in both the young and old, particularly in the area of pain communication. Young people are in the process of learning a pain vocabulary, the names of body parts, and attempting to understand sensations coming from their body. They may be unable to communicate pain in adult terms. The geriatric patient at one time had the capability of communicating pain but may have lost it due to various deteriorations associated with age and sensory alterations.

The meaning pain has for an individual flows from cultural, religious, and social expectations and from past experiences and future expectations.[18] Zborowski pioneered the systematic study of pain responses of ethnic groups. He found wide variations in overt pain behaviors that had evolved from ethnic expectations. These variations held constant through second and third-generation immigrant groups. As a result of his work, four major cultural groups and their sociocultural attributes with respect to pain have been identified. Specifically, they are Old American, Jewish, Irish, and Italian. Zborowski's work provides a general framework for understanding various groups' responses to pain.

Members of the Old American group will usually deny the existence of pain so that they may stay productive. Pain is described in an efficient, unemotional manner, and behaviors such as crying, moaning, or groaning are not seen with this group. Jewish people are very demonstrative with respect to pain and may use many affective descriptors, such as intolerable and agonizing, to describe pain. They expect family members to become involved in their suffering and are very concerned about the significance of their current pain on the future. Italian people are also very demonstrative about their pain and also expect family members to become involved in their suffering. Unlike the Jewish patient, however, pain is viewed in the context of the current sensation and not future expectations. The Irish are similar to the Old American group in their calm, unemotional response to pain. Irish patients often will not complain about their pain and frequently will withdraw from other people when in severe pain. As a group, the Irish are also very proud of their ability to fight and endure severe pain. Zborowski's work provides a framework for understanding cultural variations in pain response, but care must be taken not to expect all patients of a given cultural group to behave in exactly the same manner.

Religious beliefs may also influence current responses to pain. Members of some religious groups believe that pain is punishment for wrongdoing and may not actively seek relief from the pain until penance has been performed.[19]

Children, in the magic thinking years of four to seven, often view pain as punishment. They believe that they are hospitalized because of some bad deed they have done. Unfortunately, this view is frequently reinforced by parents during illness episodes. An example of this is the parent who threatens a child by saying, "If you don't behave, I'll have the nurse give you a shot."

Children are in the process of developing a cognitive background on which to base their interpretations of pain and do not have, as most adults have had, friends who have described pain experiences. The significance of an injection to a child is not fully appreciated by most adults. In a study by Eland,[20] 186 hospitalized children were asked the question, "Of all the things that have ever hurt you, what's hurt you the worst?" 49.7 percent of those children who were hospitalized in a large mid-western university hospital answered "shot" or "needle." Interestingly enough, six of those children, between the ages of 4 and 10, had undergone 25 surgical experiences each, and everyone of them answered "shot" or "needle" as being the most painful event. Children also lack a cognitive understanding that momentary pain of an injection will alleviate the overall hurt that they are experiencing. Younger children around the ages of four and five lack a time concept and do not associate the painful event of an injection with pain relief at a later time.

Past experiences and responses to pain can be either positive or negative. A person who has had repeated painful experiences may have developed successful ways of coping. On the other hand, if frequent painful procedures and attempts at coping have been unsuccessful, the heightened fear and anxiety over having to endure them again may elicit an entirely different response. Anticipated pain can become an overwhelming threat to this individual.

The following is the protocol developed by Eland to assess pain in children 4 through 10 years of age. Eland also has used crayons and body outlines.[21] The original idea for the use of a chromatic array of colors to represent pain was Stewart's.[22] Eland adapted the idea for this use with young children, and this particular protocol uses a felt board. Body outlines and crayons also have been used to color pain.[23–25]

In an attempt to establish rapport, children were asked about pets, school, if they like to color, and play activities. Each child was asked what their favorite color is. The child was asked the question, "What kinds of things have hurt you before?" If the child did not reply, the researcher asked the child, "Has anyone ever stuck your finger to get blood? What did that feel like?" After discussing several things that have hurt the child in the past the researcher asked the child, "Of all the things that have ever hurt you, what hurt the most?" In this study the following protocol was followed:

INTERVIEW PROTOCOL

- Present eight felt squares in a row in the exact same order to every child—yellow, orange, red, green, blue, purple, brown, black—across the bottom of the felt board.

- Ask the child, "Of these colors, which color is like _." (The event identified by the child as hurting the most.)

- Place the color square at the top of the felt board away from the other colors. (Represents severe pain.)

- Ask the child, "Which color is like a hurt but not quite as much as_." (Event identified by child as hurting the most.)

- Place the color square below the square chosen representing severe pain.

- Ask the child, "Which color is like something that hurts just a little?"

- Place the color square below the colors representing moderate and mild pain.

- Ask the child, "Which color is like not hurting at all?"

- Place the color at the bottom of the column of color squares.

- Ask the child to show on the color scale "what color is like a shot?"

PATIENTS AT RISK

Antecedent conditions of pain—physiological, psychological, and sociocultural—determine the occurrence and magnitude of pain experienced in any given individual. Many of these factors have been discussed previously. The influence that age and sex have on pain is not well documented. Traditionally it has been assumed that children and older individuals experience less pain because of lack of development or changes in the central nervous system. Research is not available to support these assumptions. Studies of children's pain done by Eland do not support the hypothesis that children experience less pain; when provided with a means to identify and describe pain they are able to do so quite accurately.

Cummings identified characteristics that have been found to signal a high potential for chronic pain in the patients treated at the Veteran's Administration pain clinic in Seattle.[26] Characteristics that have been identified include:

- Drug or alcohol abuse.

- Several previous hospitalizations or other health problems.

- Inappropriate affect.

- Depression, hopelessness, anger.

- Threatening or demanding behavior.

- Rejection of self-help measures.

- Negative feelings about job, marriage, family.

- Litigation or compensation pending.

These characteristics are not identified as causal factors of chronic pain but do suggest factors that can be considered in the initial evaluation of pain and that may influence responses to treatment.

RESPONSE TO PAIN

The potential range of individual responses to pain is both varied and complex. The labeling of pain responses or behaviors as adaptive or maladaptive is determined partially by the health care system and the culture. For example, a culture may require stoicism as an appropriate pain response. These responses become most significant when considering chronic pain, although some behaviors, such as seeking assistance and complying with treatment, are expected of patients with acute as well as chronic pain.

Lipowski has identified mechanisms that are used in coping with illness, and defines **coping styles** as the relatively enduring dispositions in dealing with stress; while **coping strategies** are those techniques used to deal with a particular stress, such as illness.[27] The strategies used will be influenced by the individual's coping style, the situational factors, and the meaning the illness has for the individual. He identified eight common meanings of illness (See Figure 17-5) that are very similar to those identified by Copp as meanings that patients use to describe pain.[28] Lipowski's conclusions about coping strategies in illness can be applied to coping strategies used with pain. The way individuals perceive pain will influence the way in which they cope or respond to pain. He states that "coping may be evaluated as either adaptive or maladaptive depending on its appropriateness to the patient's age and situation, as well as its effectiveness in achieving maximum possible function and recovery or compensation."[29]

Response mechanisms, such as addiction, manipulation of the sick role for secondary gains, and withdrawal, are usually culturally unacceptable to health care workers, as well as being ineffective for the patient. Within the wide range of culturally acceptable responses, more information is needed to identify those responses

Lipowski—Illness	Copp—Pain
1. Challenge	Challenge
2. Enemy	Struggle or fight
3. Punishment	Punishment
4. Weakness	Weakness
5. Relief	Relief (restoration of health)
6. Strategy	Self-testing (fear, anxiety, strength to cope)
7. Loss or damage	Loss or grieving
8. Value	Value

Figure 17-5. Comparison of Lipowski's Concept of Illness with Copp's Meaning of Pain

that will prove most effective for the client. A study focusing on the relationships between individual differences in coping and the course of recovery in surgical patients found that clients using avoidant modes of coping did better than those using vigilant modes of coping.[30] Avoidance modes included behaviors that showed avoidance or denial of the emotional or threatening aspects of the surgery and were demonstrated by an unwillingness to discuss thoughts about the operation. Vigilance included those responses that indicated the patient was overly alert to threatening aspects of the surgery, as demonstrated by a readiness to discuss thoughts about the operation. These findings are only suggestive of trends relating recovery and coping methods; additional research of this type is necessary to determine causal relationships.

THE NURSING PROCESS

The nurse will assess pain to provide information that will assist in making a nursing diagnosis, formulating a plan, intervening, and evaluating the effectiveness of the intervention. The nursing diagnoses will be of most value in planning interventions if the factors that contribute to the pain are identified; for example, "pain related to tension on the abdominal incision."[31] These factors will be identified as part of the assessment. Interventions may be **independent** or **dependent nursing functions** and are identified as such. The use of analgesics is a dependent function requiring nursing judgments and collaboration with the patient and physician; knowledge that will be helpful to the nurse is specifically addressed in a later section of this chapter on analgesics. Evaluation of the effectiveness of interventions may use the same protocol used for pain assessment, although general behavioral outcomes that may prove helpful are identified at the end of this chapter.

Assessment

Problems often arise with pain assessment due to the subjectivity of the pain experience. Patients should be encouraged to describe pain in their own words; however, the evaluator must recognize that pain may be difficult for patients to report accurately without assistance. Judgment must be exercised by the nurse in determining when patients need help to describe their pain. Physiological indicators of pain, e.g., redness and swelling, and behavioral responses, e.g., crying, should be evaluated in conjunction with verbal reports of pain; if the patient does not report pain, such cues may be the only indicators that the individual is experiencing pain or discomfort. In evaluating chronic pain, it must be kept in mind that the responses normally present with acute pain may be modified or absent.

A pain history should be modified to fit the needs of the usual population or of the individual patient; questions posed to the postoperative patient may differ from those asked of a person with chronic pain. The pain history should include the pa-

tient's report of pain (subjective) and physiological and behavioral responses (objective).

The report of pain includes an evaluation of location, intensity, quality, and chronology of pain. Location of pain is best described by having the person describe or trace the area of pain; the description should include the extent and spread of the pain as well as the location of pain-free areas. An anatomical diagram may be of assistance if the individual cannot describe or locate the pain or if multiple areas of pain are interspersed with pain-free areas. The use of such a tool with an individual experiencing multiple sites of joint pain is illustrated in Figure 17-6. Medical terms used to describe location include:

- Localized—confined to the area of primary focus.
- Radiating—extending outward from the area of primary focus.
- Projected—transmitted along a pathway; usually the distribution of a nerve.
- Referred—occurs in an area other than the source.

Location of the pain also should include whether the pain is deep or superficial and whether the location remains the same or changes. If the location of the pain changes, determine whether these changes are related to any factors that patients can identify.

Perceived intensity of the pain may reflect the intensity of the stimulus, the degree of tissue damage, the amount of psychological distress caused, or a combination of these factors. More precise assessments may be made by having patients rank the pain on some type of scale (See Figure 17-7). The most common method is one in which the individual ranks pain on a scale of 0 to 10; 0 represents no pain and 10 the worst pain. A 5-point ranking scale may also be used in conjunction with words

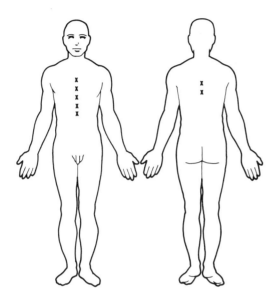

Figure 17-6. Anatomical Diagrams Can be Used to Identify Pain Locations.

does your pain feel?" The McGill-Melzack Pain Questionnaire contains groupings of words frequently used to describe pain and may be given to the patient if specifics about the quality of pain are desired.[32] The words describe sensory qualities (such as throbbing, burning, dull, tearing) and affective qualities (such as sickening, suffocating, nauseating). The presence of related sensations, such as tingling, fullness, or itching, also should be determined. The evaluator needs to determine if the quality of the pain remains constant or if changes occur; again, if the quality changes, is this related to factors the client can identify?

Chronology of the pain should be described by the client, but he may need to respond to questions in order to provide the required information. Information needed includes:

commonly used to indicate pain intensity. Having the individual compare the intensity of this pain experience with that of previous pain experiences may help the person describe his pain, if other measures are not available.

The **quality** of the pain may be the most difficult aspect for the individual to describe. You can assist him by asking, "How

- Mode of onset (sudden or gradual) and what the client was doing at the time, if related to the onset of pain.

- Pattern of the pain (steady or intermittent). If intermittent, does it follow a cycle or pattern?

- The duration of the pain, if intermittent or cyclic.

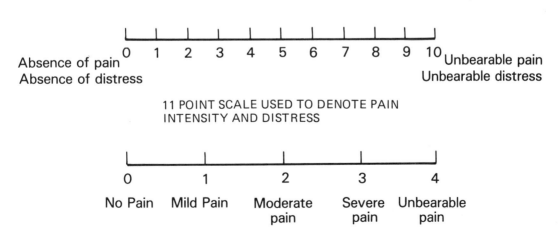

Absence of pain
Absence of distress
0 1 2 3 4 5 6 7 8 9 10 Unbearable pain
Unbearable distress

11 POINT SCALE USED TO DENOTE PAIN
INTENSITY AND DISTRESS

0   1   2   3   4
No Pain Mild Pain Moderate Severe Unbearable
                    pain   pain   pain

5 POINT SCALE DENOTING PAIN INTENSITY

Figure 17-7. Pain Scales.

- Whether this type of pain has occurred before and under what circumstances.

Associated information to be considered includes the identification of factors that precipitate or intensify the pain, as well as factors that provide relief. Does the pain awaken the patient from sleep? The amount of distress caused by the pain may be evaluated on a scale similar to the one used to rank intensity. The distress level will not necessarily be the same as the intensity level and may be anticipatory in situations that patients know will be painful, such as dressing changes. If the distress level is higher than the pain level, interventions to decrease anxiety may be of most benefit in controlling the pain.

Physiological responses may accompany acute pain and generally reflect stimulation of the autonomic nervous system. Assessing these responses is most important in situations where patients may not be reporting pain (e.g., a new post-operative patient, a person with a depressed level of awareness).

Responses to be evaluated include:

- Changes in skin color such as pallor, flushing.
- Diaphoresis.
- Alterations in blood pressure and pulse rate, increases being most common.
- Increase in respiration.
- Nausea, vomiting.

Physiological symptoms most common with chronic pain include fatigue and inability to rest, weakness, anorexia, and in some cases, faintness or syncope. Many of these symptoms are most likely to occur when the individual becomes exhausted by the pain; providing pain relief and rest may alleviate many of these symptoms.

Behavioral responses associated with pain are diverse and frequently difficult to evaluate. Body movement may be decreased, and some persons state they lie quietly as a method of controlling pain.

Body movement also may be increased and result in activities being usually carried out in an attempt to distract or alleviate the pain. Guarding or splinting body parts and rubbing painful areas frequently occurs. Facial expression may confirm or appear to contradict the presence of pain; with chronic pain, facial expression may be well controlled. The effect of pain on physical activity may be evaluated according to the degree of incapacitation. It may, however, be difficult to differentiate decreased activity related to pain from that related to other factors associated with the health problem. One method of determining the patient's perception of the effect of pain on activity is to ask what the pain has prevented the person from doing.

How the patient presently controls pain is important to assess, if the pain problem is not new. Even with acute pain, it may prove helpful in planning interventions if one knows how the person usually copes with pain. Questions such as: What relieves your pain? What increases your pain? and how do you usually control the pain? will provide some insights into the coping mechanisms used or may stimulate the client to consider methods that might be employed to alleviate the pain. The use of medication to control pain should be evaluated as precisely as possible. Information that should be assessed includes:

- The name of medication(s) used. If the patient does not know, try to ascertain if it is a narcotic. In the ideal situation, the nurse should try to physically examine the medication and its container.

- The method of administration—oral or intramuscular.

- The dose or number of pills taken at one time and the frequency of use.

- Any side effects of the drug(s) and how these are relieved. Special attention should be given to determining if constipation or gastrointestinal irritation has occurred.

A complete pain history requires that sufficient time be allowed so that the client does not feel rushed. If the cause of the pain is easily identified, the pain is acute, and temporary relief can be achieved with relative ease, the pain history can be shortened and completed quite rapidly; however, if the pain situation is complex, the time taken to do a thorough history will prove of value in planning interventions.

At the conclusion of the assessment phase, nursing diagnoses are formulated based on the data that has been gathered. Examples of nursing diagnoses for patients experiencing pain include:

- Pain due to myocardial infarction
- Pain related to labor and delivery
- Potential pain related to surgery
- Chronic pain related to rheumatoid arthritis.

Once the diagnoses have been written on the care plan, the second phase of the nursing process begins.

Planning

The next phase of the nursing process entails the preparation of a written nursing care plan. This is usually done in conjunction with the patient and his family. The patient should not be asked for information that is not to be used in planning for his care; persons with chronic pain may choose not to share information about their pain unless they believe it will be used as a basis of planning methods of controlling or alleviating the pain. Once the plan has been completed, the next stage of the nursing process can begin.

Implementation

The third phase of the nursing process is implementation of the plan. Numerous articles on nursing management of pain can be found in the nursing literature. Many of the interventions recommended are based on the experience of practitioners rather than on research, but they reflect a variety of creative techniques for assisting the client with pain. Some of the approaches are based on the gate-control theory of pain and are methods of altering pain sensation or pain reaction by "closing the gate." Other methods focus on increasing body response mechanisms, such as endorphin production. A number of physical approaches can be used for pain control. Heat and cold affect the vascular and muscular systems, but just as important are their effects on hormone production. Warmth and warm weather stimulates the production of serotonin, and cold and cold weather stimulates the production of norephinephrine.[33] Moist heat can be applied with warm soaks, compresses, or heating pads. Dry heat is applied with heating pads or as radiant heat. Cold can be applied by using ice bags, cold towels, gel packs, or as an ice massage. Cold and heat usually are most effective if applied directly to the painful area. The client may have a preference for heat or cold and should be encouraged to try both, if appropriate, to determine which method is most effective. Heat and cold are most frequently used with somatic pain, but may provide relief with cutaneous pain.

Massage, range of motion exercises, and positioning can be used to relieve pain of muscle tension or spasm. Massage should not, however, be used for calf pain or in any instance in which a thrombus may be present. The use of a menthol ointment may be included with massage. It is not known how menthol ointments relieve pain, but many persons find them effective with muscular pain.[34] Range of motion and positioning can be effective if muscle tension or spasm is reduced. The initial movement may increase the pain temporarily but this may be partially controlled with smooth, continuous motion and avoidance of sudden jerky motions. Exercise and movement may need to be planned for in conjunction with periods of decreased activity or rest. Rest may be used alone as an effective method of pain control, particularly when pain is being aggravated by fatigue or when injured tissue can heal if rest is provided. Control of environmental factors, such as noise, temperature, and light, are important considerations when providing periods of rest.

Cognitive approaches aimed at assisting the patient to gain control over the symptom or alleviating the affective distress associated with pain are recommended by practitioners. These approaches include relaxation, distraction, information distribution, and alleviation of pain apprehension. The use of relaxation in pain control is based on its effects in decreasing anxiety and decreasing muscle tension, both of which may increase the perception of pain. General relaxation techniques that are focused on total body relaxation require cooperation of the patient and adequate time to learn the technique. It is necessary to evaluate the mental and physical capability of the patient to participate. The patient must be alert and physically capable of doing the exercises. The procedures used for progressive relaxation include the following sequence.[35] The patient:

- focuses attention on a muscle group
- tenses the muscle group when a predetermined signal is given by the nurse
- maintains tension at a level that does not cause discomfort or pain for five to seven seconds
- releases tension at a predetermined signal
- focuses on the muscle group and the sensation while relaxing as completely as possible.

Relaxation also may be promoted by the use of breathing exercises, which do not require much effort or time on the part of the patient. Breathing techniques are frequently used for childbirth. The techniques require abdominal breathing to be done at a specified rate and depth. The patient assumes a comfortable position and concentrates on relaxing. A deep cleansing breath is taken, followed by slow, deep, rhythmic abdominal breathing for about 60 seconds. Relaxation is most effective if taught prior to anticipated pain or during periods of less acute pain to allow the individual to focus on learning the technique. Breathing techniques may be used without previous practice during acute pain if the nurse coaches the patient through the technique.

Distraction can be provided by any method that will successfully focus attention away from the pain. Relief will last only as long as the distraction and may be followed by increased awareness of the pain. Techniques that will provide distraction vary from person to person. Some commonly used distractors include:

- physical activities, such as pacing, visiting with others, talking on the phone
- listening to music. This is most beneficial if the patient uses a headset to allow concentration on the music and prevent distraction from other stimuli
- relating events or happenings. The nurse has the patient relate an exciting or pleasant experience. Items such as family pictures or scrapbooks can be used about the people or activities involved
- counting in a rhythmic manner, such as with a metronome, while concentrating on the activity of counting.

The distraction selected must serve as a focus of concentration strong enough to overcome concentration on the pain. The patient should be actively encouraged to use distraction and be assisted in finding those methods that will be most effective. In general, distraction will work best with brief periods and milder forms of pain. It is not as effective with chronic pain but may be used intermittently in these cases.

Discussion of pain and provision of information may reduce pain, particularly if a lack of information is increasing anxiety, or if the client does not know how he can assist in pain control. Provision of information is focused on the needs of the patient. It can include information about the source of the pain, expected course of the pain, methods that can decrease the pain, and how the individual can control the pain. Providing information about sensations that occur in situations associated with pain has been shown to decrease the amount of pain experienced.[36] Suggesting that an intervention will provide pain relief was shown to be effective in relieving pain in post-operative patients.[37] Conscious suggestion can be used to dispel anxiety and increase relaxation. The voice and attitude of the helper are crucial to the effectiveness of this technique.

General nursing care measures that decrease discomfort and distress associated with pain can be used alone or in conjunction with other interventions. These comfort measures can include touch, listening, and just "staying" with the patient. Reassurance and support can be provided by diminishing the patient's feeling of being alone with his pain.[38] Others, of the patient's choosing, also may serve the function of "staying" with the person in pain. Care must be exercised to determine the patient's wishes as well as the needs of those staying with the patient.

Nurses can administer medications as ordered by the physician to relieve the patient's pain. Some analgesics alter central control's perception of pain; some work at small-diameter (A-Delta and C fibers) or large-diameter (A-Beta) fibers. Administration of pharmacological agents with differing action sites when combined with other nursing comfort measures, such as back rubs and position changes, maximize

the potential for pain relief. The action sites of some common medications that provide a framework for combining them are as follows:

- Aspirin—small diameter fibers[39]
- Morphine Sulfate—large diameter fibers and central control[40]
- Barbiturates—central control and T-cell[41]
- Codeine Phosphate—small diameter fibers and central control[42]
- Meperidine Hydrochloride—central control[43]
- Tylenol®, Zomax®, Butazolidin®, Motrin®—small diameter fibers[44]

Aspirin remains one of the best anti-inflammatory agents and analgesics available today. It works by inhibiting prostaglandin production at the level of the small fiber.[45] For aspirin to be most effective, a blood level must be maintained in the body, and it needs to be administered every four hours.[46] Many patients have difficulty believing aspirin will work, for several reasons. It is readily available to all and does not require a prescription or special handling to acquire it. It is relatively inexpensive and side effects associated with administration are low. Many individuals believe that if a drug has these qualities, it must not be strong, and if it is not strong, it will not work. If someone believes this, the drug probably will not work.

Barbiturates have long had a recognized role in providing adequate sleep and rest for patients, but they also have a role in pain management. There is growing evidence to show that barbiturates alter the small fibers (A-Delta, C input) to the T-cell.[47,48] Additionally, barbiturates diminish the electrical activity in the midbrain reticular area, which in turn alters the pain transmitting capabilities of the substantia gelatinosa.[49]

If pain becomes extremely intense, normal doses of analgesics will not successfully alleviate it. This frequently happens when patients attempt to endure pain for a long period of time, or a nurse has not initiated pain management. As a result, the pain is excruciating before a nurse can administer an appropriate analgesic. If the usual dose of an analgesic will not eliminate the patient's pain, the patient needs to be told why, and the nurse must make attempts to secure additional medication.[50] Nurses occasionally withhold the patient's pain medication for fear of the patient's becoming addicted. In most instances, this will not occur. If the patient is promptly and adequately medicated for pain, less medication may be needed over the course of treatment. Unfortunately, the fear of creating addiction is one of the most common reasons that nurses withhold narcotics. These fears are usually unsubstantiated. Having some basic information regarding addiction will be helpful for nurses.

There is no one, recognized definition of addiction. A generally recognized definition states that addiction is an overwhelming involvement with obtaining and using drugs for their *psychic* effects rather than for medically or socially approved reasons.[51] Therefore, by definition, relief or prevention of pain is a reason to use narcotics.

Nurses also need to anticipate painful experiences and medicate patients prior to these occurrences. For example, on a postoperative surgical unit, when it it necessary for a patient to deep breathe and ambulate, a nurse needs to enter the patient's room at least one hour prior to the required activity, administer the appropriate analgesic, and allow the medication to take effect. Adequate pain control in these situations allows the patient to move more easily, to participate in care activities, and to maximize recovery.

A **placebo** is an inactive substance that resembles a medication. Placebos work be-cause of the power of positive suggestion and of the brain's power over pain.[52–55] Beecher found that 35 percent of all patients could receive benefit from chemically inert substances. This data clearly shows the power of the mind over pain. Therefore, physicians occasionally order placebos (such as normal saline for an intramuscular injection, or a flavored syrup or a pill of inert substance for oral administration) instead of a narcotic. Placebos frequently are chosen for patients whose pain has been resistant to ordinary therapeutic modalities and when health care professionals can think of nothing else to do. A nurse, when administering a placebo, tells patients everything they want to hear; that the medication is a new medication when the old ones have not worked and conveys that someone is paying attention to their pain and suffering. The patient wants the medication to work; his pain is very real to him. Placebos have no proven physiological effect, and if the patient finds out that they are being given an inert substance the nurse/patient trust relationship is destroyed. The patient feels his credibility is being questioned, and his response to other potentially successful treatment modalities during that hospitalization will be less successful and cooperative because of the deception. The use of placebos raises many ethical issues, because patients have the right (see Chapter 8) to know what treatments are being used, and dishonesty is considered unethical.

Nurses need to consider this ethical issue before they are confronted with it in the clinical area. Then, when the issue becomes a reality, the nurse can make a decision based on conscience and the individual situation. If nurses feel that they do not wish to participate in that particular part of the patient's care, they should make their stand clear to the other members on the health care team. Regardless of one's ethical stand, the ethical stand of another may be different, and it is within the other's right as a professional to choose.

Some health care disciplines provide measures for pain relief that may require coordination with nursing functions. Surgical measures, for example, may include a variety of techniques designed to interrupt the pain stimulus through destruction of part of the sensory pathway. These procedures were originally performed through open exposure of the cerebrum or spinal cord under general anesthesia. More recently, surgery has provided a means of performing these techniques under local anesthesia. Interruption of the lateral spinothalamic tract in the spinal cord (cordotomy) is the surgical procedure most commonly preferred; however, procedures that interrupt tracts at another point in the central nervous system are frequently performed. Due to the ability of the central nervous system to protect itself, suspended function may recover, and pain may recur.[56] Sympathetic blocks and sympathectomy may be of benefit in post-traumatic injuries or causalgia. A temporary block usually will be done prior to a surgical procedure to determine if relief will be obtained with interruption of these fibers.

Other forms of treatment that may be used include acupuncture, hypnosis, operant conditioning, and biofeedback. The responsibility of the nurse may range from teaching the technique, especially biofeedback, to support and positive reinforcement. Acupuncture, which is being more widely used and researched in this country, involves the insertion and rotation of metal needles in the body at specific, designated points. These acupuncture points also have been used in massage techniques that substitute hand pressure and massage for the needle.

Hypnosis can be used in the management of pain problems. Removal of pain with hypnosis should be done by one skilled in the practice of hypnosis and aware of the diagnostic and treatment problems of the disease.[57] Pain is generally reduced rather than blocked completely, so as to leave sufficient pain perception to note changes in the course of the illness. Not all persons are responsive to hypnosis, but among those who are, repeated hypnosis may provide periods of pain relief for several weeks before reinforcement becomes necessary.[58] Operant conditioning is aimed at reducing learned pain behaviors.[59] The objectives are to: reduce pain behavior by withdrawing positive reinforcement, increase activity with positive reinforcement, retrain the family to enforce well behaviors and to avoid enforcing pain behaviors, and modify deficiencies other than pain that may limit activity. Operant conditioning is most effectively provided in a controlled setting such as a pain clinic. Biofeedback is used to alter and bring under control physiological responses and may be used in conjunction with other treatment techniques. At the present time, one of the most common uses of biofeedback in pain control is for the individual with tension or migraine headaches.[60]

Electrical stimulation, although not a new concept, is another method used by physicians to control pain. The ancient Egyptians in 600 B.C. placed their gout-affected feet in buckets of water with specific electrical fish for pain relief. Recent technological advances have brought about new electrical devices for pain relief, and an increased number of physicians, nurses, physical therapists, and auxiliary personnel are finding themselves involved with them.

TNS or TENS units work by sending impulses along large-diameter fibers (A-Beta). Transcutaneous electrical nerve stimulation (TNS or TENS) units are used for acute post-operative pain, chronic pain, and as a screening device for determination of the plausibility of surgically implanting a more sophisticated unit, such as a dorsal column or a peripheral nerve stimulator. TENS units consist of two electrodes (one positive, one negative) that are attached by flexible wires to a battery pack. On the battery pack there are two or three controls that control the voltage, frequency, and pulse width of the electrical current. In an acute care setting, post-operative patients have electrodes placed along their incision lines for pain relief. In chronic pain situations, electrodes are located where large fibers become superficial over acupuncture points or sometimes geographically near the source of pain.

Nurses working with patients with nerve stimulators need to know electrode placement and taping, conductive jellies, battery changing, and adjustment of the voltage, pulse width, and frequency controls. In order for patients to receive maximum benefit, a program of nurse education needs to be undertaken. If the nurse doesn't know about the device, the placebo effect will not be operant, existing pain can be made worse, and maximum benefits will not be attained. (A discussion of all of the parameters of the care of the patient with a stimulator is beyond the scope of this chapter. Readers are referred to the reference by Sweeney, Johnson, and Eland for other details.)[61]

Evaluation

Whatever form of treatment is used to alleviate pain, the *evaluation* of its effectiveness is a necessary nursing function. Behavioral outcomes can be used to assist in this evaluation. Outcomes that can be observed and can be positive cues that some degree of pain control has been achieved include:

- Relaxation of skeletal muscles.
- Increase in normal, daily activities.
- Increased ability to rest or sleep.
- Elimination of pain postures.
- Decreased use of affective descriptors in describing pain.

- Decreased report of pain, soreness, or tenderness.
- Increased attention span.
- Focus of attention on topics other than pain.
- Verbalization that pain sensations are absent.

Once the evaluative phase of the nursing process has been completed, the cycle can begin again with a reassessment. If the established plan proved to be partially or totally ineffective, the plan has to be redesigned. It the plan was effective, then the successful outcomes need to be supported.

Through careful use of the nursing process and a firm knowledge base about pain, nurses are able to anticipate patients' needs and provide meaningful patient care.

SUMMARY

Pain is a symptom frequently encountered in the health care setting, but it is not easily defined, and there is no agreement about the mechanisms leading to pain. The gate-control theory is the most widely accepted theory at present, although it is being modified by new research. Pain may be identified as acute, long-term, or progressive. Physiological and psychological responses vary with the type of pain and may require differing methods of pain treatment. A number of variables may modify the pain experience and include such things as age, cultural background, and general coping mechanisms. Pain assessment should be thorough and include the characteristics of the pain, responses to pain, and pain history. Nursing interventions include both independent and dependent activities. The use of physical and general comfort measures, as well as the use of analgesics, are recognized nursing interventions. The role of interventions, such as teaching, suggestion, relaxation, and biofeedback, are newer and being developed at a rapid rate. The role that the nurse chooses to assume in relation to the person experiencing pain will be a vital factor in the effectiveness of pain evaluation and alleviation. The nurse can facilitate the accurate reporting of pain, the use of independent control measures, and the effectiveness of other forms of treatment. The responsibility is great, but the rewards of helping the client with pain are even greater.

STUDY QUESTIONS

CASE STUDY I

Mr. McCloskey is a 21-year-old, 120-pound male, who was involved in a motor vehicle accident 3 years ago. At the time of the accident he sustained L^{2-3-4} compression fractures. He has undergone 2 spinal fusions and 3 lumbar laminectomies to relieve his pain, but is still in pain. He is currently hospitalized for reevaluation of his pain problem.

At the time of the accident, Mr. McCloskey was employed as a steelworker. Since the accident, he has been totally disabled. (His fiancée was killed in the accident.) Mr. McCloskey now lives in his parents' home. He was forced to give up his apartment for economic reasons.

The lumbar spine x-rays, myelogram, and EMG all indicate what will most likely be permanent damage bilaterally to the nerve roots at L^{2-3-4} levels.

Medical orders include:

Regular diet
Bedrest with bathroom privileges
Laxative of choice
Patient may straight cath self p.r.n.
Intake and output
Bedboards
Overbed trapeze
Codeine 15 mg q 4° p.r.n. pain p.o. or I.M.
ASA gr X q 3–4 p.r.n. pain p.o.
Valium® 2 mg qid p.o.
2 ccs Bacteriostatic water IM q 3–4° if codeine does not relieve pain

1. Identify the data you need to assess Mr. McCloskey's pain. List the data in order of priority.

2. A new pain relief device that you have never seen before is given to the patient. What effect can your attitude toward the device have on its success?

3. List the advantages and disadvantages of using the placebo.

4. Under what circumstances would you give the placebo?

CASE STUDY II

Mr. Wesley is a 55-year-old, admitted to a unit, with intractable pain secondary to advanced heart disease. He has undergone heart surgery twice in the past two years. One surgery was for a mitral valve replacement and the other removed approximately one-third of his heart muscle because of ischemia. He is in severe congestive heart failure and will not live long. Mr. Wesley is as accepting as he could possibly be of his own death, but wants to be more comfortable than he is. During your initial interview, he admits to being suicidal over the pain.

His pain is in several locations and is present at all times. The areas of his pain include: heart, left arm, right shoulder, entire rib cage, leg pain from intermittant claudication.

Mr. Wesley has not had a good night's sleep in as long as he can remember. He lives with his two sisters in a large house he built himself. He was the head of a large university department until forced into total disability two years ago.

1. What assessment information do you need from Mr. Wesley?

2. What nursing comfort measures could you institute that would most likely make him more comfortable?

3. You have the complete resources of a large medical center at your disposal and unlimited power to take over Mr. Wesley's care. What would you do for him? What areas of the gate-theory would be affected by your interventions?

4. What is the nursing plan of care regarding pain for Mr. Wesley? (for all 3 shifts)

REFERENCES

1. Richard Sterbach: **Pain: A Psychophysiological Analysis** (New York: Academic Press, Inc., 1968) p.12.
2. Margo McCaffery: **Nursing Management of the Patient with Pain** (Philadelphia, J. B. Lippincott, 1972), p.32.
3. Ibid., p.32.
4. Ibid., p.32.
5. Ronald Melzack, Wall, PD: "Pain Mechanisms: A New Theory." **Science, 150** (1965) p.971.
6. Ronald Melzack: **The Puzzle of Pain,** (New York, Basic Books, Inc. 1972).
7. S. Kim: "Theory, Research and Nursing Practice," **Advances in Nursing Science**, 2 (1980), 43–54.
8. B. B. Wolff: "Factor Analysis of Human Pain Responses: Pain Endurance as a Specific Pain Factor," **J Abnormal Psychology, 78** (1971) 292.
9. H. Merskey, F. Spear: **Pain: Psychological and Psychiatric Aspects.** (London, Bailliere, Tindol, and Cassell, 1967).
10. Marion Johnson: "Assessment of Clinical Pain," In Ada Jacox (ed): **Pain: A Sourcebook for Nurses and Other Health Professionals** (Boston: Little, Brown, 1977).
11. H. Merskey: "Psychological Aspects of Pain." In Ada Jacox (ed): **Pain: A Sourcebook for Nurses and Other Health Professionals,** (Boston: Little, Brown, 1977), p.91.
12. J. D. Loeser: "Central Pains," **Clinical Medicine 82.** no. 4 (1975) 24–26.
13. S. H. Frazier, L. C. Kolb: "Psychiatric Aspects of Pain and the Phantom Limb" **Orthopedic Clinics of North America 1:** (1970) 481–495.
14. Ronald Melzack: "Central Neural Mechanisms in Phantom Limb Pain." In J. J. Bonica (ed): **Advances in Neurology,** Vol. 4 (New York: Raven Press, 1974) pp.333–338.
15. L. LeShan: "The World of the Patient in Severe Pain of Long Duration." **Journal of Chronic Diseases, 17** (1964) 119–124.
16. M. Schmitt: The Nature of Pain with Some Personal Notes." **Nursing Clinics of North America,** 12 (1977) 621–629.
17. W. E. Fordyce: "An Operant Conditioning Method of Managing Chronic Pain." **Postgraduate Medicine,** 53, no. 6 (1973) 123–128.
18. M. Zborowski: "Cultural Components in Response to Pain." **Journal of Social Issues,** (1952) 8–16.
19. R. Wu: **Behavior and Illness** (Englewood Cliffs, NJ: Prentice-Hall Inc., 1973).
20. J. M. Eland: "Children's Experience of Pain: A Descriptive Study." Unpublished data, 1976.
21. J. M. Eland: "The Experience of Pain in Children," unpublished paper presented to the Mid-America Sigma Theta Tau Research Conference, Kansas City, Missouri, August, 1976.
22. M. L. Stewart: "Measurement of Clinical Pain," In Ada Jacox (ed): **Pain: A Sourcebook for Nurses and Other Health Professionals.** (Boston: Little, Brown, 1977).
23. J. Eland, J. E. Anderson: "The Experience of Pain in Children." In Ada Jacox (ed): **Pain: A Sourcebook for Nurses and Other Health Professionals.** (Boston: Little, Brown, 1977).
24. S. Loebach: "The Use of Color to Facilitate Communication of Pain in Children." Unpublished Master's thesis, The University of Washington, May, 1979.
25. P. Schroeder: "Use of Eland's Color Method in Pain Assessment of Burned Children." Unpublished Master's thesis, The University of Cincinnati, 1979.

26. D. Cummings: "Stopping Chronic Pain Before it Starts." **Nursing '81** no. 1, **11**, 4 (1981) 60–62.

27. Z. J. Lipowski: "Physical Illness, the Individual and the Coping Processes." **Psychiatry in Medicine 1** (1970) 91–102.

28. L. A. Copp: "The Spectrum of Suffering." **American Journal of Nursing, 74** 491–495.

29. Z. J. Lipowski: "Physical Illness, the Individual and the Coping Processes." **Psychiatry in Medicine, 1** (1970) 91–102.

30. F. Cohen, R. S. Lazarus: "Active Coping Processes, Coping Dispositions, and Recovery From Surgery," **Psychosomatic Medicine 35** (1973) 375–389.

31. E. A. Mahoney: "Some Implications for Nursing Diagnoses of Pain." **Nursing Clinics of North America, 12** (1977) 613–619.

32. J. E. Meissner: McGill-Melzack Pain Questionnaire, **Nursing '80,** no. 10 (1980), 50–51.

33. J. E. Booker: "Pain: It's All in Your Patient's Head (or is it?)." **Nursing '82,** no. 3, **12** (1982), 46–57.

34. M. McCaffery: "Relieving Pain With Noninvasive Techniques." **Nursing '80,** no. 12, **10** (1980) 54–57.

35. J. M. Richter, R. Sloan: "A Relaxation Technique." **American Journal of Nursing,** 79 (1979).

36. J. Johnson: "Effects of Accurate Expectations About Sensation on the Sensory and Distress Components of Pain. **"Journal of Personality and Social Psychology,** 27 (1973), 261–275.

37. K. S. Billars: "You Have Pain? I Think This Will Help." **American Journal of Nursing, 70** (1970) 2143.

38. M. McCaffery: "When Your Patient's Still in Pain Don't Just Do Something: Sit There" **Nursing 81** no. 6, **11** (1981) 68–61.

39. J. Tourville: Personal Communication, 1977.

40. A. Herz, K. Albus, J. Metyz, P. Schubert, and H. Teschemacher: "On the Central Sites for the Anti-nociceptive Action of Morphine and Fentanyl." **Neuropharmacology,** 9 (1970) 539.

41. J. D. French, M. Verzeano, and W. H. Magoun: "Neural Basis of the Anesthetic State." **Archives of Neurological Psychiatry,** 69–519, 593.

42. J. Tourville: Personal Communication, 1977.

43. Ibid.

45. Ibid.

46. G. G. Gebhart: "Narcotic and Non-narcotic Analgesics and Relief of Pain." In Ada Jacox

(ed): **Pain: A Sourcebook for Nurses and Other Health Professionals,** (Boston, Little, Brown, 1977).

47. P. Hillman and P. D. Wall: "Inhibitory and Excitatory Factors Influencing the Receptive Fields of Lamina 5 Spinal Cord Cells." **Experimental Brain Research** 9 (1969) 2814.

48. L. M. Mendell and P. D. Wall: "Presynaptic Hyperpolarization: A Role for Fine Afferent Fibers." **Journal of Physiology, 172** (1964) 274.

49. J. H. Jaffe and W. R. Martin: "Narcotic Analgesics and Antagonists." In L. S. Goodman and A. Gilman (eds): **Pharmacological Basis of Therapeutics,** (ed. 6) (New York, McMillan 1979).

50. M. McCaffery and L. Hart: "Undertreatment of Acute Pain with Narcotics." **American Journal of Nursing,** 76 (1976) 1586.

51. M. McCaffery: Patients Shouldn't Have to Suffer: How to Relieve Pain with Injectable Narcotics." **Nursing, 10** (October 1980) 34–39.

52. H. K. Beecher: "Pain in Men Wounded in Battle" **Annals of Surgery, 123** (1946) 96.

53. H. K. Beecher: **Measurement of Subjective Responses; Quantitative Effects of Drugs** (New York, Oxford University Press, 1959).

54. J. B. Knowles and C. J. Lucas: "Experimental Studies of the Placebo Response." **Journal of Mental Science** 106 (1960) 231.

55. A. K. Shapiro: "The Placebo Response" In J. G. Howell, (ed): **Modern Perspectives in World Psychiatry.** (New York, Brunner/Mazel 1971).

56. D. McDonnel: "Surgical and Electrical Stimulation Methods for Relief of Pain" In Ada Jacox (ed): **Pain: A Sourcebook for Nurses and Other Health Professionals,** (Boston, Little, Brown, 1977).

57. H. B. Crasilneck and J. A. Hall: "Clinical Hypnosis in Problems of Pain". In Ada Jacox (ed): **Pain: A Sourcebook for Nurses and Other Health Professionals,** (Boston, Little, Brown, 1977).

58. Ibid, p.270

59. W. E. Fordyce: "Operant Conditioning: An Approach in Chronic Pain" In Ada Jacox (ed): **Pain: A Sourcebook for Nurses and Other Health Professionals,** (Boston, Little, Brown, 1977).

60. T. H. Budzynski: "Biofeedback Procedures in the Clinic" In Ada Jacox (ed): **Pain: A Sourcebook for Nurses and Other Health Professionals,** (Boston, Little, Brown, 1977).

61. S. Sweeney, M. Johnson and J. M. Eland:

"Pain Associated with Neurological Conditions" In Ada Jacox (ed): **Pain: A Sourcebook for Nurses and Other Health Professionals.** (Boston, Little, Brown, 1977).

ANNOTATED BIBLIOGRAPHY

Booker JE: **Pain It's All in Your Patient's Head (or is It?).** Nurs 82 12:3:47–51; March 1982. Pain can change the body's chemistry, and this article discusses techniques that will modify these biochemical responses.

Copp LA: **The Spectrum of Suffering.** Am J Nurs 74:3:491–495; March 1974. This article explores the pain experienced by 148 hospitalized persons and describes how they coped. Also suggested are ways of assisting these patients to adapt to their pain.

Granse CA: **For Control of Severe Pain, Dorsal Column Stimulation.** Am J Nurs 78:6:1022–1025; June 1978. This article describes dorsal column stimulation as a technique to manage severe, chronic pain. Some excellent nursing interventions are discussed.

McCaffery M: **How to Relieve your Patients' Pain Fast and Effectively . . . With Oral Analgesics.** Nurs 80 10:11:58–63; November 1980. This article compares and contrasts intramuscular (IM) and oral medications and proposes nursing actions to promote use of oral drugs instead of the more invasive IMs.

McCaffery M: **Patients Shouldn't have to Suffer: How to Relieve Pain with Injectable Narcotic.** Nurs 80 10:10:34–39; October 1980. This excellent article describes the issues of most concern to nurses regarding narcotic administration and proposes solutions.

McGuire L: **A Short, Simple Tool for Assessing Your Patients' Pain.** Nurs 81 11:3:48–49; March 1981. This brief article proposes a pain assessment tool.

McGuire L. Shyane D: **Managing Pain . . . In the Young Patient.** Nurs 82 12:9:53–55; August 1982. This article gives helpful tips for assessing pain in children from under two, up. It discusses some of the common problems in relieving pain in the very young.

Meissner JE: **McGill-Melzack Pain Questionnaire.** Nurs 80 10:1:50–52; January 1980. This excellent article discusses the value of a careful pain assessment and includes the unique McGill-Melzack Pain Questionnaire.

Panayotoff K: **Managing Pain . . . in the Elderly.** Nurs 82 12:8:53–57; August 1982. All patients in pain need to have nurses who are aware of their special needs. This article describes the needs of the elderly.

Wright Z: **From I.V. to P.O. Your Patient's Pain Medication.** Nurs 81 11:7; July 1981. A step-by-step procedure for the changeover from intramuscular to oral medication is discussed in this article. A patient situation is used as an example, and a pain medication flow sheet is presented.

18

IMMOBILITY

Nancie H. Pardue

CHAPTER OUTLINE

OBJECTIVES

At the completion of this chapter, the reader will be able to:

- Define immobility and discuss the various types of immobility

- List the effects of immobility on the patient's respiratory system, cardiovascular system, skin, musculoskeletal and peripheral nervous systems, elimination, metabolism, and nutrition.

- Discuss the physiological and psychosocial assessment of the effects of immobilization on a patient and identify appropriate patient needs and nursing diagnoses.

- Describe how to plan for and evaluate nursing care provided to a patient on extended bedrest.

- Specify nursing interventions that will assist the patient and family to adapt to or cope with physiological changes caused by immobility.

- Define the basic terms used in joint mobility, range of motion exercises, positioning, and problems of immobility.

- Describe potential behavioral changes that may occur in the immobilized patient.

GLOSSARY

Anorexia—loss of appetite.

Aspiration—the drawing in of foreign bodies or fluids into the lungs on inspiration.

Atelectasis—collapsing of the alveoli of the lung due to mucus plugs, excessive secretions, or obstruction by foreign bodies.

Constipation—infrequent passage of stool.

Contracture—shortening and atrophy of a muscle resulting in resistance to passive stretch due to disuse and prolonged maintenance of a flexed position.

Decubitus Ulcers—pressure sores or ulcers that are breaks in the surface skin or mucous membrane characterized by disintegration or death of the tissue.

Defecation—evacuation of the bowels.

Edema—the swelling of tissues when fluid is held intercellularly.

Embolus—a mass of undissolved matter, such as a blood clot or air, traveling through a blood vessel.

Fecal Impaction—a collection of hardened stool in the rectum or sigmoid colon.

Fowler's position—semisitting.

Hypostatic Pneumonia—an inflammation of the alveoli and buildup of secretions within the alveoli due to lack of expansion and contraction of the lung tissue.

Immobility—an intentional or involuntary limitation of activity in any sphere of a person's physical, emotional, intellectual, social, or cultural experience.

Lateral Position—sidelying.

Maceration—the reduction of tissue to a soft mass through soaking.

Mobility—the ability to move freely and easily without restrictions, in one's own environment.

Orthostatic Hypotension—the occurrence of a marked fall in the blood pressure occurring when a person rises from the recumbent to the erect position.

Osteoporosis—loss of the protein ma'rix of the bone.

Prone—lying flat with the face downward.

Reactive Hyperemia—a temporary increase in blood flow to an area of the skin that occurs just after blood flow to the area has been blocked and then released.

Recumbent—lying down.

Shearing Forces—forces that pull tissues and move one layer of tissue over another as a patient changes his position in bed.

Supine—lying on the back with the face up.

Therapeutic Bedrest—the confinement of a person to his bed to aid in the healing process and in the treatment of disease.

Thrombophlebitis—inflammation of a vein developing before the formation of a blood clot.

Thrombus—a blood clot loosely attached to the wall of a vein.

Urinary Incontinence—an involuntary release of urine from the bladder.

Urinary Retention—accumulation of urine within the bladder due to the inability to urinate.

Urinary Stasis—the pooling of urine in

GLOSSARY Continued

the urinary tract.

Valsalva Maneuver—the attempt to forcibly exhale with the nose and mouth closed, resulting in increased intrathoracic pressure

and a decreased return of blood to the heart.

Venous Stasis—pooling of blood in the veins.

ALTERATIONS IN MOBILITY

Mobility is the ability to move freely and easily without restrictions in one's own environment. An individual experiences himself and defines his health and physical fitness through his ability to be mobile. Not only does mental well-being depend on one's ability to be mobile, but the body functions best with the ability to change positions. The body organs and systems perform their functions much more easily when the person is standing. The kidneys are able to drain completely in the standing position; the lungs expand more easily; and peristaltic movements of the bowel are more effective in the upright position. The functioning and repair of joints, muscles, tendons, and bones are dependent upon the forces of motion.

Immobility may be defined as an intentional or involuntary limitation of activity in any sphere of a person's physical, emotional, intellectual, social, or cultural experience. Throughout the lifespan, individuals experience various types of immobility. Certain occupations, for example, are sedentary, requiring the body to be held in one position for long periods of time. People who practice meditation or other forms of relaxation exercises also are engaging in a limited type of immobility. Extremes of immobility are seen in nursing and medicine, and range from the unconscious or totally paralyzed patient to the person with a temporary arm sling or finger splint.

Immobility, as seen in nursing situations, is often imposed for beneficial reasons. There may be times in a person's life when healing is unable to take place or some other process prevents him from effectively adapting to changes in his environment or body. For example, being placed on bedrest will help prevent further injury or disease and will repair damage. **Therapeutic bedrest** is the confinement of a patient to his bed to aid in the healing process and in the treatment of disease. Rest reduces the metabolic needs, oxygen requirements, and body system demands of various injured and diseased organs. Certainly the heart and lungs have a reduced workload during bedrest. Immobility, by decreasing movement, enables fractures and wound edges to heal together more easily. When the musculoskeletal system is allowed to relax, this may assist in the relief of pain caused by injured muscles, nerves, and tendons. Also, the effects of gravity cause a strain on the lower circulation, so ankle edema and venous congestion are improved with bedrest.

Bedrest is also necessary for patients who are too weak or ill to remain upright and active, such as those with cancer or neurological diseases. In these situations, bedrest and immobility aid the patient's physiological adaptation to various bodily changes and stressors. Through rest, energy is freed, making it possible for the injured or diseased body systems to repair themselves.

It is often the nurse's function to assess, with the physician, a person's basic needs and adaptability, and then to determine if some form of immobility will help him to cope with his situation. It is important to look carefully at the decision to immobilize a patient because bedrest has definite hazards. Disabilities caused by immobility can affect every system and major organ of the body. Malnourished patients, the elderly, the critically ill, quadraplegics, and comatose patients, for example, are especially susceptible to the hazards of bedrest. For many years, the problems and severe disabilities associated with bedrest have

limitation of movement within his environment may be due to bedrest, a body cast, isolation, or an intensive care unit. A patient may be unable to walk due to severe emphysema or congestive heart failure.

When overstressed, a person's usual ability to adapt may be ineffective and **psychological immobilization** may occur. When a patient realizes that he has a terminal illness, for example, or is faced with paralysis or loss, the patient's responses may

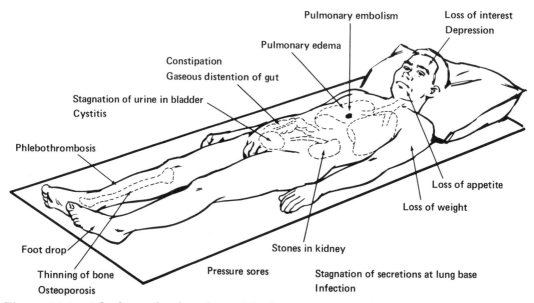

Figure 18-1.   The hazards of prolonged bedrest on various body systems.

been documented and warned against, yet we still see these complications in hospitals and nursing homes. By the completion of this chapter, the following quote from 1947 will take on new meaning.

> "Look at a patient lying long in bed. What a pathetic picture he makes! The blood clotting in his veins, the lime draining from his bones, the scybala staking up in his colon, the flesh rotting from his seat, the urine leaking from his distended bladder, and the spirit evaporating from his soul."[1]

A person experiences **physical immobility** when he has a restriction of his physical movement or bodily processes. The

consist of withdrawal, depression, crying, or denial, all of which are demonstrations of psychological immobility.

Certain persons do not adapt well to threats within their environments or injuries to their bodies, due to a lack of knowledge of how to act effectively. This is called **intellectual immobility.** This lack of knowledge may occur for several reasons. Physiological reasons include an impaired intellect caused by drugs, trauma, cerebrovascular accidents, and arteriosclerosis. Patients after surgery may be so exhausted and in pain that they are physically drained and have no mental energy left. Cultural barriers, such as language, may prevent patients from understanding their problems and how they will be treated. The nurse needs to assess a patient carefully for possible ineffective adaptation and determine if his level of knowledge or potential to learn is interfering with his ability to adapt.

Social immobility, another type of immobility, can occur when there are restrictions placed on a person's or family's normal patterns of social interaction. A quadriplegic patient, for example, will experience social immobility when returned to his home, since he is no longer able to participate in certain activities. Elderly people who gradually lose their families and friends can become socially immobile as they spend increasingly more time alone and become afraid to go out by themselves. Hospital patients with extended illnesses begin to lose touch with their friends and the community and find that their social contacts are limited to hospital personnel.

This chapter is concerned with these concepts of immobility as they apply to the practice of professional nursing.

PHYSICAL PROBLEMS OF IMMOBILITY

Immobility affects many of the body's physiological subsystems. This section will present a review of the effects of immobility on these various systems.

Respiratory System

The respiratory system is perhaps most dangerously affected by immobility, since adequate functioning of the lungs is critical to life. People who are immobile or confined to bed have decreased chest and lung expansion, and therefore respirations become slower and more shallow. As the patient uses his respiratory muscles less, they become weaker and less efficient. In addition to these changes, if there are pressures against the chest caused by bedding, restraints, clothing, or the mattress, the patient cannot take adequate deep breaths. A person in the supine position has an elevated diaphragm, a constricted chest, and a redistribution of blood flow from the legs to the chest. Abdominal distention is also a cause of restricted respiration, as is fear of incisional pain. Drugs such as morphine can prevent patients from breathing deeply.

If a patient continues his pattern of minimal lung expansion, he may develop **atelectasis.** Secretions also can block the bronchial tree, so that air is unable to enter the alveoli. The cough reflex, which is very important for mobilization of secretions, may be decreased by abdominal muscle weakness, abdominal surgery, narcotics, and anesthetics. As a result, the bronchioles become obstructed with mucus and there is a threat of **hypostatic pneumonia.**

The immobilized individual also may be susceptible to problems of **aspiration.** Aspiration occurs when foreign bodies (usually vomitus) are drawn into the lung on inspiration. This problem occurs especially among stroke, seizure, and unconscious patients. Selected medications may slow the reflex actions of the epiglottis, thus permitting aspiration of secretions from the nasopharynx. When gastric contents are aspirated into the lungs, an inflammatory reaction may occur, leading to complications.

Cardiovascular System

Changes in the cardiovascular system occur rapidly when a person decreases his activity level. **Circulatory stasis** can occur as a result of vasodilation and impairment of venous return to the heart. During muscular inactivity, the veins in the legs and other dependent parts tend to dilate. With normal activity, pressure changes on the venous bed aid venous blood to return to the right side of the heart. Changes in thoracic and abdominal pressures from movement of the diaphragm promote blood return to the heart. Pressure changes in the veins of the legs are provided by the contraction and relaxation of leg muscle, referred to as the muscle pump.

Gravity can be a factor in the impairment of venous return. When an individual is supine and inactive, the valveless veins in the legs are dependent, resulting in slow emptying of these vessels. Pressure also impedes venous return. The sitting position puts pressure on the vessels at the back of the knee, which results in pooling of venous blood. When the body is horizontal and supine, external pressure from the bed causes impairment of venous return. **Edema** can occur as a result of circulatory stasis. As the venous backup and pressure increases, fluid is forced into the tissues, and edema occurs most commonly in the legs and sacrum. This edema may cause pain, impairment of mobility, and skin breakdown.

Some immobilized patients may develop signs of **thrombus formation.** A thrombus is a blood clot loosely attached to the wall of a vein, caused by stasis of the blood, injury to a vessel, or hypercoagulability of the blood. In addition, patients on bedrest often become dehydrated and have higher calcium levels than others which contributes to increased blood viscosity and hypercoagulability. Patients susceptible are those who have a condition that increases the coagulability of the blood, and those who have had previous thrombi or recent trauma.

Calf pain may indicate **thrombophlebitis,** which is inflammation of a vein. A tender, red, swollen cord is palpable over the affected superficial vein. There will be an increased warmth of the affected extremity and a bluish mottling of the skin, particularly in the dependent position. The longer a patient is immobilized, the greater the risk of a blood clot. Factors contributing to blood clot formation begin after immobilization. If a thrombus breaks loose from a vein and enters the circulation it becomes an **embolus.** This can occur when a patient is allowed to sit or stand after prolonged inactivity. An embolus can travel to the heart and into the lung. Damage to the lung can cause a pulmonary infarct. Of those patients who develop a pulmonary embolus, nearly 40 percent die within two hours of onset.[2] An embolus may lodge in a peripheral artery of the leg and cause symptoms such as pain, pallor, coolness, and tingling.

Patients on bedrest can cause damage to their cardiovascular systems through the increased use of the **valsalva maneuver.** A valsalva maneuver is an attempt to forcibly exhale with the nose and mouth closed, resulting in an increased intrathoracic pressure and a decreased return of blood to the heart. This can occur when a bedridden patient performs a pushing, pulling, or straining movement, such as using his upper trunk muscles to turn in bed or lift himself with an overhead trapeze. Straining during bowel movements also can result in the valsalva maneuver. After holding his breath, the person releases it and the drop in intrathoracic pressure causes the blood to rush to the heart. This surge of blood causes a corresponding increase in heart rate. For individuals with heart problems, continual use of the valsalva maneuver can have detrimental effects.

Orthostatic hypotension is the inability of the autonomic nervous system to adapt to a sudden change from a lying down to an upright position. As a result, there is a rapid fall in blood pressure and increase in heart rate accompanied by dizziness, weakness, and fainting. Nearly all patients, including healthy, active people, find that they may become lightheaded when they get up too quickly after lying down, even for short periods of time. Orthostatic hypotension occurs for several reasons. Prolonged immobilization causes a decrease in blood volume due to changes in blood pressure and the redistribution of blood.[3] When the person changes position, the peripheral vessels fail to respond, and blood pools in the legs, resulting in a decreased return of blood to the heart and a subsequent decrease in blood pressure. The pressure of leg muscles against the veins is very important in helping to pump the blood back to the heart.

Prolonged immobility also can cause an **increased workload for the heart.** In a supine position, blood volume is redistributed from the legs, some of which enters the pulmonary circulation. With this increase of blood to the heart, the cardiac output and heart rate increase, so that the heart works harder. Bedrest does not harm the heart, however, and damaged or enlarged hearts do improve with a reduction in stress and muscular work.

When a person is confined to bed for a length of time with a limitation of activity, the cardiac rate, circulatory volume, and arterial pressure all decrease. This is due to the redistribution of the fluid components of the body and the unfitness of the entire cardiovascular system.[4] Without exercise, the heart does not function as well, and its efficiency deteriorates. A muscle that is well exercised is able to use oxygen from the blood more efficiently. Continual use of muscles also results in greater mechanical efficiency. When a patient does begin to get out of bed, he will experience a **decreased exercise tolerance.** His cardiovascular system will not be able to deliver adequate oxygen to perform activites that he could do easily before bedrest, and he will tire easily. It may take from days to months of gradual reconditioning before the cardiac and skeletal muscles perform as in the pre-immobile state.

Skin

Immobility can have an especially rapid and visible effect on the skin. Nurses, because of their close association with bedside care, assume a primary responsibility for inspecting and caring for the patient's skin. In addition, most of the interventions relating to the prevention of skin breakdown are carried out by the nurse. Since nurses are responsible for skin care, it is especially important for them to understand the effects that immobility can have on the skin.

The pressure that occurs when patients remain in the same position for too long can result in a **decubitus ulcer.** These pressure sores or bedsores are breaks in the surface skin or mucous membrane characterized by disintegration or death of the tissue. Pressure sores begin to form when there is a compression of skin, subcutaneous tissue, or muscle between a body prominence and an unyielding surface, so that interference with the local circulation occurs. Initially the tissues become anoxic as their oxygen is reduced. Then they become ischemic due to obstruction of the inflowing arterial blood. Finally, tissue necrosis occurs—death and sloughing of the tissue.

There are four major stages in the development of a decubitus ulcer, which correspond to tissue layers (see Figure 18-2). After the decubitus has formed, two more stages may occur that result in further fat and muscle necrosis and bone destruction. One of the severest complications that can result from these later two stages is septicemia. What is seen at the skin surface is only the top of the ulcer, since 70 percent of the ulcer is below the skin. Pressure is transmitted in a cone-shaped manner from the skin through each layer of tissue to the body prominence so that a cone of tissue destruction is created (see Figure 18-3).

Many factors contribute to decubitus ulcer formation, and it is the nurse's responsibility to be fully aware of these factors. When a patient moves in bed, he is exposed to **shearing forces,** in which the bone and underlying tissues move one way, while the

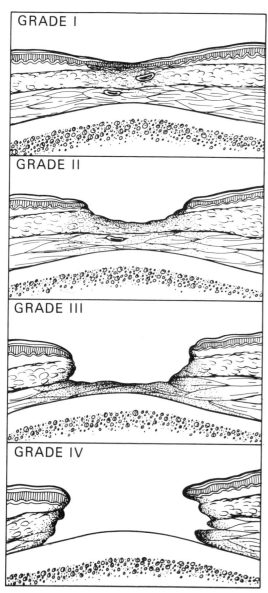

Figure 18-2. **The first stage in the development of a decubitus ulcer.** The stage of transient circulatory disturbance when pressure is applied, blocking the blood flow. As the pressure is released, reactive hyperemia of the skin occurs, displayed as a bright red flush. A Grade I pressure sore involves the superficial epidermal and dermal layers. Surrounding tissue is inflamed and swollen. Grade II pressure sores are shallow, full thickness skin injuries that involve adipose tissue. There is complete loss of the dermal and epidermal layers. Grade III ulcers have progressed into muscle tissue. Necrotic tissue must be removed before healing can take place. In grade IV, epithelial, adipose, and muscle tissue have necrosed; underlying bone or joint structures are involved. (Courtesy of Johnson and Johnson Products Inc.).

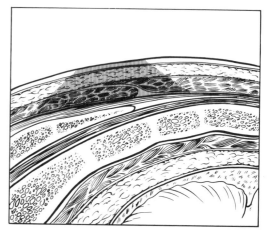

Figure 18-3. **Cone of tissue destruction. The decubitus ulcer is almost always larger than its surface would suggest.**

skin is held in place (see Figure 18.4). Shearing forces pull tissues rather than press on them. They move one layer of tissue over another. When the shearing forces are strong, the subcutaneous blood vessels can be kinked or stretched, and the soft tissues can be torn. When a patient slips down in the bed in the inclined position (see Figure 18-4), when he is pulled up or down in bed instead of being lifted properly, or if he digs his heels and elbows into the mattress, he is exposed to shearing forces. **Friction** injuries can be caused by rubbing against wrinkled sheets and over-vigorous massage with towels. The danger sites include the front of the knees, the elbows, and the inner sides of the knees and ankles. **Moisture** due to perspiration, draining wounds, or incontinence can cause skin to become swollen, soft, and easily damaged. Skin creases in fatty skin

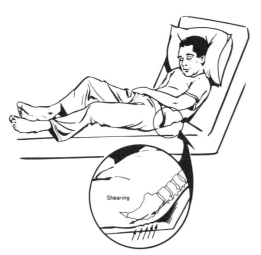

Figure 18-4. When a patient assumes a poor position in bed shearing forces occur where the bone and underlying tissues move one way, while the skin is held in place.

can develop moisture and friction resulting in sores around the genitals, between the thighs, and under pendulous breasts. **Edema** causes tissue pressure, so that cells have a reduced rate of oxygen and nutrient exchange. Edematous tissues also are more fragile and more liable to be injured.

Drugs injected into subcutaneous tissue in the same areas, without rotating sites, can cause skin breakdown. **Injuries** of the skin resulting in cracks or abrasions caused by long finger nails, poor equipment, and careless handling of patients soon lead to ulcers. **Poor hygiene** can allow bacterial invasion of ischemic tissues, increasing the likelihood of development of an ulcer. **Fever** causes a patient's metabolic rate to increase, which increases the demand for oxygen in an already compromised tissue area. **Anemia,** resulting in decreased hemoglobin, causes the oxygen supply to the skin to be reduced and can lead to skin breakdown or slow healing.

Several groups of patients are particularly susceptible to the development of pressure sores. Most pressure sores occur in the elderly. Changes in the elderly due to

the aging process include depression of resistance to infection and healing processes, hypertension, arteriosclerosis, tissue atrophy, and skin and muscle wasting. In general, the elderly have a loss of adaptability and are unable to respond to threats to their skin integrity with sufficient speed and flexibility. Other susceptible persons include thin, bony persons, and people who have peripheral edema, loss of peripheral sensation, loss of bowel and bladder control, motor paralysis, or complete immobilization. Anemia, cancer, obesity, and diabetes are examples of other precipitating factors.

When skin pressures measured over bony prominences are greater than 30 mmHg (critical value for ischemia) decubiti are likely to develop. Instruments are available to place under patients for measuring the surface pressure of weight against their skin (see Figure 18-5). When a person is on a bed in the supine position, it has been found that the highest surface pressures are recorded under six locations, in order of highest to lowest: heels, occiput, buttocks, calves, scapulae, and elbows.[5] The majority of decubitus ulcers have been found to occur over the sacrum, trochanter, heel, ischium, and ankle. The remainder of them occur on the lower leg, lateral edge of the foot, thigh, ear, scapula, iliac crest, anterior superior spine, knee,

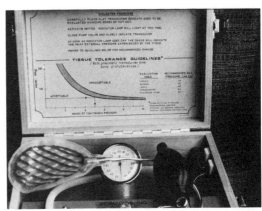

Figure 18-5. Schimedics' pressure evaluator.

spinous process, achilles tendon, sole of the foot, shoulder, elbow, and big toe[6] (see Figure 18-6).

Musculoskeletal and Peripheral Nervous Systems

Prolonged bedrest without protective measures can lead to much damage within the musculoskeletal and peripheral nervous systems. Changes occur that are not visible to the nurse until it is too late to prevent them. One of the problems that can occur is **disuse osteoporosis.** In a healthy person, bone is continually being built (osteoblastic activity) and at the same time being broken down (osteoclastic activity) at similar rates. These processes occur due to the normal stresses created by the pull of muscle on the bone. When a person becomes inactive, he has decreased stress on the bones secondary to a decrease in muscle tension, and resulting decreased stress on the long bones of the upper and lower legs. The osteoblastic and osteoclastic activities become imbalanced, and the osteoclasts break down the bone at a faster rate. The matrix of the bone becomes thin-

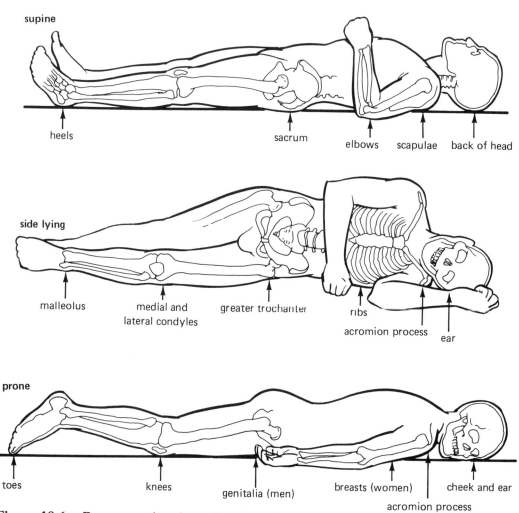

Figure 18-6.   Pressure points in various positions.

ned and porous, and calcium and phosphorus are dissolved into the bloodstream and excreted. A high blood level of calcium can result in kidney stones and the deposition of calcium in the muscles and joints, causing pain. When bones become porous and spongy, they break under weight bearing, so that a patient can develop a **pathological fracture.** This type of fracture occurs with slight or no trauma. The long bones of the lower extremities, the bodies of the vertebrae, and the heel bone are most involved in osteoporosis.

Immobility results in a **decreased muscle mass and strength,** especially pronounced during the initial period of immobilization. A muscle maintains and increases strength through frequent contractions of muscle fibers. Without activity, there is a loss of strength and mass. Muscle mass is also lost in bedrest due to the concurrent protein breakdown. The muscles that are affected the most by immobility are those that the patient uses for walking and the maintenance of an upright position.

Another major complication of immobility and bedrest is the development of contractures. A **contracture** is an abnormal shortening of muscle tissue resulting from decreased range of motion. When a joint is poorly positioned, a dynamic imbalance of muscle power may occur, as a stronger, unopposed muscle shortens and is never lengthened by its weak opponent. Once the tendons, ligaments, and joint capsule are involved, the contracture may require surgical intervention for its release.

If the foot is allowed to rest in an unsupported position, the muscles in the anterior portion of the leg become stretched. Also, the tendon of the calf muscle tends to shorten. This results in a **foot-drop** deformity. Once the patient is ready to get out of bed and ambulate, he is unable to place his heel on the floor and has difficulty walking. When patients sit for long periods of time with their knees flexed and supported by

pillows, they can develop knee-flexion contractures. At the posterior aspect of the thigh, the hamstring group of muscles, whose tendons pass under the knee, tends to contract quickly during immobility.

Patients on bedrest who are allowed to remain in the sitting position for prolonged periods of time have a danger of a prolonged outward rotation at the hips. Also, since the hips are flexed, such a patient may develop a **hip-flexion contracture.** If there is a depression in the mattress at the hip level, a contracture of the hip flexor muscles may occur, which will prevent the patient from being able to fully extend (straighten) his hips when in the upright position. Patients who are continuously turned from side to side with their legs adducted (moved towards the body) and their hips and knees flexed will also develop contractures. If pillows are not placed between the thighs for alignment of the extremities, the person may develop a dislocation of the hip that was unsupported and adducted for so long.

Patients on bedrest with very little energy frequently lie with their arms held closely to the sides of the body, their wrists crossed and dropped, and their elbows flexed at right angles. The muscles at the axillary (armpit) level, especially the pectoral group, can develop contractures. Also, patients wearing a sling who do not perform range of motion exercises may get tight pectoral muscles and an adduction contracture.

Patients confined to bedrest frequently experience backaches. When the complaint is investigated, it is usually found that the patient sits in a slumped position on his sacrum or lumbar spine with his chest caved in and his shoulders sagging forward, pulled down by the weight of his arms. Pain and spasms then occur in the muscles of the back. His hips may not be back as far as possible in the angle of the bed so that his body weight can be correctly borne on the ischia and the thighs.

Pillows are sometimes found bunched up under the shoulders and head, leaving the spine out of its normal alignment. A soft mattress also can contribute to poor support for the patient's back.

Immobility can cause damage within the peripheral nervous system. **Nerve damage** will occur from the improper use of tight restraints which causes compression of nerves. Improper body positioning and bedrest can cause compression and ischemia of superficial nerves that course around body prominences. **Wrist drop** can occur if the ulnar nerve is compressed in a wrong sleeping position. Prolonged pressure on the peroneal nerve as it courses around the head of the fibula can occur from a tight plaster cast. Foot drop or the inability to flex the foot and toes can result.

Elimination

Due to a restriction of activity and changes in body positioning from upright to lying down, patients on bedrest frequently develop problems eliminating body wastes. When not adequately treated or controlled, elimination problems can become one of the immobile patient's most trying problems.

When a patient on bedrest is in a strange environment with a changed daily routine and lack of privacy, he may suppress the desire to defecate. If a person continues to avoid defecating when he feels the urge, gradually the defecation urge will become weaker. Also, as food enters the stomach and upper small intestine, the gastric reflexes normally cause fecal material to be emptied into the colon. Recumbency and inactivity alter the effect of meals, and the passage of fecal material is delayed. Physical activity and gravity both normally contribute to the propulsive movements of the colon.

Some immobilized people do not have the muscle strength to pass stool, especially if it is hard. Abdominal and perineal muscles used for defecating become weakened by bedrest. Also it is very difficult to bear down on a bedpan while in the sitting position in bed. Many patients do not have the physical strength to position themselves and lean forward on a bedpan. The changes in intrathoracic pressure caused by the valsalva maneuver and the stimulation of the vagus nerve can cause complications such as heart block or cardiac arrest. Also, hemorrhoids, anal fissures, ulcers, and rectal prolapse can result from excessive straining at stool. Straining can increase intracranial pressure, which can cause serious damage to neurosurgical and eye surgery patients.

If the stool is allowed to become hard and dry, constipation can occur. When constipation continues, fecal impaction may result. With prolonged retention of feces in the colon, more water is absorbed and the stool becomes hard and dry. Liquid stool may begin oozing out around the impaction and mistakenly identified as diarrheal stool. A fecal impaction may result in a mechanical bowel obstruction, which interrupts the normal intestinal propulsions and movement of digested food and feces. This is a very serious situation and must be treated immediately.

Supine immobility has relatively little direct effect on the kidneys; however, when a patient is first immobilized there is an increase in renal blood flow with a subsequent increase in urine volume. Immobility also causes an increase in the volume of tissue fluid being reabsorbed into the plasma, which in turn creates a temporary increase in urinary excretion.[7] When a person is lying immobile on his back, his kidney pelvis does not completely drain. The opening of the kidney leading to the ureter is anatomically positioned to provide constant drainage of urine in the upright position. This prevents stasis of the urine. After just a few days in the supine position urinary stasis occurs in the kidney pelvis, and can result in infection and damage.

Complete emptying of the bladder occurs more easily in the upright position. Many men find it very difficult to void while lying or sitting in bed. Once they are able to stand, they find that they can urinate quite easily. When voluntary actions are not adequately carried out due to awkward positioning or embarrassment, the urination cannot be initiated. The patient may either wait too long to empty his bladder or only partially empty it. Urinary retention can cause bladder distention, which can result in a loss of bladder muscle tone, so that the patient has no desire to void even though his bladder is full. The bladder becomes distended and urine may back up into the kidney pelvis, causing damage. The patient may have to be catheterized in order to determine if there is residual urine in the bladder. Additional problems include severe discomfort, sensitivity to palpation, and restlessness.

During immobility, calcium is mobilized from the bone in the process of bone resorption and is excreted in the urine. When a patient is in the supine position, as the urine sits in the renal calices there is more time for the calcium to precipitate. As tiny particles settle out of the urine, they are the beginning of kidney or bladder stones. Alkaline urine, dehydration, infection, and a decreased citric acid concentration also contribute to the formation of renal stones. Less calcium is held in solution as the urine becomes more alkaline, while dehydration produces less urine for washout of particulate matter. Infection can provide bacteria nuclei around which stones can form. Bacterial activity may decrease citric acid levels that normally helps to maintain an acid pH. Fifteen to 30% of patients who have been on prolonged bedrest have kidney stones.[8]

Metabolism and Nutrition

Presently, very little is known about what happens to a person's metabolism, fluid and electrolyte balance, and endocrine system, once he becomes immobilized. It is well-known, though, that proper nutrition plays a very large role in maintaining crucial metabolic balances. Immobility induces a decrease in the basal metabolic rate and oxygen consumption of the body.[9] The body requires less energy to function while on bedrest, since there is less activity. Also, during bedrest the process of building new tissue from nutrients is slowed, while the processes that break down tissues are increased.

Normally, the body tissues break down nitrogen, which is lost through the urine and stool. On about the fifth to sixth day of immobilization, more nitrogen is excreted than is taken in, and a condition known as negative nitrogen balance develops. If persons are immobilized after surgery or accidental trauma, excretion of nitrogen occurs earlier. By the second week of bedrest the negative nitrogen balance reaches its peak and gradually returns to a normal state. With negative nitrogen balance, there is a depletion of stores for protein synthesis essential to healing skin ulcers and surgical or traumatic wounds. It is assumed that muscle tissue is the source of the excreted nitrogen. Patients on bedrest have muscle mass decreases although their body weight tends to remain stable. With reduced muscular activity, there is atrophy of skeletal muscle and the smooth muscles associated with gastrointestinal functioning.

Fluid and electrolyte imbalances can occur due to immobility. The kidneys respond to the changes in tissue metabolism induced by prolonged bedrest by excessive excretion of potassium and calcium.[10,11] Another change that occurs during immobility is loss of appetite, or anorexia. A patient who is inactive or immobile uses less energy and has a decreased rate of metabolism, and as an adaptive mechanism, his appetite soon decreases. The patient also may develop constipation and gas pains. Medications or other therapies may affect the patient's ability to digest, absorb, or use nutrients in the food eaten. Boredom, depression, uninteresting unpalatable institutional food, and limited chewing abilities are other causes of anorexia.

The recommended daily caloric allowance for the average person in the resting state is 1,500 calories for the male and 1,000 calories for the female.[12] Fever, stress, certain drugs, trauma, and wound healing can elevate a patient's basal calorie requirement significantly. The immediate postoperative patient requires between 2,500 and 4,000 calories per day.[13] When a patient does not eat enough, the body adapts to its lack of needed caloric intake by breaking down its own fat and protein supply. The patient then goes into a negative nitrogen balance.

PSYCHOSOCIAL ASPECTS OF IMMOBILITY

When an individual experiences immobility, he loses some of his ability to be independent within his environment. This can be a confusing and sometimes threatening situation. Frequently, the nurse tends to focus so heavily on the patient's physical problems that the psychosocial aspects of his care are neglected.

Throughout his lifespan, each person has developed needs, a self-concept, and values that are essential for his satisfaction, security, and comfort as a human being. A person may be feeling unwell and must be confined to his bed, but he still needs safety and security, love and belongingness, self-esteem, privacy, and respect from others. Needs and values relating to prestige, status, and expectations of himself do not suddenly disappear when a person becomes physically ill.

A person who experiences immobility will begin to notice that many changes—physical, internal, interpersonal, environ-

mental, social, and cultural—all of which can cause a great deal of stress for him. Changes that can occur include sensory, perceptual, and tactile deprivation (see Chapter 19). Immobility, sensory deprivation, illness, and injury also cause changes in one's body image. Patients who are immobile in some way or who are on bedrest experience a variety of feelings, perceptions, and information about their bodies. They bring with them to the hospital previously formed, culturally determined values of how their bodies should look and feel. Patients with artificial limbs, for example, experience emotional stages of loss of the body part they once took for granted. Physical changes related to immobility present a significant threat to the identity.

The social isolation and depersonalization of a health care institution also presents problems. Immobility can cause a deprivation of interpersonal relationships and other self-actualizing activities. Patients can lie in bed for days, for example, without having a meaningful conversation with anyone. Unfortunately, nurses rarely have enough time to spend talking to patients. Patients who are hospitalized and on bedrest also can experience isolation from loved ones. They are removed from close contact with family and close friends. People in the outside world may find it very inconvenient to visit. They may gradually come less frequently, as they find that they have increasingly less in common with the patient. Elderly people who live alone and have problems with mobility also may find that they are deprived of close personal relationships.

Immobility can bring about temporary or permanent interpersonal and social role changes, too. Patients are suddenly unable to fulfill their basic self-care needs and become dependent upon others. They may lose their roles in the family as breadwinner, homemaker, decisionmaker, or parent. Financial, job, and community status changes occur. The patient may have been making a large contribution to meeting the family's economic needs and providing valuable services to an employer. Patients may be painfully aware of their lowered community status and worry that their families are suffering financially. Time spent on bedrest also interferes with developmental tasks and valued goals. A patient may be losing a large block of time out of his life. Children miss school and learning of developmental tasks. Adults must delay achieving various goals in life.

There is, inevitably, a cultural dimension to patients' and families' experiences of and reactions to immobility. The American culture places great emphasis on youth, vigor, strength, beauty, and activity. A patient may feel an acute need to appear attractive and presentable for visitors. This need may not be recognized by a nurse who fails to look beyond the person's physical needs. The hospital environment can be very threatening to people who have lived in a society and culture different from that represented by institutionalized care. Men tend to have more difficulty than women in expressing their emotions, and some fare poorly in the dependent, sick role. Hospitalized men feel unproductive, for example, having been raised in a society with a strong work ethic. Foreign patients may be totally unaccustomed to being in a different cultural environment and require special foods, rituals, and religious services. Families in various cultures also react differently to the idea of caring for an immobile patient at home.

As patients experience these many threatening changes, they can develop initial emotional responses of loneliness, depression, anger, frustration, anxiety, lowered self-esteem, inferiority, worthlessness, powerlessness, and a sense of boredom, and monotony.[14,15] These signs and symptoms of psychological stress may range in severity, and their significance is related to the patient's coping patterns and support systems.

After experiencing initial psychological stress, the person goes through a phase of adaptation to his psychological stress. A patient uses adaptive measures in order to cope with and seek immediate relief from the discomfort of his initial emotional responses. His behaviors may not involve conscious problem solving or be effective unless he receives help. Ineffective adaptation behaviors exhibited by patients attempting to cope with their emotional responses to immobility include: extreme denial, dependency, disorientation, confusion, auditory and visual hallucinations, exaggerated emotional reactions, demanding and manipulative behaviors, aggressiveness, regression, withdrawal, apathy, and lessened motivation to learn and problem solve.

The psychological and physical stress of immobility also causes changes in certain mental functions and abilities. Changes include:[16,17]

- Inability to sleep
- Decreased abilities to learn and solve problems
- Diminished drives and expectations
- Inability to cooperate with treatment programs
- Decreased speed of perception
- Deteriorated perception of time and place
- Decrease in the perceptions of pattern and form, weight discrimination, and pressure
- Decrease in temperature sensitivity.

Many patients adapt well to psychological stress. They are able to direct their energies to accomplish important goals rather than to waste their time in ineffective, regressive activities. Those who adapt poorly and are unable to resolve their problems through defensive measures or problem solving tend to lose control until a state of crisis occurs. A patient experiences a crisis situation when he is no longer able to respond with adequate coping mechanisms (see Chapter 23). Patients do not always reach this phase.

THE NURSING PROCESS

The four main steps in the nursing process include assessment, planning, implementation, and evaluation. Once the nurse assesses the patient and detects his problems and needs, a nursing diagnosis can be formed. Nursing is not only problem oriented, but also is concerned with prevention, maintenance, and restoration. Nurses must plan care based not only on a patient's problems, but also on his daily needs. All of the patient's more basic needs are aimed at his ultimate desire to become a self-actualized, self-sufficient member of society. For certain patients, long-term goals may be unattainable, so the nurse should encourage them to focus on short-term needs and goals. The nurse can help the patient to attain his goals through assessment, identification of problems and needs, statement of nursing diagnoses, planning of nursing care objectives, implementation of the goals, evaluation of patient outcome criteria, and continual reassessment of all steps of the nursing process.

Assessment

During the assessment phase, the nurse performs an orderly collection of data relating to the patient's physical, emotional, family, social, and environmental needs and problems. An assessment tool may be designed specifically for the purpose of assessing the patient's responses to immobility. Refer to Figure 18-7 for an example of key components to include in such a tool. It is very important for nurses to make their assessments carefully and in sufficient detail to formulate accurate nursing diagnoses related to the patient's

independent nursing care. Because immobility can evoke such a broad range of responses, some of which develop slowly, it is important to include as much of this information as possible at the early stages of immobility. This initial baseline assessment usually is done at the time of admission or on the first home visit. In the case of hospitalized patients (or nursing home residents, etc.), a shorter version of this same type of assessment can be devised in a checklist format. Figure 18-7 can be used as a guide for either type of assessment.

The data for the psychosocial assessment of the patient can be collected gradually as the nurse provides bedside care. Of particular importance is knowledge about how a patient handles stress, what his support systems are, and how he feels about himself in general. Nonverbal behaviors, such as gestures, movements, and facial expressions, often give additional important information. A slumped body posture, for example, may indicate depression or withdrawal.

As nurses complete their assessments, they begin to identify problem areas and patient needs that will lead to nursing diagnoses and form the basis of the nursing care plan. In addition to the information found in Figure 18-7, the following data categories are presented as guidelines in the assessment of responses to immobility:

DATA CATEGORIES/PHYSICAL COMPONENTS

- Oxygenation adequacy
- Acid/base balance
- Sensory functions
- Hormonal/metabolic functions
- Body temperature regulation
- Fluid and electrolyte balance
- Nutrition of body cells
- Level of consciousness
- Elimination of body wastes
- Sleep, rest, and relaxation

Nursing Assessment for Problems of Immobility
Flow Sheet Check-List

	Date						
	Time						
Respirations regular/lungs clear							
Irregular respirations							
Shortness of breath							
Ashen/pallor/cyanosis							
Rales/rhonchi/wheezing							
Cough/sputum production							
Alert, awake, oriented							
Confused							
Restless/combative							
Drowsy/lethargic							
Comatose							
Heart sounds regular							
Peripheral pulses present							
Heart sounds irregular							
Peripheral pulse/pulses absent							
Legs unequal size/color/temp.							
Ankle edema							
Orthostatic B.P. changes							
Skin clear, warm, and dry							
Skin cool/moist							
Pressure sores/redness/edema							
Abrasions/burns/wounds							
Dry, scaly skin							
Good range of motion in joints							
Contractures							
Joint swelling							
Decreased muscle strength							
Fractures/casts/splints							
Daily stool							
Urine clear/adequate amount							
Bowel sounds absent							
Constipation							
Cloudy urine							
Burning/frequency of urination							
Incontinence							
Appetite good							
Good response to illness							
Taking nourishment poorly							
Complaints/poor coping patterns							
Sleeping poorly							
Presence of pain							
Family visited							

Figure 18-7. This assessment tool can be used each day as a guide and as a method of documenting that an assessment of the patient was done. The nurse should mark the date and time the assessment was performed and then place a check mark by the appropriate signs, symptoms, and observations.

- Hygiene and physical comfort
- Exercise, general mobility.

PSYCHOSOCIAL CATEGORY

- Protection from psychologic threat and physical harm
- Privacy and a feeling of integrity
- Dependence and stability
- A predictable, orderly environment
- Love, affection, and sexual expression
- Acceptance, approval, and companionship
- A sense of value and usefulness
- Adequacy, self-reliance, and independence
- Goal achievement and mastery of skills
- Dignity, recognition, and appreciation from others
- Attention, status, and importance
- Personal growth and maturity
- Increased learning and development of potential
- Religious and philosophical satisfaction
- Increased reality perception and problem solving abilities.

After the patient's problems and needs are identified, the nurse determines whether or not his needs are being met and if he is adapting well to his illness. The nursing diagnoses are concerned with the patient's problems and needs for the prevention of further complications and ill health, maintenance of daily care, therapy and healing of the present illness, and restoration of the patient to an independent, self-satisfied individual. The following list of nursing diagnoses represent some typical examples appropriate for an immobile patient on bedrest:

- Ineffective breathing patterns related to immobility

- Potential aspiration of food or fluid related to weakness and supine position
- Potential impaired peripheral circulation related to lack of exercise and immobility
- Real or potential impairment of skin integrity related to being on complete bedrest
- Decubitus ulcers related to prolonged bedrest
- Self-care deficits (feeding, bathing, dressing) related to severe contractures
- Decreased appetite related to decreased exercise and immobility
- Alteration in elimination related to immobility
- Ineffective coping patterns related to fear of immobility
- Role disturbance related to loss of position in family and community
- Sensory alteration related to social isolation.

Planning

Planning is the second phase of the nursing process. During this stage the nurse determines what can be done to assist the patient. This is when goals and objectives are written, priorities are judged, and methods are designed to resolve problems and meet the patient's needs. Nursing care objectives are explicit statements that describe exactly what nurses plan to accomplish with their nursing care. Examples of objectives appropriate for a patient on extended bedrest are:

Nursing Care Objectives

- To support adequate chest expansion and respiratory ventilation
- To prevent the accumulation of secretions in the respiratory tract

- To promote safety in the prevention of aspiration of gastric contents
- To prevent venous stasis, dependent edema, thrombus formation, and pulmonary emboli
- To maintain normal autonomic nervous system responses to position changes
- To promote adequate exercise tolerance of muscles
- To support the integrity of the patient's skin and mucous membranes
- To provide massage, touching, and other forms of sensory stimulation to the skin
- To provide adequate protection for maintenance of a normal body temperature
- To maintain the stability and integrity of the patient's bones
- To maintain the patient's muscle mass, tone, and strength
- To prevent joint contractures, deformities, and nerve damage
- To maintain normal functioning of the patient's gastrointestinal and genitourinary tracts
- To prevent constipation, fecal impaction, and mechanical bowel obstruction
- To prevent renal stones, difficulty in urination, and urinary stasis, retention, infection, and incontinence
- To provide adequate dietary protein and exercise for the maintenance of body protein stores
- To maintain patient's fluid and electrolyte balance
- To prevent sensory, perceptual, and tactile deprivation
- To prevent sensory overload, distortion or monotony
- To promote positive body image and self-concept

- To provide personal attention and an environment with social activities and family contacts
- To promote patient's adaptation to family, job, and community role changes
- To support needs for growth, development, learning, and spiritual satisfaction
- To support the patient's cultural needs and differences.

Implementation

After the planning stage, the nurse is ready to implement the nursing process. In the implementation phase, the plans are put into action and the actual nursing care

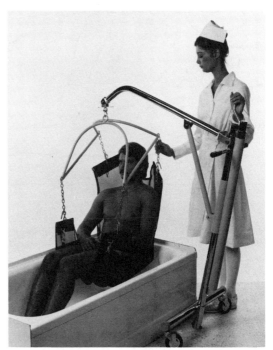

Figure 18-8.   This portable patient lifter is for lifting patients from supine to sitting and for transfer to wheelchair, commode, bath, and auto during home care. Such home aids can enable a severely immobilized patient to live at home. (Courtesy of Trans-Aid Corporation)

is given, based on defined goals and objectives. Nurses use technical, intellectual, and interpersonal skills to implement their objectives. Other members of the health care team, such as dieticians, physical therapists, and respiratory therapists, help the nurse meet goals set for the patient. Family members, and especially the patient himself, should participate during the implementation phase.

There are new products and equipment available for helping patients with various problems of immobility. Many patients are able to live at home and be cared for comfortably by family members, thanks to portable patient lifters, multipurpose wheelchairs, and well designed walking aids (see

Figure 18-8). Mechanical prostheses have been designed for useless limbs, and wheelchairs are even motorized now.

Even with the best intentions, it is not always possible for the nurse to implement all of the goals set for the patient and to prevent all of the hazards of bedrest and immobility. It is important to know, however, those nursing actions that are most likely to meet the needs of immobilized patients. The following discussion summarizes some of the most important nursing actions.

Proper positioning and body alignment are very important concepts to understand in the care of immobilized patients. In whichever position the body assumes,

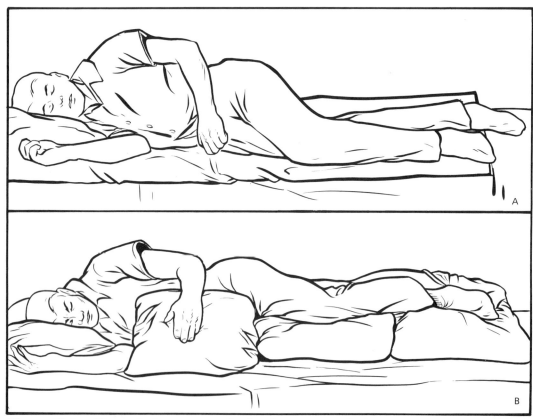

Figure 18-9.   Figure A shows a poor body alignment with the arm resting on the chest and the calf of the upper leg compressing the tibia bone of the lower leg. Figure B shows pillows placed between the legs in order to align the lower extremities. A flat pillow should be provided so that the neck is not hyperextended.

gravity continues to exert its force. Once the person lies down and is supported by a firm bed, he is pushed against the bed by the force of gravity acting at right angles or downward on each individual segment. A straight, hard bed supporting the body cannot match the normal curves of a person. Therefore, when a person is supine, the body parts that protrude posteriorly (occiput, sacrum, heels) must share most of the body weight. The segments in between them have no support and, therefore, tend to sag until the base of support is reached. These natural hollows need to be filled in or supported in order to maintain the axes of the hips and shoulders in relation to the spine. An important concept is that a good posture for a patient on bedrest to assume is the same alignment of body segments that he would assume in order to provide good posture in the vertical position (see Figure 18-9). Much equipment is available to help in positioning patients in bed, in-

cluding pillows, footboards, special boots, splints, and palm grips (see Figure 18-10).

A patient should understand his role in maintaining proper positioning and promoting adequate circulation. When a patient is on extended bedrest or in a chair, blood tends to pool in the legs. The legs may be elevated and elastic compression of the veins can be provided by using ace bandage wraps or elastic stockings. The nurse also can discuss with the physician the possibility of using inflatable leggings that provide intermittent compression of the lower legs. Certain positions cause impairment of venous return. Positions to avoid are flexion of the knees with the knee gatch or pillows, flexion of the hip with elevation of the head, leg compression from the bed, and the lateral recumbent (sidelying) position without support for the upper leg. Patients should be cautioned against crossing their legs at the knees and they should be checked for garters, tight dressings, or con-

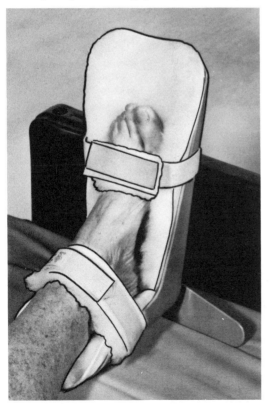

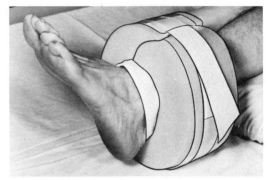

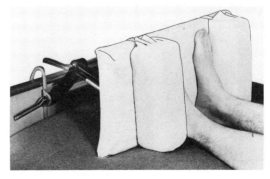

Figure 18-10. Bed Equipment.

strictive clothing above the knees. Leg massages must be avoided so as to prevent turbulence and dislodged emboli. Abdominal distention should be relieved as soon as possible, since it causes compression of the great veins. For those patients with cardiac problems, the head of the bed should be slightly elevated. This results in a decreased blood volume returning from the legs to the heart, thereby reducing the work of the heart.

Turning a patient to various positions, such as to his side, his back, his other side, a sitting position, and possibly the prone position is very important for every body system. Patients who are able to move themselves usually will shift their positions automatically when they feel discomfort from pressure, but often they lie in one

position in bed, due to heavy sedation and fear of pain. Turning patients and having them shift their weight frequently prevents the blockage of blood flow caused by external pressure on the veins in the legs and promotes gravity drainage. The body's position should be altered frequently in relation to gravity, which stimulates the postural neural reflex and prevents orthostatic intolerance. The patient should periodically ambulate, have the head of the bed elevated, and sit on the side of the bed or in a chair. One should investigate the need for a bed that allows for position changes (see Figure 18-11). The nurse can ensure that when a patient moves in bed and strains at bowel movements, he breathes through an open mouth so as to prevent the valsalva maneuver. An overbed frame and trapeze can be provided to help prevent the patient from straining. In order to protect the skin, when patients are moved in bed they should not be pushed or

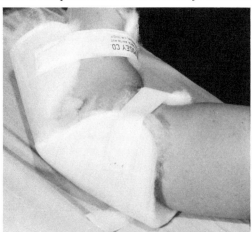

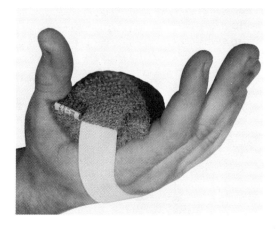

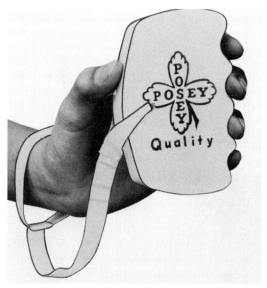

Figure 18-10. Proper supportive bed equipment can prevent a patient from developing foot-drop, contractures, and muscle wasting (Courtesy of J. T. Posey Company).

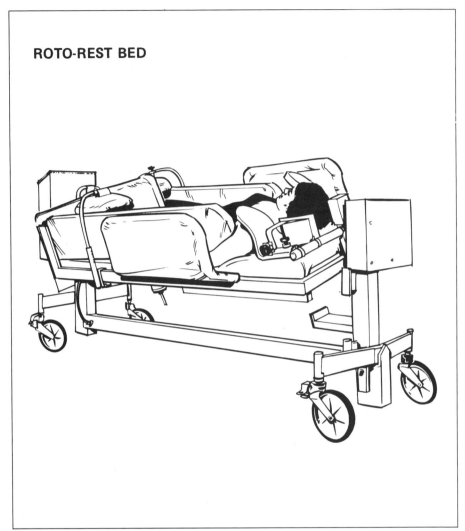

ROTO-REST BED

Figure 18-11.   Roto-Rest Bed. For kinetic care of trauma patients. The bed's silent motor slowly turns in a relaxing, continuous motion over 300 times a day. For therapeutic reasons, the immobile patient is rotated automatically in an arc of 124 degrees every 4.5 minutes. The turning is so slow it will not cause nausea or alarm; and the gentle vibration promotes sleep all night long without waking for turning. When properly positioned there is no head or neck movement which can cause further irreversible injury. Traction can be applied which is constant and the weight does not vary. The constant motion of the bed prevents stasis of urine and respiratory secretions and the occurrence of thrombosis and embolism.
(Courtesy of Kinetic Concepts, Inc.)

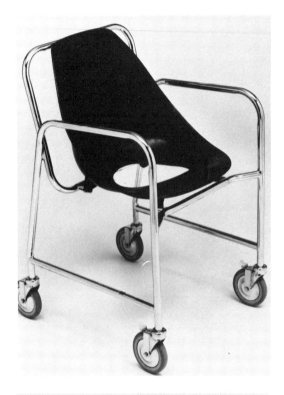

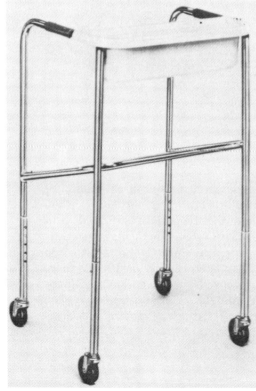

pulled along the bed surface to avoid strong shearing forces.

Since infrequent repositioning permits the same lung regions to remain dependent and at low lung volumes, it is necessary for a patient to change positions at least every two hours to allow for full expansion of all parts of the lung. Turns from side to side (120 degrees) help secretions to drain by gravity from the outer segments of each

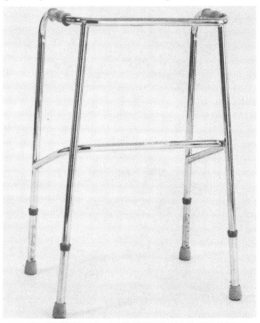

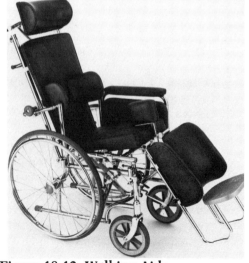

Figure 18-12. Walking Aids.

lung into the major bronchi, where they can be removed by coughing or suctioning.[18] **Postural drainage,** or "tipping," can be used to drain pulmonary secretions by gravity. To aid in dislodging the secretions, the doctor may order the physiotherapy techniques of manual percussion and vibration.

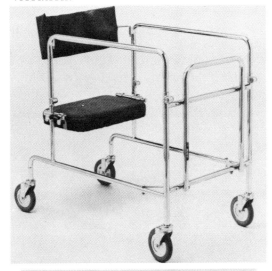

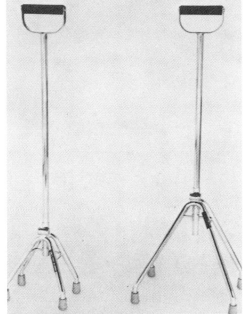

Figure 18-12a.   There are many walking aids available for patients having difficulty ambulating.

Providing exercise for one's patient is important in the prevention of contractures and muscle wasting and helps to empty the veins via the muscle pump. The various types of exercises available include an active assistive exercise carried out by the patient with the assistance of the nurse or therapist, a resistive exercise in which the muscle contracts in pushing or pulling against a stationary object, an active range of motion exercise in which the patient moves his joint through its full range of motion, and a passive range of motion exercise in which the therapist moves the patient's joints through their complete range of motion. A patient should be encouraged to perform self-care activities that cause him to use his arms in abduction and outward rotation, including combing his hair and fastening his gown. He also should perform exercises that transmit forces lengthwise along the bone shaft of the lower extremities. This slows the demineralization process. Using a footstrap or pushing against a footboard are helpful. The nurse should provide an opportunity for the patient to stand and bear weight as soon as possible. When a patient is moved from the bed to a wheelchair, he should perform a standing pivot transfer. Patients who are paralyzed also need to have their movable beds locked into a standing position occasionally in order to prevent disuse osteoporosis. For ambulatory patients with problems walking or standing, there are many walking and sitting aids available (see Figure 18-12).

Coughing and deep-breathing exercises should be taught to patients on bedrest. Coughing is the most important natural mechanism for the removal of secretions. Unless contraindicated, patients should be encouraged every two hours to take a deep breath, hold it, and forcibly cough three times. When possible, those with abdominal or chest surgery may be given pain

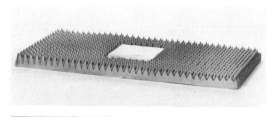

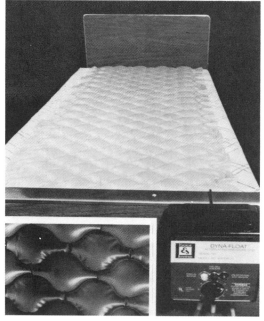

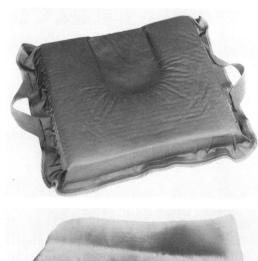

medication 30 minutes before they are to be encouraged to cough. Splinting the abdominal muscles with a pillow is also helpful in providing support. A daily fluid intake of 2,000 ml will help to prevent mucus secretions from becoming thick and viscous.[18] Humidifiers or vaporizers also are useful to prevent irritation and drying of membranes and respiratory secretions. The promotion of self-care activities will increase a patient's energy level, causing natural lung expansion and changes in position. The reasons for coughing, breathing exercises, and position changes should be explained to patients so that they will continue with their own care.

The prevention of skin breakdown is dependent on the provision of an ideal skin environment. Having a suitable room tem-

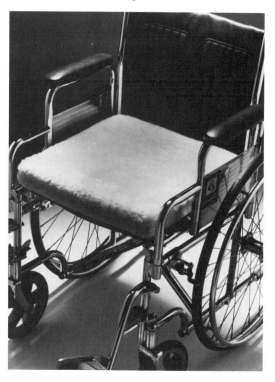

Figure 18-13.   Various beds, mattresses, and pads are available to support either specific pressure areas or the entire body surface in order to prevent skin breakdown.

perature and humidity is important. The nurse should teach the patient and family about skin care and skin inspection. A paraplegic patient who cannot shift his position can be taught to use a mirror for inspecting posterior areas. Much skin breakdown can be prevented by using good hygiene and avoiding irritating soaps or solutions containing alcohol. Skin should always be kept dry and protected from abrasions since maceration, the reduction of tissues to a soft mass through soaking, speeds the decubitus process. The need for absorbent bedpads or diapers should be investigated for incontinent patients. Casts, braces, splints, and compression bandages should be inspected, adjusted, and padded. For patients who are highly susceptible to pressure sores, the nurse should investigate the possibility of obtaining devices designed to support either specific pressure areas or the entire body surface (see Figure 18-13).

Decubitus ulcer care may become a necessity for the immobilized patient. There are several therapies available. When heat lamp therapy is prescribed, the heat pro-

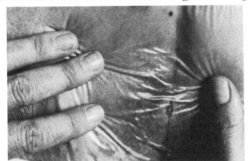

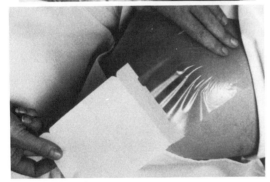

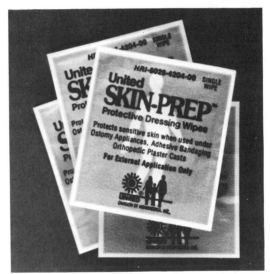

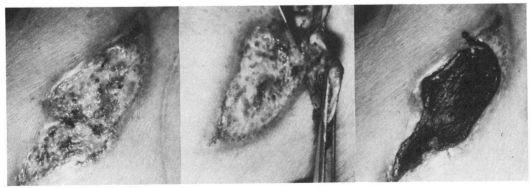

Figure 18-14. Various ointments and dressings are available to debride decubitus ulcers, support fragile tissues, and provide protection against bed clothes.

vides drying of skin salves and an increase in circulation to the area. Once skin is swollen and red or a small ulcer forms, without drainage, often the doctor will order a protective dressing or ointment to be applied. Desitin® ointment, tincture of benzoin, plastic sprays, and other special dressings all provide protection against bed clothes and support fragile tissues (see Figure 18-14). The dressings are porous, allowing hydration, and help to encourage optimal regrowth of the external cellular layer. The best method of reducing bacteria in pressure ulcers is to remove the dead tissue on which they thrive. Enzymatic agents, such as elase ointment, are used to remove this devitalized tissue. In some institutions Debrisan® wound cleansing beads are used in wet ulcers to absorb fluid and cleanse a wound area (see Figure 18-15). When a large decubitus ulcer is healing very slowly, the patient may be susceptible to infection and loses serum and protein through the sore. Surgical intervention may be necessary. Preoperatively, the ulcer frequently is debrided with irrigations and wet-to-dry dressings until a clean healthy granulating bed of tissue is obtained. Surgery includes excision of the ulcer, scar tissue, and usually the bony prominence.[19]

The prevention of problems of elimination is a major responsibility of the patient's bedside nurse. Patients need as much privacy as possible during elimination and unpleasant or foul odors should be removed from the environment. A patient should be encouraged to respond to the urge to defecate in an unrushed manner and to perform exercises in bed that strengthen abdominal and pelvic floor muscles. A plan of care can be developed to help the patient stay on his own schedule of regular bowel movements. As soon as possible, the patient should be permitted to get out of bed and use the bedside commode or bathroom, so that he strains less, and decreases energy expenditure and anx-

iety (see Figure 18-16). In order to avoid constipation in bedridden patients, they should be provided a high-fiber diet. Increased fiber in the intestinal tract speeds a slow transit time, since fiber enlarges and softens stool. A minimum fluid intake of 1,500 to 2,000 ml/day will help prevent stools from becoming hard, dry, and more difficult to evacuate. Some patients will need a daily stool softener, such as Metamucil® (bulk former) or Colace® (surface acting emollient). It is also important to check with the doctor about weaning patients off constipating narcotics and other constipating drugs, such as some antacids.

In order to aid in emptying urine from the kidney a patient should be placed in an upright position for at least part of the day. A patient with bladder incontinence may be encouraged to void every two hours. Then the interval can be lengthened as control is gained. Urine output should not be allowed to drop to less than 30 ml/hr. In order to help prevent urinary tract infections, the urinary pH can be kept acid by means of an acid-ash diet that includes cranberry juice, vitamin C, cereals, poultry, meat, and fish.

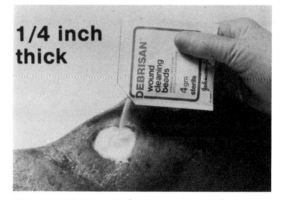

Figure 18-15. Debrisan® wound cleaning beads are tiny hydrophilic beads of a dextranomer (sugar). As the beads swell with fluid, the spaces between them form a capillary system that draws bacteria and debris up and into the bead matrix (Courtesy of Johnson and Johnson Products, Inc.).

Ensuring adequate nutrition, fluid intake, and enough calories to meet the energy requirements of the patient is an important nursing intervention. A daily calorie count can be kept with a record of exactly what the patient eats. Since protein is so vital to prevent muscle wasting, nitrogen imbalance, anemia, and skin breakdown, and to replace loss of protein through open wounds and burns, patients should be encouraged to eat high-protein foods. It also may be necessary to add extra vitamins, minerals, and trace elements, since patients are exposed to unusual stresses during illness. An adequate fluid intake of at least 60 cc/hr is necessary to provide hydration to the skin and to provide dilute, free flowing urine. Loose clothes, a comfortable room temperature, and position changes help to prevent perspiration and fluid loss. A low-calcium diet and sufficient fluids help to reduce kidney stones and blood viscosity, keeping blood clots from forming so easily.

A patient's fluid intake, vomitus, stools, urine, and wound drainage should be carefully measured. One of the best ways to monitor his progress is through daily weights. An environment conducive to eating, with a more sociable or variable set-

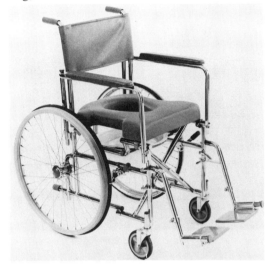

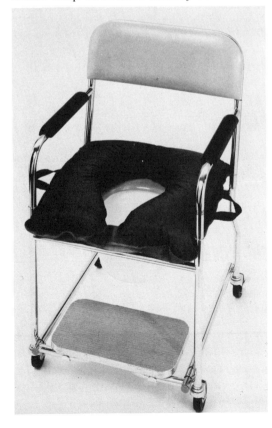

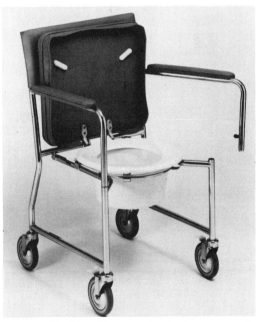

Figure 18-16.   Commode chairs are available that also can be used as shower chairs.

ting, may help the patient to eat his meals. Unpleasant procedures and the administration of sedatives prior to a meal can prevent the patient from being at his most alert and comfortable state while eating. Good oral hygiene will help a patient to retain his full range of chewing abilities. Self-help aids that include special cups and eating utensils are available for patients who lack the ability or energy to feed themselves (see Figure 18-17).

Meeting psychosocial needs is another important nursing intervention. After the nurse has assessed the threatening changes a patient is experiencing and his emotional responses to them, she must help him to adapt to his new situation. The patient will need help in learning more about his emotional reactions to problems and how to use effective coping mechanisms. One must always be alert for ineffective adaptation behaviors and should take measures to advise the patient. For the patient who is adapting well, the nurse may serve simply as a good listener. While a patient is in bed,

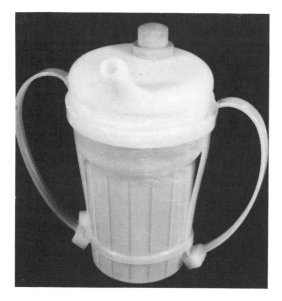

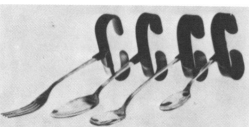

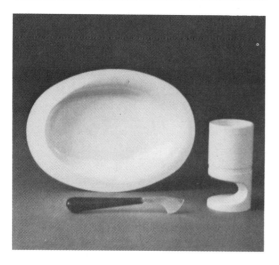

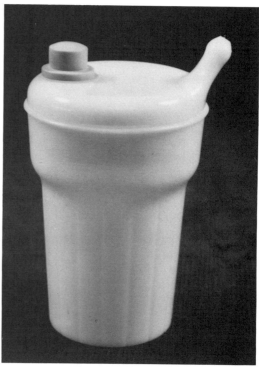

Figure 18-17. Self-help feeding aids can enable the immobilized patient to become more independent.

he may need to be provided with diversional activities and sensory stimulation. Opportunities for patients to socialize can be provided, and the nurse should ensure that patients wear their eyeglasses and hearing aids. Tactile stimulation like a back massage is important, and a sense of caring can be conveyed when a nurse touches a patient. The patient should be constantly reoriented to his environment and encouraged to maintain his normal sleep pattern. He can help to make decisions about his own care. When possible, alternatives should be provided and he should be informed of what he can expect and what is expected of him. Families also need support and encouragement to participate in the patient's care and to continue with their own lives.

Evaluation

The fourth phase of the nursing process is evaluation. The nurse wants to know how the goals have been met and to what degree the patient was maintained or restored to a level where he functions well. The evaluation process is much easier if, during the planning phase, nurses describe specifically what they expect the outcome of care to be, in terms of patient behaviors or physical characteristics. These descriptions are called expected outcomes or outcome criteria. This process of identifying outcome criteria is part of the planning stage and is written on the care plan. Once the outcome criteria are listed, the nurse should place a time limit or deadline for when the patient should be expected to exhibit the particular behavior. Some expected outcomes will need to be in effect at all times, while others, such as a healed fracture, will require a time limit in the future. The nurse then can begin collecting specific evidence to determine if the patient's progress matches the outcome criteria set for him. If he is not meeting the objectives, reassessment should occur, and

the nursing care plan should be updated. The following is a list of outcome criteria appropriate for a patient on extended bedrest. The time limits can be set by the nurse, depending on the patient's problems.

Outcome criteria

The patient evidences:

- Lungs free of heavy secretions as evidenced by normal temperature, pulse, and respiratory rate, lack of rales and rhonchi on auscultation, and absence of sputum production.

- Extremities free of blood clots or thrombophlebitis, as evidenced by lack of pain, equal and normal color, temperature, and size of both extremities, and strong pulses in all extremities.

- Adequate fluid volume and orthostatic tolerance as evidenced by urine output of at least 30 cc/hr, blood pressure higher than 90/50, pulse rate lower than 100, and lack of change in vital signs or mental status when patient rises from lying to upright position.

- Good skin condition as evidenced by clear skin with absence of redness, discoloration, blistering, increased skin temperature, dryness, cracks, abrasions, or sores under casts, at tube entry sites, near draining wounds, and at bony prominences.

- Absence of contractures as evidenced by free, complete range of motion in all joints.

- Normal bowel movements and absence of constipation as evidenced by palpation of a soft flat abdomen, lack of pain or fullness in lower abdomen, good appetite, absence of straining, and passage of soft stools every one to two days.

- Normal urinary tract functioning as

evidenced by absence of pain, urgency, or frequency of urination, presence of clear urine, and normal body temperature.

- Adequate nutrition status as evidenced by proper weight, as based on age and height tables, adequate muscle mass and strength, clear skin, moist tongue and mucous membranes, and absence of edema in ankles and feet.
- Alert and well-oriented mental status as evidenced by correct answers to questions about the time, person, and place.
- Good adjustment to body image and role changes as evidenced by positive statements about his appearance, feelings about hospitalization, and relationship to family.

Conclusions

The problems and severe disabilities associated with bedrest and immobility represent one of the nation's major health problems. Nurses must work toward maintaining and maximizing physiological and psychosocial mobility to avoid the inevitable disabilities of immobilization. When immobility and bedrest are unavoidable, the nurse is responsible for helping the patient to adapt to his situation. After a thorough assessment, nurses should determine the patient's needs and problems and specify nursing diagnoses to provide for the preventative, maintenance, therapeutic, and restorative needs of the patient. The nurse, patient, family, and health care team all should contribute to the planning phase of the patient's care. Nurses should hold themselves accountable for possessing and using updated knowledge of the most effective patient care therapies and commercial products available for the patient who is susceptible to immobilization disabilities. They must take the responsibility to ensure that the care is evaluated,

goals are met, and corrective action is taken.

SUMMARY

Immobility is an intentional or involuntary limitation of activity in any sphere of a person's physical, emotional, intellectual, social, or cultural experience. Mobility is the ability to move freely and easily without restrictions, in one's own environment. A person can be rendered immobile in many ways. Types of immobility include physical, psychological, intellectual, and social. Bedrest and immobility do have some beneficial effects, but to immobilize a person for an excessive length of time can be damaging.

Problems with the respiratory system caused by immobility include decreased chest expansion and respiratory ventilation, atelectasis, the accumulation of secretions in the respiratory tract, hypostatic pneumonia, and aspiration. Hazards for the cardiovascular system can include circulatory stasis, edema, thrombus formation, thrombophlebitis, emboli, increased use of the valsalva maneuver, orthostatic hypotension, increased workload of the heart, and decreased exercise tolerance. Nursing interventions in the care of the cardiovascular and respiratory systems include maintenance of adequate venous circulation and vascular tone, reduction of cardiac workload, frequent changes in body positioning, postural drainage and chest physiotherapy, coughing and deep breathing, mobilization and removal of secretions, hydration and humidification, and promotion of self-care and health teaching.

When a person remains too long in one position, pressure to the skin can lead to decubitus ulcers. Factors contributing to decubitus ulcer formation include shearing forces, friction, moisture, fever, edema, anemia, poor hygiene, skin creases, drugs, and injuries. Patients with malnutrition, anemia, carcinoma, obesity, diabetes, and hypotension are among those especially susceptible to skin breakdown. The areas where their ulcers are most likely to occur is over bony prominences where skin and underlying tissues are frequently compressed. Principles in the prevention and treatment of pressure sores include good hygiene, hydration and nutrition, protective dressings, topical therapy, surgical debridement, and changes of body positioning.

Immobility can lead to problems in the musculoskeletal system, such as osteoporosis, loss of muscle mass and strength, contractures, joint deformities, backaches, and nerve damage. Preventative measures include range of motion exercises and good body alignment and positioning. When a patient on bedrest is in a strange environment with a changed daily routine and lack of privacy, he also may develop bowel problems, such as constipation, fecal impaction, and mechanical bowel obstruction. Other elimination problems include those of the urinary tract—renal stones, difficulty in urination, and urinary stasis, retention, and incontinence. Measures that help to prevent elimination problems include a high-fiber diet, a good bowel regimen, exercise, and intake of sufficient fluids. Immobility also induces changes in the basal metabolic rate, a negative nitrogen balance, muscle mass decrease, fluid and electrolyte imbalances, and nutritional changes such as anorexia.

Internal, interpersonal, environmental, social, and cultural changes also can be caused by bedrest and immobility. These include sensory, perceptual, and tactile deprivation, sensory overload, distortion, and monotony, changes in body image, social isolation and depersonalization, significant-other deprivation, interpersonal and social role changes, changes in financial, job, and community status, interference with developmental tasks and val-

ued goals, and exposure to different cultural expectations. As patients realize that their goals of security and need-satisfaction are not being met, they respond with various emotions. In order to cope with their responses, patients sometimes use ineffective adaptation behaviors. It is the responsibility of the nurse to assess the patient's adaptation to immobility, to help him learn more about his emotional reactions to problems, and to teach him how to use effective coping mechanisms.

STUDY QUESTIONS

1. What are the various ways in which a person may be rendered immobile?

2. What are the stages in the development of a decubitus ulcer, and what factors can contribute to decubitus ulcer formation?

3. What is a contracture, where do contractures most commonly occur in the body, and how can they be prevented?

4. What are some of the problems that can occur within the cardiovascular system if a patient remains on extended bedrest?

5. Why should a patient avoid performing a valsalva maneuver?

6. Why can anorexia occur in an inactive or immobile person, and what are some nursing interventions you might recommend for a patient who is malnourished?

7. How might a patient develop respira-

tory problems while on bedrest?

8. What are four main problems that can occur within the urinary tract due to immobility? How do these problems occur?

9. What nursing diagnoses might be pertinent to describe ineffective psychosocial adaptation of a patient on prolonged bedrest?

10. How might a nurse help a patient to cope more effectively with his feelings and reactions to his immobility?

REFERENCES

1. Richard Asher, "The Dangers of Going to Bed," **British Medical Journal,** 2 (1947), 967–969.
2. Frances K. Milde, "Physiological Immobilization," in **Concepts Common to Acute Illness: Identification and Management,** eds. Laura K. Hart, Jean L. Reese and Margery O. Fearing (St. Louis: The C. V. Mosby Co., 1981) pp. 75.
3. F. Milde. "Physiological Immobilization." pp. 76.
4. V. S. Georgievskii and V. M. Mikhailov, **Human Physiology,** 4 (1978), pp. 703–706.
5. Steven Garvin, Stephen Pye, Alan Hargens, and Wayne Akeson, "Surface Pressure Distribution of the Human Body in the Recumbent Position," **Archives of Physical Medicine and Rehabilitation,** 61 (1980), 102.
6. N. C. Peterson, "The Development of Pressure Sores During Hospitalization," in **Bedsore Biomechanics,** eds. R. M. Kenedi, J. M. Cowden, and J. T. Scales (New York, NY: The Macmillan Press LTD., 1976) pp. 220.
7. Joan Luckmann and Karen C. Sorensen, eds., **Medical-Surgical Nursing: A Psychophysiologic Approach,** 2nd ed. (Philadelphia: W. B. Saunders, 1980) pp. 824.
8. Pamela H. Mitchell, "Motor Status," in **Concepts Basic to Nursing,** 3rd ed., eds. Pamela H. Mitchell and Anne Loustau (New York, NY: McGraw-Hill Book Co., 1981) pp. 364.
9. P. Mitchell. "Motor Status." pp. 365.
10. Aram B. Chobanian, Robert D. Lille, Ann Tercyak, and Pengwynne Blevins, "The Metabolic and Hemodynamic Effects of Prolonged Bed Rest in Normal Subjects," **Geriatrics,** (1974), 551–558.
11. A. I. Grigor'ev and others, "Effect of Duration of Bed Rest on Water and Mineral Metabolism and Kidney Function," **Human Physiology,** 5 (1979), 483–490.
12. Susan W. Salmond, "How to Assess the Nutritional Status of Acutely Ill Patients," **American Journal of Nursing,** 80 (1980), 922–924.
13. S. Salmond. "Assess the Nutritional Status." pp. 922–924.
14. Valerie McCann, "The Prevention of Depression in the Immobilized Patient," **The Orthopedics Nurses Association Journal,** 6 (1979), 433–438.
15. Carolyn E. Carlson, "Psychosocial Aspects of Neurologic Disability," **Nursing Clinics of North America,** 15 (1980), 309–319.
16. Florence Downs, "Bed Rest and Sensory Disturbances," **American Journal of Nursing,** 74 (1974), 434–438.
17. Lillian H. Parent, "Effects of a Low-Stimulus Environment on Behavior," **The American Journal of Occupational Therapy,** 32 (1978), 19–24.
18. Sharon S. Bushnell and Martha L. Morrison, "Nursing Care of the Patient in Respiratory Failure," in **Respiratory Intensive Care Nursing.** (Boston: Little, Brown and Company, 1979) pp. 28.
19. Joseph Agris and Melvin Spira, "Pressure Ulcers: Prevention and Treatment," **Clinical Symposia,** 31 (1979), 9.

ANNOTATED BIBLIOGRAPHY

Black Sister K: **Social Isolation and the Nursing Process.** Nurs Clin North Am 8:575–585; 1973. This journal article discusses the assessment, intervention, and evaluation of patients deprived of normal interpersonal contacts. Concepts of self-image, depersonalization, regression, and alienation are carefully considered.

Christian BJ: **Immobilization: Psychosocial Aspects.** In Norris CM: Concept Clarification in Nursing. Rockville, MD, Aspen Systems Corporation, 1982. A comprehensive, fairly advanced level discussion that classifies immobility into eight types of limitation of movement. Models for the sequential assessment of immobilization and the conceptual clarification of immobilization are developed.

Feustel D: **Pressure Sore Prevention.** Nurs 82 4:78–83; 1982. An excellent, concise article that discusses patients at risk for pressure sores, the areas of the body where decubiti can occur, and how to assess the patient and turn him. An extensive discussion describes positioning of the patient in supine, prone, sidelying, and sitting positions, accompanied by excellent illustrations.

Horsley JA, Crane J, Haller K, Bingle J (eds): **Preventing Decubitus Ulcers, CURN Project.** New York, Grune and Stratton, 1981. An excellent comprehensive text, written by nurses, that discusses all aspects of decubitus ulcers. Chapters include the etiology, management, and prevention of decubiti.

Jungreis SW: **Exercises for Expediting Mobility in Bedridden Patients.** Nurs 77 8:47–51; 1977. This journal article, written by a physical therapist, consists of five pages of photographs of a patient performing bed exercises. The text explains how the beginning, intermediate, and advanced exercises are performed.

Miller ME, Sachs ML: **About Bedsores, What You Need to Know to Help Prevent and Treat Them.** New York, J. B. Lippincott Co., 1974. This text is written by a nurse and physician and presents a very simple approach to the etiology and management of bedsores. The content is presented at the level of beginning nursing students and contains many excellent photographs.

Olson EV: **The Hazards of Immobility.** Am J Nurs 67:780–797; 1967. This journal article is the classic reading and first comprehensive nursing discussion of immobility in the literature. All of the body systems and psychosocial aspects of immobility are carefully considered.

Steinberg FU: **The Immobilized Patient.** New York, Plenum Medical Book Co., 1980. An advanced text, written by a physician, that summarizes the latest research on the effects of bedrest and immobility. The various organ systems are discussed with detailed physiology.

Urosevich PR (ed): **Nursing Photobook. Providing Early Mobility.** Horsham, Nursing 80 Books, Intermed Communications, Inc., 1980. This book has excellent illustrations that demonstrate in detail the technical care of the immobile patient. Topics of the chapters include body mechanics, turning and positioning, strengthening exercises, performing transfers, special equipment, and environmental considerations.

Wells T: **Promoting Urine Control in Older Adults.** Geriatric Nurs 236–269; 1980. This is an excellent comprehensive discussion of urinary incontinence and its causes. Measures for nursing interventions, bladder retraining, and available equipment are also included.

ACKNOWLEDGMENTS

ACTIVEaid, Inc.
Charles H. Nearing
Vice President
501 E. Tin Street
Redwood Falls, Minnesota 56283

Bio Clinic Co.
Jan Williams
Vice President, Education

59 E. Orange Grove Ave.
Burbank, California 91502

Cheesebrough - Pond's Inc.
Richard Ivey
Product Manager
33 Benedict Place
Greenwich, Connecticut 06830

Everest and Jennings
Edward A. Malmstrom
Rehabilitation Product Manager
1803 Pontius Avenue
Los Angeles, California 90025

Fred Sammons, Inc./Professional Self-Help Aids
LaVerne H. Norman
Advertising Manager
Box 32
Brookfield, Illinois 60513

The Jobst Institute, Inc.
Joanne Czerniakowski
Advertising Manager
P.O. Box 653
Toledo, Ohio 43694

Johnson and Johnson Products, Inc.
Nancy A. Anderson
Manager, Professional Relations
Patient Care Division
New Brunswick, New Jersey 08903

Kinetic Concepts Inc.
3417 Steen Drive
San Antonio, Texas 78219

J. T. Posey Company
Mrs. Clarice Rubin
Customer Service
5635 Peck Road
Arcadia, California 91006

Proctor and Gamble Home Service Group
J. M. Edwards
Vice-President Paper Products
P.O. Box 41713
Cincinnati, Ohio 45241

Ross Laboratories
Pat Radloff
625 Cleveland Avenue
Columbus, Ohio 43216

Scimedics, Inc.
Margaret G. Rogers, President
700 N. Valley St. Suite B
Anaheim, California 92801

Stryker Corporation
Dennis Howe
Director of Communications
420 Alcott Street
Kalamazoo, Michigan 49001

Support Systems International
P.O. Box 570
Johns Island, South Carolina 29455

Trans-aid Corporation
Lloyd J. Oye
President
1609 E. Del Amo Blvd.
Carson, California 90746

19

Sensory Alterations

Janet-Beth Flynn

CHAPTER OUTLINE

OBJECTIVES

At the completion of this chapter, the reader will be able to:

- Define the terms in the glossary.
- Discuss the sensory process.
- Compare and contrast sensory deprivation and sensory overload.
- Assess key factors contributing to sensory deprivation.
- Describe parental deprivation.
- List the levels of consciousness.
- Discuss sensory deficits and list examples from each of the senses.

GLOSSARY

Levels of Consciousness—
- **alert:** conscious, alert, and oriented
- **lethargic:** sleepy, oriented when aroused
- **semicomatose:** unconscious but may respond to pain
- **comatose:** unconscious and may not respond to pain

Parental deprivation—a state in which infants and young children fail to thrive due to parental inattention and lack of emotional or sensory stimuli.

Reticular activating system (RAS)—the portion of the brain that activates the cerebral cortex and prepares it for incoming information.

Reticular formation—an area of the brain that controls wakefulness.

Sensory alteration—changes in the ability to correctly use the sensory organs to receive information from the environment.

Sensory deficit—an alteration in one of the five senses.

Sensory deprivation—a reduction in the amount of meaningful stimuli from the environment.

Sensory overload—too much unpatterned stimuli in the environment.

Sensory perception—the ability to process data gathered by the senses into meaningful information.

Sensory process—the ability to receive information through the senses and then interpret it into meaningful information.

Sensory reception—the ability to receive information from the environment through the senses.

INTRODUCTION

Man depends on his sensory system in order to interact with the environment. Environmental stimuli are collected through the senses of vision, hearing, touch, taste, and smell, then processed by the brain into meaningful information. It is by use of these processes that man is able to adapt to his dynamic environment. Changes in the ability to accurately receive and perceive sensory stimuli can seriously affect man's ability to adapt to his environment and to maintain health.

Changes in the ability to correctly use the sensory process can be caused by a wide variety of physiological, psychological, and environmental factors. For example, an individual may become blind due to increasing opacity of the lens of the eye,

another may have a stroke that limits the ability to perceive touch. Severe depression can limit an individual's contact with the outside world, thereby narrowing sensory experiences. Environmental factors such as meaningless sounds or blinding lights also can contribute to altered perception.

Alterations in sensory input can cause individuals to become confused or disoriented. Many hospitalized patients, for example, are exposed to stimuli with which they are unfamiliar. They may be overwhelmed by a wide variety of machines, noises, light, and medical language that they don't understand.

Persons experiencing sensory alterations may demonstrate behavior that is not directed toward achieving a higher health state. An elderly patient, for example may attempt to get out of bed by climbing over the side rail, and may fall and break a hip, further adding to his health problems.

In order for individuals to be able to function in their environment, they must be able to interpret incoming stimuli into meaningful information. Too much or too little stimuli may lead to thought disorganization and confusion.

When individuals enter the health care system, they must adapt to a variety of changes in environmental stimuli. Many times, due to the unfamiliarity of the new environment, patients find it difficult to make the necessary adaptations. Patients in an intensive care unit (ICU), for example, are bombarded with a variety of incoming stimuli from the environment, but because they do not understand it, it becomes meaningless. There has been a great deal of research on why patients become confused due to alterations in the environment. The findings of these studies have shown that confused and disorganized behavior can be caused by sensory deprivation, sensory overload, parental deprivation, altered levels of consciousness, and sensory deficits.

The purpose of this chapter is to discuss selected alterations in the sensory process.

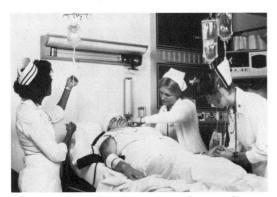

Figure 19-1. Environmental stimuli can be meaningless and overwhelming to the patient.

THE SENSORY PROCESS

Before nurses can work with patients experiencing sensory alterations, they first must understand the sensory process, which consists of an individual's ability to **receive** stimuli through the sensory organs and the ability to **perceive** or interpret the stimuli received.

Sensory reception is the collection of data through the five senses. **Sensory perception** refers to man's ability to organize and interpret environmental stimuli into meaningful information. The nervous system controls and directs the sensory process.

The human nervous system is a complex and wonderful organ system consisting of the brain, the spinal cord, the cranial nerves, and the peripheral nerves. The peripheral nerves act as gatherers of sensory information and transport it along nerve fibers. The brain acts as a control tower receiving stimuli from the senses. Then, by using highly developed mechanisms, it processes the information gathered and responds by signaling the motor nerves to act.

Thousands of pieces of information are gathered by the peripheral nerves and the sensory organs and are transmitted by the peripheral and automatic nerves through the spinal cord to higher brain centers. The spinal cord segregates incoming information into tracks and transmits it to the various appropriate sites in the brain.[1]

After reception and transmission, some information is integrated in the brain stem, which regulates many of the vital body functions and contains the reticular formation. The reticular formation is a diffuse network of neurons that extend throughout the brain stem boundaries.[2,3]

The output of the reticular formation can be divided into ascending and descending systems. The descending system influences the function of the somatic and autonomic efferent neurons, and the ascending system affects wakefulness and the direction of attention to specific stimuli.[4] This portion of the reticular formation, which coordinates input and modifies levels of awareness, is called the reticular activating system (RAS).[5]

The RAS begins in the lower brain stem and extends upward through the mesencephalon, thalamus, and the cerebral cortex.[6] The RAS activates the cerebral cortex and prepares it for incoming information. It is the RAS that coordinates input from the senses and modifies the level of awareness necessary to interpret incoming stimuli.[7]

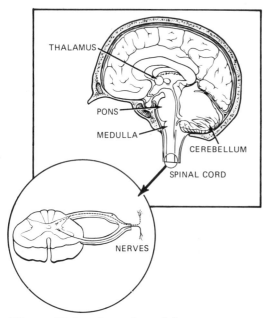

Figure 19-2.   A portion of the sensory system which transmits stimuli from the receptors to higher centers.

The cortex is the highest level of the nervous system, and its role is to process, interpret, use and store incoming sensory data in an organized and systematic manner.

Just how much stimuli is needed from the environment is highly individual. Some thrive on high amounts of sensory input, while others require much less.

Compare one teenager talking on the phone, doing homework, and listening to records simultaneously with another, reading a book in a quiet room. Each of these individuals is content in his environment and would, no doubt, be uncomfortable in that of the other. Both individuals have the same sensory apparatus but respond differently to stimuli in the environment.

The nervous system would not be at all effective in controlling body functions if all sensory information caused a reaction, therefore only about one percent of incoming information is processed and acted on. When we put on cologne, for example, we can smell it as we apply it, but shortly thereafter we become adapted to the fragrance. We can perceive it if we focus our attention to it, but if we do not, we simply do not smell it. What would happen if we attended to all of our incoming stimuli? Attention would be heightened to the world around us, but so much information would be coming into the system that the brain would be unable to sort it all and, consequently, unable to function. There is an optimal level of cortical arousal for adaptation to occur. Too high a level, for example, interferes with organizing and processing, and the RAS is unable to adapt. Too low a level does not provide enough stimuli for the RAS, and again, it may be temporarily unable to adapt.

SENSORY ALTERATIONS

Alterations in reception and perception of sensory information can lead to disorganized behaviors and can limit the ability to adapt. The most common of these alterations are sensory deprivation, sensory overload, and parental deprivation.

Sensory Deprivation

A major change in the patient's environment may produce an alteration in sensory input, which in turn upsets the balance in the reticular activating system (RAS). **Sensory deprivation** results when the sensory input is lower than the person requires to function.[8] Under conditions of decreased sensory input, the RAS is not able to maintain a normal level of activation to the cerebral cortex. The patient, experiencing less stimulation than normal, becomes more attuned to the remaining sensory stimuli and consequently receives a distorted view of reality.

Historically, the oldest report of a sensory deprivation experiment comes from the Court of Fredrick II, Emperor of Sicily, in the 13th century. The experiment was not designed to observe the effects of sensory deprivation however. Fredrick believed that individuals were born with an innate language—Hebrew. He felt that they would speak this language if they did not have another language to copy, and he conducted an experiment in which newborn human infants were placed in a controlled nursery. The nursemaids were not permitted to speak to the infants, cuddle them, or smile at them. Fredrick believed that the first words spoken by the children would reveal their innate language. The experiment proved to be a bitter failure because all of the children died.[9] They died from lack of stimulation. This study would be considered unethical by today's standards and could never be replicated. More recent studies explored this fascinating concept of sensory deprivation. In the early 1950s, political prisoners in Korea who had been brainwashed were examined. The Koreans believed that by manipulating the environment and producing the effect of sensory deprivation they could obtain confessions of wrong-doing and conversions to their system of life.

Additional studies[10-12] have investigated the effects of sensory deprivation of patients in the hospital or subjects in a simulated hospital environment. In one study, [13] researchers observed the effects of pro-longed exposure to environments with extremely limited sensory experiences. They used 22 healthy college students as subjects. The subjects were placed in beds in single cubicles for 24 hours a day. They wore translucent goggles that admitted light but prevented normal vision, and gloves and cardboard sleeves to reduce tactile stimulation. Furthermore, the cubicles were soundproofed. Sound was limited to the monotonous drone from the air conditioner. They were not told the time of day, but were permitted 2–3 hours of breaks for meals and personal needs.

Subjects found the experiment extremely difficult to endure. The researchers found that they could not keep their subjects for more than two to three days. Subjects reported that they could not stand the experience, because it was too stressful and reported that after sleeping for most of the first day, they were very bored and eager for any type of stimuli. They reported experiencing hallucinations and other types of perceptual distortions. Furthermore, they demonstrated the inability to concentrate, and their decision-making capacities were limited. If healthy experimental subjects report sensory changes within 24 hours after curtailment of sensory input, one must wonder what happens to ill individuals who are exposed to a totally new sensory environment and altered sensory input.

Hospitalized patients are certainly exposed to an altered sensory environment. Meaningless and unpatterned stimuli are present in the hospital in the form of medical equipment, sounds, lighting, and meaningless medical jargon. Limited mobility also reduces the amount of variation of stimuli and contact with significant others and medical personnel. Technical language, which the patient does not understand, is frequently used and reduces the possibility of meaningful communication. Segregation of patients to prevent spread of infection is common and increases the chance for sensory deprivation. Dying patients, belligerent patients, or confused patients often are isolated physically from other patients, so as not to disturb the others.

There are numerous occasions in which patients can suffer from sensory deprivation. It is the nurse's responsibility to identify these situations, and to manipulate the environment in order to control some of the meaningless stimuli and to provide meaningful stimuli.

Certain patients are at risk for developing the maladaptive behaviors caused by sensory deprivation. These patients include those who have diminished sensory capacities due to a physical condition or have limited interactions with others due to psychosocial conditions (See Figure 19-3).

| The isolated person |
| The person restricted to bedrest |
| The elderly person |
| The very young person |
| The terminally ill person |
| The critically ill person |
| The visually impaired person |
| The deaf or hard of hearing person |
| The dysphasic person |
| The confused person |
| The person from a different culture |
| The socially isolated person |
| The paralyzed person |

Figure 19-3.   Individuals at risk for developing sensory deprivation.

Decreased meaningful stimuli in the environment has been observed to lead to boredom, irritability, inability to concentrate, confusion and inaccurate perception of information gathered by the senses. For example, patients relate seeing dots, colors, and shapes, and hearing distorted sounds, such as wind rushing, water running, and whispers. More complex perceptual distortions include seeing people, animals, or scenes; hearing voices or music; sensations of floating or falling; and experiencing strange odors and tastes. Patients also may have vague somatic complaints or demonstrate maladaptive, noncompliant behaviors that may be harmful to them.

It is important for nurses to recognize these behaviors as they occur in order to provide the patient with the best possible care and support.

THE NURSING PROCESS

Nurses need a systematic approach to nursing care of patients experiencing sensory deprivation. The nursing process is an excellent framework for this. The nursing process has four phases: assessment, planning, implementation, and evaluation.

Assessment

The **assessment** phase is the data gathering phase. Information about the patient and the environment is gathered by observation, interviewing and history taking, examination, and record review.

The following case study provides an example of sensory deprivation.

Mrs. Kathryn Jones, an 80-year-old woman, lived in an apartment complex for the elderly until her admission to the hospital two weeks ago. She was healthy and active until her admission. She has a supportive family and many friends.

She is an active member of her church and her senior citizens group. She was also a volunteer at a local nursing home.

Mrs. Jones fell when walking to the store, broke her hip, and lost her glasses. She was rushed to the hospital in an ambulance and underwent hip pinning surgery the following day. After the surgery, she was placed in the intensive care unit, because she developed a cardiac arrhythmia during the course of the surgery.

Her room was small, containing only her bed and the medical equipment. Since she had to be watched closely, lights were left on at all times, and her room was opposite the nurses station, where there was always a great deal of activity.

Mrs. Jones began to spend a great deal of time sleeping and was becoming more and more irritable as the days went by. Finally, she became confused and couldn't remember where she was. She attempted to climb over the side rails on several occasions and had to be placed in a posey jacket restraint for safety reasons. She thought that the nurses were discussing her case at the desk and she treated them with suspicion.

Mrs. Jones was demonstrating many of the symptoms of sensory deprivation. A careful assessment of the situation yielded many weaknesses in the environment that contributed to Mrs. Jones' disorientation. Mrs. Jones was attached to a cardiac monitor, which omitted monotonous sounds and had twinkling lights. There were no windows, clock, or calendar in her room. Mrs. Jones had lost track of time, and this was reinforced by the environment because the lights were only slightly dimmed at night. Being near the nurses station also added to the noise and disruption she was experiencing.

In addition to these factors, contact with her family was restricted to a few minutes an hour. The staff were quite busy with Mrs. Jones, since she required a great deal of care and monitoring. Her vital signs were checked at least every hour around the clock, disturbing her ability to rest. Interactions with the staff were limited and not interactive on a personal level.

Her glasses were lost; therefore, her ability to see was altered. She was unable to read or watch TV.

Many features that lead to sensory deprivation can be discovered from this example, and many of the observable signs also can be assessed.

After the data are gathered in the assessment phase, nursing diagnoses are written. Nursing diagnoses related to sensory alteration for Mrs. Jones would include:

- altered sense of perception related to sensory deprivation
- alteration in vision related to loss of glasses
- confusion related to sensory deprivation
- sensory deprivation related to a large amount of meaningless stimuli in the environment.

Once the assessment is complete and the nursing diagnosis written, the planning phase of the nursing process can be started.

Planning

The written **plan** should be placed on the patient's chart or the kardex. Goals and objectives are written to direct the nursing plan, and are derived from the assessment. If possible they should be agreed upon by both the patient and the nurse. In some instances patients may be too disoriented or confused to assist in setting the goals, but they should be encouraged to participate as much as possible. An example of a goal with outcome criteria might be: After 24 hours, the patient will be able to state his name, and where he is.

When planning care, nurses should consider the potential problem of sensory deprivation and employ methods to prevent it. Prevention of a problem is always the best form of nursing care. Patients who are at risk for developing sensory deprivation need to be identified and meaningless stimuli minimized.

Meaningful stimuli should be provided in the form of clocks and calendars. Clocks that distinguish night from day by using two colors on a 24 hour face also are helpful. These patients also need access to windows to add more meaningful stimuli.

Newspapers, television, and radios are another means of providing additional stimuli. If patients wear glasses or hearing aids, they should be encouraged to wear them in the hospital.

Patients at risk for developing sensory alteration should not be placed in single rooms unless absolutely necessary (or by their own request). Assignment of staff should be adequate, so that time can be spent with these patients. Time can be spent talking with patients and letting them ask questions.

Team or staff conferences can be scheduled to discuss approaches for controlling sensory deprivation. It is important that everyone on the health care team assist in reducing the effects of sensory deprivation. Many times, the fast pace of an intensive care or other hospital unit does not give the staff time to reflect on these effects.

Implementation

Implementation of the plan is the next phase of the nursing process and is extremely important in reducing the effects of sensory deprivation. The environment can be manipulated to increase meaningful sensory stimuli. This can be accomplished in a variety of ways. Large clocks can be placed where the bedfast patient can see them, or patients can be encouraged to wear their own watch, if possible. A large calendar can be placed within the patient's view. Every evening when the patient is being prepared for the night, the nurse and the patient can cross off the present day. When entering the room, nurses on each shift can tell the patient the day, the date, and the time. Discussion of the weather is highly appropriate, too, as it helps patients orient to the season.

Clocks, calendars, and discussion of the weather are appropriate for adults, but small children do not understand time and climate changes, so it would add meaningless stimuli to the environment to discuss it. Orienting stimuli for children might include reading stories, especially ones from home that the child already knows.

Mobiles can be hung from the ceiling to add additional stimuli, and familiar toys can be placed in their beds, in most instances.

Nurses should address adult patients by their title (Mr., Dr., Mrs., Ms., Miss) and surname, and identify themselves by what they wish patients to call them. This reinforces the patient's name and reminds him of the nurse's name.

The morning bath is a good time for the nurse to spend some extra time with the patient. Problems encountered during the hospital stay and possible solutions can be discussed. Also, the morning bath is a good time to foster independence. Patients should be encouraged to do as much for themselves as they can, within the limits of their physical condition and the physician's orders. They can be allowed some control in this activity. For example, "Would you like to bathe before or after breakfast? Do you want to start with your teeth? Do you use mouthwash?" These may seem like small items but they can be quite meaningful to a patient who has had all control of the situation removed.

Environmental lighting can be controlled by opening drapes during the day and turning on lights if needed. Lights should be turned off at night to permit patients to maintain their normal biorhythms and assist them in distinguishing night from day.

Patients may distort what they hear, so talking in a whisper is not good practice. Moving the patient out of his room for a period of time everyday increases the variety of stimuli. This does not include sending him to x-ray or for a scan, where the stimuli might be as incomprehensible as in his room. If at all possible, patients can be moved to the sunroom or visiting area. Patients can meet and talk, and this provides them with a very important change of environment. Children can be taken to the playroom to play with their parents and other children.

Encouraging exercise is another important intervention. Patients can be taught to do range of motion (ROM) exercises themselves if they are bedfast. If they are able to transfer to a wheelchair, they can assist with its propulsion in the halls. Patients restricted to bed by an intravenous (IV) can be mobilized by placing their IV bag on a pole on wheels, and they can be taught to push the pole safely.

Exercise is an excellent diversion and relieves some of the boredom and daydreaming side effects of sensory deprivation. Exercise is also helpful in promoting sleep.

Interaction with family members is important for hospitalized patients. Family and friends provide meaningful stimuli for patients, and should be encouraged to visit. Patients should be encouraged to call family and friends from the room and receive calls there as well. Photographs of family, friends, and home can be displayed in the patient's room to provide additional visual stimuli. Cards from friends and family can be arranged within view of the patient. Children's drawings and letters can be displayed.

Patients in acute care settings can be encouraged to have articles brought from home to brighten their rooms. Such things as a favorite afghan, pillow, and photographs of loved ones can mean a great deal to patients. Large, breakable, or irreplaceable, expensive items should be discouraged, however. Also, if possible, patients should be encouraged to wear their own pajamas, robes, and slippers, and bring their own toilet articles.

Patients demonstrating confused or disoriented behavior should have reality reinforced constantly and consistently. All members on the staff must be consistent. Reports on what the patient has believed to be true should be discussed, as well as what the staff has done to reinforce reality. If everyone is supportive, the patient will be able to come back to reality.

Evaluation

Evaluation is the fourth phase of the nursing process. This is the phase in which the patient's present behavior is measured and compared with the goals and objectives written during the planning phase. Has the patient met these goals? Behavior before the plan was instituted should be compared with behavior demonstrated afterwards. There should be substantial evidence, if the desired outcomes were reached.

The evaluative process will pinpoint omissions that occurred during the assessment phase of the nursing process.[14] In pinpointing the omissions, the evaluation then guides reassessment, future planning, and interventions.

SENSORY OVERLOAD

Sensory overload is the opposite of sensory deprivation and can be described as a condition in which individuals receive more sensory stimuli than they can tolerate. Little research has been done in this area, so the physiological mechanism is unclear. It is believed, however, that the effects on the RAS and on behavior is similar to that of sensory deprivation.

In the hospital, the patient is exposed to many sensory stimuli—bright lights, noise, odors, scratchy sheets, pain, machinery, visits from health care staff, phone calls, visitors, TV, and the general hustle-bustle of a busy hospital unit. When individuals have trouble processing all of the stimuli, they become fatigued, irritable, and may exhibit agitation. Patients also show some of the more severe signs of sensory deprivation, such as confusion and hallucination. Think of an amusement park with all of its glaring lights, rides, noise, music, smells, and confusion. Quite a nice place to have fun for a few hours, but think of what it would be like to live there. No doubt, this would quickly lead to fatigue and irritability. There would be too many random sounds and sights to attend to, and perceptions could become distorted. Almost everyone has experienced sensory overload at one time or another—students during course orientation, or nurses when caring for a large number of patients.

THE NURSING PROCESS

Assessment

Many of the symptoms of sensory overload are the same as sensory deprivation but instead of boredom, the patient exhibits irritability and agitation. Visits from friends and family tend to increase these behaviors. Additional stimuli in the environment also adds to the patient's irritation.

The environment should be assessed. Are the lights too bright? Do they shine in the patient's eyes? Are they ever dimmed or turned off? What is the noise level? Do staff make excessive noise? Is the housekeeping department always buffing the floor? How many health care workers and support staff are in the environment at any given time?

Telephones and intercom systems contribute to the noise level and confusion on a busy unit.

There are many strange smells in the hospital, adding more stimuli for the sensory system to interpret.

At the completion of the **assessment** phase, the nursing diagnosis can be prepared. Examples of nursing diagnoses related to sensory overload might include:

- Potential sensory overload related to environment

- Irritability related to sensory overload

- Confusion related to sensory overload.

After the nursing diagnoses have been written, the planning phase can begin.

Planning

A carefully written care plan with goals and objectives should be prepared and placed on the patient's kardex. An example of a goal related to sensory overload might be: To rest in a quiet room for 1 hour every day as evidenced by sleeping or resting in the quiet, darkened room. Planning nursing interventions for patients experiencing sensory overload would include control of the environment, so that patients are exposed to less stimuli. This can be done by minimizing noise and light and by planning rest periods so that the patient can integrate sensory input.

Implementation

Once the planning phase has been completed implementation can begin. Patients experiencing sensory overload need to have a controlled environment where extreme stimuli are kept to a minimum.

The same nurses should care for patients experiencing sensory overload in order to provide consistent care and to minimize the number of health professionals involved. Establishing a routine each day is a way of providing consistency for the patient and reducing the aspect of surprise. Visitors can be limited to close friends and family and the visits kept short in order to control some of the stimuli.

Lights may be dimmed during the day and rest periods provided. Lights should be turned off at night. Reducing noise also reduces the amount of stimuli in the environment.

Odors should be kept to a minimum. Soiled linen should be changed immediately, removed from the room, and the patient bathed. Flowers with a strong fragrance can be removed or placed away from the patient's bedside.

The patient experiencing sensory overload may need to stay in the familiar environment of his room. Trips to the sunroom may not be needed. The patient can be ambulated in his room minimizing his contact with stimuli from the hospital unit. In controlling the amount of stimuli patients receive, caution should be taken so that the patient does not begin to experience sensory deprivation.

Evaluation

Evaluation is based on the behavioral objectives written on the plan. If the effects of sensory overload are decreased, then the plan and interventions are sufficient and should be maintained. If not, then the situation needs to be reassessed and the plan revised.

PARENTAL DEPRIVATION

Parental or maternal deprivation is a state in which infants and young children fail to thrive due to parental inattention or lack of emotional and sensory stimulation. Infants and children affected by deprivation present a group of symptoms that aid in nursing diagnosis. They are below the third percentile in weight, and no evidence can be found for systemic disease or congenital abnormality. Cognitive development is hampered, and language acquisition is slow. Children experiencing parental deprivation will become rigid when held and will remain unsoothed or will become flaccid by cuddling and holding. They do not smile, maintain eye contact, or respond in other ways.

Frequently there is a history of prematurity or illness at birth, which prevents parental bonding. There also may be a history of feeding problems, excessive vomiting, sleep disturbances, colic, and abnormal irritability.

Symptoms of parental deprivation decrease when the child's environment is enriched by stimulation.[15,16]

Reasons for parental deprivation are complex and have physical, psychological, emotional, and financial components. Several theories attempt to explain parental deprivation. One of these, role theory, has been advanced as an explanation for this phenomena. It proposes that the parent is too much of a child and in need of parenting to be able to nurture another. Frequently the parent had been deprived as an infant, too, and may be able to adapt if all goes well, but if additional stresses are added, is unable to continue coping. It is also common to find that other children present in the family are doing quite well and just one child is affected or deprived, which seems to be due to an infant who is more difficult to relate to. The parent is not able to give more to the infant.

Personalities of infants differ and can have definite effects on the parent/child attachment process.[17] The infant or child may be difficult to care for or may resemble someone in the family that the parent may not like.

Another theory relates to the process of reciprocity, or the regulators of cues between parent and child. Infants can cue into stimuli or block them out by nonattention or withdrawal of active attention. The person caring for the infant either attempts to reengage the infant's attention or turns away. The child responds to the caretaker's withdrawal with an even deeper withdrawal.

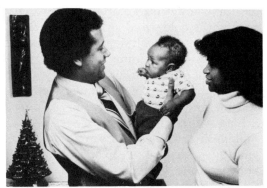

Figure 19-4.   Reciprocity is the regulation of cues between the parent and the infant.

There are two types of parental deprivation: short-term and long-term. The short-term type generally is related to a separation from parents and may be related to hospitalization. In this case, the child becomes distressed and withdrawn.

Long-term deprivation is related to prolonged hospitalization or neglect in the home. Long-term effects include cognitive retardation, conduct disorders, affectionless psychopathology and problems of dwarfism.[18]

Parental deprivation can occur across all financial and racial lines. Nurses should set aside judgmental attitudes, since these attitudes will be of no help in this situation. Prognosis for parental deprivation is at this time uncertain, but it revolves around the family's ability to change the way they relate to the infant. Families cannot do this alone. The nurse, through careful use of the nursing process, can assist these families to resolve parental deprivation.

THE NURSING PROCESS

Assessment

The **assessment** phase includes an assessment of the parents' beliefs about child rearing. Many parents believe that infants need rest and quiet to grow and will not prosper if they are disturbed.

Parent/child interaction should be observed and noted. Is the parent aware when the infant is cold, tired, or hungry? What are the parents' expectations for the infant? Many times, expectations far surpass the reality of the situation. For example, young parents might think that infants sleep all the time and may have difficulty coping with an infant who does not.

Taking a nursing history may disclose symptoms, such as sleep disturbances, vomiting, colic, difficult feeding behavior, and irritability. Since parental deprivation is a family problem, information should be gathered regarding the family system. Are there other children in the home? Do the other children demonstrate symptoms of parental deprivation? Has something stressful occurred in the family lately? Is there a financial crisis? Is the man of the household the father of the deprived infant? Is there marital discord? Does the mother have support systems beyond the boundaries of the family?

Data need to be gathered about the family's perception of the situation. Are they aware that there is a problem with the infant? Do they know what is normal? Are they aware that their infant may be behind in normal growth and development? Do they know how to stimulate the infant?

Other salient features in the nursing assessment include the measurement of the infant's length and weight and observation of the infant's nonverbal behavior, such as eye contact and body posture. The infant's temperature should be observed to determine if he is abnormally lethargic or irritable, due to a temperature elevation.

A careful Denver Development Screening Test (DDST) should be performed to assess the infant's developmental level. The DDST enables the nurse to compare the child's growth and development with standardized norms. It provides information about the child's present achievement in terms of gross and fine motor ability, social skills, and language acquisition. A sample nursing diagnosis for parental deprivation might include: inability to interact socially related to parental deprivation.

Planning

The **plan** for infants and children experiencing parental deprivation extends through the family system. If it is not possible to work with all members of the family, the infant's or child's primary caretaker should be included.

Staffing should be planned so that the same nurses care for these patients consistently, thus enabling the nurse to get to know the infant and the parents. These children should be placed in rooms with other children and require no special spatial needs. Too much stimulation should be avoided, however. The environment should be controlled to maximize planned sensory stimuli.

Planning for physical care is relatively simple in that these children do not require special physical care—they require what any child needs—to be clean, fed, dry, and safe. Developmentally, there are special considerations to be made. Care must be planned to stimulate the child on a level that is appropriate to him developmentally, not chronologically. DDST results can be used to provide this information. Planning for subsequent DDST is important, as well, to assess progress.

Implementation

Interventions should be implemented according to the plan. Physical care should be administered patiently and with care. Time for cuddling and rocking should be provided. The senses should be stimulated. During the bath and feeding, the child can be stroked and talked to. Eye contact is important too. Mobiles can add to visual stimulation. Music boxes can provide auditory stimulation.

The parent should be encouraged to participate in the physical care of the infant or child. The nurse can serve as a role model and teach the mother how to care for her child. Gradually, she can be taught about developmental and emotional needs. Time to talk with the parents is important, since they might wish to talk about their feelings. Many parents are hard to deal with, because the problems related to parenting are deep. Some of these parents continue to exhibit emotional detachment from their children.

Some families are capable of change. Through sensitive implementation of the nursing process, nurses can help fill the void that leads to parental deprivation.[19]

Evaluation

As for the other sensory alterations, **evaluation** is based on the plan. Have the goals and objectives been met? If not, why not? Thorough evaluation, reassessment can be made, and the process begins again.

LEVELS OF CONSCIOUSNESS

Occasionally, the nervous system has difficulty receiving or processing stimuli from the environment due to an altered level of consciousness (LOC). Levels of consciousness can be affected by metabolic or nutritional disturbances, neural or renal dysfunction, psychiatric conditions, circulatory failure, stroke, trauma, substance abuse, or fever.

In most cases, patients experiencing an altered level of consciousness cannot make their needs known. Every need must be anticipated by the nurses caring for these patients. Nursing interventions must be planned carefully and carried out to meet these needs.

Unconscious and semiconscious patients need total physical care. They also need to be protected from hazards in the environment. Caring for unconscious or semiconscious patients is one of the most challenging nursing experiences.

THE NURSING PROCESS

The nursing process enables nurses to provide holistic care for patients experiencing altered levels of consciousness.

Assessment

Since any change in a patient's level of consciousness may indicate underlying life threatening pathologies, all patients must

Level of Consciousness	Patient Behaviors
Alert	Conscious, alert, fully oriented to person, place, and time. Answers questions appropriately.
Drowsy (lethargy)	Sleepy. Oriented when aroused but may appear confused. May answer questions appropriately. May be oriented to person and place.
Stuporous (semicomatose)	Loss of consciousness. May be aroused but with great difficulty. Generally not oriented to place or time. May respond to painful stimuli.
Comatose	Unconscious. Cannot be aroused. May not move spontaneously. Reflexes may not be present. May not respond to painful stimuli.

Figure 19-5. Levels of Consciousness.

be carefully assessed as to their level of consciousness. Initial LOC assessment should be made and recorded for all patients when they are admitted to the health care system. Subsequent changes should be reported and recorded immediately.

There is a series of stages of consciousness ranging from alert to comatose (See Figure 19-5). Nurses need to be aware of these stages in order to distinguish among them. Distinguishing between stages is, at times, difficult and tends to be subjective, so many hospitals have begun to use flow sheets to standardize observations of level of consciousness. These flow sheets resemble temperature, pulse, and respiration (TPR) sheets and provide space for nurses to record data regarding the patient's level of consciousness. A good example of a standardized LOC flow sheet is the Glasgow Coma Scale (GCS).[20] The value of the GCS rests in its ability to help health care providers objectively document patients' LOC by focusing on measurable responses to verbal commands and painful stimuli. The GCS eliminates the more subjective descriptions of LOC mentioned above and focuses on more concrete, observable data. (See Figure 19-6).

Factors to be assessed in an LOC assessment cover a wide range of parameters. The most obvious is the patient's level of awareness, mentation, and orientation. The most important is the patient's respiratory status, because without an adequate airway, the patient will not survive. Further assessment of vital signs includes pulse, temperature, and blood pressure. Pupil size and response to light is measured for constriction, consensuality, and convergence construction.[21] Assessment includes size, rate of constriction (brisk or sluggish), and equality of the pupils and their equal response to light.

Motor response is also a part of the level of consciousness exam. Can the patient move body parts on command? Can he move against gravity or resistance? Are the movements and strength equal on both sides? Does the patient respond to pain? What other reflexes are present (cough, swallow, blink)?

In addition to the LOC assessment, nurses should assess the patient's hygiene needs. Many patients require total care, including bathing, skin, mouth, and eye care. Careful positioning is essential and turning side-to-side every two hours or more frequently is helpful in reducing aspiration and pressure damage. Bowel and bladder functioning is important to assess, too. Examples of nursing diagnoses include:

- Altered LOC related to underlying pathology

- Altered ability to perform activity of daily living secondary to altered LOC

EYES:	OPEN	Spontaneously	4
		To verbal command	3
		To pain	2
	NO RESPONSE		1
BEST MOTOR RESPONSE:	TO VERBAL COMMAND	Obeys	6
	TO PAINFUL STIMULUS*	Localizes pain	5
		Flexion—withdrawal	4
		Flexion—abnormal (decorticate rigidity)	3
		Extension (decerebrate rigidity)	2
	NO RESPONSE		1
BEST VERBAL RESPONSE**		Oriented and converses	5
		Disoriented and converses	4
		Inappropriate words	3
		Incomprehensible sounds	2
	NO RESPONSE		1
TOTAL			3–15

*Apply knuckles to sternum; observe arms.
**Arouse patient with painful stimulus if necessary.

Adapted from Upjohn, January 1980, based on Teasdale, G, and Jennett, B, Glasgow Coma Scale. *Lancet*, No. 7872, p 81

Figure 19-6. The Glasgow Coma Scale.

- Altered ability to communicate related to decreased LOC.

Planning

Once the assessment phase has been completed, the plan can be written. In the planning phase, a written care plan is detailed and incorporates the data gathered in the assessment. Due to the comprehensive care that patients with altered levels of consciousness require, adequate time must be given to perform the needed interventions. Additional support for family members is essential, because they usually are extremely concerned about their loved ones.

In the planning phase, the family should be encouraged to participate in the physical care of the patient, and touch and talk to the patient as well. Many patients who have recovered from a comatose state have related daily incidents, identified nurses by their voices, and thanked family for sitting with them and talking. Family members can be encouraged to bring tape recorders and recordings of favorite music to play for the patient, too. If they are able to hear, these actions keep the patient in contact with familiar things.

Control of the environment also should be incorporated into the plan of care.

Methods are similar to those mentioned earlier in this chapter. Safety features should be incorporated into the care plan to decrease the chance of complications. In other words, anticipating emergencies before they occur is an important step in planning the care of a semiconscious or unconscious patient. Complications can be reversed before they become harmful to the patient.

Mutual goals may not be possible for unconscious patients, but family can be encouraged to participate in preparing goals and objectives.

Implementing

Implementation of the nursing care plan is quite challenging and may vary as the patient's condition changes. Basically, nursing interventions meet all of those needs that the patient cannot meet himself. The key to intervention is prevention of complications. The airway must be kept clear, hygiene measures met, range of motion exercises performed, position changed frequently, nutritional status and elimination needs maintained. Emotional support is necessary, as is providing sensory stimulation. The patient's privacy must be maintained and his worth and dignity respected. Addressing the patient by his title (Mr., Mrs., etc) and surname is one way of demonstrating this. The nurse should always tell the semiconscious or unconscious patient who she is and what she is going to do.

Side rails should be kept up at all times and they should be padded with bath blankets in case the patient has a seizure. Padded tongue blades and plastic airways should be within easy reach in case of emergency.

Evaluation

Evaluation of the care plan will determine the effectiveness of the plan. If specific interventions are not working, they can be changed. If interventions are working to prevent complications, it is important to continue using them.

Not all patients recover from a semiconscious or comatose state, but all patients benefit from careful, caring nursing interventions.

SENSORY DEFICITS

Man depends on all his senses to adapt to his environment and actively participate in the world around him. When one of these senses is altered, man's ability to adapt may be temporarily reduced. When one or more of the five senses is limited, a sensory deficit is said to exist. For example, the blind or visually impaired individual is unable to receive clear visual stimuli, the deaf or hearing impaired individual is unable to receive auditory stimuli, and so forth. With the loss of one or more of the senses, the entire lifestyle of an individual may be threatened—even if the alteration is temporary, a sense of disequilibrium can occur. Nurses are in a key position to assist individuals as they adapt to sensory deficits.

ALTERATION IN VISION

Vision is considered by most people to be the most crucial of all the senses in terms of autonomy and independence. Loss or impairment of vision is a threat to the individual's self-concept and self-image. Vision can be affected by a variety of disease processes or conditions, for example, high blood pressure, diabetes mellitus, glaucoma, cataracts, and trauma. Through careful use of the nursing process, nurses are able to facilitate adaptation and perhaps prevent further damage to the eyes.

THE NURSING PROCESS

Assessment

Taking a careful visual history of the visually impaired patient is the first step in the assessment process. Particular attention should be given to any visual changes, trauma, previous eye conditions, and present eye diseases. Nurses should determine if the visual changes were sudden or gradual. Patients with eye conditions will probably use eye drops, so these should be noted. Noting other conditions that might contribute to visual impairment, such as diabetes, lends additional data. Inspection of the eye and surrounding tissue and structures is another step in the process, and any abnormalities, such as edema, crusting, or redness, should be noted.

Pertinent data regarding visual acuity can be gathered easily during the initial eye exam by asking the patient to read from the newspaper or a menu for near vision. A Snellen eye chart is used for assessing distance vision. If the patient wears glasses or contact lenses, he should be assessed with and without these devices. If the patient is blind, the nurse must assess if the patient can determine light, dark, shapes, and forms.

Seven danger signals indicate the possibility of eye disease, and these should be assessed.

- Persistent redness of the eyes
- Persistent pain in the eye or around the eye
- Visual disturbance, e.g. blurred vision
- Crossing of the eyes
- Growths on the eyes or lids
- Persistent discharge, crusting, or tearing
- Unequal pupils

If these signs are caught at an early stage, more severe complications may be prevented.

If the patient does have an uncorrectable alteration in vision, then assessment of the patient's degree of acceptance is essential. If the patient denies that the impairment is permanent, planning and implementing care will be difficult. Examples of nursing diagnosis are: altered vision secondary to aging, diabetes, cataracts, etc. Potential sensory deprivation secondary to altered vision.

Planning

A written care plan is essential to ensure comprehensive care of the visually impaired patient. A note should be placed on the kardex and the intercom system to alert the staff to the patient's impairment.

In addition to assistance with the activities of daily living, the nurse will have to plan an orientation to the unit for the patient. If a patient is aware of his surroundings, he will be less anxious and better able to function. Environment must be controlled to prevent injury. Precautions must be taken to eliminate electric cords, small stools, and trash baskets that might be a safety hazard to the visually impaired patient. Other safety features include keeping side rails up, attaching the call bell within easy reach and telling the patient where it is and how to use it, and placing the bedside cabinet and telephone close to the bed so that it is within easy reach. Also, if the patient smokes, he should be assisted to the lounge and supervised in order to prevent burns and fires.

Rehabilitative measures should be incorporated in the plan. Supportive measures and encouragement assist the patient in gaining his independence. Family members need support and encouragement, too. Visits from other blind patients or representatives from organizations for the blind can be incorporated into the rehabilitation plan. Referral to other agencies is easily planned, too.

Implementation

In addition to the plan, other nursing interventions can be implemented. A strong nurse/patient relationship is essential in caring for the blind patient. There are specific ways of fostering this relationship. When the patient enters the health care system, the nurse should introduce herself by name and tell the patient who she is and how she will be assisting him. Once these amenities have been concluded, she should orient the patient to the environment in detail. It is important to show him where the furniture is placed and where the bathroom is located. If the person will be an inpatient, introductions to roommates and other members of the health care team are necessary.

Helping the patient unpack may be helpful to him, but his permission should be obtained. Once unpacking has started, the patient should assist in the placement of his belongings, so that he can find them. When objects are used by the nurse, they should always be put back in the same place, as this promotes the patient's independence. Arranging the food on the blind patient's tray is another way of assisting him. An effective way is to describe the plate and tray as the face of a clock. For example, juice is at one o'clock, coffee at 4 o'clock, plate at 6 o'clock, and so on. Blind patients also need help in selecting their meals from the menu.

When performing treatments on blind patients, the nurse should call the patient by name, introduce herself, and carefully explain the treatment and equipment before starting. Telling the patient when she is about to touch him is necessary, because a sudden touch can be startling.

Other forms of sensory stimulation need to be increased for the blind patient. Frequent visits should be made by the nurse,

and visits by family and friends should be encouraged. Radios and TVs can be used to reduce sensory deprivation. Braille books can be obtained from local agencies that provide services for the blind. Interventions appropriate for the patient with sensory deprivation can be applied to the blind patient, as well. Providing a meaningful environment, rich in experiences that a blind patient can appreciate, is an essential part of caring for the blind patient.

Evaluation

Evaluation is based on the objectives that were written on the care plan. If the patient met these objectives, then the plan has been successful. If not, then the plan needs to be reevaluated. Once the plan has been successfully carried out, and problems resolved, new priorities may be determined, and the plan can be modified to reflect this.

Through careful use of the nursing process and establishment of a trusting, empathetic nurse/patient relationship, the patient can reach for his maximum potential.

ALTERATION IN HEARING

Hearing is probably the second most important of our senses because it enables us to interact with other people and the environment. Alterations in hearing can lead to social isolation and decreased self-esteem. Hearing impaired individuals sometimes conceal the fact that they are hard of hearing or deaf. It is important to identify patients with impaired hearing, so that health care can be most efficient.

THE NURSING PROCESS

Assessment

The key to working with the patient with

an alteration in hearing is accurate assessment of the patient's hearing ability. Once this ability has been established, planning of care can begin. As with the blind or visually impaired patient, it is necessary to know how long the hearing loss has been present, if there is a way of reversing it, and how the person has adapted to the loss. The patient who has lost his hearing gradually is more likely to be adapting successfully. The person experiencing a sudden loss of hearing due to trauma will experience feelings of loss, fear, and anxiety.

Patients with a minimal or gradual loss of hearing may be the hardest to assess, because they might not be aware of the loss, or they may be too embarrassed to admit to it. Ways of assessing hearing loss include the more sophisticated exam using an otoscope and tuning fork, as well as more common observation. For example, does the patient turn one ear toward the person speaking? Does the patient answer questions appropriately? Does he have trouble following orders? Does the patient answer if he does not see your face when spoken to? Does he startle if touched? Is his voice abnormally loud? Does he respond to loud noises? If several of these behaviors exist the nurse will be able to diagnose an alteration in hearing.

Communicating with hearing impaired patients can be difficult at times. There is no set way of establishing communication, because needs vary with the severity of the impairment and at what age the impairment developed. Any aids that a patient uses must be observed, as well. Does the patient lip read, use a hearing aid, or an interpreter? Ways in which patients communicate and their assistive devices must be noted and incorporated into the nursing plan. Sample nursing diagnosis include:

- Impaired hearing related to aging, ear infection, nerve damage, etc.

- Altered ability to communicate related to hearing impairment

- Altered self-concept related to hearing impairment.

Planning

The nursing **plan** for the hearing impaired patient incorporates the patient's special needs. Planning to meet these needs revolves around the amount of the loss of acuity and the patient's present state of adaptation. Family members should be encouraged to participate in the plan. If the patient is totally deaf, the nurse may need to arrange for an interpreter. One of the national service agencies for the deaf (see Figure 19-7) can refer a skilled interpreter. Additional information can be obtained by contacting local agencies and organizations.

OBTAINING AN INTERPRETER

Information regarding skilled interpreters in local areas can be obtained by contacting:

The Registry of Interpreters for the Deaf
Box 1339
Washington, D.C. 20013

or

The National Association of the Deaf
814 Thayer Avenue
Silver Spring, Maryland 20910

If the patient is deaf and blind, information about assisting these patients can be obtained by contacting:

Helen Keller National Center for Deaf-Blind
  Youths and Adults
111 Middle Neck Road
Sands Point, Long Island, New York 11050

Figure 19-7. National agencies listing interpreters for the hearing impaired.

Once the plan has been determined, the implementation phase of the nursing process can begin.

Implementation

The key to working with the hearing impaired patient is the establishment of a trusting nurse/patient relationship. Communication is the primary factor in establishing this relationship, so the first nursing interventions must be directed in this area. Assistive devices, such as glasses or hearing aids, should be used. Verbal means of communication have to be altered to maximize interaction. The nurse should face the patient at eye level when speaking and stand fairly close to the patient, particularly if the patient is lip reading.

Lip movements should not be exaggerated as this tends to make speaking more difficult to interpret. Nurses also should make every effort to keep their hands away from their lips, so that patients can easily see them.

When speaking, a normal voice level should be used, because when shouting, the voice becomes higher in pitch, and most hearing impaired patients have lost the ability to hear high-pitched tones. Eliminate competing noises from the environment, so that the patient is able to concentrate on what is being said to him.

Nonverbal cues can be used to support verbal communication, but should not distract the patient. If the patient communicates by notes, several things should be kept in mind. The first, of course, is supplying the patient with enough paper and pencils. Flash cards may be prepared for commonly used words and phrases. After the nurse and patient have communicated by note writing, the notes should be destroyed to maintain the patient's confidentiality. Most patients who communicate by notes use a child's "Magic Slate" that can be erased with a flip of a sheet.

Be calm when working with a hearing impaired patient. If both nurse and patient are anxious, the communication system can break down quickly. As mentioned before, interpreters are very helpful and arrangements should be made for one especially when the hearing impaired patient will be exposed to stressful situations, such as invasive, painful treatments or surgery.

Finally, for consistency and safe care, a note should be placed on the patient's chart and on his kardex to advise everyone on the staff that the patient is hearing impaired. Another small sign should be placed on the intercom system, so that the patient is not spoken to through it. When the patient puts on his nurse's call light, he should be responded to in person. If the nurse enters the room unseen, she should attempt to get his attention before touching him to avoid startling him by the touch.

Evaluation

Evaluation is based on the plan. If the objectives have been met, then new objectives can be written to reinforce the obtained behaviors. If the plan has not been met, then reassessment is needed.

In the health care system, it is important to determine any hearing impairments in patients, since those patients will have special needs. Without this, it may be difficult for the patient to learn to adapt to his health state.

ALTERATIONS IN SMELL AND TASTE

Olfaction, or the sense of smell, is the least developed of man's five senses. Research has demonstrated that the sense of smell arises from a small area of mucous membrane deep within the nose. Due to its location and lack of refinement, it is the hardest of the senses to study, and consequently, it is the least well understood. The sense of smell is important in man, because it contributes to our relationship with others (all of us remember how our mothers, fathers, etc., smell), protects us by detecting smells such as gas and fire, and aids in appetite stimulation.

Gustation, the sense of taste, is the function of taste buds in the mouth and on the tongue. The exact physiological mechanism of the perception of taste is not known, but it is known that there are four distinct taste sensation areas. These areas detect the tastes of salt, sweetness, sourness (acid), and bitterness.

Although smell and taste are two distinct senses, they complement each other. They are important senses, because they allow people to select their nutritional needs. If individuals are not able to smell and taste their food, they may lose all interest in eating and become malnourished and ill.

Most alterations in smell and taste result from illness or trauma. Sense of smell can be altered by nerve damage or dry nasal mucosa. Sense of taste can be altered by nerve damage, salivary gland disorders, or zinc deficiencies. Many times, a loss of sense of smell or taste is not sufficiently serious to bring individuals into the health care system. Usually, individuals will seek care because of pain or weight loss.

THE NURSING PROCESS

Assessment

Generally, the senses of smell and taste are assessed in the examination of the head and the neurological system (See Chapter on Introduction to Health Assessment). The senses of smell and taste are easy to assess by asking the patient to close his eyes and presenting him with objects to smell and taste. Responses are noted on the chart. Any changes or distortions in these senses should be measured and reported, because it may imply accelerating physiological or psychological health problems. In addition to a routine assessment, appetite and food preferences should be noted and any recent weight loss recorded. Selected nursing diagnoses are:

- Impaired sense of taste related to nerve damage, distorted sense of smell, drugs.
- Altered sense of smell related to chronic allergies, nerve damage, etc.

Planning

The nursing care plan should incorporate all of the patient's needs including the specific needs caused by alterations in smell and taste. Since altered appetite may be a problem for these patients, the dietician should be consulted in the planning phase of the nursing process. Any food preferences should be emphasized. Family can be encouraged to bring favorite foods from home, if these are unavailable in the health care setting. Smells that can be distorted should be removed from the patient's unit, because these will be disturbing. Foods that the patient finds disagreeable should be removed from his tray before it is taken into his room. All staff should be aware of the care plan, so that care is consistent. Preferences and dislikes should be noted on the kardex and on the patient's door.

Implementation

Next, the written plan should be implemented. Smells and taste that the patient enjoys should be increased. Emotional support should be given to the patient and family. Family members can learn from the dietician how to maintain a nutritious diet at home. Offending smells can be removed (where possible), and room fresheners can be used.

Evaluation

Evaluation, as always, is of the successfulness of the plan. Have the objectives been met? If not, why not?

ALTERATION IN TOUCH

The sense of touch is most closely associated with the skin and is the earliest sense to develop in the human embryo.[22]. The skin is the largest of the sensory organs.[23,24] It covers the entire body. The sense of touch comes from millions of nerve fibers located all over the skin and covers a wide spectrum of sensations, including pressure, pain, itching, and temperature.

There are two temperature receptors in the skin: cold and hot. If these are damaged, individuals may have difficulty in receiving environmental stimuli, and may be prone to frostbite or burns.

Pain receptors serve to prevent adverse effects on the environment. By this mechanism, individuals are able to prevent trauma to the body. When pain is perceived, individuals are able to withdraw and, if injured, seek help. If this mechanism is not working appropriately, injury can be sustained and left untreated, causing further injury.

There are three types of maladaptive skin (or touch) responses. **Anesthesia** is the absence or loss of feeling, **hyperesthesia** is an increase in the skin's sensitivity, and **paraesthesia** is a tingling sensation.

Alterations in touch generally are caused by impaired sensory nerve function or central nervous system dysfunctions because of disease or trauma. Alteration in the ability to perceive touch or feeling can be both physically and emotionally traumatic. There are many causes for alterations in touch—some temporary and some permanent—that may have an effect on how well the patient will adapt. A nursing diagnosis might be: Alteration in sense of touch due to lack of circulation, nerve damage, burns, etc.

THE NURSING PROCESS

Assessment

Assessment of sense of touch is based on the patient's history, observation, and other data collection methods. Superficial touch, pain, and temperature should be assessed as well.

Anesthesias, hyperesthesias, or paraesthesias should be noted. The color and condition of patient's skin should be observed and noted. At the conclusion of the assessment phase, the nursing diagnoses are prepared. A nursing diagnosis for a patient with impaired touch might include:
- Potential burns due to inability to perceive heat.

Planning

A written care **plan** is based on the assessment. Mutual goals and objectives are derived by both the patient and the client.

Implementation

Since the ability to perceive sensations is diminished, the nursing plan implemented should teach health care practices to prevent accidents, such as measuring the temperature of water before getting into the tub or shower, wearing shoes or slippers, inspecting the feet daily, and having a podiatrist cut toenails. Patients also should be cautioned about using cold applications, as they can lead to tissue damage.

Heating pads, hot water bottles, hot packs, etc., should be used with caution, if at all, and patients should be taught about their potential danger.

Patients should be positioned carefully and skin assessed frequently for breakdown. Back massage may be comforting, therapeutic, and prevent skin breakdown.

Evaluation

Evaluation of the goals and objectives should be completed to determine the strengths and weaknesses of the plan. Strengths should be fostered, and weaknesses need to be reassessed.

Conclusions

Nurses frequently encounter patients who are at risk for developing sensory alterations or who have sensory deficiencies. Through careful use of the nursing process, nurses can minimize sensory alterations and effectively communicate with patients experiencing sensory deficits.

SUMMARY

Man is dependent on his sensory system in order to interact with the environment. Stimuli from the environment are collected from the senses—vision, hearing, touch, taste, and smell. The brain interprets the sensory stimuli into meaningful information. By receiving and perceiving environmental information, man is able to adapt to his dynamic environment.

Changes in ability to receive or perceive information from the environment can be caused by physiological, psychological, or environmental changes. Alterations in sensory input may lead to confused or disoriented behavior, which may cause individuals to exhibit symptoms that are not healthful.

When individuals enter the health care system, they are exposed to a different kind of environment, and it is confusing and frightening. The stimuli may be overwhelming and meaningless. Patients may be unable to adapt under these circumstances and may demonstrate confused behavior.

Sensory deprivation results when the sensory input is lower than individuals require to function. Under these conditions, the RAS is unable to maintain normal levels of activation to the cerebral cortex, and individuals receive a distorted view of reality.

Research on healthy individuals has shown that the effects of sensory deprivation can have a rapid onset. Symptoms of boredom and irritability begin almost at once, and hallucinations appear between 24 and 48 hours. The findings of these studies are staggering. If well subjects respond to sensory deprivation as quickly as this, sick individuals may be affected at an even faster rate. Patients who are immobilized for any reason are particularly at risk.

Sensory overload is the opposite of sensory deprivation and generally is caused by too much stimuli in the environment. Behaviors demonstrated by patients experiencing sensory overload may be like those exhibited by patients experiencing sensory deprivation.

Parental deprivation is a form of sensory alteration in infants and young children who do not receive the nurturing and stimulation that they need in order to thrive and develop. These children do not respond normally and do not develop as they should. Causes of parental deprivation are complex and may have physical, psychological, emotional, and financial causes. Role and reciprocity theories attempt to provide a framework for understanding the complex problem of parental deprivation.

Occasionally, due to disease or trauma, individuals may experience an altered level of consciousness (LOC). Changes in levels of consciousness are extremely serious and should be monitored and reported immediately. There are four LOCs and these include: awareness, lethargy, semicoma, and coma. Recently, methods such as Glasgow Coma Scale have been developed to measure LOCs. These focus on measurable responses and eliminate more subjective descriptions of LOCs.

Sensory deficits exist when a sensory organ is not functioning at its optimum level. With the loss of one or more of the senses, an individual may not be able to adapt to the environment and may not be able to function adequately.

Nurses play a key role in assisting patients with sensory alterations and deficits. The nursing process provides a framework for providing systematic, comprehensive nursing care.

STUDY QUESTIONS

1. Describe an environment that might lead to sensory deprivation.

2. Put on gloves, a blindfold, cotton in your ears, and lie down for as long as you can in a quiet place. Describe your feelings during and after this activity.

3. What types of patients are most likely to develop sensory deprivation?

4. What is sensory overload? Have you ever experienced it? What was it like?

5. How do infants experiencing parental deprivation behave? Observe a healthy infant and describe its behavior.

6. Why was the Glasgow Coma Scale devised?

7. Observe a friend's pupillary response to light.

8. Put on a blindfold. Walk around. Eat lunch or a snack. Describe your feelings.

9. Wear gloves and attempt to perform normal activities such as taking coins from a purse or pocket to buy a cup of coffee.

REFERENCES

1. Laura K. Hart, Jean L. Reese, and Margery O. Fearing. **Concepts Common to Acute Illness, Identification and Management.** (St. Louis. The C.V. Mosby Company) 1981, p.152.
2. L. Hart, J. Reese, M. Fearing. **Acute Illness,** p.152.
3. Arthur J. Vander, James H. Sherman, and Dorothy S. Luciano. **Human Physiology. The Mechanisms of Body and Function.** 2nd.
4. Vander, et al. **Human Physiology,** p.168.
5. Barbara L. Conway. **Carini and Owens' Neurological and Neurosurgical Nursing.** (St. Louis, The C.V. Mosby Company), 1978, p.152.
6. Arthur C. Guyton. **Textbook of Medical Physiology,** 4th Ed. (Philadelphia: W.B. Saunders Company) 1971, p.705.
7. B. Conway. **Neurological Neurosurgical Nursing,** p.81.
8. J.P. Shelby. "Sensory Deprivation." **Image, 10,** (1978) 2. 49–55.
9. Barbara Kozier and Glenora L. Erb. **Fundamentals of Nursing. Concepts and Procedures.** (Reading, Massachusetts: Addison-Wesley Publishing Co.), 1979, p.803.
10. Leo Madow and Lawrence Snow. **The Psychodynamic Implications of Physiological Studies on Sensory Deprivation** (Springfield, Illinois: The Charles Thomas Co.) 1970, p.6.
11. Philip Solomon. **Sensory Deprivation** (Boston: Harvard University Press), 1961, p.73.
12. F.S. Downs. "Bed Rest and Sensory Disturbances," **The American Journal of Nursing, 74,** (1974) 3, 435–438.
13. W.H. Bexton, W. Herron, and T.H. Scott. "Effects of Decreased Variation in Sensory Environment." **Canadian Journal of Psychiatry, 8** (1954) 6. 70–76.
14. Helen Yura and Mary B. Walsh. **The Nursing Process.** 3rd Ed. (N.Y. Appleton-Century-Crofts), 1978.
15. Lucille F. Whaley and Donna L. Wong. **Nursing Care of Infants and Children.** (St. Louis: The C.V. Mosby Co.), 1979, pp.494–495.
16. R. Crow. "Sensory Deprivation in Children." **Nursing Times, 75** (1979), 6, 229–233.
17. K. Robinson and A. Moss. "Patterns and Determinants of Maternal Attachment." **Journal of Pediatrics, 77** (1970) 976–985.

19. L. Whaley and D. Wong. **Nursing of Infants and Children.** p.497.
20. C. Jones. "Glasgow Coma Scale." **The American Journal of Nursing, 79,** (1979), 9, 1551–1553.
21. N. Mauss-Clum. "Bringing the Unconscious Patient Back Safely. Nursing Makes the Critical Difference." **Nursing 82, 12** (1982), 34–42.
22. Ashley Montagu. **Touching.** (New York: Harper & Row, Publishers) 1971, p.1.
23. J.R. Dunn. "Regulation of the Senses" in **Introduction to Nursing: An Adaptation Model.** Sister Callista Roy (Englewood Cliffs, N.J.: Prentice-Hall, Inc., 1976), pp.133–150.
24. Ashley Montagu, **Touching, The Significance of the Skin.** (New York: Perennial Library, Harper and Row, Publishers, 1971), p.3.

ANNOTATED BIBLIOGRAPHY

Bolin RH: **Sensory Deprivation: An Overview.** Nurs Forum 8:3:240–258: 1974. A concise description of sensory deprivation citing the major concepts and interesting research findings.

Boyles VA: **Injection Aids for Blind Diabetic Clients** Am J Nurs 77:9:1456–1458; September 1977. This article discusses available aids and includes photographs of them.

Buseck SA: **Visual Status of the Elderly.** J Gerontol Nurs 2:5:34–39; September-October 1976. This article provides a framework for assessing vision status in the elderly.

Buisseret P: **The Six Senses. Part 3. The Peripheral Sensation.** Nurs Mirror Suppl 146:4:iii–vi; January 1978. This article provides basic information and enlightening drawings of the peripheral nervous system.

Chodel J, Williams B: **The Concept of Sensory Deprivation.** Nurs Clin North Am 5:3:453–465; September 1970. This article describes the sensory process and aspects of sensory deprivation.

Crow R: **Sensory Deprivation in Children.** Nurs Times 75:6:229–233; February 1979. This brief article discusses the effects of short- and long-term parental deprivation and utilizes the nursing process approach.

Downs FS: **Bedrest and Sensory Disturbances.** Am J. Nurs 74:3:434–438; March 1974. This classic article cites research on sensory deprivation and the hazards of bedrest.

Jones C: **Glasgow Coma Scale.** Am J Nurs 79:9:1551–1553; September 1979. This article describes the use of the GCS and provides an example of a completed assessment scale.

Lindenmuth JE, Brew CS, Malooley JA: **Sensory Overload.** Am J Nurs 80:8:1456–1458; August 1980. A description of sensory overload is outlined in this brief article.

Linnell C, Long Sister V, Proehl J: **The Hearing-Impaired Infant.** Nurs Clin North Am 5:3:507–515; September 1970. This article discusses the causes of hearing impairment, the importance of early diagnosis, and rehabilitation.

Lovelace BM: **The Blind Child in the Hospital.** AORN J 31:2:256–264; February 1980. This article discusses many facets of caring for the blind hospitalized child.

Mamaril AP: **Sudden Deafness.** Am J. Nurs 76:12:199201994; December 1976. Sudden deafness, caused primarily by trauma, is discussed in this article. Interesting points are raised that can be incorporated into the nursing care of these patients.

Mauss-Clum N: **Bringing the Unconscious Patient Back Safely. Nursing Makes the Difference.** Nurs 82 12:8:34–42; August 1982. This important article describes the physical attributes of unconscious patients and discusses four crucial responsibilities for nursing care.

McNamee C: **Communicating with the Hard-of-Hearing.** Can Nurse 74:3:27–29; March 1976. This short article provides very good pointers for establishing a good nurse/patient relationship with hard-of-hearing patients.

Norman S: **The Pupil Check.** Am J Nurs 82:4:588–591; April 1982. This interesting article describes the process of pupil checks and provides an illustration of pupil sizes.

Stewart LM, Dawson DF: **Blind Client-Sighted Therapist: The Interface.** JPN and Mental Health Services 31 35; November 1979. This article describes some of the difficulties in establishing relationships with blind patients and gives some interesting suggestions for nurses.

Wolf EM: **Communication with Deaf Surgical Patients.** AORN J 26:1:39–47; July 1977. This article provides an assessment tool for determining the communication profile of the deaf patient.

20

Sleep

Janet-Beth Flynn

CHAPTER OUTLINE

OBJECTIVES

At the completion of this chapter, the reader will be able to:

- Define sleep
- Compare and contrast REM and NREM sleep
- Describe the five stages of sleep
- Discuss alterations in sleep
- Discuss nursing interventions to facilitate sleep.

GLOSSARY

Circadian cycle—man's 24-hour biological clock.

Electroencephalogram (EEG)—a painless study in which EEG machines convert the electrical impulses of the brain onto a visual graph.

Enuresis—bed-wetting beyond the age when bladder control should have been reached.

Hypersomnia—periods of prolonged sleep.

Insomnia—the inability to fall asleep or to stay asleep.

Narcolepsy—uncontrollable sleep.

Nightmares—vivid dreams occurring during REM sleep and remembered upon awakening.

Night terrors—feelings of fear that occur when a person, usually a child, is awakened from NREM sleep.

Parasomnias—sleep disorders in which events occur during sleep that generally occur during the waking state.

Reticular activating system (RAS)—a neural system, located in the reticular formation, which is responsible for the wakeful state.

Reticular formation—an area in the brain that controls wakefulness.

Sleep—an adaptive recurrent state of unresponsiveness that occurs cyclically every 24 hours and has five stages.

Sleep apnea—self-limiting cessation of respiration during sleep.

Somnambulism—sleep walking.

INTRODUCTION

Sleep is a natural process important in the maintenance of physical and mental health. Human beings spend one-third of their lives asleep or approximately eight hours a day.

Almost a century ago, sleep was considered essential to human well-being. Pierce wrote in 1895,

> It is a well-established physiological fact, that during the wakeful hours the vital energies are being expended, the powers of life diminished, and, if wakefulness is continued beyond a certain limit, the system becomes enfeebled and death is the result.[1]

The amount of sleep that individuals need to feel rested and refreshed varies with age, activity, health, and emotional state. While young children need a great deal of sleep, the need for sleep decreases with age. The normal adult needs 5 to 10 hours sleep per night, with the average being around 7 to 8. A large amount of physical activity might increase the amount of sleep needed. Altered physical and emotional states might cause individuals to sleep more. Nutritional states also may influence the amount of sleep that individuals need.

Despite the common practice of sleep, an adequate definition does not exist. Definitions of sleep are present in the literature of anthropology, biology, physiology, philosophy, and many other disciplines. Definitions of sleep can be traced back thousands of years, but there has never been one definition that has been accepted by all schools of thought.

A historical definition described **sleep** as a period of profound relaxation, much like a comatose state. Current researchers have modified this definition through clinical research[2] by demonstrating that sleep is a state of consciousness, not unconsciousness, in which the individual's state of perception of the environment is decreased but not absent. Sleeping persons are able to attend to certain noises while sleeping. Some noises will awaken the sleeper, such as a smoke detector alarm, an alarm clock, or a crying baby, while other noises—traffic and birds singing—will not. This appears to occur because stimuli that are relevant to individuals will awaken them, while less essential stimuli will not.

Sleep can be considered as a recurrent healthy state of unresponsiveness that occurs cyclically and has stages within the sleep state. The 24-hour day-night or awake-sleep cycle has been referred to by scientists as the **Circadian cycle** and is a part of man's biological clock. The nature of the Circadian cycle or biological clock is still a mystery, but it appears that it is related to the light and dark cycles. It is our biological clock that causes us to fall asleep at one time and awaken at another.[3]

The Circadian cycle develops around the third month of life and appears to be inherited from the mother.[4] The site of this clock has not been determined, but several theories have been suggested.[5] The pineal gland is one of these anatomical sites, and it is located deep in the brain between the two hemispheres. It is light sensitive, and this may be how it regulates the body clock. The adrenal glands also appear to have some effect on the body clock. The hypothalamus has been considered as a location for the body clock as well.

These are just a few of the body clock location hypotheses, and there is no universally acceptable theory to date.[6]

The reticular formation in the brain has been shown to control wakefulness.[7] It consists of neurons distributed in the medulla, the pons, mesencephalon, and portions of the diencephalon (see Figure 20-1). Within the reticular formation there is a neural structure known as the reticular

activating system (RAS), which is believed to be responsible for normal wakefulness. The brainstem portion of the RAS transmits signals to the cortex to produce the awake state.

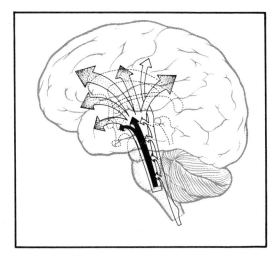

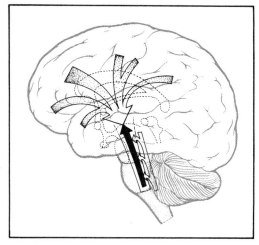

Figure 20-1.   The Reticular Formation

When people sleep, the RAS is mainly dormant.[8] It is inhibited by two neuronal systems that oppose its stimulating effect. These neuronal clusters are located in the central core of the brainstem and in the pons. The brainstem core neurons secrete serotonin (5 hydroxytrystamine), and when this level becomes high enough, the RAS is inhibited. When this inhibition occurs, the individual loses awake consciousness and is asleep.[9]

Dreams are associated with sleep, and it appears that brainstem core neurons facilitate sleep centers in the pons, where paradoxical or dream sleep originates (see Figure 20-2). Pathways ascending from the paradoxical sleep centers produce brain waves like those of the awake stage and produce eye movement.

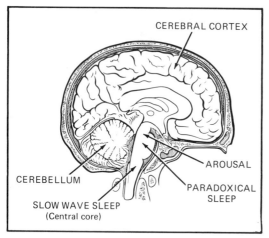

Figure 20-2.   Paradoxical or dream sleep originates in the pons.

Many studies have been done concerning wakefulness and sleep. Data in these studies have been gathered through use of an electroencephalogram (EEG) that measures the electrical activity of the brain. Researchers now have empirical, objective, and scientific data, as opposed to the highly subjective data obtained in the past.

The EEG is a painless study in which probes are placed on the scalp to measure electric potential between two points on the scalp,[10] and a mechanical printout results. The wave-like pattern of the EEG changes as a person goes from an awake state, through a drowsy state, to a sleep state. An individual who is awake and resting produces a slow wave known as the alpha wave (see Figure 20-3a). When these waves are being generated, a person, when

questioned, will verbalize that he feels content and relaxed. In the awake state, the alpha waves become smaller, but are still alpha waves.

STAGES OF SLEEP

The EEG pattern changes during the sleep state. As the individual becomes drowsy, the rhythmic alpha wave is replaced by an irregular pattern, the beta wave (see Figure 20-3b). As sleep deepens, the waves become slower, larger and more irregular—delta waves (see Figure 20-3c). These sleeping waves are interrupted through the sleep cycle by other waves that resemble the wakeful waves (see Figure 20-3d) and are generated during paradoxical sleep. In this stage, the individual still appears to be asleep, but the EEG is like the alert, wakeful pattern.

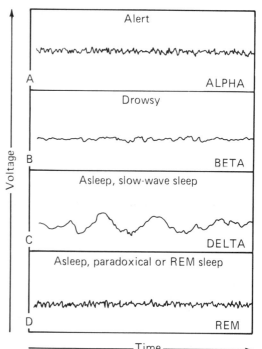

Figure 20-3.   An electroencephlogram measures the changes in electrical activity in the brain.

Based on sleep research, two types of sleep have been identified: rapid eye movement **(REM)** sleep and **non-REM (NREM)** sleep, or slow wave deep sleep. REM sleep, also known as active or paradoxical sleep, is characterized by rapid eye movements of the sleeping person, and the EEG pattern is much like the pattern of a wakeful person. NREM sleep occurs in four stages, from light, drowsy sleep to heavy, deep sleep, and it occurs in cycles, each lasting about 90 minutes.[11] Sleep is a dynamic process during which individuals move through five sleep stages.

Stage I is the drowsy state. The person still knows where he is but is relaxed. It is that pleasant transition state just before dropping to a deeper stage of sleep. Alpha waves are demonstrated on EEG tracings at this stage. Frequently, as one begins to drift into a deeper stage, the legs may jerk, causing the person to jerk awake.

Stages II and III are progressively deeper states of sleep in which an individual is not aware of his surroundings but is easily awakened. Beta brain waves are shown on EEGs in stage II sleep. Stage II sleep has been called the door stage, because it preceeds and follows REM sleep. 40 to 45 percent of total sleep time is spent in stage II. Stage III sleep is characterized on EEGs with delta waves.

Stage IV is a stage of deep, profound sleep during which individuals are difficult to arouse. There is little body movement in this stage, and vital signs and metabolic rates decrease. These EEG waves reveal slow delta patterns. This is the sleep that restores, builds, relaxes, and rests the body physically. After a day of heavy physical exercise or work, the need for stage IV sleep increases. Research has found that somatotropin or growth hormone is released during this stage of sleep.[12] It appears that some dreaming occurs during stage IV sleep. The eye movements associated with this NREM sleep are slow and rolling. NREM dreams are more realistic and thought-like than vivid REM dreams. Non-REM sleep, especially those stages that produce delta waves, is most prevelant in the first third of the sleeping time and decreases in each subsequent sleep cycle.

Stage V sleep is called the rapid eye movement (REM) sleep and is the stage most identified with dreams that are described as vivid and unrealistic. REM dreams are more often recalled than NREM dreams, and dreams that are threatening to an individual's psyche usually are repressed on or before waking.

There are four to five periods of REM sleep per night, and approximately 20 percent of the sleeping time is spent in REM sleep. As the sleep cycle progresses through the sleeping time, the REM phases become longer and occur closer together. The dreams that occur toward the end of the sleep cycle tend also to be more vivid and to be remembered on awakening (See Figure 20-4).

This stage of sleep is characterized by rapid eye movements that can be observed through the closed eyelids, and the EEG pattern resembles the wakeful pattern. Other observable behaviors include muscular twitching, and irregular breathing and pulse rates. Breathing can stop (sleep apnea) at the onset of REM sleep and the period of apnea lasts up to 30 seconds.[13] This phenomena appears to be more common in men than in women.

The purpose of REM sleep is to catalog and process the day's events, to integrate thoughts, and add to the memory storehouse. Since infants and young children have a great deal to process and store they spend a great deal of their sleep time in REM sleep. As an individual grows older, he spends much less time in REM sleep (See Figure 20-5).

REM sleep can be suppressed by use of drugs and alcohol. When this occurs, individuals lose the ability to integrate new information and process stressful events. They may begin to exhibit disorganized

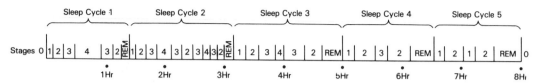

Figure 20-4.   Sleep Cycle Schema. The Sleep Cycle Schema.

Helen Yura, "The Need for Sleep," in Helen Yura and Mary Walsh. **Human Needs and the Nursing Process,** (New York: Appleton-Century-Crofts, 1978) p. 265.

Reproduced with the permission of Appleton-Century-Crofts.

behavior or the inability to cope with stressful situations.[14]

		Sleep	Dreams
Age		Hours/Day	REM Percent
Birth—30 days		16–20	50–80*
1 month—1 year		12–16	30–40
1– 3		12–14	25
3– 5		10	20
6–16		8–10	18–20
18–40		8	22
40–60		6– 8	19
65		5– 7	20–23

*higher for premature infants

Figure 20-5.   Sleep and Dream Patterns Change with Age.

ALTERATIONS IN SLEEP PATTERNS

Alterations in normal sleep patterns are frequently seen in ill patients and occasionally in those individuals who are healthy. There are a variety of reasons for sleep disturbances. Some are caused by physical discomfort, some by psychological factors, and others are environmental in origin.

The most common alteration in sleep is **insomnia.** Insomnia is the inability to obtain an adequate amount of sleep due to problems falling asleep or difficulty remaining asleep. Statistics reveal that one in three Americans suffers from a form of insomnia,[15] and Americans spend millions of dollars on over-the-counter sleep preparations. Just the thought of another sleepless night can create enough anxiety to produce the very state that the individual wishes to avoid.

Insomnia affects all of us at times, but it is not a problem unless it is chronic. Chronic insomnia deprives individuals of the needed rest and restorative functions of sleep. Research[16] has demonstrated that NREM stages III and IV are decreased in the insomniac, so not only does the insomniac suffer from decreased amounts of sleep but also from altered sleep patterns. Insomnia is related to physical discomfort, anxiety, depression, environmental conditions, and drug or alcohol abuse. Since the causes are various, treatment is diverse, ranging from exercise to sleeping medications. Treatment should be based on a thorough physical, history, and proper use of a patient-kept sleep log or diary.

Hypersomnia is the opposite of insomnia, in that periods of sleep are quite long, lasting to several days. Waking, for individuals suffering from this condition, can be difficult, and they may be confused when awakened. Hypersomnia has been reported in individuals with anorexia nervosa or obesity, causing researchers to hypothesize that hypersomnia is related to a central nervous system disorder involving the hunger-satiety center in the hypothalamus. Other conditions causing hypersomnia may include head injury, cerebrovascular accidents, brain tumors, depression, and high stress levels.

EEG tracings of individuals suffering from hypersomnia follow the normal pattern except for the long duration of the sleep period. Treatment of this condition involves limiting the amount of time spent sleeping and possibly the use of physician prescribed stimulants.

Narcolepsy is similar to hypersomnia in that individuals tend to sleep more, but the urge to sleep cannot be controlled. Sleep patterns of a narcoleptic are characterized by frequent uncontrollable periods of sleep of short duration. After these brief periods, narcoleptics report feeling refreshed. Attacks usually follow meals, are toward the end of the day, or occur in boring situations. This condition can be quite hazardous and incapacitating for individuals driving or using machinery.

EEGs performed during the daytime narcoleptic attack show REM sleep patterns. This disorder is usually treated with physician ordered drugs such as Ritalin® or amphetamines.

Sleep apnea syndrome is the self-limiting cessation of respiration during sleep. This condition is fairly common in infants up to three months of age,[17] in obese males, post-menopausal females,[18] and in all individuals during REM sleep.[19] Sleep apnea occurs during NREM sleep, too, and is associated with heavy snoring, snorting, extreme restlessness, sleepwalking, enuresis, morning headache, personality changes, daytime drowsiness, anxiety, depression, and sexual dysfunction.

Treatment includes weight reduction, abstention from alcohol and smoking, and more invasive procedures, such as tracheostomy, or removal of tissue from the oropharnyx.

Extreme care needs to be taken when administering sedatives to patients who have sleep apnea. Death can occur from this additional stress on an already strained respiratory system. If these patients are sedated, they must be closely monitored.

Parasomnias are sleep disorders in which events occur during sleep that usually occur during the waking state. Types of parasomnias include somnambulism or sleep walking and enuresis or bed-wetting.

Somnambulism is seen primarily in male children and adolescents. There is usually a strong family history of sleep walking. EEG reports show that this state occurs during NREM sleep, in stages III and IV. The child is able to get out of bed, though totally asleep, and walk around. Children have been known to get lost or into rather tricky locations such as window ledges or behind large appliances, but do not generally hurt themselves. Eyes are generally open, but the child is unresponsive when questioned, or answers briefly in a monotone. If left alone, the child generally returns to bed and sleep. Characteristically, the child has no recall of the sleep walking process. There may be an underlying emotional problem or anxiety, and the child may act this out during the sleep walking activity. Most children outgrow sleep walking. Only 1 to 5 percent of the adult population walk in their sleep, and this is usually only during periods of extreme tension and anxiety.

Treatment involves providing a safe environment for the sleep walker, and includes using side rails both at home and in the hospital.

If sleep walking continues, treatment might include administration of physician ordered medication and psychotherapy.

Enuresis is the involuntary release of urine beyond the age when bladder control should have been acquired, at around four years of age. Enuresis is the most common of parasomnias and appears to run in families. The majority of bed-wetting episodes occur during NREM sleep. Children generally outgrow this condition by the time they are 12, but it can have embarrassing effects on them until then. Causes of enuresis include psychological problems, pathology such as diabetes mellitus, and organic lesions. Treatment depends on the cause and might include exercises to enlarge the bladder capacity, psychological support for both child and parents, and limiting fluids after the evening meal. Psychological problems are treated with psychotherapy for the child and his family.

Other sleep disorders include nightmares and night terrors. **Nightmares** occur during REM sleep and can be remembered upon awaking. They are common in children but less so in adults. Adults tend to have nightmares during times of stress. **Night terrors** are most common in preschoolers. The child wakes from sleep screaming and it is difficult to console him. The cause of the terror as well as the attack generally are not remembered in the morning. Night terrors occur when the child is awakened from NREM sleep, and the attacks occur infrequently. If they become more frequent, help should be sought.

Alcohol abuse and drug use also can produce alterations in sleep patterns. Alcohol abuse decreases REM sleep and appears to disturb normal progression through the sleep cycle. The alcoholic awakens unrefreshed due to this disturbance. With the withdrawal of alcohol the alcoholic will spend much of his sleeping time in the REM stage. Drug use and abuse also can produce a decrease in the amount of REM sleep. Individuals experiencing the lack of REM sleep may not be integrated emotionally and physically. They may complain of fatigue, jitters, and a "hangover" in the morning. When drugs or alcohol are withdrawn, patients may experience vivid dreams and night terrors. In addition to this, they may become anxious about not being able to take sleeping medications or alcohol. They also suffer from insomnia and fitful sleep.

Finally **sleep deprivation,** which is the lack of sleep. Many hospitalized patients suffer from this condition due to frequent disturbances during the sleeping hours. Lack of sleep can delay the healing and recuperation processes in patients. Patients who are awakened often, such as critically ill patients and postoperative patients, lose NREM sleep that is needed for restoration, and may become irritable, anxious, and have difficulty concentrating. Total sleep deprivation can lead to hallucinations and confusion. Another interesting phenonemon can also occur in cases of sleep deprivation. Patients who need both REM-NREM sleep may drop into REM sleep during the bath and begin talking in their sleep or may appear confused until the proper nursing diagnosis is made, and they are permitted to sleep undisturbed.

Physiological conditions, such as hypothyroidism, hyperthyroidism, coronary artery disease, and nocturnal dyspnea can produce alterations in sleep patterns. Pain and discomfort can contribute to alterations in sleep, too, and need to be monitored.

The nurse can provide an environment conducive to sleeping and adequate sleeping time. Providing patients with adequate and restful sleep is probably one of the most useful services that the nurse can perform in helping patients to adapt.

THE NURSING PROCESS AND SLEEP

Adequate, restful sleep is essential for proper healing and emotional well-being. In order to meet patients' sleep requirements, the nurse should base nursing interventions on a careful sleep and rest assessment.

Assessment

A careful assessment of the patient's previous sleep habits is essential for determining general patterns. Important data to be gathered are age, number of hours slept

SLEEP ASSESSMENT

Sleep Habits

Hours slept per night _____ Number of awakenings _____
Why? _____
Hour of retiring _____ Awakening _____ Naps _____ Time _____
Awaken refreshed _____ Fatigued _____ Alteration in pattern _____
How much sleep is generally required _____ hrs.

Sleep Environment

Type of bed _____ Number of blankets _____ Number of pillows _____
Any special devices _____ TV _____ Radio _____
Sleeping companion _____
Ventilation _____ Temperature _____ Light _____ Noise _____
Music _____ Other _____

Aids

Reading, TV, Radio _____ Exercise _____
Foods and beverages _____
Behaviors (baths, showers, tooth brushing, etc.) _____
For children: bedtime rituals _____
Medications taken: _____
Alcohol _____ type _____ amount _____

Figure 20-6.   Sleep Assessment Tool

nightly, naps or rest periods taken daily, aids to facilitate sleep (reading, baths, alcohol, medication—both prescribed and over-the-counter), number of awakenings and cause, sleeping arrangements (furniture, lighting, bed linens, light, noise, etc.), whether the patient sleeps alone or with someone, amount of daily exercise, prayers or religious readings, and how much sleep the patient feels he needs (see Figure 20-6). Other data to be gathered include the patient's nutritional status, presence of stress in his environment, and the presence of noise and light in the hospital environment. Once the sleep history has been taken and observations of the environment completed, the nurse can observe the sleeping patient in the hospital over a period of several days to assess the patient's present sleep behaviors.

Nursing diagnoses are drawn from the findings of the patient assessment. Exam-

ples of nursing diagnoses related to sleep might include:

- Alteration in sleep patterns due to fever and pain.
- Alteration in REM sleep due to alcoholism.
- Potential alteration in sleep due to impending surgery.

Planning

Planning should be based on the assessment phase and should incorporate data gathered from the patient's sleep history. Planning also should include patient/family teaching when appropriate. The purpose of a sleep plan is to provide for maximum periods of sleep and to relieve sleeplessness.

Treatments, vital signs, and medications should be scheduled in such a way as to maximize the amount of time between them, so that the patient can have several hours of uninterrupted sleep. It is possible to have medications ordered for 10^{pm}, 2^{am}, and 6^{am} and treatments at 12^{am} and 4^{am}. In most instances, these times can be rearranged so that medications and treatments occur simultaneously, and the patient is allowed to sleep between these interruptions.

The nurse also should schedule her time so that she is able to spend enough time at bedtime assisting patients to meet their bedtime needs. Careful planning leads to an organized and consistent approach to facilitating sleep.

Implementation

A great many nursing interventions can be used to facilitate rest and sleep. Some are rather simple and take only a few minutes, while others are more complex and may take more time.

The simplest are the comfort measures, which involve straightening the bed linens, providing more blankets, fluffing and turning pillows so the cool side is against the patient's body. Back rubs and sponge baths are relaxing, too. Placing the patient in a comfortable position or a favorite sleeping position will facilitate sleep.

Another simple care measure is assessing the patient's physical discomfort and administering prescribed pain medication before the patient's pain tolerance is surpassed. Employing other comfort measures will aid the patient, as well.

Helping the patient maintain his normal routines promotes sleep. Providing reading materials and snacks may help, if the patient snacks or reads at bedtime when at home.

The environment should be manipulated to provide a restful atmosphere. Phones can be turned down or off, lights dimmed, and noise reduced. The patient's door can be closed as a buffer from hall lighting and noise. When checking sleeping patients, the nurse should be as quiet as possible, so that she does not disturb them.

Some patients are under a great deal of stress and are unable to sleep because of this. Talking with them and providing support is essential. If patients can discuss their problems, they may feel better and be able to get to sleep.

If the patients are not sleeping at night or are sleeping fitfully, other nursing measures can be taken. Care can be planned to leave periods of time for naps. Naps should be encouraged during the morning hours, because it has been found that individuals continue to have REM sleep during these hours. Naps should be discouraged during the afternoon, because individuals tend to drop into stage IV sleep and awake feeling more fatigued than they did prior to their nap. Elderly patients may stay awake at night and sleep all day. Efforts should be made to keep these patients awake during the day. They can be placed at the nurse's desk and walked in the corridors frequently. They may become noisy at night and disturb other patients, and have to be placed in a room alone. This adds to their sensory deprivation.

Teaching patients to relax is a good method to promote sleep. One method is to assist the patient into a comfortable position and have him concentrate on various body parts and relax them. The patient is taught to begin with the feet and work up through the calves, thighs, hips, abdomen, chest, arms, and neck while stating "Feet go to sleep," "calves go to sleep." This is a type of meditation and works for many people.

A dependent nursing action for assisting patients to sleep is administration of physician ordered drugs. These should be administered with care, usually at the patient's request. The patient should be monitored frequently throughout the night. Great care should be taken when administering sleeping medications to individuals with medical histories of respiratory problems or sleep apnea. It should be remembered that these patients will have reduced periods of REM sleep and may awaken with a drug hangover. It should be kept in mind that if sleeping medications are not administered to patients who have been taking them for a long time, they may experience vivid dreams or even night terrors due to withdrawal of the drug.

Evaluation

Evaluating the quality of the patient's sleep should be based on what the patient tells you. Many nurses have observed patients sleeping all night only to be told in the morning that the patient had a terrible night's sleep. Sleep, like pain, is a subjective experience. If the patient says that he did not rest well, then he did not. Evaluation of sleep can focus on the patient's subjective description of the activity, the nurse's objective observation, and on the waking behavior of the patient, such as irritability or dropping off to sleep at odd times.

Once careful assessment planning and intervention has brought about restful sleep, the patient is well on his way to regaining his optimal health level.

SUMMARY

Sleep is a natural, recurring process important in maintaining physical and mental health. The amount of sleep individuals need to feel rested depends on age, activity, health, and mental state. Most normal adults need between 5 and 10 hours sleep per night, and children need from 10 to 12.

At this time, no completely acceptable definition of sleep has been advanced, but it seems safe to say that sleep is a recurrent healthy state of unresponsiveness that occurs cyclically and has several stages. The day-night cycle which man adheres to, is referred to as the Circadian cycle, and it is a part of man's biological clock. The Circadian cycle appears to be controlled in part by the pineal gland and the reticular formation.

Within the reticular formation is an area known as the reticular activating system (RAS) that appears to control sleep and wakefulness. Brainstem core neurons facilitate sleep centers in the pons, where paradoxical or dream sleep, originates.

Researchers have used electroencephalograms (EEG), which measure the brain's electrical activity, to obtain empirical data on sleep. This research has shown that an individual's EEG changes as he goes from an awake state to a sleep state. Based on this research, two types of sleep have been identified: rapid eye movement (REM) sleep and nonrapid eye movement sleep (NREM).

Sleep has five stages. Stage I is the drowsy state. Stages II and III are progressively deeper stages of sleep. Stage IV is a stage of deep profound sleep, which individuals need for physical restoration. Stage V is REM sleep and is associated with dreaming, and its EEG pattern resembles the wakeful pattern. The purpose of REM sleep is to catalog and process the day's events, to integrate thoughts, and to add to the memory storehouse. Infants and young children have a great deal of information to store and process, and they spend a great deal of time in the REM sleep, while older people need less REM sleep. Lack of REM sleep can produce disorganized behavior and mental confusion.

Alterations in normal sleep patterns are common and can be caused by a wide variety of factors, including physical discomfort, emotional disturbances, and environmental factors. The most common sleep disorder is insomnia. Other disorders include hypersomnia, narcolepsy, sleep apnea, parasomnias, nightmares and night terrors, REM deprivation, and sleep deprivation.

Adequate sleep and rest are essential for

adaptation, and by using the nursing process, the nurse can facilitate sleep. Careful sleep assessments are necessary in order to determine the problem. Then the plan can be determined, implemented, and evaluated.

STUDY QUESTIONS

1. What is sleep?

2. What is NREM sleep? Why is it necessary?

3. What is REM sleep? Why is it necessary?

4. What stage of sleep is essential for psychological well-being?

5. How can the nursing process be used to help patients with alterations in sleep patterns?

6. How can the nursing process be used to promote sleep?

REFERENCES

1. R.V. Pierce, M.D. **The People's Common Sense Medical Adviser in Plain English: or Medicine Simplified.** 50th ed. (Buffalo, N.Y.: World's Dispensary Printing Office and Bindery, 1895), p.278.
2. Karen C. Sorenson and Joan Luckman. **Basic Nursing. A Physiologic Approach.** (Philadelphia: W.B. Saunders Company, 1979), p.540.
3. K. Adams. "A Time for Rest and a Time for Play." **Nursing Mirror,** 150, (1980).
4. M. Walsh. "Prologue: Biologic Rhythms and Human Needs" in Helen Yura and Mary Walsh. **Human Needs and the Nurs-** ing Process. (New York: Appleton-Century-Crofts, 1978), pp.1–33.
5. Arthur L. Guyton. **Textbook of Medical Physiology,** 4th ed. (Philadelphia: W.B. Saunders Co., 1971), p.705.
6. M. Walsh. "Prologue." **Human Needs.** p.8.
7. A. Guyton. **Medical Physiology,** p.705.
8. Ibid.
9. A. Vander. **Human Physiology,** p.557.
10. A. Vander. **Human Physiology,** p.553.
11. J. Hayter. "The Rhythm of Sleep." **The American Journal of Nursing,** 80 (1980) 457–461.
12. Harriet C. Moidel, Elizabeth C. Giblin, and Bernice M. Wagner. **Nursing Care of the Patient with Medical-Surgical Disorders.** 2nd Ed. (New York: McGraw-Hill Co.) 1971, p.272.
13. C. Guilleminautt. "State of the Art Sleep and Control of Breathing." **Chest,** 73 (1978) 293–296.
14. H. Yura. "The Need for Sleep" in **Human Needs and the Nursing Process.** Helen Yura and Mary Walsh. (New York: Appleton-Century-Crofts, 1978), pp.259–318.
15. Pamela H. Mitchell and Anne Loustaw. **Concepts Basic to Nursing.** 3rd Ed. (New York: Mc-Graw Hill Book Co. 1981), p.612.
16. I. Oswald. "Drug Research and Human Sleep," **Annual Review of Pharmacology,** 13 (1973), 213.
17. A. Kales and J. Kales. "Sleep Disorders," **New England Journal of Medicine, 290** (1974), 9, 478.
18. J. Washburn. "Sleep Disorders," **American Journal of Nursing,** 82 (1982), 6, 936–940.
19. K.C. Sorenson and J. Luckman. **Basic Nursing,** p.548.

ANNOTATED BIBLIOGRAPHY

Bassler SF: **The Origins and Development of Biological Rhythms.** Nurs Clin North Am 11:4:575–582; December 1976. This article discusses the body rhythms of sleep, wakefulness, and physiological rhythms, and uses a nursing process approach to relate rhythm research to nursing.

Grant DA, Klell C: **For Goodness Sake— Let Your Patients Sleep!** Nurs 74 4:11: 54–57; November 1974. This article discusses the Circadian cycle and the need for all stages of sleep, and offers suggestions for nursing interventions based on day, evening, and night hours.

Hayter J: **The Rhythm of Sleep.** Am J Nurs 80:3:457–461; March 1980. This excellent article discusses the stages of sleep and implications for nursing practice.

Long B: **Sleep.** Am J Nurs 69:9:1896–1899; September 1969. This article discusses how knowledge of sleep can help nurses assess the sleep needs of hospitalized patients.

Tom CK: **Nursing Assessment of Biological Rhythms.** Nurs Clin North Am 11:621–630; December 1976. This interesting article proposes an assessment tool for assessing Circadian cycles.

Yura H: **The Need for Sleep.** In Yura H, Walsh M: Human Needs and the Nursing Process. New York, Appleton-Century-Crofts, 1978. This comprehensive chapter discusses all aspects of sleep and cites current sleep research. In addition, it uses the nursing process as a framework for patient care.

Zelchowski GP: **Helping Your Patients Sleep: Planning Instead of Pills.** Nurs 77 7:63–65; May 1977. This article suggests alternative methods for assisting patients to sleep without medications.

21

Anxiety, Fear, and Stress

Marie Rawlings

CHAPTER OUTLINE

OBJECTIVES

At the completion of this chapter, the reader will be able to:

- Define the concept of anxiety.
- Define the concept of fear.
- Define the concept of stress.
- Describe physiological responses to anxiety, fear, and stress.
- Describe the four levels of anxiety.
- Identify four defense mechanisms.
- Discuss the importance of the nurse/patient relationship in regard to nursing intervention for anxiety.

GLOSSARY

Anxiety—tension caused by an imagined threat to the self that affects physical and mental functioning.

Fear—tension caused by a real threat to the self that affects physical and mental functioning.

Fight or flight response—the physiological response to a threat that consists of autonomic nervous system activation to provide strength and resourcefulness to fight or flee the threat.

General adaptation syndrome—physiological pattern of response to stress consisting of an alarm reaction stage, stage of resistance, and the final exhaustion stage.

Intrapsychic—pertaining to or originating from the mind.

Stress—the body's physical, mental, and chemical reaction to any change in adaptation.

INTRODUCTION

Anxiety, fear, and stress are terms most people are aware of, because they describe feelings that are commonly experienced by everyone. To many, they are dreaded conditions that hopefully will not have to be encountered. Avoidance of anxiety, fear, and stress, however, is not only impossible but also undesirable, as they can contribute to growth and productivity. On the other hand, they can have a detrimental effect on one's functioning ability and need to be controlled.

All three concepts have been studied extensively under the realm of the physical and social sciences, and the findings indicate that there is a mind-body relationshp associated with anxiety, fear, and stress. **Anxiety** is tension caused by an **imagined** threat to the self that affects physical and mental functioning. **Fear** is tension caused by a **real** threat to the self that affects physical and mental functioning. **Stress** is the body's physical, mental, and chemical reaction to any change in adaptation. Nurses must be aware of these mind-body relationships and interactions if they are to provide total nursing care.

ANXIETY

Anxiety is a factor the nurse frequently encounters. It is a natural response to situations in which one feels insecure. By definition, anxiety is tension felt in response to an anticipated threat to self-integrity. The awareness of the threat is perceived consciously or unconsciously, but the perception is vague and nonspecific, as opposed to the real or specific threat associated with fear. The feeling of tension from anxiety can be described as an uncomfortable feeling of uneasiness, of impending danger, nervousness, or panic. The stimulus for anxiety may originate from psychic conflict when ideas, thoughts, or feelings threaten the individual's self-integrity. Consider, for example, a woman uneasy with close relationships, because unconsciously she thinks she is unlovable and that men eventually will reject her. The stimulus also may originate outside the psyche, when something in the individual's biological or social environment threatens self-integrity. Examples would be an airline pilot faced with failing eyesight, or an individual with minimal education feeling anxious at social affairs where others are highly educated.

Throughout the lifespan, we experience anxiety in varying degrees. For most people, anxiety usually remains within the range of normal limits. For others, it is the basis of severe mental and emotional disturbances, some of which are situational and relatively short-term, while others last for years. Most patients in the health care system experience some type of anxiety, since illness, hospitalization, medical tests, and procedures can all provoke feelings of insecurity. For example, surgical removal of a limb may threaten the security a patient has with body image. Confinement to a wheelchair may threaten the role of a parent of small children. A lengthy recovery from an illness could threaten one's financial security. Patients may imagine countless ways that their future will be affected, as well as fantasies about how their medical plight came about. For example, a woman awaiting the results of fertility testing may be anxious that she will lose her husband if she cannot have children, or that infertility would be punishment for past promiscuous behavior.

The discomfort and energy that anxiety arouses motivates action in search of relief. Nurses may observe uncommon or fluctuating behaviors, such as anger or sudden crying outbursts, as a patient attempts to cope with or avoid anxiety. The attempts can be adaptive, such as the tension relief provided by crying, or maladaptive, such as angrily throwing things or destroying property. Understanding anxiety enables the nurse to provide an environment conducive to the patient's maintaining self-integrity, and to aid the healing and learning processes.

Theories of Anxiety

Probably the widest known theories of anxiety originate in psychoanalytic theory, with Freud's the most famous. Initially, Freud conceptualized anxiety as a state of unpleasure caused by repressed or pent up sexual energy. Thus, the experience of anxiety originated within the individual. In later years, he viewed anxiety as tension resulting from internal or external threats to the ego. (Refer to chapters 11 and 14 for readings on Freud's psychic apparatus—the id, ego, and super ego.) He viewed the occurrence of anxiety as a response to anticipated danger, based on an individual's past experience with traumatic events that remain with the individual on a conscious or preconscious level. Once the ego receives a threatening cue, it mobilizes protective measures to ward off danger. Freud believed anxiety resulted when the ego did not adequately defend against danger, and fears were externalized in symptoms such as phobias or obsessive compulsive behavior. In psychotic states, the failure of the ego to defend against danger is even more complete, so that the ego is overwhelmed or destroyed, with a resultant loss of contact with reality.[1]

Harry Stack Sullivan, another psychoanalyst, also believed that an individual's past experiences influence present behavior. His concept of anxiety, however, pertained only to interpersonal relationships. He believed that the self-developed, to a large extent, in relationship to approved, acceptable social norms and behavior patterns. An individual's self-esteem is incorporated in his acceptance of society's norms. When he experiences disapproval by significant others, his interpersonal security decreases. When he disapproves of his own behavior or thoughts, the result is a decrease in self-esteem. A decrease in interpersonal security or self-esteem is called **anxiety tension.** Sullivan viewed it as human nature that individuals constantly strive toward euphoria, or absence of tension. Subsequently, in the presence of anxiety tension, an individual will strive to modify his behavior in attempts to achieve an absence of tension.[2]

Portnoy speaks of anxiety as a normal reaction when we face our limitations, or the degree of our vulnerability. These traits are said to be inherent in the nature of man. They are brought to awareness in the face of realities such as death, old age, and illness. Portnoy points out that we also experience anxiety as we expand or move forward from the sheltered, the known, or the certain, to the new, unknown, untested, and uncertain. In this view, anxiety is an inevitable accompaniment of healthy growth and change. To Portnoy, a healthy involvement with normal anxiety would be to fight or flee to maintian the self. A neurotic involvement with anxiety would be to shrink or vanish as a self.[3]

Peplau views the cause of anxiety as any threat to an individual's security. Such threats fall mainly into two categories:

- threats to biological integrity—threats to maintenance of homeostasis through such processes as temperature control, vasomotor stability, and through actions taken to meet bodily needs,
- threats to the self-esteem—threats to maintenance of established views of self and the values and patterns of behavior used to resist changes in self-view.[4]

The theorists mentioned all agree that anxiety is the result of a threat to one's self-integrity. The theories differ in what they regard as precipitating a threat. Threats can arise from within the individual's psyche, from the social environment, and from loss of biological integrity.

Levels of Anxiety

Anxiety can be useful to an individual, depending on the amount or level, and whether behavioral responses are adaptive or maladaptive. Theorists see anxiety as a continuum similar to that in Figure 21.1. At each level, one's behavior is affected by the amount of tension because tension causes changes in perceptual awareness, the ability to concentrate, and the ability to reason.

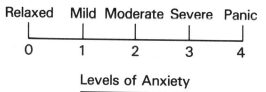

Levels of Anxiety

Figure 21-1. Levels of Anxiety

When **relaxed,** the individual is comfortable, unconcerned, and has a sense of well-being. This is the optimal state for healing to take place. During this state, however, one may lack motivation to change, learn, or expend energy.

With **mild anxiety,** there is slight tension and an accompanying increase in energy. The senses are more alert, and the perceptual field is widened. Thus, the individual is attentive to his own concerns as well as his environment. He is able to concentrate and reason to his full capacity. One is capable of effective problem solving with mild anxiety. During an average day, most people probably fluctuate between being relaxed and mildly anxious.

With **moderate anxiety,** the individual is more alert and tense. The perceptual field is narrowed. One is able to focus on events important to him in the environment, but is less aware of peripheral details and forgets or ignores less important details. One can effectively reason or problem solve when moderately anxious, although usually not for prolonged periods of time. The average person is uncomfortable during this state, but some people can function effectively with moderate anxiety for prolonged periods of time without discomfort.

With **severe anxiety,** the perceptual field is gravely narrowed. The individual will focus on details, unable to see the larger picture of events in the environment. He also is unable to make reasonable associations between the details of which he is aware. The person will be mostly unaware of anxious behavior, but very aware of the discomfort from tension. The individual with severe anxiety cannot focus attention to problem solve and has difficulty reasoning. Severe anxiety is detrimental to the healing process, and always should be considered a problem necessitating intervention.

In **panic** the perceptual field is com-pletely disrupted. The individual focuses on detail, but the perceptions are enlarged or distorted. Consequently, perception of what is going on around the person is frag-mented and distorted. Thinking is disor-ganized, and behavioral responses will be inappropriate. Individuals in panic feel overwhelmed and frightened. In essence, they are in a crisis state (see Chapter 23).

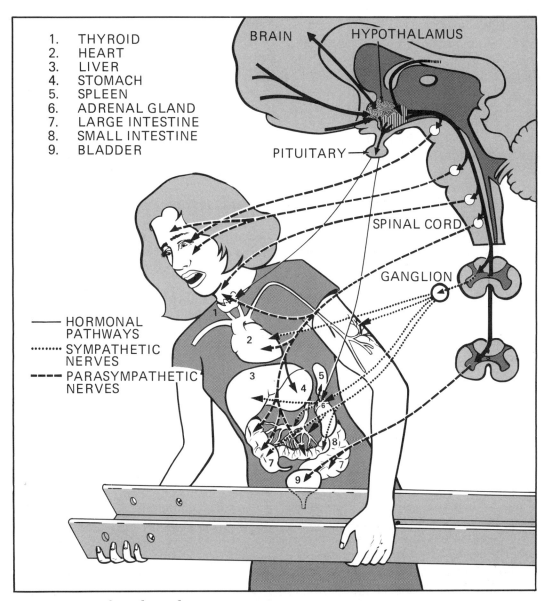

1. THYROID
2. HEART
3. LIVER
4. STOMACH
5. SPLEEN
6. ADRENAL GLAND
7. LARGE INTESTINE
8. SMALL INTESTINE
9. BLADDER

BRAIN   HYPOTHALAMUS

PITUITARY

SPINAL CORD

GANGLION

——— HORMONAL PATHWAYS
·········· SYMPATHETIC NERVES
– – – PARASYMPATHETIC NERVES

Figure 21-2. Physiological Response to Stress

Physiological Response

When an individual is faced with a threat, the body systems adjust to provide the individual with more energy to confront or get away from the threat. This is known as the "fight or flight response." This physiological response is a result of autonomic nervous system activation aided by pituitary stimulation, which together provide far greater strength and resourcefulness than is usual.

The autonomic response is activated once the brain perceives a threat. The brain, by way of the hypothalamus, triggers the sympathetic portion of the autonomic nervous system, which increases visceral and mental functions by stimulating increased secretion of adrenalin from the adrenal medulla. Simultaneously, the sympathetic nervous system increases functioning in those organs that aid the fight or flight response. The functioning of organs that do not aid the fight or flight response is inhibited. This process of stimulation/inhibition results in the following physiological changes.

Activation of cardiopulmonary functioning results in increased heart rate, arterial pressure, and respirations, to provide greater blood supply to the tissues. Increased nerve enervation and cellular metabolism to muscles of the motor system result in greater strength and agility. Pupils are dilated to widen visual perception. The gastrointestinal and genitourinary systems are generally inhibited as they are not important to the fight or flight response. Increased blood flow to the brain increases mental alertness. Increased sympathetic nervous stimulation to the liver results in increased release of glucose for energy. Stimulation to the spleen increases the amount of red blood cells in circulation. The increased autonomic nervous system functioning is aided by hypothalamic stimulation of the pituitary, which triggers production of hormones that act on the thyroid to produce growth hormones and on the adrenal cortex to produce hormones that aid in glucose production (see Figure 21-2).

Signs of the internal physiologic response may be observed externally. Because of the circulatory changes, the vital signs may increase. The increase in adrenalin and autonomic nervous system enervation may be observed in behaviors like trembling, restlessness, and dilated pupils. Dry mouth, perspiration, and menstrual changes are indicative of changes in glandular activity. Inhibition and stimulation of particular areas of the gastrointestinal and genitourinary systems may cause vomiting, loss of appetite, diarrhea, constipation, and urinary frequency.

Internal and External Behavioral Responses

Many internal and external responses typically are associated with anxiety. In order to gather data that indicates internal behavioral responses to anxiety, the nurse must rely solely on the patient's subjective account of what he is experiencing. The external behavioral responses to anxiety may be directly observed or measured. Figure 21-3 lists the internal and external responses typically associated with anxiety. These responses reflect the physiological and psychological adaptation to anxiety.

Adaptive and Maladaptive Behaviors Related to Anxiety

Individuals experiencing anxiety consciously or unconsciously adapt their behavior to avoid, minimize, or eliminate the anxiety. The method depends on the intensity of the threat, current circumstances, and one's established repertoire for coping. Possible adaptive and maladaptive behaviors may be observed in the physiological, psychological, and social areas of the indi-

Internal Behavioral Responses to Anxiety	Jittery or tense	Heart pounding
	More alert	Nausea, heartburn, gas
	Headaches	Dry mouth
	Chest pain	Loss of appetite
	Tightness in muscles	Inability to concentrate
	Comprehension difficulty	Confusion
	Apprehension	Guilt
	Shame	Doubtful
	Depression	Helplessness
	Jealous	Suspiciousness
	Uncertainty	Isolation or loneliness
	Worthlessness	Anger
	Hallucinations	Delusions
External Behavioral Responses to Anxiety	Elevated blood pressure	Increased pulse rate
	Increased respiration	Sleep disturbance
	Trembling	Restlessness
	Vomiting	Diarrhea or constipation
	Urinary frequencey	Perspiration
	Pupils dilated	Appearing hypervigilant
	Appearing worried or preoccupied	Appearing sad
		Angry outburst
	Crying	Talkativeness
	Joking	Inquisitiveness
	Withdrawn	Dependent, clinging behavior

Figure 21-3. Internal and External Behavioral Responses to Anxiety.

vidual's self-system. Each of these areas of the self-system can be a cause of anxiety as well as the basis for adaptation.

The **physiological** adaptive response to the energy and tension of anxiety may be observed in disturbances in sleep (see Chapter 20). Some individuals may complain of insomnia, which is usually not a problem for short periods. Over prolonged periods, however, insomnia interferes with the healing process and can limit a person's reasoning and problem solving abilities. Other individuals may sleep excessively in an attempt to avoid tension or in response to exhaustion from tension. This may serve to "recharge batteries" and allow one to subsequently cope from a stronger position. Excessive sleeping for days, however, may indicate pathological withdrawal, such as that accompanying severe depression.

Many anxious patients experience headaches or vague aches and pains, as the body goes through the circulatory and musculoskeletal changes of the adaptive fight or flight response. The patient's awareness of anxiety and taking appropriate measures for relief are an adaptive response. However, constant complaining may indicate a maladaptive response, as the patient focuses on detail, and an inability or reluctance to focus on the broader source of tension.

Adaptive behaviors such as picking at clothing, twirling or pulling hair, and pacing the floor are indications of restlessness or anxious energy. Constructive responses are directed toward effectively dealing with or avoiding the source. It also is constructive to work off excess energy through exercise or hard work. A maladaptive response may be observed in hostile aggression toward others or destruction of property.

Behaviors associated with anxiety can be constructive or destructive to the **psy-**

chological integrity of the self-concept. Anxious persons, for example, may be observed to be deep in thought or daydreaming. This behavior is adaptive when it results in the individual gaining awareness of his feelings and accurate perception of threatening events. However, excessive fantasizing ("what if—" or "if only—") and withdrawal from reality are maladaptive responses.

Verbal and emotional expression of feelings can be helpful in relieving psychic tension. Expression of feelings may be noted in behaviors such as crying, laughing, and swearing; verbalization of guilt or anger. Resistance to expressing intense feelings generally increases or maintains psychic tension.

Attention to the physical and personal self can be constructive to the anxious person. Examples of adaptive responses in this area would be taking necessary physiological precautions during an illness, and attention to grooming and hygiene to preserve body image. Maladaptive responses would be self-destructive behaviors, such as suicide or mutilation attempts, apathy or avoidance behavior towards problem solving, and behaving in a manner that is contraindicated to one's own well-being, such as abuse of alcohol or drugs.

Adaptive and maladaptive behaviors can stem from anxiety affecting the **social** realm of the self-image. Anxiety often affects an individual's role. For example, a project engineer may be unable to complete a project because of his inability to problem solve. A student may be unable to study because of inability to concentrate. The failure to perform a role in a usual manner can contribute to anxiety. One may, at times, have to make adjustments in role functioning, in order to cope with anxiety. Maladaptive responses would be inability to make choices regarding role functioning, rigidly maintaining roles when adjustments should be made, or feeling alienated from established roles.

Many people turn to others to provide care and emotional support when they are anxious. The care and support of others can relieve tension by increasing an anxious person's self-esteem, lessening the burden of problem solving by offering different perspectives, or by handling stressful situations until the anxious person is better able to handle them. Maladaptive responses to these dependency needs could be behavior that is demanding of attention or rigidly denies the need for help.

Coping/Defense Mechanisms

Anxiety can result from intrapsychic conflict as well as from external threats. This conflict generally arises when an individual has desires, fears, or motives that threaten his concept of self. To defend against the pain and tension from the anxiety these conflicts cause, people learn to develop certain behaviors over time, to conceal these threats to self from their awareness. Hence, **defense mechanisms** are usually unconscious behaviors. Individuals may be aware that they use such mechanisms at times, but during the process of employing them, they are unaware. Figure 21-4 lists the most commonly known defense mechanisms with examples of the desires, fears, or motives that may cause intrapsychic conflict.

Everyone uses defense mechanisms to some degree as a means of coping with anxiety. Individuals may unconsciously choose a particular mechanism for consistently defending against anxiety if it was successful in the past. However, occasions may arise when usual mechanisms of defense are ineffective. Panic or poor mental health can result when the usual mechanisms fail.

In summation, anxiety is an intense emotion that can be constructive as well as destructive. Awareness of anxiety expands the role of the nurse beyond "hands on" care, and is inclusive in total care of the patient.

- **Compensation**—Emphasizing or excelling a certain personal feature to defend against anxiety stemming from perceived personal deficiency in another area. Example—a boy with below average intellectual capacity may compensate by being the "class clown."

- **Denial**—Refusing to accept, on a conscious level, the presence of a threatening event or personal attribute. Example—a person who is clearly alcoholic may insist that drinking is not a problem.

- **Displacement**—Transferring the emotional feeling toward something or someone to a substitute, because it would be too threatening or unacceptable to express them toward the originating source. Example—a child who is angry with a parent for refusing to grant permission to go out subsequently goes to his room and kicks his bed or smacks a stuffed animal.

- **Identification**—When one incorporates attributes of someone he admires into his own behavior to increase self-esteem. Also, when one is unusually sympathetic with someone else's plight because of his own sense of guilt, conflict, or similar experience. Example of the latter—a student organizing a protest against the expulsion of another student found guilty of cheating because of his unconscious sense of guilt.

- **Projection**—When one attributes his own unacceptable motives, thoughts, or feelings to someone else. Example—a husband accuses his spouse of being unfaithful when actually he is defending against his own desire to be unfaithful.

- **Rationalization**—When one gives a reason for behavior other than the real motivating desires or thoughts one feels guilty about. Example—a failing student withdraws from college early with the excuse that it was not a good college, rather than admit a personal failure.

- **Regression**—Reverting to earlier successful methods of coping that have been outgrown in an effort to cope with a currently overwhelming situation. Example—an adult whose parents took responsibility for childhood difficulties when she cried and looked helpless, cries and looks helpless when the nurse coaches her to self administer an insulin injection for the first time, as a way of coping with overwhelming conflict about having diabetes.

- **Repression**—Not allowing undesirable thoughts or feelings to come to awareness. Example—a man who hates his father and has no awareness of it.

- **Sublimation**—Gratification of an impulse through socially acceptable channels. Example—directing the energy from aggressive (anger) impulses into aggressive sports activities.

- **Suppression**—The conscious or subconscious disallowance of undesirable thoughts to come to awareness. Example—a woman who has strong feelings against divorce pushes from awareness any feelings of her own marital discontent.

- **Reaction formation**—Handling the tension from undesirable thoughts by behaving in a manner that is the direct opposite. Example—a person who has a lot of hate and anger, constantly behaves as a kind, polite, friendly person.

- **Introjection**—Incorporating into the ego system the standards and values of someone who is regarded with love, hate, fear, or guilt, in an effort to control the tension resulting from these feelings. Example—a woman begins to dress and act like her deceased mother in an effort to stay close to her.

- **Conversion**—Relieving the tension of emotional conflict by symbolically expressing it through physical symptoms, thus drawing attention away from the conflict. Example—a person overwhelmed by guilt and shame, resulting from having committed a theft, develops paralysis in the hands for which there is no physiological basis.

Figure 21-4. Defense Mechanisms.

FEAR

Fear is another emotion that nurses observe during patient care. It is similar to anxiety in many ways, yet different enough to warrant exploring. Understanding the difference between the two can help maximize the possibility of effective nursing interventions.

Definition of Fear

Fear is a strong emotional response to the threat of danger to one's well-being. The threat associated with fear is specific and consciously perceived. This means that one who is fearful would be able to recognize what is causing the discomfort and why. This differs from anxiety, wherein the perception of threat is most often unconscious and vague. The experience of fear can be characterized as a feeling of dread, doom, or panic.

Types of Fear

Most fears are rational; that is, fear is a reasonable reaction to certain stimuli. For example, a woman who finds a lump in her breast may fear she will die from cancer. The reality may be that the lump is not cancerous and, if it is, the prognosis for her surviving may be excellent. However, since lumps in the breast can be cancerous, with the possibility of metastasis and death, her fears are not without basis. Our awareness of fearful or dangerous events is learned from past experiences with dangerous events, or from observing or learning of the danger associated with particular situations.

Sometimes fears are irrational—i.e. the fearful response seems unreasonable to the specific stimuli. This type of fear is exhibited in panic associated with phobic fear (of heights, germs, enclosures). These fears are the result of the projection of anxiety from inner conflict to external objects and are neurotic in nature. Illness, surgery, medical tests, and procedures all can signal a response of fear. There may be danger of pain, death, disfigurement, and loss of usual mode of functioning. Fear can be a useful emotional response, if the energy alerted is focused on preparing for the dan-

ger. If there is no preparation for danger, fears may be heightened and interfere with the healing process.

Responses to Fear

Fear triggers the same **physiological response** as that associated with anxiety. When the brain perceives a threat, it does not distinguish whether the threat is real (as in fear) or imagined (as in anxiety). In either case, the individual's need for "fight or flight" is the same.

The observable **behaviors** associated with anxiety are also associated with fear and are a result of the anticipation of danger. (Review internal and external behavioral responses to anxiety.) The behaviors that will be particularly associated with worry and feelings are those of helplessness (agitation, preoccupation, dependency). The emotional responses associated with inner conflict (guilt, anger, shame) also may be observed in patients who ponder the origin of the danger. It is not unusual for patients with fear to initially "freeze" or respond with panic in a psychological attempt to deny or flee the danger. Anxiety may be a response to fear when the individual anticipates a danger before actually experiencing danger.

Adaptive responses to fear foster preparation for the threat of danger and subsequently defend against overwhelming anxiety. Patients who ask questions about their illness or medical procedures and make plans for how they will deal with them are adapting to fear. Calling upon past experiences with similar dangers and appropriately applying learned methods of coping also show adaptation to fear. For example, a patient recently diagnosed with a cardiac condition may plan to have his wife attend his next visit to the doctor for emotional support and to gain knowledge to help with their future life adjustments. Another patient, who has learned that taking deep breaths and relaxing muscles decreases pain, may apply that principle to a painful testing procedure. These adaptive responses assure that the patient will be able to cope with the threat.

Maladaptive responses are those that do not prepare patients for danger and threaten to overwhelm them with anxiety. Those who deny or suppress worries about the danger are more apt to be anxious, overwhelmed, and helpless when confronted with the danger. Those who ruminate over frightening rumors and their own imagined exaggerations are likely to be overwhelmed with anxiety. These maladaptive responses do not prepare the patient with mechanisms for coping, which further compromises psychological and physiological integrity. The nurse's understanding of and appropriate intervention regarding signs and symptoms of fear are important responsibilities for providing total nursing care.

STRESS

Definition and Introduction

As noted with anxiety and fear, stress is also a result of adaptation to events in the social, physical, and emotional environment. Socially we are often confronted with stress when changes are made in our political, ethical, and technological systems. The impact of these changes causes disruption in our usual mode of living. We are confronted with stress due to events such as maturation (i.e., change from one developmental stage to another), and family or interpersonal relationship difficulties. Stress also can be caused by physical difficulties. It can be caused by the physical environment, such as skin and temperature changes due to extreme weather conditions, air and noise pollution, and trauma to the body from injury or disease. These events can disrupt psychobiological functioning. Thus, a broad definition of stress is the body's physical, mental, and chemical reaction to any stimulus that causes change in adaptation.

Stress can be caused by events in our lives that are pleasant as well as those that are unpleasant. Getting married, for example, is a pleasant event, and getting divorced is an unpleasant event, but the process of accomplishing either is stressful. Stress has a positive aspect, in that it keeps us creative and productive. Therefore, a goal is not to eliminate stress, but to manage or adapt to it successfully.

How one reacts to stress is an individual matter. It would depend on how one perceives the stressful event, the stressor, or the degree of change caused by it, and the individual's ability to adapt, such as one's health, genetic endowment, and available coping mechanisms. When the level of stress is more than the individual can handle, well-being is threatened. The nurse can play a significant role in helping patients avoid poor mental and emotional health by teaching effective stress management.

Theories of Stress

A theory of the biology of stress was introduced in the 1920s by Cannon. It was Cannon who discovered the "fight or flight" response as he observed responses to emergency situations, such as pain, fear, anger, starvation, and inadequate supply of oxygen. He saw the fight or flight response as the body's adaptive process to maintain homeostasis.[5]

In the 1930s, Hans Selye's research concluded that fight or flight was only the initial alarm reaction to stress, and that two other stages follow.[6] He identified these responses to stress as a syndrome. A syndrome is a group of signs and symptoms occurring together that characterize a disorder. Selye called the first stage of the stress syndrome the **alarm reaction;** the second stage, **resistance;** and the third stage, **exhaustion.** His theory describing these stress responses is known as the General Adaptation Syndrome (GAS), which is described in Figure 21-5. Selye also brought attention to the fact that, although the physiological response to stress is a specific syndrome, the stimulus for stress is nonspecific. This means that whatever the stressor is, the physiological response is the same.

Stage 1—**Alarm reaction** is the "fight or flight" response. Selye emphasized the process of enlargement of adrenal cortex, enlargement of the lymphatic system, and increase in hormone levels, because these activities are responsible for disease symptomatology. The extent to which these activities are increased depends on the perception of the stressor.

Stage 2—**Resistance** is reached when the body fails to resist stress any longer. This stage is characterized by enlargement and dysfunction of the lymphatic structures and an increase in hormone levels with eventual depletion of adaptive hormones.

Stages 1 and 2 are repeated throughout life. If an individual cannot sustain resistance to stress, exhaustion will occur with accompanying psychophysiological alterations.

Figure 21-5. General Adaptation Syndrome.

Harold G. Wolff, in the 1940s and 1950s, studied life situations and emotional stages associated with certain illnesses. He concluded that disease can be precipitated by stress in combination with other predisposing factors, such as genetic endowment, individual needs, and past experiences. This combination of stress and the aforementioned predisposing factors affect the body organs in stereotypical ways, and if the stress persists, the physiological changes become chronic.[7]

Holmes and Rahe conducted some interesting studies on thousands of patients. They noted that a number of significant life events tended to occur in a brief period prior to the onset of major illnesses. They gave a numerical value to each of these events to represent the amount, duration, and severity of change required to cope with the event. From their observations, they devised a scale, whereupon adding the values for recent life events, one could determine what percent chance there was for the occurrence of a major illness in the next two years.[8] See Figure 21-6.

Behavioral Responses to Stress

The behavioral responses to stress are the same as those associated with anxiety. The most common of these are listed below as follows:

● Increased vital signs
● Sleep disturbance
● Appetite disturbance
● Fatigue
● Tension
● Concentration difficulties
● Decreased ability to problem solve
● Irritability and emotional liability
● Body aches and pains
● Depressed mood.

Physiological Response to Stress

The general changes that occur in the body during adaption to stress were noted in the discussion of the "fight or flight." However, if stress continues without remission, the body becomes exhausted, which can lead to structural changes in the organ systems. Consequently, many of the diseases the nurse comes in contact with are stress-related. The determinant for which organ system is particularly affected by prolonged stress is mainly based on genetic load. For example, if one's ancestors had cardiac problems, one is more likely to have distress in the cardiovascular system, if stress is prolonged. Figure 21-7 lists disorders that may be caused by stress.

Adaptive Responses to Stress

Many of the stressors in life can be positive, and, if managed appropriately, provide one with a sense of self-satisfaction and increased ability to cope. Examples of such stressors are career tasks, developing intimate relationships, political or academic pursuits, and any type of contest. Negative stressors, such as death of a loved one, may be unavoidable, but in the pro-

FIGURE 21-6. THE SOCIAL READJUSTMENT RATING SCALE*

Life Event	Mean Value
1. Death of Spouse	100
2. Divorce	73
3. Marital Separation	65
4. Jail Term	63
5. Death of Close Family Member	63
6. Personal Injury or Illness	53
7. Marriage	50
8. Fired at Work	47
9. Marital Reconciliation	45
10. Retirement	45
11. Change in Health of Family Member	44
12. Pregnancy	40
13. Sex Difficulties	39
14. Gain of New Family Member	39
15. Business Readjustment	39
16. Change in Financial State	38
17. Death of a Close Friend	37
18. Change to Different Line of Work	36
19. Change in Number of Arguments with Spouse	35
20. Mortgage	31
21. Foreclosure of Mortgage or Loan	30
22. Change in Responsibilities at Work	29
23. Son or Daughter Leaving Home	29
24. Trouble with In-laws	29
25. Outstanding Personal Achievement	28
26. Wife Begins or Stops Work	26
27. Begin or End School	26
28. Change in Living Conditions	25
29. Revision of Personal Habits	24
30. Trouble with Boss	23
31. Change in Work Hours or Conditions	20
32. Change in Residence	20
33. Change in Schools	19
34. Change in Recreation	19
35. Change in Church Activities	18
36. Change in Social Activities	17
37. Mortgage or Loan Less than $10,000	16
38. Change in Sleeping Habits	15
39. Change in Number of Family Get-Togethers	15
40. Change in Eating Habits	13
41. Change in Schedule (Vacation)	12
42. Christmas	11
43. Minor Violations of the Law	

Scores of 150–199 indicate a 37% chance of physical illness
Scores of 200–299 indicate a 51% chance of physical illness
Scores of 300 indicate a 90% chance of physical illness

*Reprinted with permission from Journal of Psychosomatic Research, Vol. II, Holmes, T, and Rahe, R "The Social Readjustment Rating Scale," 1967, Pergamon Press, Inc.

Figure 21-6. Rating Scale.

Cardiovascular disorders—arrhythmias, hypertension, coronary occlusions, migraine headaches

Gastrointestinal disorders—chronic constipation or diarrhea, colitis, gastritis, ulcers, unhealthy weight loss or gain

Genitourinary disorders—urinary frequency, nocturnal enuresis, disturbance in sexual functioning, menstrual difficulties

Musculoskeletal—torticollis, back pain, arthritis, rheumatism, bruxism

Endocrine disorders—menstrual irregularities, thyroid conditions, diabetes, fertility problems, excessive sweating, hirsutism

Skin disorders—acne, hives, eczema, psoriasis

Respiratory disorders—asthma, chronic bronchitis, emphysema

Figure 21-7. Classified List of Stress Related Disorders.

cess of adapting positively to them, one's self-esteem and ability to cope are enhanced. Since stress is inevitable, an adaptive response would be to effectively manage what can be controlled, such as:

- **Regular exercise**—strengthens the cardiovascular system, promotes healthy breathing for better cell oxygenation and metabolism, helps to regulate hormonal activity, and increases muscular strength. Exercise provides energy and well-being to help cope with stress.

- **Nutrition**—proper nutrition provides strength and energy to resist stress.

- **Regular relaxation**—helps to decrease stress and cope by providing diversion from stress. Examples of techniques for relaxation include:

Yoga	Spectator sports
Biofeedback	Crafts
Meditation	Vacations
Hypnosis	Leisure interests
Progressive	Self-help groups
relaxation	Psychotherapy
Hobbies	

- **Self-awareness/acceptance**—self-awareness regarding one's strengths and limitations is helpful in order to use available skills and avoid, if possible, those things one cannot cope with. Whenever possible, it is also helpful to control life stressors by setting priorities for accomplishment, scheduling or managing time well, and to some degree, regulating the amount of stress allowed into one's life. Self-awareness includes becoming familiar with body cues, such as tight muscles or headaches, that might indicate stress. These cues can alert one to the need for control measures.

Maladaptive Responses to Stress

Maladaptive responses to stress are responses that do not help a person cope with or minimize stress. We have mentioned the physiological maladaptive response in the discussion of the exhaustion phase of the General Adaptation Syndrome. Stress-related illnesses also have been mentioned as physiological maladaptive responses to stress.

Behavioral manifestations of maladaptation to stress are, primarily, anxiety, depression, and mental confusion. There may be drug and alcohol abuse. Bizarre behavior, such as severe hostility, suspiciousness, and suicide attempts, also may be seen. These maladaptive behavioral responses do not necessarily mean that the individual has an emotional or mental disorder. Prolonged stress, however, can lead to emotional or mental disorders as well as physiological disorders.

THE NURSING PROCESS

The nursing process is the basis for effectively identifying and intervening in problems of anxiety, fear, and stress.

Assessment

Assessment is the first step in the nursing process. It involves collecting subjective and objective data for formulating a nursing diagnosis. The most important tools the nurse can use to assess the presence of anxiety, fear, or stress is skill in observation and interviewing. Indications of anxiety, fear, or stress may be noted in five general areas of the patient's behavior and appearance:

1. Motor activity—physical signs of agitation, such as pacing back and forth, rapid limb movements, increased restlessness.

2. Mood—angry, sad, anxious, pensive.

3. Vegetative signs—changes in sleeping habits, appetite, or elimination.

4. Thinking processes—forgetfulness, concentration difficulties.

5. Perceptual awareness—loss of ability to see things clearly or realistically.

(Review the list of internal and external responses in Figure 21-3.)

Once the nurse has observed behavior indicating anxiety, fear, or stress, interviewing skills must be used to determine what factors are influencing the patient's behavior. Thus, interviewing must be geared toward determining:

1. What the internal or external threat to the patient's self-integrity is.

2. Other factors present in the patient's life that may be relevant to the present experience.

3. What past experiences or beliefs might help the patient to cope with anxiety, fear, or stress, or what might hinder adaptation.

After the aforementioned data has been gathered, the nurse must identify and rank the problems that necessitate intervention. To do this, the level of anxiety, fear, or stress must be known, whether the behavior observed is adaptive or maladaptive, and what behaviors are most threatening or destructive to the patient's self-integrity.

It is important for nurses to share with patients their nursing assessment. This provides them some understanding of what they are experiencing, which helps to decrease any feelings of hopelessness, help-lessness, or powerlessness. The patient's understanding of their maladaptive behavior also encourages change.

After gathering the data, a nursing diagnosis is made for problems necessitating intervention. The following are examples of possible nursing diagnoses:

- Loss of appetite in response to anxiety

- Insomnia due to stress

- Fear related to feelings of helplessness regarding illness.

Once a nursing diagnosis has been formulated, goals for intervention must be planned.

Planning

Planning is the second stage of the nursing process. In planning for intervention in problems, the goals should be client centered and focused on behaviors that maintain the client's self-integrity. In some situations of anxiety and fear, this may be accomplished with goals aimed toward eliminating, diminishing, or encouraging adaptation to the threat provoking the anxiety or fear. With stress, the focus of planning may be on avoiding, minimizing, or managing the stress. The goals may be to change maladaptive behavior to adaptive behavior. The following are examples of appropriate goals using the previously stated nursing diagnoses as reference:

Nursing Diagnosis	Goal (Outcome Criteria)
Loss of appetite in response to anxiety	Patient will verbalize understanding of this response and its hazard to illness
Insomnia due to stress	Patient will sleep 4–5 hours at night
Fear related to feelings of helplessness regarding illness	Patient will discuss a plan for increasing his sense of control in managing his illness

After goals are established, the nurse is ready for the next stage of the nursing process, which is implementation.

Implementation

The most important tool for implementing the goals for intervention in problems of anxiety, fear, and stress is the nurse/patient relationship. By providing a warm, trusting atmosphere, patients can be helped to talk about their concerns and recognize how these concerns affect their behavior. The nurse's skill in observation, listening, interviewing, and teaching will help guide patients toward understanding the dynamics of anxiety, fear, and stress. The nurse's presence, strength, calmness, and control may help patients manage their own behavior. The nurse must use expertise and judgment in offering alternatives to maladaptive means of coping, taking into consideration individual patient needs and circumstances. In instances of fear, a careful explanation of what the patient can expect when confronted with a threat, as well as suggestions for how it may be dealt with, is often helpful. Implementation of plans for relieving stress most often will involve education regarding what caused the stress and how it can be managed. (Review adaptive responses to stress.) The client's self-integrity is supported by offering praise and encouragement for adaptive behavior.

Evaluation

To determine whether the interventions were effective or not, the nurse must do an **evaluation** of the care plan. This last stage of the nursing process entails applying the outcome criteria to the continued observations of the patient's behavior. Criteria for evaluating outcome should include the following:

1. Is the patient able to express concerns related to anxiety? (fear? stress?)

2. Is the patient able to discuss the connection between concerns and behavior?

3. Can the patient verbalize adaptive methods of coping with anxiety? (fear? stress?)

4. Did the patient feel the nurse's interventions were helpful in changing maladaptive behavior?

5. Was anxiety decreased? (fear decreased? stress decreased?) as evidenced by. . . .

6. What goals were not met?

For those goals not met, the nurse must go through the nursing process again to reassess the problem and reformulate goals and interventions where necessary.

SUMMARY

Anxiety, fear, and stress result from man's psychological and physiological interaction with his environment. The adaptation response to anxiety, fear, and stress is behavioral and physiological. The initial physiological response is the same with anxiety, fear, or stress, and is known as the fight or flight response. This physiological response is a result of autonomic nervous system activation aided by pituitary stimulation, which together provide far greater strength and resourcefulness to the individual than is usual.

Certain behaviors are associated with certain levels of anxiety. The same behavioral responses are associated with fear and stress, with some variance in incidence and intensity. These behaviors reflect changes in perceptual awareness, the ability to concentrate, and the ability to reason. Maladaptive responses intensify and prolong anxiety, fear, and stress. This interferes with the healing process and can lead to poor mental or physical health. Adaptive responses relieve anxiety, fear, and stress. This aids in the healing process, and promotes individual growth by increasing coping skills. Nurses commonly encounter all three of these concepts in all types of clinical settings. The nursing process provides a basis for intervening in maladaption to anxiety, fear, or stress, and for supporting adaptive responses.

STUDY QUESTIONS

1. Identify personal sources of anxiety over a 24- or 48-hour period and rate your behavioral responses according to the levels of anxiety.

2. You are assigned to medicate a 13-year-old adolescent who begs you to stay away from him because he is afraid of needles. How would you use your knowledge of fear to intervene effectively?

3. Discuss specific ways that nurses can help patients understand how stress and illness are sometimes related.

4. Explain what is meant by the "fight or flight" response.

REFERENCES

1. A. Freedman, H. Kaplan, B. Sadock (eds): **Comprehensive Textbook of Psychiatry**, 2nd ed. (Baltimore: The Williams and Wilkins Co.) 1976.
2. Ibid.
3. I. Portnoy: The Anxiety States. In Arieti S (ed): **American Handbook of Psychiatry**, (New York: Basic Books, Inc.) 1959.
4. H.E. Peplau, "A Working Definition of Anxiety," In Burd S., Marshall M. (eds): **Some Clinical Approaches to Psychiatric Nursing** (New York: Macmillan) 1963.
5. W.B. Cannon, **The Wisdom of the Body.** (New York: Norton) 1932.
6. H. Selye, **Stress Without Distress** (New York: Lippincott) 1974.
7. H. Wolff, **Stress and Disease** (Springfield, Illinois: Charles C. Thomas) 1953.
8. T. Holmes, R. Rahe, "The Social Readjustment Rating Scale," **Journal of Psychosomatic Research,** 2, Vol. 4, pp.213–217, 1967.

ANNOTATED BIBLIOGRAPHY

Peplau HE: **A Working Definition of Anxiety.** Burd S, Marshall M (eds): Some Clinical Approaches to Psychiatric Nursing. New York, MacMillan, 1963, 323–327. Provides a working definition of anxiety formulated by a nurse author "from the experiences of experts." It is an operational definition presented in outline form.

Perley NZ: **Problems in Self-Consistency: Anxiety.** In Roy Sister C: Introduction to Nursing. Englewood Cliffs, Prentice-Hall Inc., 1976. Discusses the behavioral manifestations of anxiety and underlying states of mind usually associated with the threat that causes anxiety. Emphasis is on the nursing process, based on the adaptation model.

Sidelau BF: **Stress and the Mind-Body Interrelationship.** In Haber J et al: Comprehensive Psychiatric Nursing. McGraw-Hill, New York, 1978, 407–417. An excellent resource for the historical perspective on stress and understanding the stress syndrome.

Sidelau BF: **Physiological Maladaptation to Stress.** In Haber J et al: Comprehensive Psychiatric Nursing. McGraw-Hill, New York, 1978, 421–439. Discusses physiological maladaptations to stress from a psychosomatic illness point of view. Considerable attention is given to nursing care planning, and particularly to primary, secondary, and tertiary prevention in stress management.

Wilson H, Kneisl C: **Disturbed Personal Coping Patterns.** In Psychiatric Nursing. Menlo Park, Addison-Wesley, 1979, 291–301. Distinguishes anxiety from fear and provides data that indicate fear. Good diagrams of autonomic nervous system responses.

22

Loss

Sally Laliberté

CHAPTER OUTLINE

OBJECTIVES

At the completion of this chapter, the reader will be able to:

- Define the terms loss, grief, mourning, anticipatory grief, maladaptive grief.
- Describe various types of losses that affect persons at different points in the lifecycle: age/development; life experience; illness; death.
- Describe the physical and emotional responses that occur as part of an uncomplicated grief reaction.
- Describe the stages of the mourning process along with characteristic responses of the person moving through each stage.
- Identify factors that influence the type and severity of the grief reaction and mourning process.
- Describe the nurse's role in dealing with persons experiencing a loss.
- Identify factors that influence the nurse's ability to work effectively with persons experiencing a loss.
- Describe basic nursing interventions useful in assisting persons suffering from a loss.

GLOSSARY

Anticipatory grief—The experience of a grief reaction and movement, either partially or completely, through the mourning process while under **threat** of a loss.

Bereavement—The period of grief following the death of a loved one.

Grief—A series of intense physical and emotional responses that occurs following a loss; an adaptive response.

Loss—Any situation either actual, potential or perceived in which a valued object is rendered inaccessible to an individual or is altered in such a way that it no longer has qualities that make it valuable.[1]

Maladaptive grief—A grief reaction complicated by an abnormal psychological response to a loss; the inability to allow oneself to experience grief or resolve a loss.

Mourning—The period of time in which the grief reaction is expressed and resolution and integration of the loss occurs; an adaptive process.

INTRODUCTION

In our modern world, we are constantly confronted with loss. Through advanced communication systems, we hear frequent reports of terrorism, war, and natural disaster. There is also a growing potential for loss through depletion of natural resources, advancing technologies, and the increasing stress of living in an advanced society. It can be overwhelming to contemplate real and potential losses. As members of a helping profession, nurses must be aware of the potential for loss in today's world, as well as the processes by which man adapts to them. These two factors, potential for loss, and man's adaptive processes, become part of the environment surrounding each individual who must deal with a specific and personal loss.

At every point in the lifespan, we are faced with loss. Loss is an essential part of the human experience, for without it, we cannot continue to grow. With every loss there is always the potential for some gain. Just as a young man leaving home to begin a new job loses the security and support of his family, he also gains status in his new position and a sense of pride and accomplishment in his new role.

Often the concept of loss is linked only with illness and death. In reality, loss occurs daily. In fact, certain losses are necessary for man to maintain adaptation and to grow physically, psychologically, socially, and spiritually. For example, each day, the human body uses nutrients and disposes of wastes. Millions of cells are turned over daily, and through this process the steady state within the body as a system is maintained. Likewise, a toddler will gain an increasing sense of independence with his ability to manipulate certain parts of the environment. As he gains in mastery, he also loses a sense of security that came from dependence on parents to maintain control over the environment. It is crucial to interpret the concept of loss in this broader context in order to understand that man deals with loss daily, and in so doing, establishes certain patterns of response in an attempt to adapt to specific losses.

The study of loss as a concept for nursing

is twofold: as a knowledge base from which to proceed, and in the context of our own personal experience with loss. How we have dealt with loss in our own lives will certainly impact on the nursing care we are able to give. In reading this chapter, be aware of your own feelings about loss. Reflect on your own experiences with loss and recall your responses.

Loss is defined as:

"any situation either actual, potential or perceived in which a valued object is rendered inaccessible to an individual or is altered in such a way that it no longer has qualities that make it valuable."[1]

It is important to remember that a loss can be potential or perceived as well as an obvious or actual loss.[2] It is easy to understand the severity of the loss when a family member dies. It may be much less obvious when the loss involves an ideal, a life goal, or one's self-perception. For example, a young woman gives birth to her first child after a long, tiring labor. She had planned to use no medication but ended up having taken several injections during her labor. She and her infant are healthy and recovered, yet no one can understand why she feels a sense of loss within herself. She was not able to have the kind of experience she envisioned and so it is a loss of what might have been.

The various types of loss with which the nurse must be familiar are divided into four basic categories: **loss related to age and development, loss related to life situation, loss related to illness, and loss related to death** (see Figure 22-1). Figure 22-1 is certainly not an exhaustive list, but recounts many common losses that occur within each category. Review them and see if you can add any more, given your own personal experience with loss.

I. Loss Related to Age/Development:	
Age	*Related Loss*
Infants	—protective, warm environment in utero —breast or bottle and comfort of sucking
Toddlers/ Preschoolers	—immediate and consistent meeting of needs as the toddler grows in independence and begins testing the environment —spontaneity of bodily function that comes with toilet training and acquisition of other social skills —familiar environment when leaving the home for daycare or nursery school —special place in family as the only child or the youngest child, with birth of sibling —first set of teeth
School age	—friends and significant others (teachers, coaches, ministers) as they move through grades at school or as the family moves —loss of body function at various times with normal childhood illness and injuries
Adolescent	—spontaneity and freedom of childhood with increasing social pressures to act "grown up" —child's body with advent of puberty and secondary sexual characteristics —first boyfriend/girlfriend with adolescent "crushes" —virginity with first sexual encounter —known, safe environment of family, friends, and community, with leaving home to work or continue education

Young Adult	—loss of financial security through parents when leaving home —friends, through leaving school, changing jobs, or moving —childhood dreams, fantasies, expectations, and ideals —freedom, with increasing responsibilities of adulthood (e.g., marriage, family, job) —sexual partner for any reason —a job
Middle Adult	—spouse, through divorce or death —physical capacities with increasing age (especially stamina and strength related to athletic abilities) —children as they grow up and leave home —friends through moving, changing jobs, death —spouse, through divorce or death —"youth," especially related to physical appearance, changes in libido, and physical capacities —fertility in women, with menopause —parents through death
Older Adult	—sensory acuity —hair and teeth —sexual desire or function —intellect and memory —control over some bodily functions —job, through retirement —independence in living (moving in with children or to retirement home) —spouses and friends through death

II. Loss Related to Life Experience:

—Death of a spouse, child, relative, or friend
—Separation or divorce
—Breakup of a love affair or friendship
—Loss of a job
—Financial loss
—Move away from friends, family, professional contacts
—Change of teachers, school, neighborhoods
—Loss of a personal goal or ideal
—Robbery, assault, rape
—Fire, flood, or other natural disaster
—Status
—Hope
—Control
—Self-confidence

III. Loss Related to Illness:

Loss of:
    —Good, general health due to chronic illness or repeated episodic illnesses
    —Bodily function and control
    —A body part or part of a body system
    —The perception of oneself as whole and integrated
    —The perception of oneself as independent and functional
    —A positive self-image
    —Independence and the ability to make choices about one's care and life
    —Control over one's environment

IV. Loss Related to Death:

Loss of:
—A cherished, significant person
—An interdependent relationship
—A significant support
—A defined role (in relation to the space left by the loss one)
—Sexual partner
—Chance to work out areas of conflict
—Hope (for future relationships)

Figure 22-1. Categories of Loss.

COPING WITH A LOSS

Grief

Loss of a significant and valued object is considered to be the precipitating factor for the state of acute grief. Grief is defined as a series of intense physical and emotional responses that occur following a loss. The lost object is defined as any person, place, or other entity (job, dream, hobby) that has significant value to the person suffering the loss. It is important that the nurse be aware of common responses in an individual dealing with a loss in order to accurately assess the behavior indicative of the normal grief state.

It has been postulated that even the use of the term "normal grief" is an erroneous one. Engle states that the grief reaction corresponds to many other entities commonly regarded as diseases and fulfills all the criteria of a discrete syndrome."[3]

- There is a common etiologic factor (i.e., the loss)

- There is a predictable symptomatology and course

- There is impairment of capacity and function for a considerable time period

- The stricken person is acutely distressed and disabled.

Engle offers the term "uncomplicated grief" to specify a grief reaction that normally occurs following a significant loss. This reaction runs a fairly consistent and predictable course and ends in the relinquishing of the lost object and the return to the patient's previous, although not unaffected, life.[4]

Some of the common responses encountered in a person suffering from a recent loss are listed in Figure 22-2. Remember that not all people may experience all symptoms; however, those listed have been validated as the responses most often seen in individuals suffering from a recent loss.

Lindemann's[5] classic paper on the manifestations of acute grief led the way for other clinicians working with grieving patients to validate and expand on his observations. During Lindemann's interviews, patients who had recently lost a loved one described "waves" of discomfort that were precipitated by the mention of the lost one. These waves lasted about 20 minutes to an hour and including feelings of tightness in the throat along with a choking sensation, a need for sighing, shortness of breath, an empty feeling in the stomach, muscle weakness, and an "intense subjective distress described as tension or mental pain."[6]

Symptoms that are manifest in the acute grief reaction are both physically and emotionally draining. They are also variable in intensity and frequency and tend to be self-

Physical Reactions	Psychosocial Reactions
• Loss of appetite	• Helplessness
• Digestive intolerance	• Hopelessness
• Insomnia	• Severe "pangs" of loneliness
• Decreased libido	• Extreme sadness
• Loss of weight	• Denial
• Increased susceptibility to illness	• Guilt
• Lack of strength/physical exhaustion	• Hostility
• Restlessness	• Anger
• Inability to initiate or complete activities	• Tension
• Weeping	• Disturbing dreams/fantasies
• Other physical complaints (i.e., headache, backache, muscle tension)	• Feelings of emptiness
	• Preoccupation with lost object
	• Need for solitude mixed with need for social contact
	• Inability to concentrate

Figure 22-2. Common Reactions to Loss.

limiting. As the person experiences grief and begins to work through the loss, life takes on its previously normal patterns. The uncomplicated grief reaction related to death averages approximately six months.[7] That is, the period in which the most intense physical and emotional reactions are felt, and disorganization of the person's life occurs. This time frame should be interpreted with great flexibility, since it varies depending on many different circumstances. The length of a grief reaction related to other types of loss is not well documented but also would depend on the specific loss, its meaning to the individual, and many other influencing factors.

Mourning

Many terms have been used to describe the period of time in which grief is expressed. **Mourning** and **bereavement** commonly are associated with the period during which one expresses grief, when the loss is through death. However, it is important to remember that a person will express grief with any significant loss and will move through a process of mourning

no matter how tragic or trivial the loss may seem. The difference is only in the length of time grieving takes and the intensity of the feelings expressed.[8] A very simple example might be when a person misses the bus to get to work. Although this may seem trivial, the process is the same as for a major tragedy. The man who misses the bus for work one morning expresses **shock/disbelief** ("I can't believe I missed it, I ran all the way . . ."), a **developing awareness** ("If only the driver had slowed down I would have made it"), and **restitution/recovery** ("Oh well, I'll have to call a cab now"). Again the only differences are in the intensity of feelings expressed and in the length of time needed to resolve the loss. The process will always be the same.

Other important terms to keep in mind are **survival, healing,** and **recovery,** because they are three processes that mingle to produce growth through the experience of loss.[9]

Stages of the Mourning Process

The process of mourning traditionally has been associated with death; however, it will be used here in its broadest context, that is, **the period of time in which the grief reaction to some specific loss occurs, as well as the time it takes to integrate and resolve the loss.** We are faced daily with minor losses, and periodically with major ones. Each loss that occurs adds to our experience in dealing with loss and forms the basis of our ability to cope with future ones.

Separate and distinct stages characterizing the process of mourning have been documented.[10—13] Although the occurrence of a major loss is usually the precipitating factor for triggering a grief reaction and the mourning process, clients may experience these under only threat of loss. This is known as **anticipatory grief.** This phenomena was first observed in the spouses and other family members of military personnel who were stationed overseas during World War II. In anticipatory grief, a person experiences symptoms of grief and moves through the mourning process while anticipating a major loss. The advantages of anticipatory grieving is that it allows a client to begin working through an inevitable loss (i.e., a person who is terminally ill) or may prepare a person for the news of a possible tragic loss. The disadvantage is that sometimes a person may have worked so completely through the process and resolved the loss that they are unwilling to accept, for example, a loved one home again.[14]

This is a phenomenon seen today in the families of chronically or terminally ill clients. With advances in treatment modalities, many clients can live for long periods of time following diagnosis. Since they usually are under constant threat of death, families have considerable difficulty with prolonged grief and mourning periods. This can become a major nursing care problem when members of the family go through anticipatory grieving. The family may then isolate the client, sometimes so completely that the client's entire support system is gone.

The three stages of the mourning process, according to Engle[15] are an initial stage of **shock and disbelief,** a second stage of **developing awareness,** and a final stage of **restitution and recovery.** Usually stage one is the shortest, lasting an average of six to eight weeks. Stage two is somewhat longer, six months to a year, and stage three, the longest, lasting possibly several years.[16—19] It is important to remember that not only is there a progression from one stage to another, there is also movement within each stage. Progression occurs, but only with many periods of regression. In other words, measurement of progress must be flexible and take into account the many variables that influence how each person may react to a loss.

Stage One—Shock and Disbelief. In this initial stage, the person discovers the loss. He is unable to acknowledge that the loss is threatened or has occurred. People react to shocking news in a variety of ways, such as, sitting or standing abruptly, fainting, crying out, moaning, pacing, wringing hands, inability to speak, or rhythmic body movements. The person usually will feel dazed, disoriented, and helpless.

The initial phase can be a time of intense physical and emotional pain, depending on how shocking the loss is. However, some patients find that they are numbed, as if they cannot feel anything. This can be quite upsetting and may cause a person to feel abnormal or "crazy." This period is a crisis point in which a person needs a lot of caring from family, friends, and professionals.[20]

During this stage and well into the second stage of developing awareness, a person may find himself excessively preoccupied with the lost object. If a loved one has died, the person suffering may find himself "searching" for that lost individual.[21] "I keep expecting her to come through the front door." "I see his face everywhere I go, but it's never really him."

Parkes believes that this searching behavior is found in anyone who has lost a loved one. It has been observed that a person in an acute grief state is restless and seems to move about aimlessly. He is unable to begin or finish any activity, and is "continually searching for something to do." Parkes contends that there is a purpose to such behavior: the recovery of the lost one. Since recovery is usually irrational, especially in the case of death, many people will not admit to this need, for fear of sounding crazy.[22]

Part of this searching process may be manifest in the need, on the part of the patient, to review over and over again the details of the time immediately preceding the loss. Trying to remember what happened, who was there, and what was said can be useful in helping the person begin to believe that the loss is real. In fact, intense preoccupation with a lost loved one is considered essential in eventually resolving the loss.[23,24]

Denial is an important and frequently found component of this stage of the mourning process. "Denial functions as a buffer after unexpected shocking news, allows the patient to collect himself, and, with time, mobilize other, less radical defenses."[25] Denial is used throughout each stage of the mourning process in various ways and to different degrees. In an uncomplicated grief reaction, denial is generally a temporary defense. When reality testing is done, the patient knows that the loss has occurred. The patient also realizes that he cannot realistically hold onto the belief that the loss is temporary.

Separation anxiety is also common in the stage of shock and disbelief. The death of a loved one naturally will evoke anxious feelings. The client may wonder how he will ever survive. A death is especially anxiety producing due to the concommitant loss of a defined role, within which the patient is used to functioning. Separation anxiety can occur with other losses, such as loss of a job or loss of friends, as one moves to a new place. In fact, it has been postulated that separation anxiety is at the very core of the grief experience.[26]

Stage Two—Developing Awareness. The stage of developing awareness, in which the patient must come to terms with the fact that the loss has occurred, may be the most painful psychologically. The patient not only will have to recognize the reality of the loss, but attempt to understand the meaning of the loss in relation to the rest of life. As this happens, many of the feelings previously described will be experienced. Overwhelming feelings of helplessness and frustration are common at first. The realization of having no power to change the loss contributes to these feelings.

Anger and hostility are common during this stage. The person often will try to blame others for what has happened. Many times, health professionals take the brunt of such hostility when loss is related to illness and death. Family members are often blamed, not only directly related to the loss, but indirectly in day-to-day living situations. The patient may feel that no one can do anything right. "If only the doctor had operated two years ago." "He never gave me a chance, that's why I was fired." "Don't talk to me like that, I don't need your pity." Statements like these reflect a patient's need to let someone else take responsibility for the loss, at least for a while.

Feelings of guilt also emerge during this stage and are closely related to anger. The client may feel guilty about something he said or the manner in which he behaved. He may perceive these as somehow contributing to the loss. Clients also may feel very guilty about any anger or hostility that was shown to health professionals, family, or friends who were trying to help him.

Extreme sadness and feelings of isolation and loneliness are other components of this stage. Grief "pangs,"[27] which are periods of intense feelings of anxiety and psychological pain, are also common. This is especially true with clients who have lost someone close to them through death, or with clients who are terminally ill and anticipating their own death. These pangs are extremely uncomfortable and are evoked when the lost one is mentioned or when the patient is alone and thinking about the lost one. It is significant that a person feels such sorrow in order to be able to move toward integration of the loss. Initially, grief pangs occur quite frequently and are usually most acute in the months following the loss. Later they may occur around anniversaries of the loss or at other special times that remind the patient of the loved one, such as holidays, birthdays, or vacations. This may happen for years following a major loss.

There is usually great variability in mood states during the time of developing awareness, since clients experience many intense feelings. Relatively normal behavior, in terms of daily living, alternates with periods of immobility and helplessness. Weeping and expressions of loneliness are common. There may be variable levels in activity, appetite, libido, and sleep. The client may also experience changed needs for solitude and social interaction. There will be many days when clients feel as if they have made no progress and that they never will recover and be able to live their lives normally.

Stage Three—Restitution and Recovery. In this final stage of the mourning process, the client continues to deal with the loss and its effect on his life. However during this time, he also does much of the work involved in the true healing process.

> "Normal grieving involves a reintegration process which brings together the intellectual awareness of a loss, its implications and consequences, and the physical and emotional experience of deprivation, mourning, and healing."[28]

The goal of this stage is the acceptance of the altered state and the relinquishing of the lost object. This is signaled by the formation of new relationships and patterns

of social interaction.[29] Preoccupation with the loss continues but on a different level. There are no longer such extremes in emotion, but gradually a detachment and intellectualization of the loss. This is not to say that the lost object is forgotten or any less meaningful to the patient, but rather that the client is coming to terms with the loss and managing to continue a normal life.

As this growing away from the loss occurs, less acute pain is felt. The client can allow himself to tolerate ambivalent feelings about the loss. For example, a man who is fired from his job initially may be full of anger and resentment toward his boss. Only after he resettles into a new job and has had time to reflect and grieve does he allow himself to experience mixed feelings. Perhaps his former boss taught him many skills that helped him acquire his current job. He is now able to have positive as well as negative feelings about his loss.

How and when a client is ready to do this work depends on the type and severity of the loss. If the loss is related to the death of a loved one, for example, it may take considerably longer and be that much more difficult to tolerate such ambivalent feelings. We can probably each recall someone in our lives who has lost someone close, who can think only of the good qualities and good times related to the lost one. The importance of being able to experience ambivalence must be stressed, because a large portion of the work of integration and recovery is related to developing a realistic perception of the loss and its meaning for the future.

Another crucial part of the recovery has to do with the formation of new relationships and patterns of social interaction. This must be interpreted in a broad context. A person suffering a loss must be able to get on with life. This means interactions with family, friends, neighbors, co-workers, and others, that are changed as a result of the loss. This is not as easy as finding a new mate or simply getting a new job. It also means being able to see oneself as a normal, whole, worthwhile human being. A loss can and will affect any of these self-perceptions, and, in turn, with social interaction.

> A 19-year-old woman training to be an olympic skater lost her leg in an accident. She recovered well physically but had a great deal of trouble establishing friendships with anyone her own age for about two years following her accident. She worked in a preschool day-care center and volunteered occasionally in a nursing home. She found that she could not relate to her former friends, and she never dated. She said the reasons were because they didn't want to be around a "cripple" and because she could no longer skate. Only through the establishment of new relationships was she able to see herself more realistically. She subsequently went to work as a skating coach for handicapped children.

The client has to be willing to take some risks and look at the loss realistically. It can be quite painful to acknowledge what a particular loss means in terms of one's future. When this is done, however, comfort and relief usually follow, and movement toward recovery occurs. Sometimes it takes trying to establish new social patterns to force a person to look at the loss more realistically. Letting go may then be easier in light of the reward of new relationships.

Since a loss causes such tremendous changes in a client's daily life, at least for a period of time, his opportunities for renewal of relationships and establishment of new ones may be quite limited. The social networks we build center mainly around our likes and dislikes, physical abilities, jobs, and family or other personal ties. When a loss occurs, these networks can be severely disrupted. Many adjustments and perhaps major changes will have to be made. In light of the disruptions caused by a major loss, changes may be very difficult tasks to accomplish.

> A 34-year-old man lost his wife and was left with their three young children. He con-tinued working but had to cut back his hours somewhat due to the demands of his children. This caused quite a bit of friction at work. He was unable to socialize with friends from work because of his new responsibilities at home. He rarely saw any of the friends he and his wife used to associate with. He and his children lived some distance from both sets of grandparents, so he became isolated from his family, friends, and coworkers.

Due to this man's life situation, including responsibilities to his children and need to continue working, his "normal" life was severely disrupted. Not only did he have to deal with losing his wife and missing an intimate and interdependent relationship with another adult, but also with very little opportunity for any new, adult social interaction. Even if a client can reach a point where he is willing to try to renew normal relationships or to develop others, he may truly be hindered by either limited opportunities or limited knowledge of opportunities. This can be a source of considerable frustration and may require professional intervention.

During this process of attempting to adjust to the loss and form new relationships, the client also may be dealing with periods of denial, anger, guilt, and sadness. Although these are certainly less acute than in the stage of developing awareness, they may still be present. This is especially true around times that remind the client of the loss, such as birthdays, anniversaries, and holidays. It is important to remember that mourning is not simply a gradual, one-way process, from shock to recovery, but rather is full of "ups and downs, progression and regression, dramatic leaps and depressing backslides."[30] For the client, adjustment in this stage can be difficult, because on the surface his life appears to be back to normal, when in reality he is still dealing with many feelings and changes in his life brought about by the loss. This is why restitution and recovery may be such a slow process, and indeed, why it is the longest stage of mourning.

FACTORS INFLUENCING THE GRIEF RESPONSE

Numerous factors influence the type, severity, and length of a specific grief reaction. Since these factors play a key role in how a particular client will experience and cope with grief, it is important that the nurse be aware of them.

One basic influencing factor will be the client's self-concept. Self-concept is how a person sees himself in the world; what he values about himself. It is a constantly evolving phenomenon, and just as the self-concept will affect how a person copes with a loss, so too will it be further shaped by the loss. The major components of a client's self-concept are his **physical self** and his **personal self.**[31]

The physical self encompasses the client's body image, which includes both physical appearance and functioning. Other important components are sexual identity and general health state.[32] Body image is developed over the course of a lifetime and will vary depending on age, developmental task mastery, and life experience. When the loss of a body part or function occurs, a threat to the physical self follows. A loss of this type will have profound implications, depending on how positive or negative the client's body image is. For example, the self-concept of a 43-year-old woman who loses her breast following diagnosis and treatment for cancer may be severely threatened because of the impact of the loss on her physical self: her appearance and function, sexual identity, and perception of herself as ill.

The personal self encompasses the client's moral values, self-expectations, regulatory behaviors, and self-esteem.[33] This part of the self-concept is involved in every experience of loss, especially in a client's coping mechanism. For example, expression of emotion during the grief reaction may be distasteful to certain men. For many years society has dictated that men should be "strong" and unemotional, and so men traditionally cry much less than women. A man may feel inhibited about weeping following a loss because his value system tells him men should not cry, therefore his expectation of himself is not to show emotions publicly. Self-regulation requires that he "be in control," so his self-esteem will be maintained only if he can refrain from weeping.

Another important component of the self-concept is the mastery of age-appropriate developmental tasks. Depending on where a client is along the age/development continuum, the impact of a major loss will be experienced differently. Children may be able to adapt to changes in their lives more easily than adults, provided the adults around them handle the situation and the child's feelings in an appropriate manner. This means recognizing the child's or adolescent's level of understanding and helping him to express, not repress, his feelings about the situation. However, certain kinds of loss at key developmental points in life may have a profound effect on a person's progression through task mastery.

It has been observed that both children and adults can regress or fixate at a level of development as a result of certain types of loss.[34] This is especially true with children and adolescents, since they are still in the process of mastering basic tasks necessary for positive ego functioning.

When a major loss occurs, such as the death of a parent or sibling, or parental divorce, the potential for maladaptation in a child or adolescent can be great. This will depend on the developmental level, family functioning, and how the situation is handled by key adults in the child's or adolescent's life. Unfortunately, problems may go unnoticed for many years, because feelings may be repressed, or because adults around the child do not recognize the child's needs. Only when a situation such as some other major loss (or potential loss) triggers recall of feelings can a problem be discovered.

A 25-year old woman became pregnant with her first child. She and her husband were excited and had planned the pregnancy. Yet during her fourth month she developed hyperemesis, a syndrome of severe vomiting in pregnancy. She was then hospitalized for dehydration, and eventually went home apparently well. She was subsequently readmitted twice, for the same problem. During a psychiatric evaluation it was discovered that her mother had died during the birth of a sibling when the patient was five years old. She had never resolved her grief over her mother's death and it took becoming pregnant herself, to trigger those feelings. With some counseling, she was able to work through her delayed grief reaction and go on to have a healthy pregnancy and birth.

It is important to understand how a child's concept of death develops, since it is tied to developmental task mastery and is different at various levels. There is a wide variety of opinion related to exactly when a child becomes cognizant of death and is able to grieve. It is generally recognized that children are aware of death after the age of at least two years, but are not cognizant of the finality of it. From then until age five or six, the child's understanding is at the level of a temporary separation.[35] A child understands that there is something special and significant about death, probably due in large part to the behavior of adults around them. However, at this age a child cannot acknowledge the inevitability or finality of death. Preschool children may be especially apprehensive about death because they are increasingly aware that it is both an important and disruptive event. The child searches to find causes of death and may misinterpret certain phenomena as being involved with death.[36] The formation of unrealistic associations are common. For example, going to sleep may mean that the child will die. An all too common response of parents when children ask what happened to someone who

died is, "She's sleeping with God in heaven." Often, when a child's pet dies he is told that the pet was "put to sleep," and then sees that the pet never returns. It is crucial that the issue of death be handled with reassurance and realistic explanations in order to prevent the formation of completely erroneous ideas about death. This would certainly be true of other major losses, such as separation of a child and parent or sibling through divorce or illness. Pre-schoolers also tend to blame themselves, and this can have tremendous effects on their feelings of self-worth, unless they are reassured that they are not responsible for the loss.

For children between the ages of 5 and 10 a gradual understanding that death is both inevitable and final develops. During this time the child tends to personify death. The child fantasizes that death is a person who has the power to take the child away. This personification has been called the "deathman."[37] Children will devise all sorts of ways of avoiding the deathman. Behaviors such as hiding under the bed covers, looking behind doors and in closets may be indicative of this avoidance behavior.

After about age 10, the child is able to recognize death as the final cessation of body function and the ultimate outcome of human life.[38,39] As children move towards adolescence and its many new developmental tasks, they develop their concept of death more fully. Death becomes an issue as adolescents begin to intellectually analyze the world and understand where they fit in it. Kastenbaum[40] believes that the intellectual tasks of adolescents are important to their developing concept of death:

"At the very time that everything is changing inside and around him, the adolescent must begin to develop a comprehensive and stable conception of the adult-world-with-him-in-it."

This includes thoughts about his ultimate end. As the adolescent begins to take on

Age	Perception/Developmental Disruptions
Birth–2 years	Not aware of death. Can react to parent and family's emotional response to death. Can appreciate disruption in normal routines. May have significant psychosocial problems if mother or surrogate is lost in first two years of life.
2–6 years	Sees death as a temporary separation. Can understand and react somewhat to the gravity of death, but this is greatly influenced by the reaction of parents or other caretakers. Many have significant psychosocial problems if either parent is lost at this stage, especially from ages 4 to 6 and with parent of same or opposite sex depending on where child is in relation to sex patterning and identification.
6–10 years	Can appreciate that death is inevitable and final. Fantasizes and tends to personify death (i.e., the "death-man"). May have nightmares normally, even without experiencing death firsthand. Deathman avoidance behavior common, such as leaving on lights at night, closing closet doors, hiding under covers. At this age a child may feel intense guilt surrounding a loss and responsibility for death of a close relative (parent or sibling).
10 years— adolescence	Able to recognize that death means the cessation of bodily functions and is the ultimate outcome to human life. Adolescents tend to deny that death could ever happen to them, whereas preadolescents may still worry about death to some extent. Loss of a parent at this stage may have a profound effect on the adolescent's movement into young adulthood and their ability to form intimate relationships with members of the opposite sex.

Figure 22-3.   Children and Adolescent's Perceptions of Death.

increasingly adult responsibilities and thoughts, he begins to see loss as a potential in many life situations. (See Figure 22-3 for a summary of the child's and adolescent's perception of death.)

Any type of major loss that occurs at key points in the lifespan has the potential for interferring with the mastery of specific developmental tasks. Children and adolescents can be quite vulnerable to complications following a loss, due to the number of age-specific tasks to be accomplished. However, in adult life, the self-concept continues to evolve with increased responsibilities and life experience. In addition, during the adult years the potential for loss through illness and death are much more profound especially in middle and late adulthood. Thus, age appropriate developmental task mastery as an integral part of the evolving self-concept is crucial to assess when looking at factors influencing loss.

Another factor that influences a person's

reaction to a specific loss is his perception of the magnitude of the loss. This perception will be influenced by self-concept and developmental level, religious and cultural orientation, and relationship to the lost object. Self-concept and developmental level have been discussed as the basis on which a person perceives himself and his world and will not be further delineated here. See Chapter 15 for further discussion of self concept.

Religious and cultural orientation as well as previous experience with loss can have a significant effect on the perception of all types of loss, especially major ones, such as death or separation from a loved one and illness. Each culture and the religious sects within it have certain beliefs about birth, death, and illness. Many dictate mourning rituals and, to a certain extent, normal conduct for men, women, and children at various points in the lifecycle. Beliefs in God, after life, and redemption of the soul have been observed as important components in helping patients move through the mourning process when the loss is or will be death.[41] Depending on the type of loss and when it occurs, cultural and religious orientation has varying degrees of influence.

Finally, the patient's relationship with the lost object will have profound influence on perception of the loss. It is also important to understand that the loss may be replaced, to some extent, in the patient's life. Certainly people and our interactions with those we love can never really be replaced. However, the needs met by key people in our lives can be met in other ways and by other people. Of course, this issue is at the very core of the grief experience: enough healing must take place so that new relationships can be initiated.

The amount of interdependence involved with the lost object will influence the perception of the severity of loss. The change in a client's daily life may be great depending on the amount of daily interaction and interdependence.

> Mr. and Mrs. J. had waited until their late 30s to begin their family, and after a few years of infertility problems, had a daughter, C. Mrs. J. stayed out of work for 11 months to be home with C. She was ambivalent about leaving her with a sitter, but finally decided to return to work on a full-time basis. She was called home one day by her frantic babysitter. The woman had been carrying C. down the stairs and accidently dropped her. Upon arrival at home, Mrs. J. found her daughter barely conscious. The child was immediately helicoptered with her parents to a regional trauma center, and underwent surgery for several hours. She never regained consciousness and died two days later.

The loss of a child will have a tremendous impact on the parents' lives. So much of everyday living is centered around young children, since they are dependent on parents for meeting basic survival needs. In the above example, there are additional factors to consider, such as the couple's infertility problems, their age (a factor in

considering future children) and the mother's ambivalence about leaving her child in the care of another person. A high degree of interdependence with the lost object is usually associated with a more severe although not necessarily a more complicated grief reaction.

Other important factors that influence the grief reaction are the meaning of the loss in relation to past experience with loss and the client's normal methods of coping with any crisis. Clients nurses work with experience numerous kinds of loss in their lives. In addition, they may have had vastly different life experiences and have formed methods of coping that have been significantly influenced by those experiences. A client's usual methods of coping with any stressful life situation will serve him during the mourning process. This is why, for some people, denial works best initially, and for others hostility is encountered first. Some people need to be close to others immediately following a loss. Some need space and time.

Resolution of a loss is a painful process and must be done by the client in his own way. As professionals, nurses can care, assess, advise, and assist, but the client will have to follow his own course, depending on many influencing variables, as he moves through the process of mourning.

THE NURSING PROCESS

Nurses in all specialties will deal with patients recovering from many different types of loss. In almost any situation that requires nursing intervention, loss of control and independence will be manifest. In addition, many other situation-specific types of loss will be encountered. Hospital based nurses generally will deal with patients experiencing loss through acute, episodic illnesses or through acute phases of chronic or terminal illness. On the other hand, community health nurses more often deal with loss related to chronic ill-

Assessment Tool for Loss

A. **Type of Loss** (describe) _____
_____

When did it occur? _____
B. **Client Characteristics**
Name: _____
Age: _____ Sex: _____ Occupation: _____
Place of employment: _____
Developmental Stage: _____
Cultural Orientation: _____
Religion: _____
Affiliation (church/synagogue) _____
C. **Support System**
1. Family members: _____
_____
_____

2. Friends: _____
_____
_____

3. Other Relatives: _____
_____

4. Religious: _____
5. Problems: _____
D. **Activities of Daily Living** (note specific problems)
Diet: _____
Exercise: _____
Sleep: _____
Elimination: _____
Social Interaction: _____
Personal Hygiene: _____
Sex: _____
Work: _____
E. **Community Resources** _____
_____
_____

F. **Assessment** _____
_____

1. Problem Areas to Address _____
_____

Figure 22-4   A written assessment tool can aid the nurse in assessing loss.

ness and loss of function, as well as those types of loss related to life situations resulting from poverty. The nursing process is an excellent framework for the delivery of nursing care.

Assessment

The initial patient assessment should be quite thorough in order to make an adequate care plan. Figure 22-4 offers the major areas in need of assessment for a client suffering a loss. When describing a client's loss, try to see it from his viewpoint, because that is crucial to the planning phase.

In addition to assessment of the adaptive grief reaction, the nurse must look for signs of maladaptation. Differentiation may be very difficult at times. Since a major loss causes such disruption of the patient's daily routine, minor physical illnesses may be precipitated. Due to problems, such as insomnia, poor appetite, and lack of exercise during the period following a loss, the patient will not maintain his regular activities. He may then be more susceptible to colds, intestinal problems, headaches, and muscular aches and pains. The patient's weight may increase or decrease depending on how food is used in times of stress. This can lead to an even further susceptibility to physical problems and decreased self-esteem due to a change in body image.

Certain diseases have been specifically associated with the stress following the death of a loved one. These include ulcerative colitis, rheumatoid arthritis, and asthma.[42] Exacerbation of other illnesses diagnosed previously, such as hypertension, diabetes, heart disease, stomach ulcers, migraine headaches, skin problems, and various neuromuscular disorders may occur in patients under stress.[43,44] These will cause additional problems to be dealt with in planning care.

Important components in the differentiation of adaptive from maladaptive behaviors involves the duration and intensity of the reaction as well as the perception of resolution on the part of the client. Some basic behavior patterns that are indicative of a prolonged or maladaptive grief reaction include:

- Gross disruption of the patient's daily life, lasting longer than about six months.

- Serious suicidal thoughts or any suicide attempt.

- Acquisition of symptoms belonging to the last illness of a deceased loved one.

- Extreme weight changes; a loss or gain of 30 to 50 pounds.

- Extreme social isolation. Inability to renew and maintain relationships or to form new ones.

- Extreme hostility toward a person or group.

- No apparent reaction in relation to the loss.

- Severe insomnia with early morning waking.

- Extremely low self-esteem.

- Inability to see lost object as really gone.

- Use of present tense in speaking of loss.[45-48]

If any of these behaviors are noted, and they more often are groups of behaviors, the patient may need additional intervention by someone experienced in handling a maladaptive grief reaction.

An important reminder here is that, when confronted with a client suffering a major loss, the nurse needs to consider her own feelings about the specific loss. Those feelings can either positively or negatively affect how the nurse is able to care for the client.

A 22-year-old graduate nurse was reassigned from the surgical floor where she usually worked to the pediatric unit due to a staff shortage. The first day was enjoyable for her, since she liked being around children and usually worked exclusively with adults. On her second day on the new unit, she was assigned a 10-year-old boy who was dying of leukemia. She was able to finish her morning care of the child, which took almost three hours, since he was unable to do very much for himself. At lunch time she told the head nurse that she was feeling too ill to finish her shift, and requested to be sent home. She was unable, however, to tell the head nurse that she had had a younger brother who had died of leukemia when he was 8 years old.

Many times in your nursing career, you will be confronted by clients with such tragic personal losses that they seem almost overwhelming. All the factors that we assess in our clients, such as age, sex, developmental stage, religion, etc., also have an impact on us as nurses and the care we are able to give. There may be many times when feelings of anger, frustration, hopelessness, and guilt must be first worked through in order to help our clients. Many times these feelings are subtle, and since it is not really our loss, they are difficult to recognize. Sometimes we may notice a simple resistance to going into that one client's room, or putting off that one home visit until next week. It is helpful to think about loss in its broadest context, so that in our dealings with all clients, we are cognizant of loss as an issue each one deals with to some extent.

At the conclusion of the assessment phase of the nursing process, nursing diagnoses are formulated. Examples of nursing diagnoses for loss include:

- Loss related to amputation of a leg
- Grief secondary to impending death
- Grief reaction related to a loss of a significant other.

Planning

In order to effectively develop a plan of care for a client experiencing loss, the nurse must be familiar with the types of interventions appropriate for such clients. Three main categories of intervention are: physical and psychological assessment, education and guidance, and mobilization of resources.

Goals should be developed within these three categories. Mutual goal setting with the client may be difficult in the initial phase following a loss. However, after the initial shock period, goal setting may be helpful, for example, helping a client learn to resocialize, find a new job, or join a therapy group.

Use knowledge of the normal grief reaction and phases of mourning in the nursing care plan. Take into account regression as well as progress toward adaptation. The care plan is dynamic and needs to be flexible to account for this.

Implementation

Intervention within the three categories identified above will be discussed. In addi-

tion, since communication is at the very core of any type of intervention, techniques specific to intervening with clients suffering a loss also will be delineated.

Intervention is generally not needed in the course of an uncomplicated grief reaction. Usually a caring, understanding approach is sufficient. The nurse's demeanor is important in allowing the patient to feel comfortable to discuss feelings related to the loss. Above all, the natural healing process must be allowed to progress.

Listening and attending skills are useful in dealing with grieving patients, especially in the initial period following a loss. When a great personal loss does occur, or is threatened, there is really not much anyone can say, although most caring people will feel the need to do so. At this point, the client needs empathy and understanding offered within his own frame of reference.[49] At times, silence and just being with a client is all that is necessary and communicates effectively the notion of not knowing what to say, but still caring.

Denial is a reaction that emerges initially following a loss and warrants special attention in discussing communication. It will continue throughout the mourning process in varying degrees. Since it is an important defense against intense feelings of separation anxiety, the client may need to experience denial, depending on the loss and its meaning to him. Vigorous confrontation of the person experiencing denial may be harmful, because he may not be ready to confront the reality of his loss. The nurse should not, however, support unrealistic ideas or fantasies. Most grieving clients understand that their loss is real. Denial is used simply as a way of insulating themselves from the initial shock.

Some clients deny a loss because they were never able to realistically experience it. For example, a woman delivered a stillborn infant under general anesthesia and was never allowed to see her child. Perhaps the family held the funeral while she was in the hospital, or perhaps there was no formal acknowledgment of the infant's death through a funeral. Too often, in an effort to make the client "feel better" or "feel less pain," family, friends, and health professionals deny someone the chance to acknowledge their loss and begin the healing process.

In fact, it is inappropriate at any time to try to suppress normal expressions of grief, which involve many feelings and defense mechanisms. Often clients are given the message that their feelings are abnormal or, at the very least, that other people cannot tolerate such expressions. An example is overmedication of clients because the health professionals caring for them are unable or unwilling to deal with their feelings. This deprives the person of full awareness and of experiencing the real significance of his loss.[50] This is a good opportunity for the nurse to act as a role model for the client, family, and other health professionals, in order to facilitate attitudes of acceptance toward expression of the pain associated with loss.

Along with role modeling, another communication technique that may be helpful is appropriate sharing of personal experience. There are times throughout the mourning process when this technique is very useful. Having personally experienced a similar loss may enable the nurse to understand more fully the intense pain associated with a client's specific situation. The nurse may be aware of certain resources, such as a particular type of support group that could be of benefit to the client. Certainly, through both personal and professional experience, the nurse will be able to share experience and resources for dealing with specific problems associated with certain types of loss.

Another communication technique that is often used is facilitation of decision-making. This is more often done during the stage of restitution and recovery, since this is the time when the patient has to deal most concretely with the effects of his loss. The patient may need to make many decisions. He also will experience many changes in his life that will require some additional problem solving. Exploration of the problem begins the process, followed by focusing on the various alternatives available. The nurse then assists the patient in evaluating each separate alternative and facilitates the patient's choice of the best one.

Reflection and clarification are also important communication techniques. See Chapter 11 for examples of using reflection and clarification techniques. One of the goals of the mourning process is to assist the client and family to express their feelings of anger, guilt, doubt, and sadness. Reflection and clarification can be useful in encouraging such expression. It may be extremely uncomfortable and threatening for many people to be able to express such intense feelings. It has been observed that although great relief usually follows weeping and expression of feelings, the patient often feels compelled to apologize for letting go in front of another person.[51] The nurse must communicate a sincere attitude of personal acceptance and respect for the client and family in order to facilitate emotional expression.

Communication patterns between nurse and client are best facilitated by the establishment of rapport, by a caring, empathic attitude, and by allowing the patient to progress through this mourning process at his own pace based on his special needs. It is important to point out that nurses are not always able to follow a patient through the entire mourning process, due to limited contact and the length of the mourning process. We usually only see patients at certain points in the process. Knowledge of normal progression through the process will help the nurse to use the most appropriate, situation-specific patterns of interaction, within each category of intervention.

Category One: Physical and Psychological Support. In nursing care, we usually strive for complete physical independence (or as much as possible) on the part of the clients with whom we work. Generally, we can more readily accept the need for psychological dependence. However, the person who is grieving following a loss may need substantial physical and psychological support for a period of time following the loss. As in any major crisis, the impact may immobilize some individuals. It is not uncommon for a person to forget to eat, to be unable to maintain even the simple activities of daily living, or to take care of other family members who are dependent on them. The nurse must make an adequate assessment of the client's physical needs and then plan for meeting those needs either through direct action or delegating certain tasks to family, friends, or other health care workers. For example, many people lose their appetite during the early traumatic period following a loss. Taking the client for a walk prior to meals and keeping the menu simple but nutritious may encourage a lagging appetite. Eating with the client or sitting with him during meals may also be helpful.

Personal hygiene is another area that may be neglected. This can be harmful to a client if severe. Skin and scalp problems and even breakdown of the skin barrier allowing for entry of pathogens can occur. This also perpetuates a cycle of a negative body image and low self-esteem. Assisting a client in maintaining adequate personal hygiene tells him that he is a person worth caring about. It also gently lets the client know that life continues after a loss, and that it is important that he move on. This is a subtle but powerful suggestion.

Adequate rest is another area in which a client may be lacking. Certain individuals deal with trauma by sleeping much of the day. Others find it difficult to fall asleep. Rest is crucial, since the body and mind are healing. So much emotional energy is being spent that even though a person may be "doing nothing," he will feel exhausted for some time. Suggesting the time honored remedies for insomnia may be helpful. Warm baths, warm milk, relaxing music, or reading can aid insomnia.

There are many conflicting opinions regarding the prescription of tranquilizers and sedatives to induce relaxation and sleep. Certainly there are advantages for certain patients, depending on the type and severity of the loss. However, this must be weighed against the idea that sleeplessness is very common to the grief reaction and in essence may represent the extra emotional work being done in an effort to adapt. Medications are more often used with inpatients and are frequently prescribed on an outpatient basis. The nurse's observations may be extremely important to a physician managing the client's medical care and in deciding for or against the use of drugs as an adjunct to other therapies.

Another physical problem that may occur is changes in pattern of elimination. Diarrhea and constipation are frequent developments. They are probably due to a combination of change in diet, exercise, and sleep patterns. Certain people notice gastrointestinal problems whenever they are under stress, such as stomach pain, gas, cramping, and change in stools. Helping the client return to as normal a pattern of daily living as quickly as possible usually will relieve these problems.

Clients who are ill or who have suffered exacerbation of a previously diagnosed illness concurrent with a major loss may need substantial physical support for some period of time. A diabetic, for example, may need to be given insulin injections, even though normally, he manages his own care. An elderly man living alone may need a male home health aide to assist him with personal care following his loss of sight. These clients are especially susceptible to the development of complications to their illnesses and need to be closely monitored for adverse signs and symptoms.

> A 37-year-old woman was just finishing divorce proceedings after a struggle of several months regarding child custody and support. She had been diagnosed with multiple sclerosis several years earlier during her first pregnancy, but had been quite well with only a couple of mild flareups of her symptoms. She now began to notice increasing weakness in her right leg and some occasions of urine incontinence. She eventually had to be hospitalized for stabilization and was successfully treated with steroids. She was referred for counseling to assist her in transition to single parenthood, her return to full-time employment, and working through her feelings surrounding the divorce.

In this case, the woman's M.S. symptoms were aggravated as a direct result of the loss that occurred with its concurrent stress.

When a client's loss involves any physical limitation, such as loss of a body part of body function, the nurse needs to assist in adaptation to a new body state as well as maintaining and increasing body function. In this type of loss situation, the client not only must accept and integrate the loss, but also must learn many new skills that will be strange and awkward at first. There may need to be a period of considerable physical dependence during this learning phase.

At times, it is difficult to separate physical and psychological support. Much is conveyed in the nurse's physical actions that can be viewed as supportive. A client will feel understood and helped as the nurse offers physical support when necessary, encourages and accepts expressions of feeling, and is able to anticipate the client and family's need for information and guidance.

Category Two: Education and Guidance. Education, along with anticipatory guidance, are necessary to help the client understand the normal grief reaction and period of mourning. Many people who suffer a major loss and consequently go through an uncomplicated grief reaction feel that they are abnormal. They may never have experienced such extremes in emotion or such disruption of their personal lives. Some patients express feeling "crazy," or worse, feel crazy and are not able to tell anyone. Educating the client and family about common reactions to loss may offer them reassurance. Including family and friends is also important, because they then may be even more sensitive to the patient's needs. Anticipatory guidance about what to expect in the months to follow a loss also will be helpful.

Some specific information that will be useful to share with any patient or family suffering from a loss follows:

- The healing process takes time. Allow yourself time to experience the pain you feel. It is healthy to do this.

- Use your family and friends. Let them know how you are feeling and how they can best help you.

- Try and stick to your normal schedule. Make certain you eat right. Allow yourself some extra time off from work or school, if possible.

- Do not make any major changes in your life right now. Keep decisionmaking to a minimum. Your judgment won't be what it is normally.

- Many people experience thoughts that they would be better off dead, rather than feeling such emotional pain. If you seriously consider hurting yourself, talk to someone immediately.

- Don't be afraid to let out your emotions. Crying is useful to some people. Screaming in the shower or in your car can be good ways to let out feelings of anger and frustration. Beating up pillows is another.

- Physical exercise can also be helpful. You have a right to feel terrible, a terrible thing has happened to you.

- Avoid addictive behaviors, such as smoking, drugs, or overeating. These are escape mechanisms.

- It's a healthy idea to seek help from a counselor if you feel the need for more support than you're getting from family and friends.

- Some people find keeping a journal of thoughts, feelings, and dreams helpful in working through this disruptive time.

- Prepare yourself for changes in your life that may be frustrating, sad, or scary. As you heal, the changes may become exciting or fun. Allow yourself to feel good. Sometimes you may feel guilty about feeling good again. When this happens, you are truly recovering.[52]

These suggestions should not necessarily be given to patients as a list. The patient may be ready to hear them only at different points in his own process of recovery. Keep them in mind and be ready to share them appropriately.

Category Three: Mobilization of Resources. Mobilization of resources is an important component of caring for clients suffering a major loss. It includes using family, friends, relatives, church and civic organizations, other health care professionals, and appropriate community resources. Planning for and use of additional resources must be an integral part of total care to provide the client and family ongoing support once the crisis is past. Very often, the only time a client receives help is during this initial trauma, when he simply cannot function alone. As we have seen in the discussion of mourning stages, once a person has recovered from this early period of shock, the true healing process begins. Significant and ongoing physical and emotional support is critical in the client's making an adaptive response.

Mrs. J., a 63-year-old, insulin-dependent diabetic was sent home from the hospital after a below-the-knee amputation of her left leg. She was to be fitted for an artificial limb two months after surgery, but never kept her appointment. Six months later she presented through the emergency room with multiple skin ulcerations of her right lower leg. She was brought in by a neighbor who said he found her hopping around the ground of her apartment. Her physical exam revealed a thin, poorly kept, woman who was unable to follow the physician's questioning. Mrs. J. was readmitted to the hospital for stabilization, and it was subsequently discovered that her son, who was her only relative, had died in a car accident three months earlier. Mrs. J. had no support system.

In this case, many preventive measures should have been instituted prior to Mrs. J.'s discharge following surgery. Referring her to a visiting nurse association or the public health nurse in her area could have prevented the problems that followed. Most communities have some sort of "meals-on-wheels" program and public nursing service facilities for elderly, homebound people. A little educational planning along with referral to the appropriate agency can make all the difference in assuring clients some continuity of care and prevention of further disability.

Evaluation

The ultimate evaluation of the impact of nursing care given to clients suffering from a major loss is that the client moves through the process of mourning. Although the general symptomatology relative to grief and mourning have been documented in the literature, it is impossible to generalize any specific time frame in which all people suffering all types of loss will adapt. The broad range of influencing factors that contribute to anyone's private experience with grief and mourning make specificity impossible.

However, in order to evaluate a client's progress, we must have some criteria by which to measure the reaction. The estimate of six months to one year following a sudden, major loss has been postulated[53] as a time frame in which an otherwise healthy person is well on the way toward integration of the loss. It must be emphasized that this estimate requires great flexibility relative to the individual, the type of loss, the perception of loss in relation to the client's specific life situation, and any concurrent physical or psychological illness. If, after that time, any symptoms previously described under maladaptive grief response are exhibited along with or in addition to signs of depression or extreme anxiety, professional psychiatric help is warranted.

Some general criteria to evaluate movement through grief and mourning from the onset related to a major loss are:

- Grief symptomatology—i.e., extreme sadness, depression, anxiety—in which the client is in a crisis state. This should be close to the time the loss occurred.

- Requests for help from family, friends, health professionals. Most people will ask someone for help.

- As time progresses following the loss, the client should be returning to his more normal pattern of living. Most people can verbalize that they feel less pain.

- There are definite periods of regression when the client feels awful again, but these are usually brief and happen less frequently with the passing of time.

- Establishment of new patterns of social interaction is a crucial signal that the client is adapting to the loss.

Evaluation of a person moving toward adaptation of a loss is critical throughout the entire recovery period. By continual evaluation and reassessment, we can anticipate and prevent problems from occurring and better deal with maladaptive behaviors as they do occur.

SUMMARY

The concept of loss has been presented in a broad context, affecting clients at all points along the lifespan. A sound knowledge base related to the concept and its manifestations in the people we care for will help us to assess, plan, intervene, and evaluate our nursing care.

Methods of coping with a loss involve the acute grief state and the process of mourning. This process is divided into three overlapping stages: shock and disbelief, developing awareness, and restitution and recovery. The many factors that influence the type and severity of a particular grief reaction were delineated and are important in helping us to maintain a flexible approach. The nursing process framework was used to outline the basic approaches to nursing intervention with clients suffering a major loss. The three categories of nursing interventions are physical and psychological support, education and guidance, and mobilization of patient resources.

Coping with loss has become so much a part of our existence that, as health care professionals, we must be aware of the many types of loss that our clients face. The relationship between loss as a stressor and resulting physical illness is a critical area to pursue, both in clinical practice and in the promotion of research. Through these efforts we may be able to make the grief experience easier to bear and can maintain and enhance a high level of wellness in the populations we serve.

STUDY QUESTIONS

1. Identify at least three types of loss an 18-year-old boy might experience following amputation of his lower leg due to a bone cancer.

2. Name two major losses that occur dur-

ing the life experience of a 45-year-old woman.

3. What is meant by an "uncomplicated" grief reaction?

4. Denial is used throughout the entire process of mourning. In which stage is it most common?

5. Describe a "grief pang."

6. Acceptance of the altered state and relinquishing the lost object is the goal of which stage of the mourning process?

7. How do age and developmental level affect the type and severity of the grief reaction?

8. What is probably the most significant influencing factor that affects the severity of the grief reaction?

9. Describe the three categories of interventions used with patients suffering from a loss.

10. Identify five behaviors that are indicative of a maladaptive grief reaction.

REFERENCES

1. Baccalaureate Curriculum Committee, Catholic University of America. "Adaptation as a Model for Nursing Curriculum and Practice," Unpublished, Catholic University of America, Washington, D.C., 1978, p. 16.
2. M. Colgrove, H. Bloomfield, and P. McWilliams. **How to Survive the Loss of a Love,** (New York: Bantam Books, 1976), p. 16.
3. G. L. Engle, "Is Grief a Disease?" **Psychosomatic Medicine, 23,** (1961), p.18–22.
4. **Ibid.,** p.18.
5. E. Lindeman, "Symptomatology and Management of Acute Grief," **American Journal of Psychiatry, 101,** (1944), p.141–148.
6. **Ibid.,** p.141.
7. V. Volkan, "Re-grief Therapy," in Schoenburg, Carr, et al (eds), **Bereavement: Its Psychosocial Aspects,** 1975.
8. Colgrove, et al, Loss of Love, p.16.
9. S. Freud, "Mourning and Melancholia" in W. Gaylin (ed), **The Meaning of Despair,** (New York: Science House, 1968).
10. Lindeman. "Symptomatology," p.147.
11. Eagle, "Is Grief a Disease," p.18–22.
12. Elizabeth Kubler-Ross, **On Death and Dying,** (New York: MacMillan Publishing Co., Inc., 1969).
13. Lindeman "Symptomatology," p.147–148.
14. **Ibid.,** p.148.
15. Eagle, "Grief," p.18–22.
16. Volkan, "Regrief."
17. Lindeman "Symptomatology," p. 147–148.
18. J. M. Schnieder, "Clinically Significant Differences Between Grief, Pathologic Grief, and Depression," **Patient Counseling and Death Education, 2,** 161–166.
19. Collin M. Parkes, **Bereavement: Studies of Grief in Adult Life,** (New York: International Universities Press, Inc.), 1972.
20. **Ibid.** Chapter 4.
21. Lindeman, "Symptomatology," p.42.
22. Parkes, **Bereavement.**
23. Lindeman, "Symptomatology," 147–8.
24. Schneider, "Significant Differences," 161–166.
25. Kubler-Ross, **Death and Dying,** p.39.
26. David K. Switzer, **The Dynamics of Grief,** (New York: Abington Press, 1970) p.105.
27. Parkes, **Bereavement.**
28. Schneider, "Significant Differences," p.166.
29. Lindeman, "Symptomatology," p.148.
30. Colgrove, **Loss of a Love,** p.16.
31. Baccalaureate Curriculum Committee, "Adaptation" pp.16–17.
32. **Ibid.,** p.16.
33. **Ibid.,** p.16.
34. Perihan A. Rosenthal, "Short-term Family Therapy and Pathological Grief Resolution with Children and Adolescents," **Family Process, 19** (1980), 151–159.
35. Robert Kastenbaum, "The Child's Understanding of Death: How Does it Develop? in E. A. Crolhonan (ed), **Explaining Death to**

Children. (New York: Springer Publishing Co., 1967), p.89–108.

36. **Ibid.,** p.101.
37. Maria Nagy, "The Child's View of Death," **Journal of Genetics and Psychology, 73** (1948) p.3–27.
38. Kastenbaum. "Child's Understanding of Death," p.103.
39. Sharon Roberts, **Behavioral Concepts and Nursing Throughout,** the Life Span, (Englewood Cliffs, N.J.: Prentice-Hall, Inc., 1978), p.145–171.
40. Kastenbaum. "Child's Understanding of Death," p.105–106.
41. Kuhler-Ross. **Death and Dying.**
42. Lindeman, "Symptomatology," p.145.
43. R. Rabe, "Social Stress and Illness Onset," **Journal of Psychomatic Research,** 8, (1964) 35–43.
44. Hans Selye. The Stress of Life, (New York: McGraw-Hill Co., 1956).
45. **Ibid.,** p.144–46.
46. Volkan. "Regrief."
47. Parkes, **Bereavement.**
48. Schneider, "Significant Differences," 161–166.
49. Lynette Long and Sr. Penny Prophit, **Understanding/Responding: A Communication Manual for Nurses,** (Monterey, California: Wadsworth Health Sciences Division, 1981), p.19.
50. Schneider, "Significant Differences," p.162.
51. Maurice J. Barry, "The Prolonged Grief Reaction," **Mayo Clinic Proceedings, 48,** (1973), 329–335.
52. Colgrove, et al. **Loss of a Love.**
53. Schneider, "Significant Differences."

ANNOTATED BIBLIOGRAPHY

Colgrove M, Bloomfield HH, McWilliams P: **How to Survive the Loss of A Love.** New York, Bantam Books, 1976. This superb book offers ways of dealing with loss.

Engel GL: **Grief and Grieving.** Am J Nurs 64:9:93–96; September 1964. This classic article discusses the adaptive grief process and suggests ways to help individuals suffering loss.

Grollman EA (ed): **Concerning Death: A Practical Guide for the Living.** Boston, Beacon Press, 1974. This book presents a collection of classic articles relating to grief and death and dying.

Jackson PL: **Chronic Grief.** Am J Nurs 74:7:1288–1291; July 1974. This article discusses the concept of death through use of a care plan.

Johnson-Soderberg S: **Grief Themes.** Adv Nurs Sci 3:15–26; July 1981. This article uses examples from literature to provide examples of the grieving process.

Kubler-Ross E: **On Death and Dying.** New York, MacMillan Publishing Co. Inc., 1969. This excellent classic book identifies and describes the five stages of dying and gives many examples.

Kubler-Ross E: **Death: The Final Stage of Growth.** Englewood Cliffs, Prentice-Hall, Inc., 1975. This book is a collection of articles about death and dying.

Lindeman E: **Symptomatology and Management of Acute Grief.** Am J Psychiatry 101:141–148; September 1944. This classic article discusses grief and the grieving process.

Mandel HR: **Nurses' Feelings About Working With the Dying.** Am J Nurs 81:6:1194–1197; June 1981. This article discusses the psychological impact of working with the terminally ill.

Miles HS, Hays DR: **Widowhood.** Am J Nurs 74:2:280–282; February 1974. This article describes the formation of a support group for widows.

23

Crisis, Crisis Intervention, and
Suicide as a Response to Crisis

Linda Manglass Shapiro

CHAPTER OUTLINE

OBJECTIVES

At the completion of this chapter, the reader will be able to:

- Define crisis
- Discuss theoretical development of crisis and crisis intervention
- Identify elements of a crisis
- Differentiate between maturational and situational crisis
- Identify factors that indicate crisis
- Use a crisis intervention model in providing nursing care for clients experiencing a crisis state
- Identify suicidal behaviors as a maladaptive response to crisis
- Recognize prodromal clues to suicide
- Assess client lethality when presented with suicidal behavior
- Describe steps taken when intervening with suicidal clients
- Predict behaviors in family members and significant others following a suicide attempt
- Describe resources available on a primary, secondary, and tertiary level for the client in crisis

GLOSSARY

Adventitious crisis—accidental, uncommon, and unexpected crisis that results in multiple losses and environmental changes.

Anticipatory guidance—a process that aims to help persons cope with a crisis by discussing the details of the impending difficulty and intervening before the event occurs.

Anxiety—a diffuse apprehension that is vague in nature and is associated with feelings of uncertainty and helplessness; an emotion without a specific object, subjectively experienced by the individual and communicated interpersonally. Anxiety occurs as a result of threat to a person's being, self-esteem, or identity.

Crisis—a situation in which customary problem solving methods are no longer adequate; a state of psychological disequilibrium. A crisis may be a turning point in a person's life.

Crisis intervention—an intervention process aimed at reestablishing the individual's functioning to a level equal to or better than the precrisis level.

Developmental crisis—a crisis that occurs in response to stresses common to all people in particular phases of human development and transition.

Grieving—a process of separating from a highly valued person, place, object, or ideal.

Lethality assessment—an estimation of the probability that a person experiencing suicidal impulses actually will succeed in an attempt based on the method described, the specificity of the plan, and the availability of means.

Primary prevention—biological, social, or psychological intervention that promotes emotional well-being or reduces the incidence and prevalence of mental illness in a community by altering the causes before they have an opportunity to do harm.

Situational crisis—a crisis that occurs when a person is confronted with a stressful event of unusual or extreme intensity or duration and habitual methods of coping are no longer effective.

Survivors of suicide—individuals, usually family or close friends, who are at risk following the death by suicide of someone close.

Tertiary prevention—the elimination or reduction of residual disability following illness.

INTRODUCTION AND DEFINITION

Individuals vary in their ability to adapt adequately to anticipated and unanticipated events in their lives. Most of the time, people live in some degree of balance or homeostasis. Individuals usually are able to cope with the everyday stressful events that occur and maintain an adaptive balanced state. Sometimes, however, there is an imbalance between the problem facing an individual and his perception of it and the repertoire of adaptive behaviors available to him. In such situations a crisis may be precipitated.

A crisis is defined by Gerald Caplan as "a psychological disequilibrium in a person who confronts a hazardous circumstance that for him constitutes an important problem which he can, for the time being, neither escape nor solve with his usual problem solving resources."[1] A crisis occurs "when a person faces an obstacle to important life goals that is, for a time, insurmountable through utilization of customary methods of problem sovling. A period of disorganization ensues, a period of upset during which many abortive attempts at solution are made."[2] A person in crisis is at a turning point. His usual methods of coping are not available or are not working for him. He experiences helplessness and increased anxiety. In the search for a solution, which is considered to be time limited to four to six weeks, and relief, the individual may move toward healthy adaptation or increasingly maladaptive behavior.

Crisis intervention is a direct, goal oriented approach to help the individual resolve the crisis as quickly as possible and return to a level of functioning at least as functional as prior to the crisis.

THEORETICAL DEVELOPMENT

The study of crisis, crisis theory, and the crisis intervention approach to the treatment of emotional disturbances is relatively new when compared to psychoanalysis, psychotherapy, and other traditional approaches of providing care.

The theory of crisis intervention rests heavily on the early formulations of Erich Lindemann[3] and the subsequent works of Gerald Caplan.[4] In 1944, Erich Lindemann studied 101 individuals in crisis. These were survivors and the families of those

killed in the Coconut Grove nightclub fire in Boston. Hundreds of people lost their lives in this fire, and Lindemann's observations of and work with survivors and families provided the basis for crisis intervention theory and practice. Lindemann believed that the concept of intervention during bereavcment could be applied to intervention during other kinds of crisis situations.

Also of significance in the development of the crisis approach was the report of the Joint Commission on Mental Illness and Health published in 1961.[5] A result of this publication, which was based on massive analysis of the nation's mental health services and resources, was the Community Mental Health Centers Act of 1963. Between 1963 and 1972, the population of state institutions across the nation declined by almost half. Local community mental health centers were to be created to meet the mental health needs of communities. This act was supposed to create several thousand such centers. In fact, fewer than 500 were formed by 1973. Thus, a direct, brief, cost-effective treatment approach based on the concepts and principles of crisis intervention began to be used in an effort to meet the demands of this increased population in need of mental health services.

Gerald Caplan's preventive approach to psychiatry was instrumental in the articulation of key definitions, terms, and concepts of crisis intervention. According to Caplan, a crisis is composed of the following characteristics:

- It is a threat or danger to life goals.
- It creates mounting tension or anxiety and the effects of fear, guilt, or shame are felt subjectively.
- It evokes or awakens unresolved problems from the past.
- It is a turning point in which the person may achieve emotional growth or

become further disorganized.[6]

A crisis does not occur automatically as a result of a particular set of circumstances, nor does it develop quickly. There are identifiable phases of development that lead to an active state of crisis. Caplan describes four phases in the development of extreme anxiety and, finally, crisis. Recognition of these phases can help prevent a full-blown crisis.

Phase I—The individual is faced with a crisis provoking situation. He tries coping with the anxiety and tension by using behaviors that have worked for him successfully in the past.

Phase II—The crisis provoking situation continues to cause anxiety and tension as usual coping mechanisms and problem solving techniques fail. The person feels increasingly upset and perplexed. At this state, since there is greater stress, the possibility of a crisis state occurring increases, but is still not inevitable, depending on what happens next.

Phase III—Emergency problem solving mechanisms are brought into play; the individual searches for assistance and calls on all reserves of strength. As a result, the problem may be solved and equilibrium restored.

Phase IV—If the problem is not solved, an active crisis state will result. A person in crisis feels helpless and does not know where to turn or what to do. Internal strength and social supports are unavailable or lacking. He experiences unbearable anxiety and tension.[7]

Howard Parad and Harvey Resnik identify a crisis sequence that involves three time periods—pre-crisis, crisis and post-crisis. An individual in pre-crisis functions in his usual manner to ensure the achievement of needs. The person in crisis experiences a period of disorganization and disequilibrium. Attempts are made to reduce the discomfort and anxiety experienced.

The resolution of the crisis or post crisis period can result in either an increase or decrease in the person's level of functioning or a return to a pre-crisis level of functioning.[8] The three periods of crisis sequence are pictured in Figure 23-1.

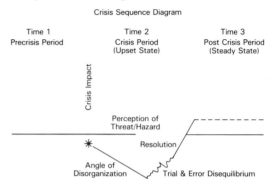

Crisis Sequence Diagram

| Time 1 | Time 2 | Time 3 |
| Precrisis Period | Crisis Period (Upset State) | Post Crisis Period (Steady State) |

*The asterisk indicates the onset of crisis.

Figure 23-1.   Crisis Sequence Diagram.

Source: Parad, H. and Resnick, H., "A Crisis Intervention Framework" in *Emergency Psychiatric Care*, eds. H. Resnick and H. Ruben (Bowie, MD: Charles Press, Pub., Inc., 1975) p. 4.

Obviously a person cannot stay in crisis indefinitely. The feelings experienced are far too uncomfortable and distressing. It is generally accepted that there is a limitation to the amount of time an individual can remain in a crisis state. The emotional discomfort stemming from the extreme anxiety moves the person to reduce the anxiety to a more manageable level as quickly as possible. Experience with persons in crisis has led to the observation that the acute emotional upset lasts from a few days to a few weeks.[9] Several outcomes, as described by Lee Ann Hoff, are possible for the individual experiencing a crisis state.

● The person can return to his pre-crisis state. This happens as a result of effective problem solving, made possible by one's internal strength and supports.

● The person may not only return to the pre-crisis state, but can grow from the crisis experience through discovery or new resources and ways of solving problems.

- The person reduces intolerable tension by lapsing into maladaptive patterns of behavior. For example, the individual may become very withdrawn, suspicious, or depressed. Others in crises may reduce their tension, at least temporarily, by excessive drinking or other drug abuse, or by impulsive, disruptive behavior. Still others resort to more extreme measures by engaging in suicidal or homicidal behaviors.[10]

TYPES OF CRISES

In an attempt to differentiate types of crises, two broad categories are considered. Developmental crisis, also referred to as maturational or internal crisis, is one, and situational or external crisis is the other.

Developmental Crisis

Maturational crises are expected life events that occur in most individuals' lifespans. They have been described as normal processes of growth and development. As an individual grows and develops, he constantly is faced with new situations, challenges, and influences to which he must adapt biologically, psychologically, and socially. Potential crisis areas occur during these periods of change and stress.

Eric Erikson's psychosocial maturational tasks provide a theoretical framework for the understanding of maturational crisis (see Figure 23-2) and developmental task achievement.[11] Others, such as Piaget's development of intellectual abilities; H.S. Sullivan's stages of personality development, and Maslow's basic human needs theory, also provide frameworks for assessing maturational growth and task achievement.

Facing the challenges of developmental task achievement can be and, in fact is, usually somewhat stressful and anxiety provoking. Coping behaviors that until now have been adequate and appropriate are no longer effective. Adjusting to previously unexperienced biological changes in adolescence or old age, for example, may precipitate concern over body image and physical functioning. Adjusting to new societal expectations regarding role changes—from single to married, childless to parent—requires energy, understanding, and nurturance from others.

With adequate support, individuals usually are able to successfully meet the tasks required in the normal process of growth and development. It is in this sense that maturational crises are considered normal. Because maturational crises are expected, there is opportunity to prepare for them. No amount of preparation can eliminate the crisis, but preparation can increase control over the event, thus reducing the amount and severity of disequilibrium experienced. This kind of preparatory education is an important aspect of crisis intervention.

Situational Crisis

Situational crises occur when a specific external event upsets an individual's psychological equilibrium. Some situational crises may stem from anticipated life events, such as beginning school, changing schools, success or failure in school. Family-related events may be the addition of a family member through birth or adoption, separation, divorce, remarriage, or a change in the family's financial status. Examples of anticipated events related to self are outstanding personal achievement, beginning to date, the breakup of a relationship, an unwanted pregnancy, physical deformity, or involvement with drugs or alcohol.

Unanticipated life events (sometimes referred to as adventitious crises) are distinguished from anticipated life events by the variable of prediction. Caplan defines unanticipated life events or situational crises as chance events that are viewed by the person as unpredictable.[12] It is often a traumatic event that is beyond one's control. Some common situational crises are loss of a loved one through death or divorce, loss of financial security, imprisonment, rape, assault, hospitalization, and natural disasters. The occurrence of one of these events does not automatically mean that a crisis will occur. As is true of developmental crisis, much depends on the individual's personal and social resources. Another factor influencing whether a crisis results is the person's stage of development. An individual confronting a major developmental task is already vulnerable. It is more likely that the added stress of a traumatic event will precipitate a crisis.

Developmental Stage	Area of Resolution	Basic Attitudes and Behaviors
Infancy (0–18 mos.)	Trust versus mistrust	Developing a sense of trust in oneself and others; hopefulness
		Withdrawal from others
Early Childhood (18 mos.–3 years)	Autonomy versus shame and doubt	Ability to express oneself and cooperate with others; self-control without loss of self-esteem
		Defiance; compulsive self-restraint or compliance
Late Childhood (3–5 years)	Initiative versus guilt	Purposeful behavior with a sense of reality; beginning ability to evaluate one's own behavior
		Self-denial and self-destruction
School Age (6–12 years)	Industry versus inferiority	Believing in one's abilities and competencies; perseverance
		Self-doubt and a feeling that one can never do well at things; withdrawal from school and peers
Adolescence (12–20 years)	Identity versus role diffusion	A clear sense of self; plans to actualize one's abilities
		Confusion and indecisiveness about oneself; a crisis of identity; may lead to antisocial behavior
Young Adulthood (18–25 years)	Intimacy versus isolation	Capacity for reciprocal love relationship; commitment to work and relationships
		Impersonal relationships; prejudices
Adulthood	Generativity versus stagnation	Capacity to care for others; creativity and productivity
		Impoverishment of self; self-indulgence
Old Age (65 years–death)	Integrity versus despair	Acceptance of one's life as worthy and unique
		Sense of loss; contempt for others

Figure 23-2   Erikson's Eight Stages of Man

PREDICTING CRISIS

Herbert Schulberg identified a number of factors helpful in predicting the probability of a crisis occurring. According to him, several factors should be considered in assessing which persons are crisis prone and at risk:

- The probability that a disturbing and hazardous event will occur. For example, death of a close family member is highly probable, whereas natural disasters are very improbable.
- The probability that an individual will be exposed to the event. For example, every adolescent faces the challenge of adult responsibilities, whereas only some face the crisis of an unwanted pregnancy.
- The vulnerability of the individual to the event. The mature adult, for example, can more easily adapt to the stress of moving than a child in his first years of school.[13]

In looking at the probability of any one individual experiencing a crisis, one needs to consider the degree of stress stemming from a hazardous event, the risk of being exposed to the event, and the person's vulnerability or ability to adapt to stress.

IDENTIFYING INDIVIDUALS IN CRISIS

Nurses, by virtue of where they work, and as health care providers, are often in positions of meeting individuals experiencing crises. Hospitalization has the potential to provoke crisis because of the many changes with which the individual is confronted. It is always an anxiety provoking and stressful experience. The reason for the hospitalization itself has crisis potential—loss of physiological integrity, loss of independence, or a change in role and functioning, as examples.

Individuals experiencing maturational crisis can be identified in settings such as maternal-child health, pediatrics, young adults, and gerontology. It is in these age groups where individuals make transitions in life style behaviors. Nurses in emergency units frequently see people experiencing unanticipated events, such as disasters, suicide attempts, unexpected life threatening accidents, and illnesses.

Nurses who work in the community are in a position to recognize maturational and situational crises occurring in the home—the child who refuses to go to school, the parents of a new baby, the family that has experienced a recent death.

The ability to accurately assess and intervene with individuals' crises is a learned skill, and it is invaluable for nurses in almost every health care setting. Nurses in positions of assessing and providing care to clients experiencing crisis can use the crisis intervention model, which is a problem solving approach, and closely follows the steps in the nursing process.

THE NURSING PROCESS

The crisis approach to problem solving, articulated by Morley, Messick, and Aguilera, involves an assessment of the individual and his problem, planning of therapeutic intervention and resolution of the crisis, and anticipatory planning.[14] This model is pictured in the paradigm depicted in Figure 23-3 and in Figures 23-4 and 23-5.

Assessment

Assessment begins before or upon initial contact with the person. It is often possible to anticipate that an individual is experiencing crisis behaviors by being familiar with events surrounding his contact with the health care system. For instance, an emergency unit receives a call from the

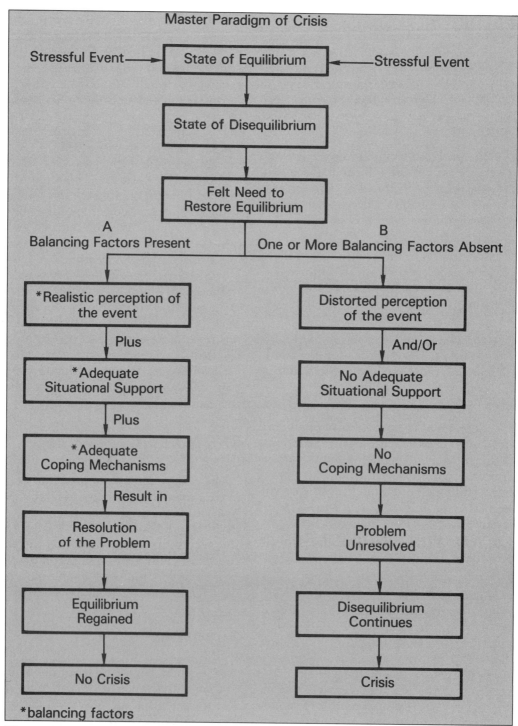

Figure 23-3.   Master Paradigm

Source: Donna Aguilera & Janice Messick, **Crisis Intervention** 4th ed. (St. Louis: The C.V. Mosby Co., 1982)

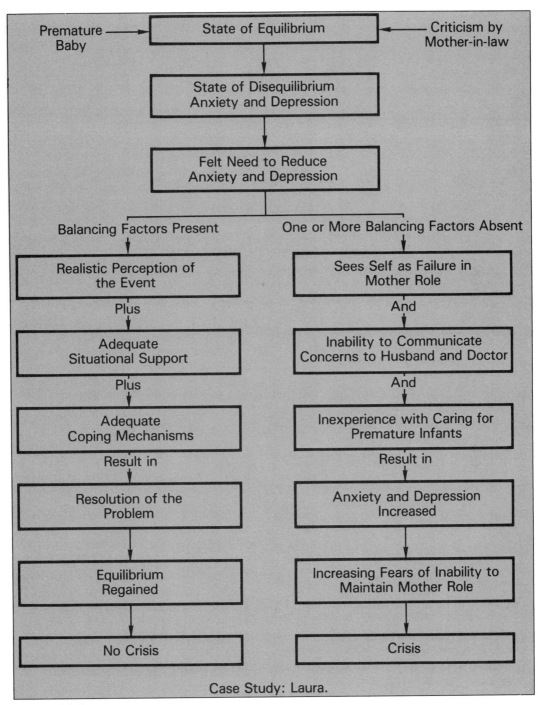

Figure 23-4.

Source: Donna Aguilera & Janice Messick, **Crisis Intervention** 4th ed. (St. Louis: The C.V. Mosby Co., 1982)

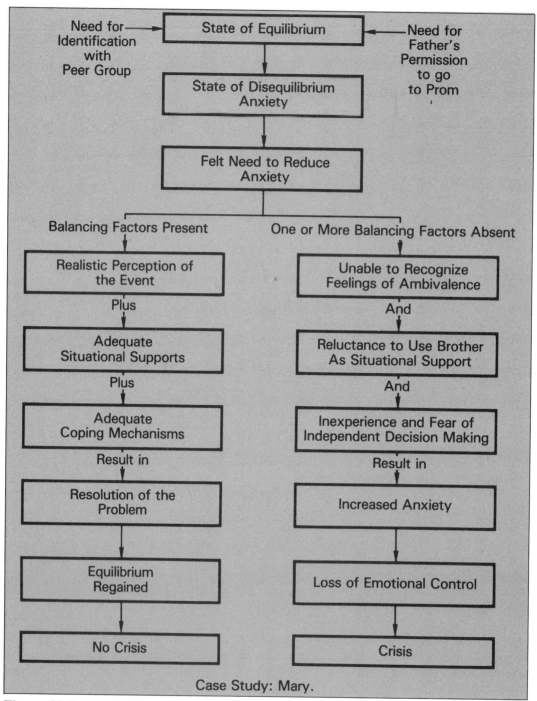

Figure 23-5.

Source: Donna Aguilera & Janice Messick, **Crisis Intervention** 4th ed. (St. Louis: The C.V. Mosby Co., 1982)

highway patrol that persons will soon be arriving who have been in a serious accident. Family or friends accompanying these persons may also be in need of crisis intervention. The news of serious illness, injury, or death always brings with it the possibility of difficulties in adaptation. A phone call to the community health nurse may reveal a distraught mother of a new infant who is having problems with breastfeeding. An adolescent confides to his nurse practitioner that he is failing in school and can't seem to make any friends. These are all situations nurses face that call for careful assessment and intervention.

Basic to carrying out the steps in the nursing process is establishing an alliance with the individual. This is facilitated by conveying to the client that you want to help him. It is useful to remember that the goal of crisis intervention is to reestablish psychological equilibrium as quickly as possible. The first step in crisis assessment is to identify events that led to the person's distress. A workable differentiation has been made, by Naomi Golan, between the hazardous event and the precipitating factor, both important concepts in crisis intervention.[15]

The **hazardous event** is the initial shock or internal rise in tension that sets in order a series of reactions leading to the crisis. The hazardous event may be anticipated or unanticipated, and may be related to maturational or situational events. In order to determine the hazardous event, the question, "What happened?" should be asked. The process of talking about the event and recalling time sequences, circumstances surrounding it, and others involved is often helpful for the individual. The opportunity to put the events in order and make some sense out of what is often chaos has a calming effect and gives the person a sense of control. Simple, direct questions and clarifying comments are useful in assisting the individual.

The **precipitating event** is the "straw that broke the camel's back." It is usually the focal point that prompted the person to seek help at that particular time. It is not always clear to the person what the precipitating event is, and the question, "What happened today that made you seek help?" is often a useful one. In crisis, the precipitating event usually has occurred within 10 to 14 days before the individual seeks help. In many situations where nurses are involved, the situation is one that just occurred at that very moment. In attempting to identify the precipitating event, look for themes of loss. Often a recent loss (i.e., threat of a boyfriend breaking off a relationship) will precipitate or reawaken feelings of another loss (death of mother a few months earlier).

It is imperative, in the assessment process, to determine the individual's perception of the event. How does the individual (or family) view the event? What significance does it have for him? What is the impact of the event on the rest of his life and his future? How this event fits into the client's view of his world may be very different from how the same event would fit into the nurse's world. Nurses will not be able to intervene in a manner that is useful or helpful to the client unless they are able to establish meaningful communication with their clients. It is necessary to develop an awareness and understanding of what needs (particularly developmental needs) are important in the client's life and how these needs and values influence his perception of the event and his response to it.

A thorough assessment of the client in the crisis also includes identifying other **balancing factors** that influence an individual's response to the crisis provoking event. Identification of these balancing factors also aids the nurse in planning intervention strategies.

Aguilera and Messick state that between the perceived effects of a stressful situation and the resolution of the crisis are three recognized balancing factors that may determine the state of equilibrium. Stress or weakness in any one of these areas can be directly related to the onset of crisis or its resolution. These are:

- perception of the event
- available situational supports
- coping mechanisms.[16]

By assessing these stimuli, the nurse identifies areas in which to intervene.

Perception of the Event. In addition to the individual's perception, it is necessary to determine whether the individual views the event realistically or in a distorted manner. If the event is perceived realistically, there will be recognition of the relationship between the event and the distressed feelings. In this case, intervention can be directed toward relief of anxiety and tension, and successful resolution will be more probable.

Available Situational Supports. Identification of situational supports is important in assessing the individual or family and planning for intervention. Who are the significant people in the person's life? Has he discussed the event with them? If not, why not? If so, how have they responded so far? Is there anyone with whom he feels safe and comfortable at this time? It is not unusual for individuals in crisis to be underutilizing the support systems they do have. This, in fact, may be a determining factor in whether an individual handles a situation adaptively or goes into crisis, and is valuable information for planning interventions.

Coping Mechanisms. The third set of balancing factors are related to coping mechanisms. What kinds of coping mechanisms does the individual usually use to handle stressful situations? How has he handled stressful situations in the past? Coping mechanisms are conscious and unconscious ways of relieving and dealing with anxiety and tension. An individual, because of the newness of the situation or the severity and shock of the event, may not be able to use those coping mechanisms that have worked for him in the past. Exploring with the client what has worked for him previously, how he can try using those behaviors again, or what other kinds of coping behaviors he could try (i.e., patients confined to bed in a hospital often are not able to use mechanisms that have worked for them in the past), is a nursing intervention strategy. (For more information on coping behaviors and intervention strategies see Chapter 21 on Anxiety.)

After the assessment has been made, nursing diagnoses can be formulated. Examples of nursing diagnoses that may arise in crisis situations include:

- Anxiety related to mothering role
- Potential crisis state related to lack of support systems
- Ineffective coping related to developmental crisis.

Planning

Throughout the process of assessment, plans should be formulated as to how to intervene with individuals experiencing a crisis state. It should be kept in mind that the goal of crisis intervention is the reestablishment of equilibrium and a return to the precrisis state. Plans should, therefore, be specific and time relevant. Examples of planning goals for an individual in crisis might be as follows:

- The client will experience a decrease in anxiety by the end of the interaction as evidenced by:
  —verbalization of an increase in comfort level and a decrease in restlessness
  —ability to state what he is going to do and with what kind of support, over the next 24 hours
- The client will identify one person who can be contacted as a support system.

Once the plan has been developed it should be written on the client's chart or kardex, and the implementation and evaluation phases of the nursing process can begin.

Implementation

Intervention in crisis actually begins with the establishment of an alliance with the client. Conveying a caring, concerned attitude is, in itself, helpful and reassuring. Providing an opportunity for the client to verbalize, clarify, and organize is useful in gaining a sense of control over the situation. General principles of crisis intervention include:

- Decrease the intensity of the crisis experience. This is accomplished primarily through anxiety reducing techniques (see Chapter 21 on Anxiety), reassurance, and support.

- Keep intervention brief and goal oriented. The goal is to reestablish equilibrium and return the client to at least a pre-crisis level of functioning as quickly as possible. This is not the time for in-depth intrapsychic exploration or resolution of chronic emotional problems. It is not unusual to have to differentiate the crisis the client is experiencing from other more chronic kinds of emotional difficulties the client brings up.

- Identify and use client strengths. How has the client been coping with the situation so far? He may, in fact, be dealing with the situation very well. The emotional pain and distress he is experiencing can easily get in the way of his recognizing that he is doing alright. Reassuring the client that the grieving process he is going through, although very painful, is in fact normal and necessary, is an invaluable tool in helping the client cope with the situation. Focusing on strengths helps raise self-esteem, making the person feel more confident and capable of coping.

    Another aspect of using strengths has to do with support systems. As soon as significant others can be brought in and those ties cemented, the nurse may assume a less active role and move out of the situation. Ways to achieve this may include calling a family member or friend to be with the client or making sure he can name someone to contact, and have him do so. Before you leave the crisis situation, you must replace yourself, depending upon the severity of the situation, with another person or with the availability of another person to help the client, should he need it.

- Environmental manipulation is an intervention aimed at altering the environment that is influencing the client in crisis. It usually involves changing the individual's personal or interpersonal situation, which in turn will decrease stress and provide support. For example, moving people into the home environment temporarily may provide support (as in the case of an individual alone during crisis), or moving some children out of the home to relieve the pressure on a mother may be appropriate.

Throughout the process of assessment and intervention, the nurse conveys an attitude of concern and caring. Crisis intervention requires that expertise, responsibility, and knowledge be communicated to the client. Specific communication skills necessary in working with a client in crisis include:

- Listening. Listen to find out what the crisis is and the meaning it has for that person. Putting your perception of the situation into words and summarizing for the client is a way of assuring you have an accurate understanding.

- Focusing. Keep the client focused on issues relating to the problem causing the disequilibrium.

- Questioning. Ask questions to clarify, to find out details, and to refocus.
- Observe and acknowledge feelings. This aids the individual in sorting out feelings, expressing them, and having them validated as normal and acceptable.
- Solve problems and explore alternatives. Discuss new ways to deal with the problem. Offer suggestions and provide opportunities to try new behaviors, if possible.

In many situations, the nurse's involvement with a client experiencing crisis may stop when the nurse assesses a client is in crisis and needs further help. In such situations, a referral made for the client is appropriate. Referrals for clients in crisis should be expeditious, with as much help from the nurse as is necessary to ensure follow through.

Evaluation

The evaluation phase of crisis intervention is fairly simple. The client should be experiencing a more tolerable level of anxiety as evidenced by his verbalizations of such and his ability to use effective coping mechanisms. There should be other people actively involved with him in offering support and problem solving. He should be functioning minimally at his pre-crisis level. Crisis have inherent growth producing potential. People who master crisis situations have the opportunity to develop a broader repetoire of coping skills that will help them deal more effectively with life situations in the future.

SUICIDE AS A RESPONSE TO CRISIS

There are instances when an individual responds to crisis by attempting to commit or committing suicide.

In an attempt to standardize terms and definitions, the Conference on Suicide Prevention, in the 1970s, agreed on the following definition and three broad categories of suicidal behaviors:

Completed suicide—includes all deaths in which a self-inflicted, willful and life threatening act has resulted in death.

Suicide attempt—includes situations in which an individual has performed a seemingly life threatening act or actual behavior with the intent of either giving the appearance of or actually jeopardizing his life, but which do not result in death.

Suicide ideas—includes behaviors that may be directly inferred or observed that are concerned with a move in the direction of a possible threat to a person's own life.[17]

Suicidal behavior is a form of self-destructive behavior. There are many other forms of self-destructive behaviors in which an individual may engage, particularly in times of crisis and as a response to stress. Self-destructive behavior includes any action by which a person damages or ends his life emotionally, socially, or physically. Examples of self-destructive behaviors range from smoking cigarettes to reckless driving, obesity, and suicidal acts. Individuals from any social or economic class, age group, location, religion, race, or sex may respond to crisis with suicidal or self-destructive behaviors.

Nurses, as health care providers, find themselves in situations where an individual is responding to crisis by engaging in suicidal thinking or behavior. A knowledge of facts about suicide, demographic characteristics of suicidal individuals, how to assess suicide lethality, and intervention approaches is, therefore, necessary.

There are numerous myths regarding suicide that influence how we think about and act with suicidal individuals. The following statements are examples of some of the myths about suicide. True or False?

1. __ An individual serious about kill-

ing himself leaves a note.
False. A note may or may not indicate seriousness of intent.[18]

2. __ At one time or another almost everyone contemplates suicide.
True. Suicide is common enough that everyone is familiar with it as a behavior and thinks about it at some point, although not necessarily with intent.

3. __ Only "crazy" people or those with weak moral characters attempt or commit suicide.
False. Suicide, as a response to crisis, is used by all kinds of people.

4. __ People who talk about suicide never do anything about it.
False. People who give verbal indications of suicidal feelings and intentions should *always* be taken seriously. Studies have shown that as many as 75 percent of persons who commit suicide have contacted their physicians for some reason within three to six months prior.[19]

5. __ Suicidal persons are fully intent on dying and nothing you can do or say will stop them.
False. Suicide is a behavior, and there is communication in any behavior. Persons who engage in suicidal behaviors are attempting to communicate their helplessness and despair. Suicidal people are ambivalent; they are struggling with a desire to live and a desire to die. As long as an individual has ambivalent feelings, it is possible to work with him in considering alternatives. Individuals who are no longer ambivalent seldom come into contact with others willing and able to offer help.

6. __ Asking a person if he is suicidal only puts ideas into his head.
False. Even if you have no indication that a person is considering suicide as an alternative to crisis, you should ask about it as part of your assessment. "Sometimes people under a lot of stress have thoughts of hurting themselves. Have you had any thoughts like that?" "Are you so upset you're thinking of killing yourself?" Comments made by individuals that should be explored include such statements as, "If it weren't for the children, I wouldn't be going through this," "Sometimes I wish I'd just fall asleep and never wake up," "I can't live with myself," or "There's nothing left for me now."

Behavioral clues that should be addressed are actions such as giving away possessions, taking out a life insurance policy, and a "tidying up" of one's personal affairs. Asking a person outright about how he is feeling, if he is experiencing any self-destructive thoughts, is appropriate and necessary. Having someone pick up the cues he is sending and provide an opportunity to talk about it can be helpful and reassuring.

Suicide has been recognized as a serious problem in the United States for many years. In 1962, a grant from the United States Public Health Service was awarded to the University of Southern California to open a suicide prevention center in Los Angeles. Much of what is known about suicide has been discovered through the research done at this center.

A major task in preventing suicide is accurate assessment of the seriousness of suicidal intentions. This assessment of **lethality** is the process of determining the likelihood of suicide for an individual. The nurse's first goal in working with an individual responding to crisis with suicidal thinking is to determine how likely the person is to engage in suicidal behavior in the immediate future, so that appropriate action can be taken. Lethality assessment techniques are based on knowledge obtained from the study of completed suicides. Research about suicide is a difficult area, and the knowledge available, although extremely useful, is by no means absolute.

THE NURSING PROCESS

Assessment

The following information is a compilation of the results of much research done in the area. Most notably, Edwin Schneidman, Robert Litman, and Norman Faberow[20] from the Suicide Prevention Center in Los Angeles, California, and also Beck, Resnick, and Lettieri,[21] and Linden and Breed.[22]

It is known that men commit suicide three times more frequently than women and are higher risks. This risk increases with age until age 85. The exception to this is among urban black males between the ages of 20 and 25. The suicide rate among this group is twice as high as for white males of the same age group. Women, however, attempt suicide three times more frequently than men.

Certain population groups are higher risks than others. The elderly (over age 65) constitute an estimated 25 percent of all suicides. Considering that the elderly only account for 10 percent of the total population, this is a disproportionate number. The elderly can kill themselves in ways not likely to be detected as suicide; e.g., neglecting to take life-sustaining medication, falls, or accidents. The crises of old age that lead to suicidal behavior in some elderly individuals have most to do with irreversible losses. The least likely to be able to deal successfully with these crises are white males, 70 to 74. Their suicide rate is three times higher than non-white males of this age and five times higher than women of the same age group.

Suicide is the third leading cause of death in the 15 to 19 age group, and the second leading cause of death among 19- to 24-year-olds. The crises of adolescence and young adulthood are among the most difficult.

For many years, experts questioned whether young children could really suffer emotional pain to the point of intentionally seeking relief through death. Recent research shows that they do. The data available has shown suicidal thinking most often associated with depression and related to the crises of loss (loss of parents), fear of loss, and abandonment. It is important to know that the wish to die for some children may be a misconception, since most children do not comprehend the finality of death before age eight.

Influencing Factors. Time is relevant to the onset of crisis. If there has been an acute onset in relation to a specific stress, that usually represents a higher, more immediate danger than would a condition of recurring crises with several prior events similar to the one being described.

A crisis that involves a loss is a very significant indicator for risk. This is particularly true among adolescents.

Contact with others is critical in crisis situations involving suicidal behavior. If a person has family, friends, job, therapist, the danger is reduced. Studies have shown that people are less likely to commit suicide while in contact with others. Suicide occurs less frequently among the married and people who have never been married. The risk is higher for divorced or widowed people who live isolated lives, either emotionally or physically.

The state of an individual's health is an indicator in predicting suicide. People who are physically ill, particularly those with recently diagnosed illnesses that affect self-image or lifestyle, are a high risk.

Alcohol and drug usage increase the risk of suicide. It is estimated that at least one in five suicides is alcohol related. Suicide among drug abusers is three times as high as for the rest of the population.

Personality structures and degree of emotional health are important influencing factors. An individual who is depressed or experiencing emotional problems such as psychosis (hearing voices telling him to kill himself), an alcoholic, or drug addict may be a high risk.

Probably the most significant factor in assessment of suicide lethality is the individual's plan. Suicide is rarely an impulsive act. Studies of complete suicides show deliberate planning. If it is determined through questioning that the person is not considering suicide as a response to crisis, or if he has thought of it but has no plan or intent, there is probably no need for further assessment in this area. If the person says he has a plan, you must find out what it is by asking, "What are you thinking of doing?"

The methods by which individuals choose to commit suicide fall into high-lethal and low-lethal categories. High-lethal methods include guns (a plan to shoot oneself in the heart or head is more lethal than planning to shoot oneself in the abdomen), jumping out of a window ("What floor do you live on?"), drowning (determine nearness to water), carbon monoxide poisoning, barbiturates, aspirin, or Tylenol® in high doses, or automobile accidents. Low-lethal methods include wrist cutting, house gas, nonprescription drugs, and tranquilizers.[23] The person's knowledge about the lethality of the chosen method is important. For instance, does he know how many pills it will take to kill him?

The availability of means or access to a lethal method may be the single most alarming criterion. Does the person have a gun; does he know how to use it? The more available the method, the higher the risk and the more lethal.

How specific are the plans? Has the person thought out how he is going to do it, where, and when? A plan that includes pre-cautions against discovery, for instance, is more lethal than one that takes no precautions.

Does the individual have a previous history of attempts? Has he ever acted on suicidal feelings? How? A move from a history of low-lethal to high-lethal indicates seriousness of intent.

The following case studies are examples of the significance of demographic factors, method, plan, assessing suicide potential, and intervening appropriately.

Carol (age 28) was brought to the emergency unit of the community hospital by her husband. When he had arrived home that evening at his usual time, he found Carol asleep and only partially responsive. There was a half-empty bottle of Valium® in the bathroom. After medical intervention, more information was obtained from Carol. It was learned that she had recently discovered that her husband was having an affair with another woman. She felt alone and helpless to deal with this. She was embarrassed to share with friends and has no family available to her. She said she does not want to die, but wanted to be able to talk with her husband about her despair and knew of no other way to communicate. She was responsive to an appointment made for the next day at the crisis service.

Carol is a low risk. She expected her husband home at the usual time. Timing made discovery likely. There was little planning involved, the intent being to bring about a change in her environment.

Warren (white, age 54) has recently been diagnosed as having metastatic cancer. His wife died six months ago, unexpectedly, and he had had a difficult time adjusting to that change. He has not been able to use support systems available to him because of his depression, and now the news of his illness is "the last straw." He lives alone, and called a crisis hotline because he is thinking of going to a cabin he owns and shooting himself. He has been drinking.

Warren is a moderate-high risk. He has

experienced a recent loss. He has a plan with available means. He is a high risk in terms of age, sex, race, and marital status. The influence of alcohol is involved.

Beck and associates developed a scale for assessing the seriousness of suicide intent.[24] This scale ranks various categories from zero to 20. Examples of some of the categories are shown on the continuum in Figure 23-6.

High Risk _____ *Low Risk*
gravely serious .... **extreme ambivalence**
Timing and Isolation
no one near or   someone nearby
expected .... **and in contact**
Precautions Against Discovery
extensive precautions .... **no precautions**
Acting to Gain Help
no attempt .... **attempt to get help**
Plans for Attempt
elaborate plans .... **no plans; impulsive**
Communication of Intent
note, letter, message .... **no note, no message**
Purpose of Intent
remove self from   bring about change
environment .... **in environment**

Figure 23-6. Circumstances Related to Suicide Attempt.

Before going on to the planning and implementation phases of the nursing process, nursing diagnoses should be formulated. Examples of nursing diagnoses for the two previous case examples might be as follows:

- Ineffective coping, with suicide attempt secondary to low self-esteem (Carol).
- Depression, with suicide attempt secondary to loss and alcohol abuse (Warren).

Planning

Once the assessment phase has been completed, a written care plan can be prepared and placed on the client's chart. In the case of suicide prevention, implementation may be going on during the plan formalization stage in order to prevent harm to the client.

Implementation

Intervening with clients who are thinking of suicide as a response to crisis situations requires knowledge of assessment techniques including demographic characteristics and use of lethality scales. It also requires that the intervenor has access to expert consultation.

As beginning practitioners of nursing, you should be able to accurately determine whether an individual is experiencing suicidal thoughts and assess the seriousness of intent and suicidal lethality. Unless you have an opportunity to become confident of your skills in this area through experience and supervision, these judgments should always be made in consultation with an experienced clinician. Occasionally, a situation may occur when it is necessary to intervene in some way even before consultation can be sought. Some general guidelines that are helpful in immediate intervention follow. All the techniques for intervention in crisis are applicable in intervening suicidal crisis.

An attitude of acceptance, hope, and encouragement may help offset the hopelessness and despair the person is experiencing. It is important to recognize that the hostility and anger that may be expressed are a reflection of the despair and have probably pushed everyone else away.

Involving others (other professionals, family members, friends, coworkers) in the identified client's crisis situation is imperative. Suicide is a solitary act and the more quickly others become involved, the faster the risk is decreased. In some situations, this may involve getting a friend or family member to remove the lethal weapon.

Encourage the person to avoid making such a final decision during this time of crisis. Maintain contact with the individual until a plan is worked out.

There may be occasions when a nurse must use **telephone intervention** with an individual who is expressing thoughts about suicide. Intervening when face to face contact is not possible is very difficult, since the benefits of nonverbal attending behaviors (See Chapter 11) are unavailable. Norman Faberow outlines a plan for telephone intervention that is a useful guide:

- Establish a rapport with the individual as quickly as possible. Maintain contact and obtain as much information as possible in a nonthreatening, accepting manner.

- Identify the central problem and maintain the focus on this concern.

- Evaluate the potential for action.

- Assess the individual's strengths and resources; an improvement of mood during the call, even the ability to listen to you and focus on the conversation.

- Formulate and initiate plans; call an ambulance, get him to go to an emergency unit or crisis center, arrange for an appointment the next day. Contact should be maintained until a plan is worked out and some change has occurred in his mood or tone.[25]

Survivors of Suicide

The survivors of a suicide—those left after someone commits suicide—are a crisis prone population. In addition to the usual feelings associated with loss, there is the tragic aspect of it, the anger at the individual that he is no longer a part of one's life, and the surviving person's guilt about the experience. The guilt is over not having been able to prevent it from happening or even seeing it before hand. Sometimes there is a sense of relief, especially if the individual had been having difficulties for a long time.

Some suicide prevention centers have established programs for survivors of suicide. One plan developed is termed **"postvention"** and occurs in three phases.

The first phase is **resuscitation.** This occurs within 24 hours of the suicide. Usually the survivors are in shock at this time and another follow-up visit is in order within three days. At this point, the intervenor can expect to deal with feelings of guilt and blame.

The second phase lasts two to three months and is **resynthesis.** Explaining grief reactions—Are the survivors grieving appropriately? How are they adjusting?—is the focus at this time.

The last phase is **renewal.** This is the period, from six months on, when the survivors will be forming new relationships and finding substitutes for the loss. This phase ends with the anniversary of the death. This can be a particularly vulnerable time for survivors, and a last contact should be made at this time.[26]

Crisis Prevention

Nurses are offered many opportunities to intervene with individuals facing crises or crisis provoking situations, including suicidal crises. The first step in helping individuals and their familes deal with such situations is through anticipatory guidance and education. This is an aspect of primary prevention. Primary prevention is designed to reduce the occurrence of mental disabilities in a community through education, consultation, and crisis intervention.[27] Examples of ways nurses can be involved in primary prevention are educative groups such as prenatal classes, parenting groups, groups formed to deal with major life events like adolescence and aging. Community health nurses and those in schools are in unique positions to engage in primary prevention. These types of situations afford nurses opportunities to recognize and intervene with individuals at risk.

Secondary prevention includes early recognition and detection with prompt, timely intervention, such as offering support and guidance to the newly bereaved spouse (the postvention approach previously described), or intervening with the patient who has recently been diagnosed with a life threatening illness. Emergency units, outpatient departments, and occupational health settings are just a few places where early recognition and intervention is appropriate and necessary to prevent the client from harm.

The tertiary level of prevention includes intervening to prevent any further maladaptation and helping the individual to achieve or regain his maximum level of adaptive functioning. This usually occurs in inpatient settings, but also occurs in the community and some outpatient settings.

Evaluation

Evaluation of suicide prevention is obvious, in that the client should demonstrate and verbalize a reduced desire to harm himself. Evaluation should be based on the goals and objectives delineated in the planning stage of the nursing process. If the client is meeting these, then the plan is working. If not, the client needs to be reassessed and the plan altered, implemented, and reevaluated in a cyclic process until positive outcomes of interventions can be measured.

SUMMARY

This chapter has discussed the development of crisis intervention historically and theoretically. Crisis as a concept, the elements of a crisis, and characteristics of individuals in crisis were presented to provide the basis for using the nursing process in assessing clients in crisis, planning and implementing nursing care for clients experiencing crisis, and criteria for evaluating the effectiveness of nursing strategies implemented.

As we have seen, crisis can be viewed as an opportunity for growth and the development of new, more effective problem solving skills, or may be a time when individuals resort to maladaptive, growth inhibiting behaviors.

STUDY QUESTIONS

1. Describe characteristics of a crisis state including feeling, state, and sequence of events.

2. How does crisis intervention differ from other intervention methods?

3. Under what circumstances and in what types of settings might a nurse see individuals or families in crisis and utilize a crisis intervention model?

4. Differentiate between maturational and situational crisis and give examples of each.

5. Describe factors necessary to adequately assess and plan in a crisis.

6. Discuss goals and intervention strategies in helping an individual in crisis.

7. State demographic characteristics useful in assessing suicide potential.

8. Discuss the concept of lethality.

9. Describe intervention strategies in helping the individual experiencing suicidal thoughts and feelings.

10. Discuss and give examples of primary, secondary, and tertiary prevention.

REFERENCES

1. Gerald Caplan, **An Approach to Community Mental Health.** (New York: Grune and Stratton, 1961).
2. Caplan, **Community Mental Health**
3. Erich Lindemann, "Symptomatology and Management of Acute Grief," **American Journal of Psychiatry,** 101, (September 1944), pp.101–148.
4. Gerald Caplan, **Principles of Preventive Psychiatry.** New York: Basic Books, 1964).
5. **Action for Mental Health, Report of the Joint Commission on Mental Health.** (New York: Basic Books, 1961).
6. Caplan, **Preventive Psychiatry.**
7. Ibid.
8. Howard Parad and Harvey Resnick, "A Crisis Intervention Framework" in **Emergency Psychiatric Care**, ed. Harvey Resnick and H.L. Ruben (Bowie, Maryland: Charles Press, 1975).
9. Lindemann, "Management of Acute Grief," pp.101–148.
10. Lee Ann Hoff, **People in Crisis: Understanding and Helping,** (Menlo Park, California: Addison Wesley Publishing Co., 1978), p.21.
11. Erik Erikson, **Childhood and Society,** 2nd ed. (New York: W.W. Norton and Co., Inc., 1963), pp.247–274.
12. Caplan, **Preventive Psychiatry.**
13. Herbert Schulberg and Alan Sheldon, "Probability of Crisis and Strategies for Preventive Intervention," **Archives of General Psychiatry,** 18, (May 1968), p.558.
14. Wilbur Morley, Janice Messick and Donna Aguilera, "Crisis, Paradigms of Intervention," **Journal of Psychiatric Nursing,** 5, (November–December 1967), pp.538–540.
15. Naomi Golan, "When is a Client in Crisis?" **Social Casework,** 50, (July 1969), pp.389–394.
16. Donna Aguilera and Janice Messick, **Crisis Intervention,** 2nd ed. (St. Louis, Missouri: The C.V. Mosby Co., 1974).
17. Committee Meeting on Nomenclature and Classification, Conference on Suicide Prevention in the Seventies, (Phoenix, Arizona: January 1970).
18. Robert Litman, Edwin Schneidman, Normal Faberow and Tabachnick, "Investigation of Equivocal Suicides," **Journal of the American Medical Association,** 184, (June 1963), pp.924–929.
19. Robert Litman, "Actively Suicidal Patients: Management in General Medical Practice," **California Medicine,** 104, (1966), pp.168–174.
20. Edwin Schneidman, Norman Faberow and Robert Litman, eds., **The Psychology of Suicide.** New York: Science House, 1970), pp.165–228, 259–292.
21. Aaron Beck, Harvey Resnick and Don Lettieri, eds., **The Prediction of Suicide.** (Bowie, Maryland: The Charles Press Publishing, Inc., 1974), pp.59–141.
22. Leonard Linden and Warren Breed, "The Demographic Epidemiology of Suicide," in **Suicidology: Contemporary Developments,** ed. Edwin Schneidman (New York: Grune and Stratton, Inc., 1976).
23. Hoff, **People in Crisis,** p.119.
24. Aaron Beck, Dean Schulyer and Ira Herman, "The Development of a Suicidal Intent Scale," in **The Prediction of Suicide,** pp.45–56.
25. Norman Faberow, Samuel Heilig and Robert Litman, "Evaluation and Management of Suicidal Persons," in **The Psychology of Suicide,** Chapter 16.
26. Harvey Resnick and Berkley Hawthorne, eds., **Suicide Prevention in the 70's.** (Washington, D.C.: U.S. Government Printing Office, Department of Health Education and Welfare, Publication No. (HSM) 72-9054, 1973).
27. Gerald Caplan and Henry Grunebaum, "Perspectives on Primary Prevention: A Review," **Archives of General Psychiatry,** 17, (1967), pp.331–346.

ANNOTATED BIBLIOGRAPHY

Chapman AH: **Harry Stack Sullivan: The**

Man and His Work. New York, G.P. Putman Sons, 1976. This is a readable work about the foremost developer of the interpersonal approach to psychiatry. It is intended to increase understanding of interpersonal relationships and their bearing on emotional health and social living.

Faberow N, Schneidman E (eds): **The Cry for Help.** New York, McGraw-Hill Book Co., 1961. Somewhat of a "classic" in the field of suicide, this work covers all aspects of suicide and is highly recommended reading.

Hall J, Weaver B (eds): **Nursing of Families in Crisis.** Philadelphia, J.B. Lippincott Co., 1974. A valuable resource for nurses covering many different types of family related crises.

Maslow A: **Toward a Psychology of Being.** Princeton, D. Van Nostrand Co., 1962. This psychologist presents a theory of human functioning based on needs. It is an easily used theoretical framework and is highly applicable to nursing.

Piaget J: **The Origins of Intelligence in Children.** New York, International Universities Press, 1952. Piaget developed a theory of cognitive development in children that has become classic. The book defines developmental stages as defined by Piaget.

Russianoff P (ed): **Women in Crisis.** New York, Human Sciences Press, 1981. Addresses aspects of and issues relevant to women in crisis, including intervention problems and approaches.

Soreff SM: **Management of the Psychiatric Emergency.** New York, John Wiley and Sons, Inc., 1981. This book presents different psychiatric emergencies and how to deal with them. It is addressed to those who work in emergency departments, but is useful for others.

Section 4

Social Systems, the Environment, and Nursing

In nursing, family and community concepts have traditionally been viewed apart from concepts related to the individual in the acute care setting. Likewise, the importance of understanding global environmental issues and group dynamics has often been directed toward specialty areas such as community and psychiatric nursing. Clearly these concepts are unique and expand beyond the scope of the individual. Equally clear is the fact that the health status of the individual, whether on the illness or wellness end of the continuum, is profoundly affected by family and community relationships, and their importance cannot be minimized in the delivery of quality nursing and health care in any setting.

This section provides an awareness of how group and family concepts and community and environmental issues can be used in the nursing process. Community concepts are presented both generally and in the context of community health nursing, giving the reader an understanding of community roles and responsibilities as well as broadly applicable concepts. The family chapter presents selected historical aspects of the American family as well as therapeutic concepts and techniques that provide a base from which to understand and work with present day families. Environmental issues such as air pollution and the control of toxic substances are presented in the context of significance to health and disease prevention. Factors of environmental control and safety within the hospital are explored.

24

Group Concepts

Nancy S. McKelvey
Sally Laliberté
Phyllis B. Heffron

CHAPTER OUTLINE

OBJECTIVES

At the completion of this chapter, the reader will be able to:

- Define the following terms: group, group process, group cohesion, and group dynamics.
- Discuss the contributions of at least two group dynamics theorists.
- Explain the purpose for nurses working with groups.
- Describe the group as a system.
- Differentiate between formal and informal group structure.
- Describe the communication processes that occur in groups.
- Compare and contrast the three main types of group leadership.

- List the task and maintenance functions in a group.
- Describe typical member behavior in each of the three phases of group process.

- Identify four types of groups nurses work with.
- Discuss the application of the nursing process to working with the group as the client.

GLOSSARY

Group—a system composed of two or more individuals engaged in repeated interaction within an interdependent relationship and sharing a need or goal.

Group Boundary—delineation that separates members and nonmembers of a group (external boundary), or that differentiates between the members of a group (internal boundary).

Group Cohesiveness—the attractiveness of a group for its members; the force that develops to give a sense of belongingness and a desire to participate in the group.

Group Dynamics—scientific study of groups; the forces in group situations that are determining its nature and the behavior of the group and its members.

Group Norms—rules or standards about appropriate behavior in a group.

Group Process—conflicts of forces that result from attempts to disrupt or change the structure of a group; the stages that a group moves through.

Maintenance Functions—actions that encourage harmony and meaningful social interaction between members in the group.

Primary Group—informal social group that generally functions with spontaneous communication; e.g., family group.

Secondary Group—formal group generally existing for a specific purpose; e.g., post-mastectomy support group or a professional association.

Task Functions—actions that encourage the group to do the work necessary for goal achievement.

INTRODUCTION

Groups have always been important in society. Beginning with the earliest experience of the family group, all persons become naturally and increasingly associated with friendship groups, school and church groups, work groups, and other clusters of people.

The family group is known as a **primary group.** Primary groups are generally established through involuntary means, such as common heritage or geographic location.[1] Members communicate over long periods of time in face-to-face interactions and have a high degree of influence over the behavior of individuals within the group. Neighborhood cliques and adolescent peer groups, as well as families, provide examples of these informal groups.

Individuals also function within **secondary groups.** These groups usually are established for a specific purpose, and they involve a more formal pattern of interaction. They generally exert less influence on their members than primary groups do. Examples of secondary groups include committees, therapy groups, and professional associations.

A simple definition of **a group** is two or more people engaged in repeated interaction, who are in an interdependent relationship and share a need or goal. Various disciplines and people who have studied group concepts have given definitions relative to kinds of groups or to group functions. Lewin, a psychologist and imminent researcher in group therapy, defines a group as "a dynamic whole based on interdependence."[2] Bion, another major group researcher, defines a group as "an aggregate of individuals who have a specific function or set of functions."[3] Murray and Zentner, nurse authors, define a group as an "assembly of people who meet over a period of time."[4]

An important concept regarding the definition of group is the differentiation between a group of people and an aggregate of people. A group refers to associations between people in an interdependent relationship.[5] This chapter addresses the ways that people organize this interdependence and how they accomplish their goals as a result of their interactions.

The use of groups in the general population has mushroomed in recent times. There are, for example, groups designed to help people lose weight and control eating behaviors, groups that teach stress management and assertiveness, groups to help recently divorced or widowed persons cope with loss, and groups to assist smokers quit their habit. The intensiveness of the group experience movement in the United States has made it a social phenomena.[6]

The concept of working with groups in the health care setting also has expanded, particularly in the past decade. Nurses have worked therapeutically with groups in the inpatient psychiatric setting for many years. In addition to working with hospitalized patients, nurses in the mental health field who have additional training and supervision also work as group psychotherapists. Community health nurses work with family groups, either as health counselors or family therapists.

There are vast opportunities for group work with patients in all types of clinical settings, and both hospital and community health nurses are increasingly taking advantage of this. Examples of group work by nurses include prenatal teaching groups, groups for post operative patients such as amputees and persons who have undergone colostomies and mastectomies, groups to prepare post-heart attack patients for discharge from the hospital, and motivational groups for patients in extended care facilities.

In addition to direct clinical involvement with groups, nurses frequently participate in other personal and professional groups, such as leading team conferences and serving on planning committees. Because so much of the nurse's personal and professional time is spent with groups, it is highly desirable for them to develop skills and knowledge about group dynamics. Knowing how to participate effectively with groups enables nurses to facilitate behavior change and to accomplish goals in the group setting.

This chapter provides an overview of the theoretical basis of group study, identifies types and characteristics of groups, and discusses the use of groups in carrying out the nursing process.

THEORETICAL FOUNDATIONS OF GROUP CONCEPTS

One of the first recorded research efforts on groups took place in the health field in 1905. Dr. Joseph Pratt, a Boston physician, worked with a group of tuberculosis patients and recorded his observations of their behavior and reactions over time.[7]

Early sociological investigations of groups centered around behavior in crowds (mobs, fads, cliques, and public gatherings) and approaches toward understanding the dynamics of groups have evolved since that time.[8]

Jacob L. Moreno introduced the term **group psychotherapy** in 1932 and developed a special kind of therapy called psychodrama, which was group theory and dramatic techniques to achieve psychotherapeutic goals.[9] During World War II and since that time there has been tremendous growth in the use of groups for psychotherapy.

Kurt Lewin, a German psychologist and gestaltist, conducted early research on group dynamics and group behavior in the 1940s. His research demonstrated that learning occurred productively in groups, and that groups assisted active participants to develop new attitudes, learn new skills, and make behavioral patterns more effective.[10] Lewin developed what is known as field theory and did considerable research on group leadership style.

Small group theory, as a conceptual entity, has been widely studied in education, business, and industry for a number of years. The term small group is generally referred to in the literature as stemming from the basic training group (T-group), which was a group experience invented by the National Training Laboratories in 1947 for the purpose of helping persons become more sensitive to social reality.[11] Bion, a British psychiatrist, contributed to small group theory by studying group leadership and extending group concepts to institutions and organizations.

The study of groups draws on a wide range of theoretical frameworks. The practice of group therapy, for example, can be based on any of the theoretical approaches to psychotherapy—Freudian, transactional analysis, or gestalt.[12] The scope of this book limits a comprehensive listing or indepth discussion of all the contributions to research on groups and group dynamics. **Group dynamics** is the scientific study of groups.[13] The term describes the forces in the group situation that are determining the behavior of the group and its members.[14] Group dynamics is the net result of what has been learned about groups through research and, through an understanding of this knowledge, nurses will increase their effectiveness as they participate in group activities.

CHARACTERISTICS OF THE GROUP

The group is a system composed of elements or individuals who are its members. These individuals come together because of a common interest or need, to accomplish a task, or because of situations they find themselves in (e.g., work place, neighborhood, family groups).

Holistic Character of Groups

As individual members interact and develop a sense of interdependence, a group begins to form. The members acting together become greater than and different from any individual member. The group is thus said to exhibit the property of **summativity,** in which the whole becomes more than the sum of its parts.[15] Members of a task group attempting to influence legislation on the use of seat belts may be willing to behave more aggressively than any individual. This group would be acting in a different way than any of the individuals would act.

Boundaries

As group members continue to meet, communicate, and work together, the group gradually assumes its own character. Goals become apparent, special communication patterns develop, and behavior standards are established. The group members grow more interdependent and the group values and limits become apparent. While this is happening, the group is increasingly developing its own identity. Boundaries separate members of the group from nonmembers. "We" and "they" can be delineated.

Equilibrium

Not only do unique communication patterns and behavioral norms help to maintain the group's identity, but they provide the basis for sustaining the group's **equilibrium, steady state,** or sense of **balance.** Members will adapt to changes that occur within the group. If the psychotherapy group member who usually assumes a scapegoat role is absent, the other group members will adapt their behavior to adjust to this situation. For instance, the remaining group members may keep their communication superficial at that meeting because they fear unpredictable circumstances. The group maintains its equilibrium when an internal change occurs.

Open Versus Closed Systems

Groups also attempt to maintain their equilibrium in response to external influences. A group is said to be an open system, since it engages in an exchange relationship with the environment.[16] It responds to input from the environment, uses that input for change, and then produces output that affects other groups in the environment.

Input, throughput, and **output** are referred to as the three major processes of groups.[17] **Input** involves bringing energy or information into the group from outside its boundaries. **Throughput** refers to the process that occurs within the group in response to the input. **Output** is the result of accomplishing the group goal and provides the purpose for the group. The group's output provides input for groups in the environment as well as for the original group. When the output comes back and provides input to a group, we call that input **feedback.** Characteristics of the group as an open system must be remembered as one examines group structure, function, and process factors in greater detail.

GROUP STRUCTURE, FUNCTION, AND PROCESS

The three major components of groups, as a concept for nursing, are **structure, function,** and **process.** It is important to have a clear understanding of each of these major aspects of group before using the nursing process in group work. From a system's perspective, structure, function, and process are inseparably linked and serve to maintain equilibrium within the group as a system. However, for clarity, the three will be discussed individually.

Group Structure

Structure provides a system within which a group can meet its goals in some fairly predictable fashion. It offers the group an operational form from which relationships and boundaries within the group will develop. The relationships and boundaries occur between group members individually and between the group and the outside environment in which it functions.[18] Structure maintains constancy within a group over time so that, even as members move in and out, the basic group structure remains the same.

Members can and do have an impact on group structure. Again, structure is dynamic and constantly evolving; therefore, a change in membership or leadership will have some effect on structural aspects of the group. There are certain constants relating to structure, however, that need to be understood.

Group Boundaries. Berne has identified important sets of group boundaries.[19] The **major external boundary** separates the group leader and members from the outside environment. The **major internal boundary** separates the group leader from the group members. The **minor internal boundary** establishes vertical communication patterns between members, in which a type of hierarchical class system for interrelating develops. Assessment of group boundaries reveals important information about group roles, power, prestige and ability of members, group identity, stability, and group communication patterns.

Structural Forms. Group structure can be divided into two basic forms: formal and informal. A **formal** group structure consists of the explicit or readily apparent arrangements of the group. These include who the members are, the meeting time and place, length of group meetings, agendas, specific rules and duties, and responsibilities and rights of both the membership and the leadership. The formal structure is open, visible, and quite easily assessed.[20]

Informal group structure refers to the implicit or less readily apparent networks within the group, especially those related to power, prestige, and ability.[21] This informal group structure differs from the formal in that it pertains to how individuals within the group see themselves in relation to other members. Depending on members' perceptions of their own needs and goals within the group, as well as their past experiences, informal structures can be similar to formal structures, but more often are quite different. They also may be important to group functioning and development.[22] For example, in many groups, certain individuals are seen as quite powerful, perhaps due to personal qualities such as assertiveness or aggressiveness. The formal structure may delineate the leadership as rotating each week, but the informal structure reveals one member consistently taking on the leader's role. Assessment of

structure necessitates looking beyond the readily apparent formal structure, or much valuable information will be lost in the process.

Group Roles. The role network of a group is another important aspect of group structure. It has been described aptly as an interlocking network formed by many different roles.[23] Each group member will take on various roles over the lifetime of a group, depending on his own needs and past experience. The interaction of these roles within the role network of a group serves as a basis for the group to function and develop.

Many roles are inherent in any group. These will become manifest at various times depending on the type of group and the specific work being done. Three basic categories of roles have been identified.[24–26] **Individual roles** meet the individual member's personal needs and are not aimed at group task and maintenance functions. **Task roles** deal with the actual work of the group, i.e., accomplishing group tasks and working toward meeting group goals. **Maintenance roles** deal with the social and emotional aspects of group work, such as support and nurturing of members, easing communication, and socialization of group members. Specific task and maintenance functions within the group will be delineated under group function.

Communication Patterns. Communication structure forms the basic patterns by which group members will interact. In addition, communication within a group is significantly different than communication between two individuals due to the number of possible interactions between group members. The basic axioms of communication, however, apply within the group format.

There are two levels of communication: verbal and nonverbal. Communication involves four components: sender, receiver, message, and context. (Refer to Chapter 11 on communication for greater detail.) It is impossible not to communicate. Communication patterns are learned. These factors are critical. Since communication patterns are learned, they also can be unlearned and replaced with more effective ones. In fact, learning how to communicate effectively can be one of the greatest advantages of group work.

There are four basic structural patterns of group communication networks (See Figure 24-1). In analyzing group communication patterns, a key concept is **centrality**.[27] This is the position of dominance in a communication network from which and through which most communication flows. For example, the most central position in the chain is C, whereas in the circle all positions are equally central, since all are equidistant.

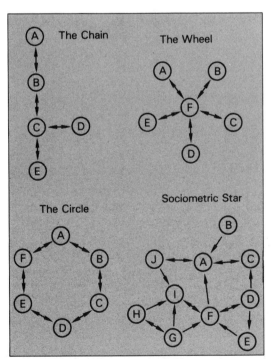

Figure 24-1. Structural patterns of group communication networks.

Research on group communication structures has shown that the more highly centralized group communication structures (chain, wheel) are most efficiently used in simple task oriented groups. When the task is very complex, a more decentralized structure (circle) is more efficient.[28] For example, in a group of people conducting a telephone poll, the wheel would be quite effective. Each member is given a list of numbers to call and a tally sheet for recording the results. By having one person in a central position to give information, make sure members get their calls done, and then collect tally sheets, the task can be accomplished in an organized, efficient manner. On the other hand, in a support group for overweight adolescents, the circle would be a more effective communication structure to meet the group's goals.

Another important type of communication structure within groups is the sociometric star.[29] This will be noted more in the informal structure, since it is based on attraction of group members to others in the group.[30] Generally, one member is known as the **sociometric star**, or the person chosen most often with whom to communicate. In Figure 24-1, that person is A. There is also a member known as the **sociometric isolate**, who communicates with A, but with whom no other member communicates. Within this type of structure, we also can see different pathways and subgroupings. Certain individuals may communicate with each other, but not other members, such as E, who communicates with H, I, and F, but no one else.

The communication structure of a group may involve overlapping of one or two structures. This is especially true in therapeutic groups, which are more process oriented. Evaluation of the communication structure yields valuable information, and the formation of **dyads** (two individuals who interact exclusively) and **subgroups** (three or more individuals who interact excluding other members) can be assessed by looking at both formal and informal communication structures. These components are extremely helpful in evaluating the group's progress.

Leadership Structure. Group leadership is a critical factor in the overall structure of a group. It helps guide, direct, and develop the group's progress. Depending on the leadership model and style, it is crucial to an adaptive group process.

There are three basic models for group leadership. In the **single** leader model, a group functions with the same leader throughout all group sessions. In the **co-leader** model, two persons share the leadership, and in the **rotating** leader model, a different leader is designated from the membership at each group session. There are advantages and disadvantages to the three models, and each will influence a group in different ways depending on the specific type of group. Figure 24-2 compares the advantages and disadvantages of the three different models of group leadership.

Leadership Model	Advantage	Disadvantage
SINGLE LEADER	Leader gives total attention to the group; does not need to concentrate on a co-leader relationship. Timing of intervention and follow through is facilitated. Economical	Entire burden of responsibility for leading and evaluating group falls on one person.
CO-LEADER	Leaders can model effective communication patterns. Interpretation and evaluation of the group is improved with two leaders combining impressions. Complementarity of styles may increase effectiveness of group. Permits working through anger at one therapist. Facilitates training for an inexperienced therapist. Simulates the family group situation and allows members to work through problems. One leader may work intensively with a member of a group problem, while the other monitors the general group process.	May be difficult for co-leaders to develop a egalitarian or good working relationship. If strain between co-leaders, group may exhibit tenseness and inhibition. Widely divergent styles can cause problems. Subgrouping may occur if a small group aligns itself to one therapist or if a "splitting" arrangement occurs. Expensive.
ROTATING LEADER or LEADERLESS	May foster independence and responsibility of group members. In self-help groups, members feel a particular affinity to a leader who has the same type of problems.	Generally, little opportunity for working through conflict or authority issues. Difficult to facilitate behavior change.

Figure 24-2. Advantages and Disadvantages of Three Leadership Models

Style is another important component of leadership structure. Three basic styles have been described.[31] The **democratic** leader operates within a member centered framework. This type of leader acts primarily as a facilitator of the group's participation in forming goals, decisionmaking, problem solving, and evaluating member participation. The democratic leader sees the strengths and resources in group members and tries to develop a climate in which these qualities can flourish and thereby accomplish the work of the group.

The **autocratic** leader is very much leader centered. This type of leader assumes the position of "leader knows best." He determines group goals, tasks, norms, and frequently the roles members should take within the group. This type of leader is not necessarily aggressive or hostile. The autocratic leader may also foster excessive dependency, hostility, passive-aggressive behavior, and apathy in group members.

The third style of leadership is the **laissez-faire** approach. This is the least active type of leader. He takes a very passive role in the group, allowing members to do what they will, when they want to, for whatever reasons they choose. The laissez-faire leader believes the group will produce without intervention. The effects of this style on group interaction tend to be confusion and frustration or dissatisfaction with the group. The group may never form goals or be able to function.

Some characteristics of an effective leader are:[32–34]

- Conveys security and acceptance of own limits; in turn, accepts others and helps them feel safe.

- Demonstrates friendliness, empathy, and concern for others.

- Listens carefully for unspoken as well as verbal messages.

- Insists on freedom rather than perfection within the group.

- Is capable of using humor kindly and appropriately.

- Permits dissent from group members.

- Does not resort to and does not permit blaming or persecution of members.

- Does not anticipate immediate release from conflict but strives to cope with and gain meaning from the conflict as part of the resolution.

- Does not permit himself to be used as a means to an end and does not use others in this manner (manipulation).

- Does not assume superiority over others.

Functions of Groups

Purpose and Goals. A group originates and continues for some specific purpose. That purpose generally defines, and to some extent is defined by, the type of group. For example, one type of task group may have a purpose of developing a patient classification system for direct reimbursement for nursing care. A therapeutic group's purpose will be very different; to prevent excessive emotional trauma to a group of elderly patients who are relocating to a new resident facility. The purpose of any group should be understood clearly at the beginning of group work.

Again, we see the interdependence of structure and function. Purpose gives form to function; without it, there is no reason for the group to function and grow. Purpose is also linked to structure; it is a key element that allows the group to form, develop, and eventually terminate.

Purpose will remain fairly constant throughout the life of the group. Goals and tasks, which flow directly from purpose, are dynamic and will continually change as they are met, and subsequently new goals and tasks evolve.

Whereas purpose is explicit at the beginning of a group's life, goals and tasks are not. Part of the initial phase of group interaction and development is definition of group goals. This should be a joint enterprise between membership and leadership.

One factor that will certainly influence group goal setting is the personal goal orientation of both members and leaders. These need to be clearly identified and articulated in the beginning phases of group work. Unfortunately, this is not always done, because either members are not consciously aware of their personal goals or are not comfortable enough in the group to share them. In task oriented groups, a lot of personal needs sharing is not usually tolerated, so this may be a problem in these groups. Group process can be severely inhibited if personal goals are not identified early, because members' needs will not be met, and members may not be able to fulfill the task and maintenance roles required for adaptive group functioning. For example, Nurse X agrees to become a member of the above mentioned task group to set up a nursing classification system. Her personal goals include acquiring expertise in nursing classification systems and fulfilling requirements of committee work for a promotion from staff nursing to nursing administration. She knows that two influential administrators are also on this committee and wants to impress them. She chooses to share only her first goal, the acquisition of expertise. During the initial meeting, she is assigned the duty of collecting patient records from nursing units and reviewing them for certain data. To do this, she will have very little contact with the influential administrators she is trying to impress. Her group role assignment does not meet her needs, and so in her group work, she may actually hinder the group process toward meeting its goals because she is too busy trying to meet her own.

Group **goals** are related to and develop from the purpose. They are objectives defined by the group to be met within the group. Group **tasks,** on the other hand, are the actual work that must be done in order to meet the group goals. The purpose, goals, and tasks of the nursing classification system committee are differentiated in Figure 24-3.

Purpose:	The development of a patient classification system in order to receive direct reimbursement for nursing care.
Goals:	1. To develop a patient classification system ready for pilot testing within one year. 2. To develop an operational definition of professional nursing care. 3. To identify various levels of professional nursing care. 4. To define outcome criteria for evaluating different levels of nursing care. 5. To identify two nursing units that are best suited for a pilot study of the newly developed system.
Tasks:	1. Hold biweekly group meetings to share information and report on progress. 2. Send out a memo to all nursing units to inform them of group purpose. 3. Meet with nursing unit coordinators to share ideas. 4. Review the literature related to nursing classification systems. 5. Spend time on each nursing unit and chart observation of direct nursing care. 6. Review medical records of patients in the last year to identify levels of care used.

Figure 24-3.   Purpose, Goals, and Tasks of the Nursing Classification System Committee.

The distinction between purpose, goal, and task is important to an understanding of group process and evaluation of the ability to function as a group.

Another related functional issue is motivation, which has been described as a system of internal tension that is aroused within a group member and is not relieved until the group goal has been met.[35] The need for congruence between a member's personal goals and the overall group goals has been addressed. The key point here is that without such congruence, a member will lack the motivation needed to perform tasks necessary for goal achievement. Commitment of members to accomplish group goals will be influenced by several factors:

- The desirability of the goal.
- The likelihood of group accomplishment.
- The challenge of the goal—what is the risk of failure?
- The abilities of the group to delineate when and if the goal has been achieved.
- The satisfaction or reward the group will receive with goal achievement.
- The working relationship among members necessary to achieve goals.

Task and Maintenance Functions. Once goals are developed by the group and the tasks are identified, certain functions are necessary for the actual work of the group to proceed. These have been described as task maintenance functions. **Task functions** encourage the group to do the work necessary for goal achievement. **Maintenance functions** encourage harmony and meaningful social interaction between members. A summary of task and maintenance functions follows:[36]

Task Functions
Information and Opinion Giver: Offers facts, opinions, ideas, suggestions, and relevant information to help group discussion.
Starter: Proposes goals and tasks to initiate action within the group.
Summarizer: Pulls together related ideas or suggestions, and restates and summarizes major points discussed.
Energizer: Stimulates a higher quality of work from the group.
Evaluator: Compares group decisions and accomplishments with group standards and goals.

Maintenance Functions
Encourager of Participation: Warmly encourages everyone to participate, giving recognition for contributions, demonstrating acceptance and openness to ideas, is friendly and responsive to group members.
Tension Reliever: Eases tensions and increases the enjoyment of group members by joking, suggesting breaks, and proposing fun approaches to group work.
Evaluator of Emotional Climate: Asks members how they feel about the way in which the group is working and about each other, and shares own feelings about both.
Process Observer: Watches the process by which the group is working and uses the observations to examine group effectiveness.
Trust Builder: Accepts and supports openness of other group members, reinforcing risk taking and encouraging individuality.

Process

Group process refers to the stages through which a group passes during its existence. These stages are characterized by specific group behaviors and feelings.[37] They also are influenced by the structural and functional properties of the individuals who comprise the group. The three basic stages that all types of groups go through are beginning, working, and termination.[38]

The **beginning** stage is an initial orientation period for the group. Generally, the formal structure is delineated early, usually by the leader. Expected behavior related to group norms and roles, as well as general operational components of the group, are dealt with during this time. Goals and tasks are developed, and members become acquainted, at least superficially.

Initial sessions may be uncomfortable for group members because of fears of exposing their inner feelings and thoughts. These may be even more pronounced in therapy groups, in which the basic purpose is self-disclosure. In task oriented groups, members may be better able to hide behind the tasks to be accomplished.

During this stage, several important group themes arise. **Themes** are the issues underlying specific content being discussed. Some of those important to this stage of group development are:

- Exclusion versus inclusion
- Trust versus mistrust
- Control
- Safety
- Resistance.

A new member will be concerned about being accepted as a member. Can he trust members not to reveal what he discloses in the group? Will other members or the leader recognize his vulnerability? Will the group like him and care about his participation? Will he lose control of his emotions? What will happen if he does? Will he find out that he is abnormal? Should he risk any of these?

The idea of group work is frightening to many people, therefore anxiety is common to this stage. Generally, the group will look to the leader as an authority and sit back waiting to be told what to do. Members also tend to be unable to focus on themselves. Situations outside the group are discussed at length, but there is resistance to concentrating on their own feelings and

perceptions within the group.[39]

There is no sharp dividing line between the stages of group development. It is, therefore, somewhat arbitrary to divide them into distinct entities. Nevertheless, there are behaviors that signal a transition from the beginning to the **working** stage.

Trust is a crucial issue for a group, for without a sense of trust among the membership, the true work of a group can never take place. There are many indications of trust. When members begin to take risks by sharing their feelings and reacting to others in a "here-and-now" focus, they are trusting the group.[40] When conflict is recognized and resolved or members can agree to disagree, trust is operational within the group and it is truly in a working stage.

In addition to the themes underlying group work in the beginning stage, ambivalence and caring emerge in the working stage of a group. Members are now sharing more of themselves, yet they may have ambivalence about just how far they can go. At this time members also begin to really care about the feelings and perceptions of the rest of the group. The problem of one member becomes the problem of the entire group. Members are able to give of themselves without necessarily needing to receive anything. A sense of belongingness is present. The work of the group progresses, and members seem to care about it. Attendance at group meetings is good and in-group participation is high. At this point the group is said to be cohesive.

Cohesion may take quite a while to develop depending on the type and purpose of the group. It is essential, if a group is to continue to grow and to be able to effectively meet its goals. Cohesion also allows the membership to work with less dependence on the leader. Members can deal with difficult issues with much less leader participation. Qualities that promote positive group interactions are recognized in members within the group, and task and maintenance roles are operational over and above individual roles.

As the group moves along, the third stage of group development is recognized. The **termination** stage is not simply the last meeting or two. It is really a distinct process in its own right. In reality, termination begins with the first few group meetings, when goals are developed. There is always an end in mind, a place where the group members want to be eventually. Dealing with issues surrounding termination usually begins at some point during the working stage of the group. As members develop a sense of cohesion, dependence becomes a major theme. With dependence also comes the idea of loss. What happens to me in the future, without this group? Many times, this issue comes to the surface when the first member or leader leaves the group. Separation anxiety is present due to the loss of a significant, interdependent relationship with its concomitant role. At this point, the group tends to revert back to needing more direction from the leader, because termination can be a painful process. In a highly cohesive, well-adjusted group, termination also can be a very important growth experience.

Other behaviors noted in this stage are a need to review what has been accomplished in the group, expression of caring and appreciation of group members and the leader by group members, as well as resistance to termination. This stage may be marked by regression of members and the entire group in an attempt not to have to deal with goodbyes.

In very task oriented groups, there may be a celebration party or formal dinner to acknowledge the completed work of the group. Certain psychotherapy groups may be ongoing, and the group never completely dissolves. Members may come and go. In other therapeutic groups, final termination may be simple, with each member expressing to the group what the group has meant to him, prior to disbanding.

TYPES OF GROUPS

Nurses work with clients and colleagues in many types of groups. They can be categorized into four types, according to purpose.

A **task group** has the purpose of accomplishing a designated task. For example, the rehabilitation team meets to develop discharge planning protocols for patients with spinal cord injuries. The group has a particular task to complete.

A second type of group has been termed a **therapeutic group** by Marram.[41] The purpose of this type of group is to support and maintain adaptive behaviors for people involved in change or crisis situations. A therapeutic group for newly diagnosed diabetics, for example, may have the purpose of preventing maladaptive coping behaviors while adjusting to the idea of having a chronic disease that requires medication, dietary changes, and so forth. Therapeutic groups also may be used for clients experiencing developmental or situational crises. Groups for new parents or recently widowed men provide examples of groups where support, sharing of feelings, and developing new coping behaviors would be stressed.

The third type of group is the **therapy group,** intended for clients needing treatment for an emotional disturbance.[42] The purpose of the therapy group is to provide the group members with insights into themselves and help them change their behavior. Therapy groups are used in psychiatric hospitals, mental health clinics, and in the community. Groups of narcotic addicts or depressed individuals may meet for psychotherapy in the group situation, for example.

A fourth type of group is called the **training group,** or T-groups, developed in the early 1960s. They were designed to teach people about developing interpersonal skills and about group processes. Members participate in the group and gain cognitive and experimental knowledge about group processes. Encounter groups, such as those associated with the women's movement, also foster self-awareness and development of interpersonal competence.

This classification of groups provides a convenient way to identify the purpose of any group the nurse might work with. The classification is not rigid, however, and many groups overlap in purpose, and fall into more than one category. Figure 24-4 provides a summary of the types of groups with their purposes, membership, and leadership characteristics.

THE NURSING PROCESS

Once nurses have obtained knowledge and experience with groups, they may wish to use group intervention to assist their clients. Nurses use the nursing process to guide their practice with groups just as they use it with individuals. The nursing process provides a framework for the nurse, once she perceives a problem amenable to nursing intervention. The four phases of the nursing process provide a systematic way to proceed.

Assessment

After the nurse perceives a problem, she enters into the assessment phase of the nursing process. In this phase, the nurse systematically reviews the situation in order to make a nursing diagnosis.

Maxine Loomis provides the following set of questions that can be used during assessment to determine whether the use of group intervention would be appropriate:[43]

- What are the client needs I am attempting to meet?
- Can these needs be met in a group?
- What are my expectations for the group?

- What are the expectations of the system relative to the proposed group?

If the answers to these questions are consistent with group intervention, the nurse formulates appropriate nursing diagnoses. For examples of group relevant nursing diagnoses see the clinical example at the end of this chapter. Once the nursing diagnoses have been established, the planning phase begins.

Planning

The planning stage for group intervention first involves clearly articulating the purposes or objectives for the group. The purposes will determine what type of group is being planned.

The nurse then must decide who will be admitted to the group. One should avoid a very large or a very small number of members. Six to ten members is thought to allow for a variety of interactions, experiences, and opinions, but is not so large that it prevents all members from fully participating in the group.

Planning also involves deciding on an open or closed group structure. Will members be permitted to join as others terminate, or will there be a predetermined number of meetings that all members are expected to attend?

Planning the physical arrangements for the group must include a convenient and consistent meeting place with adequate space, ventilation, and lighting. Any special requirements, such as access and additional space for a group involving clients in wheelchairs, should be planned for.

Other planning activities have to do with leadership. What will the role of the leader be, and what are the leader's goals? What reimbursement if any, will the leader receive?

In addition, planning involves preparing the clients for what will happen in the group. Some leaders prefer to have a

	Task Group	Therapeutic Group	Therapy Group	Training Group
PURPOSE	Accomplish designated task.	Support and maintain adaptive coping behaviors.	Provide intrapersonal insight; reeducate, remotivate, or support behavior change.	Learning cognitively and experientially about group process.
MEMBERSHIP CHARACTERISTICS	People assigned or volunteer for job.	Emotionally healthy. Experiencing stress related to physical illness or maturational or situational crisis.	Individuals experiencing emotional disturbance. Desire to learn new ways of coping.	Basically healthy individuals desiring to improve knowledge and skills in interpersonal relations.
LEADER ROLE	Facilitates progress toward desired goal. Maximizes problem solving capabilities of the group.	Facilitates group process; Provides supportive climate; Information giver; Role model; Select and prepare clients.	Stimulate member interaction; reinforce appropriate behavior; select and prepare new clients.	Facilitates group process. Resource person, catalyst. Maintain educational focus.
REQUIREMENTS FOR LEADERSHIP	Knowledge of task. Acceptable to members.	Knowledge and skills for group therapy; Ability to identify appropriate levels of intervention and interaction.	Knowledge and skills for doing psychotherapy in group; knowledge of group and individual dynamics.	Knowledge of group, interpersonal, and individual dynamics. Ability to maintain appropriate level of interaction and focus.

Adapted from the following references: Spradley, *Community Health Nursing*, pp. 289–298; Hall & Weaver, *Distributive Nursing*, pp. 120–124; Marram, *Group Approach*, pp. 9–72.

Figure 24-4. Types of Groups

pregroup interview with each member to discuss group goals. The interview can explain generally what goes on in a group, what is expected of members, and what members can expect to gain from the group experience. A group contract may be used to formalize this part of the planning process.

Finally, deciding how to measure whether the group objectives are being met must be considered. Documentation may be necessary before the group begins. For instance, it may be very important to document the members' blood pressure prior to the group experience, if one is expecting to lower the blood pressure through a group stress reduction scheme.

Implementation

After the planning phase is complete, the nurse will begin implementation of the group intervention. The implementation phase involves use of leadership skills and knowledge of group processes. Relying on her knowledge of the three stages of group development, the nurse acts as the leader in the implementation phase.

In the "beginning stage" the nurse attempts to provide both caring and stimulation to group members. She aims to provide enough structure to allow both the members and herself to become acquainted with each other in order to build a sense of trust, and to protect members from the embarrassment of divulging too much information. In addition, she teaches members how to use the group to redirect their questions and focus their attention on the group.

As the group moves into its "working stage," the leader encourages the members to express their feelings, be aware of their behavior patterns, respond to one another, share experiences, work through conflicts, and turn to the group for help.

Another leader role in the implementation phase is to prepare the group for ter-

mination. This process must begin before the last session, and group members should be encouraged to recognize what has been achieved.

Evaluation

The final phase of the nursing process is evaluation. Plans for measuring the objectives for the group is started in the planning phase, when the nurse states goals and outcome criteria. At this time, the nurse appraises the changes experienced by group members as a result of the group experience and applies outcome criteria.

CLINICAL EXAMPLE

The following situation describes how one nurse used the nursing process to work with a group of new parents.

Miss Marcus teaches childbirth education classes. When she talks to her former students after their babies are born, she consistently perceives a need for support and further education for new parents. Some of these new parents seem frightened about the responsibility of caring for a new infant; others just seem to need reassurance. Because our society is transient, extended family support systems are frequently missed. Also, since family size continues to decrease, the chances are increased that one or both of the parents have had no experience with or exposure to new babies. The parents may have no friends with babies.

Assessment. The nurse, Miss Marcus, has recognized potential client problems that she feels may be helped by nursing intervention. She begins assessing the problem in order to determine how to proceed. Miss Marcus uses the questions proposed by Loomis to begin her assessment.[44]

What are the client needs I am attempting to meet? Miss Marcus reviews what she knows about the needs of new parents. She considers their developmental stage. From her studies about human development, she realizes that new parenthood may initiate a maturational crisis if the couple is not supported in acquiring the adaptive behaviors necessary for this developmental stage.[45]

She decides that the new parents need information about infant development and the wide range of normal infant behavior. They may need practice with infant care skills. In addition, the parents may need an opportunity to express their feelings about being parents. The mother and father may need help in communicating and working on their own relationship.

On the basis of the feedback she receives from new parents and her knowledge of the new parents' developmental tasks, Miss Marcus feels the major client need is for support and education: support with developing adaptive coping behaviors to their new situation, and education about the new baby.

Can these needs be met in a group? Miss Marcus feels that group intervention would be the best approach to meeting the new parent needs. She recognizes that as group members share information about their own parenting experiences, they will realize the commonality of their situation and difficulties, as well as the different approaches that can be used in problem solving.

The needs of the parents may be more economically met in the group situation. In addition, the couples have already demonstrated willingness to work in groups by participating in childbirth preparation groups.

What are the objectives for the group? Miss Marcus decides that she wants to focus on learning and practicing communication skills and expression of feelings. Learning about the infant will be secondary. She feels that other resources are available for learning about infant care. Also, the nurse can give information when the

situation is appropriate.

Client objectives for the group are as follows:

- Parents will communicate their feelings about the baby, being a parent, and their own relationship, as evidenced by verbalization.

- Parents will feel support and maintain good parenting behaviors, as evidenced by verbalization and observation.

- Parents will feel more confident about their ability to care for their child, as evidenced by parenting behaviors.

- Parents will be able to identify age-appropriate behaviors for their child in his first year of life, as evidenced by their ability to discuss these behaviors.

These objectives will all be met by group members by the termination of the group.

What are the expectations of the system relative to the proposed group? No conflict exists in this situation. Miss Marcus feels that congruence exists between the answers to her questions.

One nursing diagnosis applicable to this situation is as follows:

- Potential alterations in good parenting behaviors due to lack of knowledge and experience regarding infant development and care.

Planning. Based on her assessment, Miss Marcus decides to lead a therapeutic group for new parents. Its purpose will be to maintain adaptive or healthy coping behaviors during this new developmental stage. The group also will have an educational component. Using this model for assessment of group needs provides a framework which includes purposes and objectives. Many nurses use a planning framework that includes these and, if so, purposes and objectives are a part of the planning phase. An outline of Miss Marcus' plan for the group follows:

A. Structure
1. Group member characteristics
   - Male/female couple with an infant who is two weeks to three months of age at the beginning of the group.
   - Couples will attend group voluntarily.
   - Selection of appropriate couples.
2. Closed group to meet for eight weeks.
3. Physical variables
   - Meet for two hours one evening per week.
   - Group size—five to six couples.
   - Meet in a well-lighted, comfortable room, large enough to accomodate six couples with their babies, the leader, and infant care equipment.
4. Leader reimbursement: $80.00/couple/8-week series.
5. Leader role
   - Support.
   - Facilitator of group process.
   - Educator/information giver.
B. Function—the nurse will prepare each couple for what they might expect from this group.
C. Process—the nurse and the couple will agree on a contract with mutual goals and designated responsibilities.
D. Plan how to measure whether the objectives are being met.

Implementation. Miss Marcus identifies the following steps and actions in carrying out her plan:

A. Demonstrate awareness of the three phases of the group process, and the leader and member roles in each phase.
B. Attempt to have the group exhibit balance of task and maintenance functions.
C. Promote group cohesiveness.
D. Act as supporter and information giver.

Evaluation. The following plan for evaluating the nursing instruction was devised:

A. Administer pre-test and post-test to measure knowledge about infant development.
B. Obtain verbal or written feedback on an ongoing basis about progress toward meeting objectives.
C. Observe factors, such as attendance, prompt arrival, and participation, for information on member attachment to the group.
D. Keep anecdotal records on observed couple communication and infant handling so that behavior change can be measured.
E. Have a colleague review tapes of selected meetings to provide feedback on the effectiveness of leadership skills.
F. Obtain written information about each group members' perceptions of his ability to communicate with his partner and about feelings of being understood by the partner. Measure this information before and after the group experience.

SUMMARY

Everyone participates in groups throughout their lifespans. Nurses can be more effective as group members and as group leaders if they use more than "intuitive" knowledge as a basis for participation and actions.

Group dynamics is the scientific study of groups. Utilizing knowledge from this study and from other theoretical frameworks provides a basis for practicing with groups.

One of the major theoretical frameworks

used in group work is systems theory. The group is an open system which engages in constant interchange with its environment. It is composed of members who, when they behave independently, provide the group with its own identity and boundaries. Input, throughput, output, and feedback are the group's processes.

Each group exhibits structure, function, and process characteristics. Structure provides the group with an operational form or system that allows the group to meet its goals in a particular fashion. Structural components include group roles, communication patterns, and leadership roles.

The function component of a group includes the group's purpose, tasks and goals. The group member's motivation and performance of appropriate task and maintenance functions help the group to achieve its purpose.

The process component describes the stage of the group. Beginning, working, and terminating stages have definite characteristics which group members and leaders should be aware of.

Four types of groups are described. The task, therapeutic, therapy, and training groups are classified according to their main purpose. Leadership and membership characteristics may differ or they may overlap from group to group.

In all types of groups nurses use the nursing process. This approach provides a systematic and comprehensive process for nursing intervention. The assessing, planning, implementing and evaluating steps supplies the framework for the process of working with groups as clients.

STUDY QUESTIONS

1. Identify five groups that you belong to. Classify each group as a primary or secondary group. Specify the purpose of each secondary group.

2. Explain the difference between group process and group dynamics.

3. Describe how your clinical nursing group works as a system.

4. Observe the communication that occurs in your next group meeting (study group, social group, dormitory unit meeting). Describe the nonverbal communication patterns you observe.

5. Think about a task group that you have participated in recently. Did task or maintenance functions predominate? What happened to goal achievement as the result?

6. Differentiate between the role of the leader in the task, therapeutic, therapy, and training groups.

7. Identify three health problems that you feel need nursing intervention. Assess each problem to determine whether group intervention would be appropriate. Plan an implementation strategy for one problem with a potential group solution.

8. Describe the evaluation methods you could use if you were leading a support group for homesick freshman students.

REFERENCES

1. Joanne E. Hall and Barbara R. Weaver: **Distributive Nursing: A Systems Approach to Community Health** (Philadelphia: J.B. Lippincott, Co., 1977), p.122.
2. Kurt Lewin: **Resolving Social Conflicts** (New York: Harper & Row, 1948).

3. Margaret Rioch: "The Work of Wilfred Bion and Groups," in **Group Relations Reader,** Arthur D. Coleman and W. Harold Bexton, eds., (San Rafael, Calif., Associates Printing and Publishing Co., 1975), pp.3–8.

4. Ruth Murray and Judith Zentner: **Nursing Concepts for Health Promotion,** 2nd ed., (Englewood Cliffs, NJ: Prentice-Hall, Inc., 1979) p.189.

5. Edward E. Sampson and Marya Marthas, **Group Process for the Health Professions,** 2nd ed., (New York: John Wiley and Son, 1981), p.120.

6. Ann W. Burgess: **Psychiatric Nursing in the Hospital and the Community** (Englewood Cliffs, NJ: Prentice-Hall, Inc., 1979), p.189.

7. Murray and Zentner **Nursing Concepts,** 1979, p.191.

8. Malcolm and Hildar Knowles: **Introduction to Group Dynamics** (Chicago: Follet Publishing Co., 1972), p.18.

9. Holly S. Wilson and Carol R. Kneisl: **Psychiatric Nursing** (Menlo Park, Calif.: Addison-Wesley Publishing Co., 1979), p.435.

10. D. Johnson and F. Johnson: **Joining Together: Group Theory and Group Skills** (Englewood Cliffs, NJ: Prentice-Hall, Inc., 1975).

11. L. Solomon and B. Berson (eds.): **New Perspectives on Encounter Groups** (San Francisco: Jossey-Bass, Inc., 1972).

12. Darwin Cartwright and Alvin Zander: **Group Dynamics Research and Theory** (New York: Harper and Row Publishers, 1968) p.19.

13. Marvin E. Shaw, **Group Dynamics** 3rd ed. (New York: McGraw-Hill Book Co., 1976) pp.14–15.

14. David H. Jenkins, "What is Group Dynamics," in Leland Bradford (ed.), **Group Development** (LaJolla, CA: University Associates, 1974), p.5.

15. Sampson & Marthas, **Group Process,** p.121.

16. Ibid., p.120.

17. Hall & Weaver, **Distributive Nursing,** pp.123–124.

18. Eric Berne: **The Structure and Dynamics of Organizations and Groups** (New York: Grove City Press, 1963), pp.53–64.

19. Ibid., pp.54–56.

20. Hall and Weaver, **Distributive Nursing,** p.124–126.

21. Ibid., p.124.

22. Ibid., p.125.

23. Sampson and Marthas, **Group Process,** p.52.

24. Kenneth Benne and Paul Sheats, "Functional Roles of Group Members," **Journal of Social Issues, 4** (1948).

25. Robert F. Bales, "Task Roles and Social Roles in Problem-Solving Groups," in **Readings in Social Psychology,** 3rd ed., eds. E.E. Macoby, T.M. Newcomb and E.L. Hartley (New York: Holt, Rinehart and Winston, 1958).

26. Hall and Weaver, **Distributive Nursing,** p.128.

27. Marvin E. Shaw, **Group Dynamics,** 3rd ed. (New York: McGraw-Hill Book Company, 1976), p.140.

28. Ibid., pp.139–142.

29. J.L. Morens, **Sociometry, Experimental Method and the Science of Society** (New York: Beacon House, 1951).

30. Sampson and Marthas, **Group Process,** p.62.

31. Ronald Lippitt and Robert White, "An Experimental Study of Leadership and Group Life," **Readings in Social Psychology,** 3rd ed., eds. E.E. Macoby, T.M. Newcomb and E.L. Hartley (New York: Holt, Rinehart and Winston, 1958).

32. Ruth Murray and Judith Zentner, **Nursing Concepts for Health Promotion** (Englewood Cliffs, NJ: Prentice-Hall, Inc., 1979). pp.194–195.

33. Edward Lindman, **The Meaning of Adult Education** (Montreal: Harvest House, 1961).

34. Robert Wicks: **Counseling Strategies and Intervention Techniques for the Human Services** (Philadelphia: J.B. Lippincott Co., 1977).

35. Johnson and Johnson: **Joining Together,** p.88.

36. Ibid., pp.26–27.

37. Gerald Corey and Marianne Corey, **Groups: Process and Practice** (Monterey, California: Brooks/Cole Publishing Co., 1977).

38. Hall and Weaver, **Distributive Nursing,** pp.137–141.

39. Corey and Corey, **Groups,** pp.92–94.

40. Ibid., p.102.

41. Gwen D. Marram, **The Group Approach in Nursing Practice** (St. Louis, C.V. Mosby Co., 1978), pp.18,19.

42. Barbara W. Spradley: **Community Health Nursing: Concepts and Practice** (Boston: Little Brown and Co., 1981), p.298.

43. Maxine Loomis, **Group Process for Nurses** (St. Louis, C.V. Mosby, Co., 1979). pp.18,19.

44. Loomis: **Group Process for Nurses.**

45. Donna C. Aguilera and Janice M. Messick, **Crisis Intervention: Theory and Methodology,** 3rd ed., (St. Louis, C.V. Mosby Co., 1978), p.151.

ANNOTATED BIBLIOGRAPHY

Adrian S: **A Systematic Approach to Selecting Group Participants.** J Psychiatr Nurs 18:2:37–41; February 1980. Nurses may use this article to assist in selecting or referring clients for participation in health care groups. An assessment tool is presented and can be used to determine appropriate candidates for group participation by using inclusion and exclusion criteria.

Corey G, Corey M: **Groups: Process and Practice.** Monterey, Brooks/Cole Publishing Co., 1977. The first section of this book reviews information necessary for working with groups in a leadership role. The second section provides examples of various therapeutic groups one would use for clients throughout life. Each of these latter chapters describe the leader's considerations for the particular type of group.

Johnson D, Johnson F: **Joining Together.** Englewood Cliffs, Prentice-Hall, Inc., 1975. This is a general book about working with groups in a membership or leadership role. It contains many assessment tools used to gain knowledge about how one functions within the group setting.

Johnson R et al: **The Professional Support Group: A Model for Psychiatric Clinical Nurse Specialists.** J Psychiatr Nurs 20:2:9–13; February 1982. This article describes how psychiatric clinical nurse specialists use the group intervention model to provide practical help to one another, stimulate ideas, and share personal and professional information. The description suggests how nurses can use groups to support their professional and personal growth. This journal issue is devoted entirely to group therapy.

Larson M, Williams R: **How to Become a Better Group Leader.** Nurs 78 8:8; 1978. Nonfunctional problem behaviors are identified and illustrated in this article. Suggestions of how the leader may deal with the "smoke screener," "interrogator," "rescuer," etc., are provided. The authors also describe the situations in which the behaviors are likely to occur.

Llewelyn S, Fielding G: **Under the Influence.** Nurs Mirror 155:4:37–39; July 1982. The authors describe how groups influence the beliefs, behavior, and attitudes of their members. They emphasize the impact of group influence on student nurses and on health care situations. Group membership, as well as leadership factors are noted.

Loomis M: **Group Process for Nurses.** St. Louis, C.V. Mosby Co., 1979. This is a very helpful book for nurses who plan to work with groups. It provides frameworks for the nurse to follow from the time she perceives a problem and determines that it may be appropriate to intervene through leading a group.

Marram GD: **The Group Approach in Nursing Practice.** St. Louis, C.V. Mosby Co., 1978. This book describes the scope of group work in which nurses may function effectively as group leaders. The first section examines four types of groups, their objectives, and indications for nurses as leaders. The second section outlines various theoretical frameworks that guide the nurse's interventions and interpretations. Finally, there are sections on the application of theory to practice, common objectives, and on group membership.

Sampson E, Marthas M: **Group Process for the Health Professions.** New York, John Wiley and Sons, 1981. The book deals with why health professionals need to understand the group's role in health promotion and illness. It describes the group process and the health professional's role as member and leader in groups. Change theory and its relationship to the group process is discussed.

Yalom ID: **The Theory and Practice of Group Psychotherapy.** New York, Basic Books, Inc., 1975. This is a comprehensive but easily read book on group psychotherapy. The nurse who is just beginning to study group work will find the sections on the curative factors in group, group process, group cohesiveness, and problem patients particularly enlightening.

25

The Family as a System

Phyllis B. Heffron
Eliza M. Wolff

CHAPTER OUTLINE

OBJECTIVES

At the completion of this chapter, the reader will be able to:

- Describe briefly the history of the family.
- Identify four distinctive approaches to family study.
- Discuss the relationship of systems theory to family study.
- Describe at least six organizational structures of families.
- Describe three types of boundary regulations in families.
- Identify at least six major roles families must perform for effective family functioning.
- Identify two types of role conflict in families.
- Identify six bases of power in families.
- Describe at least six major functions performed by the family.
- Identify the major components of the family assessment.
- Discuss at least four general methods of nursing intervention with families.

GLOSSARY

Ecomap—a family assessment tool that consists of a graphical representation of a family's relationship with its environment.

Extended Family—a nuclear family group with the inclusion of additional related members such as grandparents, aunts, and uncles.

Family of Orientation—the family group into which a person is born.

Genogram—a family assessment tool that consists of a familytree diagram depicting family dispersals, losses, roles, and organizational patterns over three or more generations.

Monogamy—the practice of being married to only one spouse at a time.

Nuclear Dyad—a husband and wife with no children.

Nuclear Family—a family grouping that consists of a husband and wife and their children.

Polyandry—a family unit in which there is one wife with two or more husbands at the same time.

Polygamy—the practice of having two or more spouses at a time.

Polygyny—a family unit in which there is one husband with two or more wives at the same time.

Single Parent Family—a family grouping consisting of only one parent; the single parent may be the mother or the father who may be widowed, separated, divorced or never married.

INTRODUCTION

The **family system** is the most basic and primary unit of every human society. It is universally recognized as primary because of its reproductive and parenting functions. In addition, it is the most stable of primary groups and endures the longest. All of us, as newly born infants, are first received by the family group, and we develop and experience many crucial "firsts" within its boundaries.[1]

Families have been studied by several disciplines, most notably sociology, biology, anthropology, and psychology. At the most fundamental level, a family can be defined in terms of its biologically central members, the mother, father, and dependent children. Called the **nuclear family,** this baseline bio-social definition is what many people think of when thinking about families. However, many different kinds of

family groups exist within our society and in other cultures.

Beyond the very traditional definition of the nuclear family, families can be defined in terms of domestic living arrangements, roles, functions, and personal relationships. These criteria, among others, may vary even further from culture to culture and within geographic or religious boundaries within the same culture.

Some communal families, for example, may be characterized by several nuclear families that share a common household, while others may include a group of unmarried men and women with or without children, who share a similar group living arrangement. In Western societies, such as the United States, people are increasingly mobile and separated from the families they are born into and may describe selected friends and neighbors as their family.

Despite all the definitions, viewpoints, and structural and functional variations of families that will be discussed in this chapter, there are certain basic concepts and assumptions applicable to almost all family groups. These assumptions and concepts have been derived primarily from the social sciences and help to illustrate why family study is so important to the nursing profession.

- The family is a complex social system and is the basic unit of all societies.
- The family is a primary group in the sense that it gives the individual his earliest and most complete experience of social unity and initiates self-concept formation.
- The family is an adaptive open system that is constantly influenced by exchanges with its environment.
- All family systems have goals in the areas of reproduction and the meeting of physical needs, love and affection, economic survival, and socialization.
- The family is the locus of health beliefs, practices, values, and attitudes and is often the greatest single influence on the health of the individual.[2–5]

Throughout its history, the nursing profession has maintained an interest in families, particularly in the areas of public health nursing, community nursing, and, maternal and child health nursing. As the holistic approach to health and health care has increasingly advanced, nurses in all specialties have found a need for family study.

Consumers of health care are asking for more personalized and individualized attention from health care professionals. The cost of hospitalization and specialized health services has contributed to a shift of many health care activities from the hospital to the community and home settings. Clients are very interested in learning about illness prevention and self-care; they are aware of pursuing health and wellness through self-directed activities such as exercise, nutrition, and stress management for the whole family. The hospice movement, which is very dependent on the interest, support, and care of families by nurses is another illustration of the importance of family study by nurses.

Nurses are taking responsibility for coordinating and giving expert professional services in other areas about which families have special needs and concerns. Home birthing experiences, family planning services, and the provision of adequate parenting skills are some of the topical issues that maternal-child health nurses and nurse-midwives are helping families with. In traditional hospital settings, for example, the impact of the birth of a new baby on family members has long been ignored. Staff nurses are encouraged to foster the importance of family interaction at this time by facilitating the opportunity for sibling visitation.[6]

Psychiatric nursing is increasingly involved with families and their mental health concerns. These concerns may range from relatively mild situational anxieties or depressions related to a role change by one family member to more serious issues of coping with chronic alcoholism or child abuse. The community mental health movement, which began in the 1960s, has led to nurse involvement with families of newly discharged former psychiatric inpatients, and the services may include family therapy as well as individual and marital counseling. Community mental health nursing has been described as favoring a holistic approach of which family analysis is a vital part.[7]

The next section of this chapter is concerned with the historic events relative to family concepts and provides an overview of what has been written and thought about families over the ages. Theoretical approaches to formal family study will be presented in terms of major, accepted frameworks and pertinent research.

The greater portion and remainder of the chapter concentrates on two areas: a descriptive discussion of types, characteristics, and functional processes of families and the nursing process as it relates to both family nursing and the nursing of individuals as family members. A systems adaptation view of the family is further described and expanded in these two sections and is used to illustrate and unify related concepts throughout.

HISTORICAL PERSPECTIVES

Families have existed in one form or another since the beginning of time. Duvall categorizes family history in terms of four major transition periods. The first period, which took place about 10,000 years ago, describes families as hunters and food-gatherers until the time when they became dwellers in farming villages. The growth of cities some 5,000 years later marks a second transition period, followed by an industrial and technological growth period. The fourth and present transition period is marked by profound advances in science and technology, and changing ideas, attitudes, and beliefs.[8]

The family system can be traced back at least 3,000 years, though there is no written comprehensive account or recorded models of family behavior prior to the 20th century. Much of the early information on family issues is derived from historic documents, folklore, and myths.

Only recently have efforts escalated, and research is underway to look more specifically at resources that can help build a composite picture of the history of the family.[9]

Early Family History

Anthropologists and archeologists give very early evidence of the family as the center of individual and community life, regardless of its form.[10]

These early sources show the focus of family systems and their functions shifting. The ancient family, for example, was strongly patriarchal, with the father the supreme head of the household and family heritage traced through his lineage only. The practice of polygamy was common. This patriarchal orientation has shifted back and forth through the ages to a nearly egalitarian, monogamous, and conjugal family situation.[11,12]

In early family sociology, there were several different models or frameworks proposed as ways to view the family. They were based on various political, religious, and philosophical ideologies, and fostered studies that sought to uncover whether human societies were originally matriarchal or patriarchal, whether they were monogamous or promiscuous, etc. These early studies failed to produce any concrete patterns or widely accepted viewpoints, and posed conflicting ideas and issues—actually helping to create more interest in the family.[13]

The rapid social changes that took place in Europe, and later in America, brought attention to the family—through the many problems created by poverty and its resulting suffering. Mass immigration to the United States led to overcrowding in urban areas, and the family faced increasing problems with juvenile delinquency, crime, and disease. Industrialization and specialization began to affect the family profoundly, as technological advances mushroomed and the family, as a unit of production, began to disappear. The following discussion of the impact of industrialization on the family is based largely on material presented by Hawley,[14] Gordon,[15] Goode,[16] and Murray and Zentner.[17]

The Industrial Revolution

The industrial revolution, which began to flourish in America in the latter part of the 19th century, was characterized by centralization (from home to factory) of the production of goods and services, growing reliance on machines and other technological advances, and a shift away from an agrarian way of living to an urbanized society. Factories, the primary institutions of this movement, were uniquely specialized and market oriented. They created many new consumer goods and services, particularly in the areas of food-processing, garment manufacturing, recreational facilities, home construction, education, and health care.

The functional role of the family changed dramatically from a production unit (producers) to a unit of consumption (consumers). As producers, families had spent all of their time together working jointly toward the prosperity of the household. With the introduction of the factory, the father began to work outside the home and contribute finances to the family system. Women were freed from some of their domestic chores, e.g., they no longer had to spin cloth and sew everything from scratch, do all the laundry by hand, or harvest and prepare food on a daily basis. Children were no longer viewed as a valuable resource to the family prosperity, as future members of the household labor force, but as a charge against a wage or salary income.

The role of the elderly changed with the coming of industrialization, and the family was faced with a number of new problems in this area. Prior to industrialization, the extended family was more common. Elderly members remained a part of the family household and contributed as they were able. Young adult children remained at home, and generations shared a common base. As work options increased, young people had greater independence and could go outside the family to work and live. The organization of factories, along with the growth of corporate industry and government regulations led to forced retirement and an altered role of senior family members. Burnside presents a listing of some 43 psychosocial needs of the elderly today in which things such as role reversal, isolation, fear of being unwanted and no longer useful, no interested family, loss of status, difficulty in adjustment to institutional living, boredom, and self-devaluation are major headings.[18]

During this same time, other social problems affecting families became apparent. The middle class was increasing and family forms changing. Divorce and separation increased and the birth rate declined. Babies, on the average, were born earlier and were more closely spaced, leaving more leisure time for the parents. Families became mobile due to greater choices in jobs and industry controlled moves, and it was uncommon for families to stay in one community permanently. Thus, kinship ties were potentially weakened. Within communities and neighborhoods, the higher turnover rate of residents lessened the probability of emotional friendships developing through long-term associations. The family had to devote a great deal of energy in constant adaptation to new surroundings.

Families were affected by numerous new stresses and strains that were imposed on participants in the industrial workforce. Mass production, for example, required workers to become specialized in a single task and perform it over and over in the course of a workday. Closely aligned were the concepts of assembly line production and automation, all of which tended to result in workers becoming bored and frustrated as they were denied the pleasures of creativity and a sense of fulfillment in completing a whole task. In addition, automation led to the reduction of some jobs, as machines became more sophisticated and able to perform tasks previously done by hand. Increasingly, the primary responsibility for relieving these stresses and strains and satisfying the emotional needs of the worker rested with the family.[19]

Because the employed adult became one of the primary supportive structures of the family, there emerged a great deal of pressure to compete for favorable jobs, perform in a satisfactory manner, and seek avenues for upward mobility. When job security became threatened in any way, workers were highly susceptible to depression and emotional and physical illnesses, all of which affected the family system.[20]

Industrialization and modern technology have contributed to changes in traditional family value systems. Achievement of the individual is highly valued in our society and often takes precedence over birthright. As young people moved to jobs outside the family, jobs were no longer passed down from father to son or to other family members, and the individual was forced to make his own way. Johnson states that technology has influenced the nature of contemporary social organization by substituting more individualistic striving to gain a paycheck in place of duty to the family group.[21] Materialism has been identified as a central value in American life and, theoretically, an individual with enough money can live a life completely apart from his family.[22] There is great pressure to purchase and consume and to judge others by their ability to do the same; family relationships are easily manipulated under these circumstances.[23]

A great deal more has been written about the industrial revolution and its relationship to the evolution of the family. There has been considerable debate on the causes, and whether the technological advantages outweigh the disadvantages.

Most scholars agree that it is a very complex relationship. Although it is clear that the industrial revolution fostered many changes from family behaviors and organization, it is still unclear as to the **degree** of change that it has contributed.[24]

The Space Age Family

The effects of social changes on the modern 20th century family have been so vast, particularly since 1950, that characteristics and lifestyles between one family generation and the next are often totally dissimilar. The rapidity of these changes has been unparalleled in human history and has required the family to be extremely adaptive and flexible.[25]

Economic and educational changes, technological advances, and political shifts all have contributed to changes in family structures, roles, attitudes, and lifestyles.

Economic change, and in particular the economic relationship between families and society, continues to be a central factor in shaping family life today. The basic changes in economic patterns that industrialization brought to the family have become more and more complicated. Production and distribution of goods have increased, and there is more to buy. In nuclear families, not only does the father go outside the home to work everyday, but he may commute an hour or more each way and be accompanied by his working wife. Economic welfare for the family becomes the focal point of the family's existence. Families feel pressured to consume material goods, as perpetuated in advertising and other media communications, and competition with other families often produces stressful consequences. Frequent relocation to new communities has become a way of life, and the cause of this mobility is most often job related. Family stability and security, especially for school age children, can be severally jeopardized.

The changing roles of women in American society, particularly in regard to employment, has had far reaching effects on the family. More women are working than ever before, and many have children and maintain a family life, as well. In 1975 for the first time in American history, a majority of the nation's mothers with school age children held jobs outside the home.[26] The rise of single parent families has nearly doubled since 1950 and is associated with increasing statistics of divorce, illegitimacy, and desertion. In 1975 more than 7 million American families were headed by women, a 44 percent increase since 1965.[27] These statistics account for growing concerns about modern day childrearing, child abuse, and an increase in depression among children. Stress is greatly increased in both single parent families and families in which both parents work, and children often end up spending less and less personal contact time with parents.

Much has been written about the effects of such stressors as economic uncertainty, dual career family situations, single parenthood, and high technology on the stability and quality of family life. Some authors are very pessimistic about what is happening to the American family and feel its strength and unity is declining.[28] Others take a more conservative view and look at the enduring history of the family as a guide for predicting the future.[29]

One thing is certain: throughout the ages, and very much in evidence today, is the need for adaptation in families. Today, families' adaptive abilities are being tested, perhaps more than ever before, as they cope with the impact of changes in functions and roles within the context of our urban society.

THEORETICAL APPROACHES TO FAMILY STUDY

The study of families and the theoretical approaches used to describe how they function are many and varied. These approaches can be classified in a variety of ways. One method is to look at family study in terms of the disciplines within which they were developed. In this context, anthropological, sociological, psychological, and psychoanalytic family frameworks can be delineated. Other frameworks for family analysis that have been identified include the structural/functional approach, the interactional approach, the systems approach, and the institutional approach. Family study has been viewed from a purely developmental approach, as well as philosophical and legal points of view.[30,31]

This chapter focuses on the family as viewed from a systems and structural/functional approach. An overview of other selected theories and conceptual frameworks of the family appear in Table 25-1.

THE SYSTEMS/ADAPTATION APPROACH

The family as an adaptive system gives us an orderly and structured way of describing families and their characteristics. It allows us to "break down the whole" and look singularly at each part as well as learn how the parts relate. In this approach, the "parts" of the family system are viewed in terms of individual members of the family and in terms of traditional system parts, such as boundaries, roles, and subsystems. By looking at families in this way, nurses can focus on one member in relation to the whole group or on the entire family.

The systems approach defines a family as an open, living, social system.[35] It has distinct structures, functions, and patterns of communication, power, and decision-making. Family systems are adaptive by nature and continually communicate with environmental subsystems in the community and world. Within the context of being

Framework	Key Features
INTERACTIONAL	• the family is defined as a set of interacting personalities, each having self-defined roles • the general approach is psychosocial, in which personality and socialization are key • the family is studied by assessing roles and relationships within the family system • intervention is based on analysis of communication patterns and other internal family dynamics as they affect relationships
STRUCTURAL/FUNCTIONAL	• the family is defined as a social system whose members have specific roles geared toward maintaining internal and societal stability • family functions are defined primarily in terms of societal needs • the nuclear family and traditional sex roles are seen as universal and timeless • families are assessed in terms of fulfillment of roles and functions
INSTITUTIONAL	• the family is defined as a social unity that functions in accord with established social institutions • primary concerns of family study are cultural values and how family functions have adapted in response to societal changes
SYSTEMS	• the family is viewed holistically as an open system made up of various subsystems, all working toward common goals • family members are interdependent and relate through communication and feedback • adaptation is ongoing in families, and there is a tendency toward growth and differentiation • family study and assessment depend on analysis of all the parts of the system, patterns of communication, and adaptive abilities
PSYCHOANALYTIC	• the family is defined as a natural group whose members have complementary needs • the family is seen as the root of human behavior, and there is a strong correlation between individual personality development and the growing up exieriences in the family • there is emphasis on the importance of intrapsychic conflict between individual needs to remain close to the family group versus establishing self-identify • feelings, attitudes, and values are transmitted from one family generation to the next through an unconscious process of assimilation
DEVELOPMENTAL	• the family is viewed as it evolves over time • families have a predictable life cycle that can be divided into chronological stages of development • specific tasks and role assignments are associated with each developmental stage • assessment and family study is based on analysis of task fulfillment with major considerations given to physical maturation, social and cultural factors, and individual personality and values

Table 25-1.   Overview of Theoretical Frameworks for Family Study[32-34]

a social system, families have certain tasks, such as biological reproduction, socialization of members, and maintenance of order.[36] Within an adaptive framework, family systems continue to grow and change.

Although the family is viewed in this chapter as an adaptive system, selected ideas and research findings from other family studies using other approaches are included.

Types of Family Organization

As we have noted earlier, there is a wide range of definitions of a family. Friedman says that "a family is a group of people emotionally joined together who live in close geographical proximity."[37] Nye and Berardo write that a family is "two or more people related by blood or marriage who customarily maintain a common residence."[38]

Scientists who have studied the family have noted a variety of forms families may take. These include the **nuclear family,** the **extended family,** the **nuclear dyad,** the **single-parent,** and the **single adult.** Other varieties of family forms include **homosexual pairings, common-law marriages, communes, group marriages,** and **cohabitation without marriage.** Nurses may encounter any of the above family forms in their nursing practice, and understanding of the organizational arrangement is important. Stresses and health needs may be very different in a single parent family than in a homosexual pairing.

The **nuclear family** consists of a husband and wife and their children. This is the family form with which most people have had the most experience. "Although the classic form continues to, and most probably always will exist, there are now many variations of the nuclear model as well as emerging new patterns of family structure. Each requires recognition and acceptance by the professionals who wish to help actualize family health potential."[39]

The **extended family** includes the nuclear family and other related members of the family, such as grandparents. Other people who may be included are siblings of the husband and wife and the siblings' children. Extended families living together were once common in America, but mobility, industrialization, and a changing economy have led to a decline in this pattern. The extended family in several households, however, is an important part of family life in Native American culture. Non-kin may be incorporated into Indian family life through formal and informal processes. Non-kin for whom a child is named participate in a formal ritual. That individual is expected to participate in childrearing and role modeling.[40]

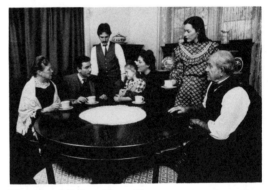

Figure 25-1. Family structure varies within and across cultures.

When clients have special health needs, members of the extended family may be able to offer care and support if they live with the family or nearby.

The **nuclear dyad** refers to the husband and wife with no children. This may become an increasingly common family form, as more couples choose to remain childless. The nuclear dyad also refers to the couple whose children have moved away.

The **single-parent family** is becoming increasingly common. Single parents include divorced, widowed, unmarried, and adoptive parents, as well as step and foster parents. The most common type of single parent family is that headed by a woman.[41] In the United States, this family form comprises 12 percent of households.[42] The single-parent family may be subjected to unusually high stress levels. This parent often works and combines the role of mother and father in caring for children at home. The parent may have to curtail social life because of other responsibilities. According to the 1980 census, about one-half of families below the poverty line were composed of women and children with no husband present in the home. The poverty rate in this type of family was 32.7 percent. For single men with children, the poverty rate was 11.1 percent, while the rate for couples was 6.2 percent.[43]

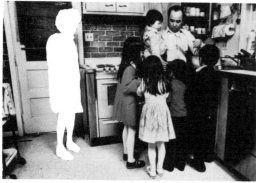

Figure 25.2   The role of a single parent may pose special stresses.

Single adults are another family form. Approximately 6 percent of adults live alone.[44] Although they live by themselves, they are part of a family referred to as the **family of orientation,** the family into which the person is born.[45] Single adults may be young and recently separated from their parents, or they may be elderly and without any immediate family left. They may be lonely and may not have ready support systems available. Nurses need to be alert to these possibilities. People who live alone may have no one to care for them if they are sick or disabled, or they may have no one to talk with in times of crisis.[46]

Additional family forms include **common-law couples, communes,** and **group marriages. Common-law couples** are those who are eligible to marry but don't. They maintain a common residence. Such couples are recognized in a number of jurisdictions by the law as a family.[47] **Communes** refer to households where adults live together but are not necessarily monogamous. The latter example is a group marriage.

Characteristics of family structure are affected by cultural norms and values. Nye and Bernardo describe the kinship system in the United States according to the following characteristics:

- There is an incest taboo.
- Monogamy is the prevailing pattern.
- As far as location of household, choosing a mate, or inheritance patterns are concerned, there is no preference shown to maternal or paternal kin.
- No particular preference is shown to lines of descent of either the husband or the wife.
- Major emphasis is on the immediate conjugal unit (the mother, father, and children).
- The nuclear family is a fairly autonomous unit.
- The family is a consumptive rather than a productive unit.
- There is relatively little emphasis on tradition because of the emphasis on the nuclear family and the multilineal kinship system.
- Free dating and mate selection is the norm.
- There is widespread dispersion of adult children.[48]

These characteristics of our society may vary considerably among families in other countries and cultures. The one exception is the incest taboo. This characteristic is common to family life in nearly all societies. Whereas **monogamy** is a common feature in our culture, **polygamy** (plural spouses) may be a common feature of other cultures. **Polygyny** refers to one husband with two or more wives at the same time. **Polyandry** refers to one wife with two or more husbands at the same time. This latter form has been recorded in only four societies.[49] Murdock studied 565 societies of the world; he found that about 75 percent favored polygyny and 25 percent favored monogamy. Less than 1 percent favored polyandry. No society practiced group marriage.[50]

It is important for nurses to understand as much as they can about the structure of the families under their care and of the families of their specific clients. With more and more people living in family structures other than the nuclear or extended type, the kind of and need for nursing services is changing. Support groups and needs differ from one type of family to another, and some of these family types are more dependent on the health care system than others.[51]

Stresses, health needs, and health practices may vary considerably according to these structures, and an organizational knowledge will help guide the nurse in carrying out the nursing process.

Family Processes

All family systems, regardless of their structure or stage of development, possess certain characteristics that help define them and maintain their viability. These characteristics or processes, make it possible for families to function as whole units and include the basic systems concepts of boundaries, roles, power, decisionmaking, energy, communication, and feedback. Various subsystems exist within the family system. Some of these subsystems include dyads, such as husband-wife, parent-child, or sibling-sibling. In any subsystem, the individual learns interpersonal skills, performs roles, and has varying levels of power. Adaptation is constantly taking place within families, and through an interplay between family coping mechanisms and family processes, equilibrium can be maintained and growth can take place.

Boundaries. All subsystems have semipermeable boundaries, and clarity of these boundaries in families is very important. Boundaries are the rules that define how participation takes place in subsystems.[52] Boundaries also serve to foster differentiation of family members.

All families are involved in distance regulation in order to attain goals of affect (love and intimacy), power (freedom to decide what they want and the ability to get it), and meaning (a philosophical framework by which to order events). Families attain these goals as they regulate boundaries applying to space, time, and energy.[53]

Regarding the issue of space, family members are continually engaged in the task of developing and maintaining spatial relationships with one another. As they interact, decisions must be made about how close to be.[54] The desire for and tolerance of close physical proximity varies from person to person and culture to culture.[55] Much has been written about how individuals communicate through body language. Boundary and distance regulation are important facets of this communication. Physical space boundaries may be quite specific in families—a person's bedroom or favorite spot at the dining table. Every individual also maintains what is called "personal space" which can be violated when there is poor communication or a lack of sensitivity among family members. Assessment of a family's use of space may be very helpful in the overall analysis of family interaction and function. Such things as the actual physical design of a house may have a strong effect on how much closeness or distancing is attained by the members.[56]

In addition to spatial boundaries, families erect temporal boundaries in order to help them attain their goals.[57] Aspects of boundaries concerning time include frequency, rate, sequencing, duration, calendar time, and clocktime. How individual members use their time and how the family uses time together give clues to these kinds of family boundaries. Schedules for going to bed, getting to work or school, and going shopping are also examples of time boundaries. Family members all need a certain amount of solitude or "private time." This kind of privacy involves temporal as well as spatial boundaries. Other types of temporal boundaries involve feelings and thoughts about past experiences and future plans. Information such as this can be helpful in assessing family functioning and in helping families organize their time efficiently.

Boundary Maintenance. An important role for nurses working with clients and families is to support clear and appropriate boundaries within subsystems of the marital dyad, the parental dyad, and the sibling dyad. Where there are problems with boundaries, enmeshment (diffuse boundaries) or disengagement (rigid boundaries) may occur.[58] An overprotective mother who keeps her son home from school when he is able to go is an example of enmeshment. In some chaotic families, there are no links between members and boundaries are rigid. They come and go with no regard for others in the family system. Both types of families may need counseling to alter their boundaries. The psychiatric nurse who has specialized in

family therapy has special skills in helping families attain more satisfactory boundaries.

Energy is defined as the capacity to do work. All family activities require the expenditure of energy in order to attain goals. Energy within a family system refers to psychic and physical energy. Psychic energy refers to attitudes and feelings of motivation that precede the action. The capacity to show an interest, to want to get involved in something, or to go through the mental steps of organizing and managing an action are some general examples of psychic energy. The mother who takes the initiative, for example, to call for an appointment with the pediatrician, find out how to get to the office, call the bus for a schedule, and arrange for a change in her own work schedule is expending considerable psychic energy. How the family obtains energy and with what frequency are important for nurses to understand when they are working with families.[59] Chronic illnesses, depression, and situational crises within families can affect family energy levels.

The regulation of energy flow to attain energy balance or imbalance is the major energy issue in families.[60] Community nurses and others who work with families in depth often can provide this kind of intervention.

Roles. How are duties or roles in families assigned? Who takes out the trash, cooks the meals, works outside the home, and cares for the children?

Role refers to an expected set of behaviors. It is a dynamic family aspect, the acting out of behaviors expected of the occupant of a particular status or position. "Role is referred to as more or less homogeneous sets of behavior which are normatively defined and expected of an occupant of a given social position."[61] Nye emphasizes that these expectations are based not just on present day role behaviors, arising out of social interaction, but on the behavior of those previously occupying the roles.[62] Roles include not only behavior but attitudes and values.

Role enactment is necessary for the fulfillment of family functioning.[63] Roles we commonly think of in families include those of husband-father, wife-mother, and child-sibling. These roles are associated with expected behaviors. Some of Mrs. Jones' roles as wife and mother include housekeeping, child care, child socialization, and sexual partner. Because Mrs. Jones works, she shares the provider role with her husband.

Types of roles. Roles must be negotiated. They may be decided on the basis of tradition, competence, or what the husband and wife each like best or least. Families commonly perform the following roles:

- **Provider**—The occupant of this role provides income to secure material resources.

- **Housekeeper** —Cleaning house, obtaining food, and preparing food are some of the expected behaviors of this role.

- **Sexual partner**—In addition to the act of sexual intercourse, part of the expected behavior of this role for both men and women today is to provide pleasure to the partner.

- **Therapeutic** —Role behavior in this category includes the provision of emotional support, sustenance, and reassurance.

- **Child care**—Providing the basic needs of a child through feeding, changing, and clothing are components of this role.[64]

- **Recreational and kinship**—Providing recreational activities and keeping in touch with relatives.[65]

Women traditionally have been involved in housekeeping, child care, and child socialization roles, while men have filled the provider role. More and more women, however, are entering the work force. In the 20 years from 1960 to 1980, one-earner households decreased by 27.2 percent. These households declined from 49.6 to 22.4 percent. At the same time, the percentage of married working women increased from 32 to 51 percent. While 26.3 million mothers stayed at home, 31.8 million went to work.[66]

In a study of attitudes and practices of roles among 1,518 cases (759 husbands and their wives), Albrecht, Bahr, and Chadwick found greatest acceptance of the female provider role among younger study participants (under 30 years of age). Most respondents favored the traditional role of greater wife involvement in the child care and housekeeper roles. A majority of participants felt that kinship roles should be shared.

When role enactment (the actual carrying out of a role) was investigated, a higher percentage of older respondents (over 65) shared the provider role. Women of all ages were more likely to have a larger role in housekeeping, kinship, and child care. Most role sharing was seen in the kinship role. Some was seen in the child care role.

Women made decisions about housekeeping and child care. Some shared decisionmaking was seen in the child care and provider roles. Husbands under 30 were more likely to be involved in decisionmaking about children. Most shared decisionmaking was seen in the kinship role.[67]

Smith states, "Research indicates that although dual career couples may have egalitarian attitudes, women are still responsible for the majority of domestic tasks. Further, both partners generally relegate the wife's career to secondary status—second to her husband's career and second to her roles as homemaker, wife, and mother."[68]

Formal and informal roles. Roles may be

formal or informal. "Whereas formal roles are explicit, roles which each family role structure contains (father-husband, etc.), informal roles are implicit, often not apparent on the surface, and are played to meet the emotional needs of individuals and/or to maintain the family's equilibrium."[69]

Examples of informal roles include the following:

Encourager	Harmonizer
Initiator-contributor	Compromiser
tor	Follower
Blocker	Recognition-seeker
Dominator	The Great Stone
Martyr	Face[70]
Pal	

Role variation. Families may base their roles on the pattern the culture provides. They also arrive at decisions about roles through interaction, negotiation, and trial and error.

Roles may vary considerably, within and across cultures. This is true for the husband-father, wife-mother, and child-sibling roles. Expectations concerning role performance may be strong or weak. To determine importance of role expectations, sanctions applied for not meeting expectations are a good indicator.[71]

Example
Lisa was supposed to be in from her date at midnight on the weekend. While attending a party, she didn't notice the time and arrived home at two hours past her curfew. Her parents had waited up for her. Lisa was grounded the following weekend.

Role complementarity is the match between role performance and the expectations of the partner in the role relationship. When complementarity doesn't exist, conflict occurs.[72] This conflict may arise from within or outside the person. Intrarole conflict occurs when there are conflicting expectations about one role the individual holds. Interrole conflict occurs when two or more roles of the individual conflict with each other.[73]

The concept of roles is important in understanding and promoting adequate family functioning. There is wide variation in the way families enact roles. Roles can be changed if they are not satisfying and if the family is willing to negotiate. A frequent nursing role is to help families maintain healthy roles and to learn new ones when they are needed. Families can be helped to learn new roles by teaching, role modeling, and role playing.

Power. When boundaries and roles are decided, the method of decisionmaking is an indicator of power in the family. Various authors have described power as the ability to influence the behavior of another, to influence a decision, to achieve intended outcomes or goals, or to influence the emotions of others.[74–77] Power is a concept with multiple dimensions. In all systems, it is dynamic, not static.

Friedman says that there are six bases of power.[78] **Legitimate power,** also called primary authority, is the shared belief that one person in the system has the right to make decisions for others in the system. Such power is traditionally based. The power of elected members of Congress to enact laws for the health of the nation is legitimate power. Another example is found in the Smith family. Mr. Smith, the breadwinner, makes all the decisions. Mrs. Smith regards this decisionmaking power as her husband's right. This is a traditionally based power, which has the status of legitimacy in such a family. In families where women work, it is less commonly seen.

Referent power is the influence of one person over another. This occurs through positive identification with the person possessing power. In this situation the person with less power adopts behaviors and attitudes similar to those held by the person in power. Referent power may be seen when clients positively identify with good role models in the health care system. This can be a sound influence in fostering the adoption of positive health behaviors such as stopping smoking.

Expert power, based on the perception that a person or group has particular knowledge or skills, is important in the health care system. One of the reasons Mrs. Stokes consented to having her baby delivered by a nurse-midwife is because of her belief in the knowledge and skill of the nurse-midwife.

The expectation that a person has the resources to reward others is **reward power.** In the practice of nursing, the nursing supervisor will have reward power because of her ability to grant time off and to recommend promotions and merit pay increases. Patients may be vested with a certain amount of reward power in their appreciation of the nurse's efforts, although this should not influence quality of care.

Coercive power is the expectation that punishment will occur if something is not done. Husbands and wives who physically abuse one another are using coercive power. Nurses may have to use it when telling a mother that her child is not allowed in school without immunizations.

Informational power is the power of a message to convince the recipient of the message that change is necessary. Television commercials have strong informational power. Health brochures may have informational power.[79]

Decisionmaking. An important way to gain understanding of the dynamics of family power is to analyze decisionmaking within the family. Decisionmaking is necessary for the family to fulfill its functions. Areas of decisionmaking include:

- Who decides who will be involved in the decision?
- Who is actually involved? How did this come about?
- What is the relative power of each member?
- What processes are used in decisionmaking? (Processes may include assertiveness, control, persuasion, negotiation, and influence.)
- Who makes the final decision?
- What is the significance of the decision?
- How is it implemented?
- What are its effects on relationships?[80,81]

Decisionmaking reflects how the family meets the needs of its individual members. In the Stokes family, members felt very differently about a decision made on the basis of discussion and consensus as opposed to a decision made on the basis of threatened punishment.

Types of decisionmaking. Families may arrive at decisions through consensus, accommodation, or just by allowing things to happen. **Consensus** is a type of decisionmaking achieved through discussion and consideration of all viewpoints. Everyone agrees on the course of action. There is equal commitment to and satisfaction with the decision made. This kind of decisionmaking is seen more in families where power is shared. It requires the ability to communicate and problem solve.[82]

Accommodation, another type of decisionmaking is "always an agreement to disagree, to adopt a common decision in the face of irreconcilable differences."[83] Accommodation may occur through coercion, bargaining, or compromise.

In **coercion,** one or more family members agree because of an implied threat if they don't go along with the decision. When Suzanne angrily refused to join her family for Thanksgiving dinner unless her boyfriend was invited, she was using coercion to influence decisionmaking.

In **bargaining,** the decision reached may

involve each side's giving up something, but there are elements in the final decision that are satisfying to all concerned. Each party expects his sacrifice to be reciprocated. It is a tit-for-tat arrangement. Joanna and her mother agreed that if Joanna helped her mother with housework in the morning, her mother would take Joanna shopping in the afternoon.

Compromise involves a decisionmaking process where involved parties agree on a course of action that was not the original one. The new course of action has satisfying elements for all. In the Parson family, everyone agreed on a movie to be seen that was not one first choice; compromise had been reached.

Defacto decisionmaking occurs when things are just allowed to happen. Archer refers to decisionmaking by default where all options except one are exhausted. Only one recourse is left open to the family. This leads to crisis management. Those involved can only react and not participate, in shaping events.[84]

Factors influencing decisionmaking. What factors influence decisionmaking? Cultural norms and social class can both play a part. Power may increase, for example, as the husband or wife's income increases. The family life cycle also influences decisionmaking. Women with young children have less power. Their power increases when the children leave home. When men retire, women's power also increases.[85]

Other factors that affect decisionmaking include:

- **The communication network in the family.** If members talk to each other only through a mediator in the family, the person in the mediating role has more power.[86]

- **Implementation control.** Power resides in the person who must implement the decision.

- **Interpersonal resources.** These resources can be influential in the decisionmaking process:

—**Self-confidence.**

—**The meaning and importance of the issue to the individuals involved.** People who are more emotionally involved in the decision will put more energy into bringing about a resolution they want.

—**Restrictive norms.** Cultural norms may inhibit certain kinds of behavior in individuals.

—**Attitudes toward conflict.** Where conflict is viewed as wrong, families may not work at decisionmaking.

—**Importance of relationships.** An individual may avoid conflict or alter his behavior in situations where the relationships are important to him.

—**Formation of coalitions.** Where the majority side on an issue, this may influence the outcome of the decision.

Decisionmaking may be autocratic (decisionmaking for the group by only one person), syncratic (shared), autonomic or atomistic (making decisions for oneself alone or independently of one another), or chaotic.[87]

Power in the family may be demonstrated by decisionmaking. Culture, the family's ability to communicate with each other, the importance of the decision to various family members, and the influence and numbers of those involved in the decisionmaking process influence family decisionmaking.

Adaptation and Communication. All of the processes that take place in a family system are related. Adaptation, as a process, is dependent on the existance of boundaries and how they are maintained, on the availability and use of energy, and on the use of power and decisionmaking within various role structures. Adaptation in the family is the ability of members to change their responses to one another and to the outside environment as the situation dictates.[88] Adaptation is essential in the survival of any system, and in family systems it often makes the difference between functional and dysfunctional families.

Communication processes in the family are closely aligned with adaptation and are frequently the single most important factor influencing equilibrium. Communication in families can be viewed as a subprocess of adaptation.[89] Family communication is the giving and receiving of messages among family members and between members and the environment.

Chapter 11 presents the classic communication theory and gives insight into successful and unsuccessful communication patterns. Communication in families has the same basic characteristics as human communication anywhere, and much of the content of Chapter 11 is applicable here.

In addition, communication in a family tends to take place within the context of its structures. Family members have a tendency to communicate in terms of their roles and how much power or status they have.[90] Families also have distinct styles of communication that can be related to cultural norms, social class standing, and age.[91]

Nurse therapists and community health nurses who work in depth with families can draw more specific conclusions about communication in families from authors such as Virginia Satir. Satir uses communication theory as a basis for her practice in family therapy and outlines many assessment and intervention techniques for working with communication problems in families.[92] Later in this chapter some further examples of assessment of communication in families is given.

Growth and Differentiation. The term differentiation is a systems concept that describes the systems tendency toward growth and advancement.[93] Families, particularly those that are well adapted and functioning within a healthy environment, are continually in a state of change and growth. This growth and change may be manifested physically, emotionally, and socially. Families vary in their ability to grow and change, and the rate of change is particularly affected by various life crises. Each time a family goes through a developmental crisis, such as a birth in the family, new roles are formed, new methods of coping are learned, and behavior and communication patterns change. In therapeutic situations where the nurse is in the role of family counselor or therapist, growth can take place similarly through changes in communication style, lifestyle, interpersonal relations, and interpersonal transactions.[94]

FAMILY FUNCTIONS AND THE FAMILY LIFE CYCLE

Family Functions. Most families have specific and fundamental functions in common. These functions can be broadly categorized into biological, economic, educational, affectual, status conferring, recreational, religious, and protective.[95] Friedman views family functions as outcomes or consequences of the family structure and identifies the following additional and more specific functions: socialization of children and social placement function, family coping function, and physical and health care function.[96] Basically, functions describe what the family does in order to meet its goals and maintain a balance, both within itself and in relation to outside systems.

The biological function of the family is primarily reproductive and provides for the creation of family members, the society, and continued human survival. This most basic function traditionally has been seen by many families and groups of people as a moral obligation to society, a requirement or necessity in which all families participate. Increasingly, however, the birth of children is not viewed within such rigid boundaries, and families feel more freedom to choose whether or not they will participate in this function.

Meeting the sexual needs of adult partners in the family is also part of this biological function. In the past, the sexual relationship was taken somewhat for granted and often not identified explicitly as a responsibility. Heightened public and professional awareness about sexuality and sexual functioning have been very positive in regard to understanding this function and promoting its healthy adaptation in families.

The economic function of the family is to provide financial resources to meet the needs of the family. As discussed earlier in this chapter, American families are extremely dependent on financial income. With few exceptions, most goods, services, and other resources needed by the family are obtained through financial arrangements. This function entails allocation of resources as well as attainment of them. Family values, educational level, personal needs, and a host of other circumstances contribute to how families decide to spend their money and balance income with expenditures. There are considerable health care implications related to the economic situations of families, such as the high incidence of disease and prevalence of ill health among poor families.[97] Unemployment and work related disabilities also have health care implications and pose great threats to this vital function.

The educational function of the family pertains primarily to the socialization of children and helping them to fit into the structure of society. The socialization process helps children form acceptable behavior patterns and skills, develop a personal value system, learn about cultural traditions, and learn to live satisfactorily with their fellows. More specifically, this function provides children with a sense of right and wrong, of what is normal and appropriate, and what is accepted in the way of role and status.[98] This crucially important process is one of the most significant family functions and provides influences that mold basic attitudes and personality characteristics for life.

The family function of protecting and nurturing is interrelated with all other functions of a family. In the United States, this function is recognized legally as well as traditionally; all states have laws requiring parents to support their children, and many laws broadly support parental authority.[99] Families function to provide a safe environment for their members, especially young children. Physical and mental health is protected by meeting basic nutritional needs, a safe and warm shelter, love, affection, emotional interaction, and health care. Another term used to describe much of the essence of the protective function is **parenting.** Parenting behaviors are functions passed down from generation to generation and include roles of teaching and modeling as well as protection.[100] Also, adult members of the family frequently need protection, particularly from some of the stresses and strains of modern life. The family unit can function as a haven or safe retreat where people can feel trust and regain their equilibrium.

Meeting recreational needs is another function that families perform. Recreation refers to activities that take place during leisure time and that are not connected to obligations of work or school. These activities vary greatly from family to family and within families and may include religious, educational, civic, cultural, sports, or entertainment activities.[101] Helping younger family members to use their free time constructively and develop special interests or hobbies is an essential aspect of this function. The fostering of pleasurable and diverting activities also helps the family to relax and reduce day-to-day stresses. Whether quietly reading alone, enjoying a family picnic, or playing a vigorous game of handball, it is important that the family sanction and support these kinds of activities.

The religious functions of a family vary according to individual beliefs and cultural traditions within the family's history. Many families are members of a particular religion and identify strongly with its teachings and practices. Other families may not espouse a specific religion but follow a special philosophy of life or set of beliefs. An exact definition of the religious function in families is difficult to generalize. It is a function that centers around maintaining a faith or philosophy of life that allows for growth beyond one's personal and immediate needs; it gives a more futuristic and comprehensive framework from which families and individuals view themselves.[102] A religious environment can support and encourage growth and service to mankind.[103] The religious or philosophical element in a family can be a strengthening bond that helps people cope with and understand more about peak life events such as birth, death, serious illness, marriage, and divorce.

Families function to provide each other with love, affection, and emotional support. All human beings have strong needs to be cared for and nourished by others. Just as young children need affection and nurturance for their development, adults need it for continued feelings of security, self-esteem, and emotional growth. From earliest infancy to the most advanced age, the feeling of being deeply loved and valued is an important precondition to meeting life's challenges and expectations, to doing one's best without unhealthy stress.[104] Families carry out the affective function by demonstrating caring and trust through verbal communication, touch, empathy, and numerous other gestures that convey messages of love.

All of the above family functions are related and interdependent. They are all part of a system that works together to achieve goals and relate to other environmental systems and subsystems. In addition, these functions are highly individualized and vary from family to family and culture to culture. They are subject to unique situations, such as economic circumstances, natural disasters, health, and illness. The amount of energy available and the type of decisionmaking in the family system also affect functions and what priority is given to each of them. One of the most helpful ways to understand family functioning is to consider the natural life cycle of families, their predictable stages, and related tasks.

The Family Life Cycle. Families are dynamic social systems that go through predictable stages of development and rhythmic cycles of behavior and activities. As two people come together to share their lives, a family is born. Typically, the family increases over time with children, and each child, along with the parents, continue growth and development patterns. Chronologically, there are births and deaths in the family, and the cycle is repeated. "The family life cycle is a composite of the individual developmental changes of its members and the cyclical changes of the marital relationship itself."[105]

Duvall has identified an eight-stage family life cycle framework that has corresponding developmental tasks. (See in Figure 25-3.)[106]

Although this framework is limited to families with a nuclear structure, it can be very useful in understanding family dynamics and assessing family functioning. It begins by identifying a young couple as they establish their relationship and adjust to forming a household. The second stage begins with the first pregnancy, and the next four stages correspond to events in the developmental years of the children

Stage	Developmental Tasks
1. Married couple	a. establishing a mutually satisfying marriage b. adjusting to pregnancy and the promise of parenthood c. fitting into the kin network (in-laws)
2. Childbearing	a. having, adjusting to, and encouraging the development of infants b. establishing a satisfying home for parents and infant
3. Preschool age	a. adapting to the critical needs and interests of pre-school children in stimulating growth-promoting ways b. coping with energy depletion and lack of privacy as parents
4. School age	a. fitting into the community of school age families in constructive ways b. encouraging children's educational achievement
5. Teenage	a. balancing freedom with responsibility, as teenagers mature and emancipate themselves b. establishing post-parental interests and careers as growing parents
6. Launching career	a. releasing young adults into work, college, marriage, military service, etc., with appropriate rituals and assistance b. maintaining a supportive home base
7. Middle-aged parents	a. rebuilding the marriage relationship b. maintaining kin ties with older and younger generations
8. Aging family members	a. coping with bereavement and living alone b. closing the family home or adapting it to aging c. adjusting to retirement

Reprinted by permission from E.M. Duvall, *Marriage and Family Development*, 5th ed., Lippincott, 1977, p.179.

Figure 25-3.   Developmental Stages in the Family Life Cycle.

until they marry or leave home. The last two stages focus on the couple after all the children have gone.

In families with more than one child, the stages will overlap, and tasks from several stages may be going on simultaneously. Other factors and situations result in variations of the order of stages or completion of tasks. Among these are foster families, families who adopt older children, or those who wait until later in life to have their first baby. A couple may have a 10- or 20-year age difference, for example, and the husband may be planning retirement at the time of the first pregnancy. Divorce, single parenthood, remarriage, and changes in child custody also affect the order and emphasis of the family life cycle. Some individuals or groups never do fit into Duvall's framework. Among these are most homosexual pairings, nontraditional group marriages, communal households without children, and childless couples.[107]

THE NURSING PROCESS

The nursing process is equally applicable in the care of individuals, families, or communities. An understanding of family processes and family dynamics helps nurses to care for family units, to assess the role of the family in caring for ill individuals, and to be aware of the impact of an individual's illness on the family.

Each subsystem in the family influences the other subsystems. Because of these influences, the family is an important determinant in health care practices. Families decide when members are ill, whether care will be sought, and what care will be sought. The family also decides whether to implement prescribed health care. Friedman states that 75 to 85 percent of health care provided is given by the family.[108]

The following discussion of the four components of the nursing process, as it applies to family theory, focuses primarily on the whole family as the unit of care.

Assessment

Family assessment is the collection of data that give a comprehensive and graphic description of a family's structure and cultural makeup, conditions of living, financial resources, communication and emotional support systems, and physical and mental health status of each member. The family is assessed in terms of its internal functioning and its relationship to the external environment. This serves as an important guide in formulating nursing actions, based on family strengths as well as needs or imbalances in the family system.[109] The family assessment is an ongoing process requiring a great deal of trust and open communication between the nurse and the family. Community health and visiting nurses are usually fortunate enough to assess the family in the home setting over a period of time. Each time there is contact with the family, the health status continues to be assessed; the information base grows and changes over time, and the nurse-family relationship deepens.

Information sources. Information sources for the family assessment include the family interview, physical examination of members or the identified patient, information in the family or patient record, videotapes of family interaction, and staff and other community agencies that have worked with the family.[110] An important principle in the ongoing process of conducting a family assessment is to obtain available information before the family interview, if possible. This will help to organize the interview, save the family time, and avoid repetitious reporting of information.

Information for the family assessment can be gathered in any setting, but every effort should be made to interview the family at least once in the home. In this way, the nurse can observe living conditions, the neighborhood, and community characteristics on a first-hand basis and acquire a better understanding of family values and priorities.

Making a Home Visit. Making a home visit is quite a different experience from interviewing a client in the hospital or clinic setting. For nurses who are accustomed to caring for clients in these latter settings or for student nurses making their first home visit, there may be feelings of role reversal or confusion. A person's home is his private domain, a space where he is usually in control, and where he exercises power over who visits and what they do there. On the contrary, the hospital or other health care facility is the domain of the health care worker, and the client is subject to power and control by nurse and doctors. Being aware of some of these feelings and using guidelines presented in the following discussion will help to make home visiting experiences more successful.

Preparatory guidelines that can help organize the home visit and increase chances for things to go smoothly include the following:

- Call the family ahead of time to verify the convenience of the time and make sure they will be at home.

- Verify the family's address and directions for getting there.

- Review the purpose of the visit and make notes regarding your goals.

- Assemble any equipment including health and family assessment forms and educational materials.

Upon arrival at the family's house, observe the neighborhood. Look for such things as safety, conditions of the buildings, and accessibility to shopping and transportation. Are there rodents? Is play space available? Are there trees, grass, and flowers? If so, are they well-tended? Look at the family's house. Is it a single family dwelling, a group home, or an apartment building? Are window panes knocked out? Are screens broken? Such factors are important, because they enhance entry of disease carrying vectors as well as cold and rain.

It is important to ensure that initial contact with the family is as nonthreatening as possible and starts off positively. An amiable introduction to the person who answers the door sets the tone for establishing trust and cooperation. The nurse's attitude should reflect the fact she is a guest in the client's home and considers it a special privilege to visit.

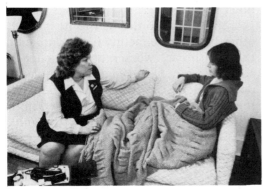

Figure 25-4. An appropriate introduction helps set a good tone for the home visit.

In beginning the interview, it is important to let the family know the purpose of the visit in terms they can understand. The nurse "contracts" with the family regarding what she would like to do in the assessment process, why the actions are necessary, and what expectations and outcomes there are for all involved.

Information obtained from the family interview is a combination of subjective and objective data. Subjective data are all the things the family verbalizes. Objective data are observable things, such as skin color, household odors, and patterns of communication. Family assessment tools are constructed in varying formats, but they all contain basic categories of subjective data (biographical information, family history, family health practices, income data, and so forth) and sections for the nurse to record her observations and other objective data. The remainder of this section discusses the important categories of family assessment as carried out in the ideal setting—a home visit where the nurse can interview family members and observe them interacting.

The Household Roster. The household roster is a listing of all the members of the family and any other persons residing permanently in the home. Biographical information, such as sex, date and place of birth, education, and occupation are included for each person. It is customary to identify the heads of the household first, followed by children, in order of birth. Other relatives and individuals who live with the family are listed last. It is important to clarify the first and last names of each member of the household. Children of divorced or remarried parents often have different last names. Also, mothers of illegitimate children may give the child the last name of his father.[111]

The Family's Health Picture. In order to begin determining areas of nursing need, it is necessary to find out about illness in the family and about health practices that are health promoting. This will help draw conclusions about what the nurse and the family see as problems, needs, and strengths. The questions below serve as guides for assessment:

- Who is currently ill in the family?
- What is wrong with them?
- How long have they been ill?

- What medicines and treatments are being used in their care?
- What is the family pattern of care giving?
- What feelings has the family expressed about their situation?
- What is the frequency of illness among various family members?
- What symptoms of poor health are present in the family—chronic fatigue, pain, abuse, or neglect?
- Are children immunized?
- What is the family's source of medical care? Dental care?
- When did family members last have a physical exam?
- When did family members last have a dental exam?
- Who smokes?
- Is there alcohol or drug abuse of which you are aware?
- What plan of care does the family have in case of emergency?[112, 113]

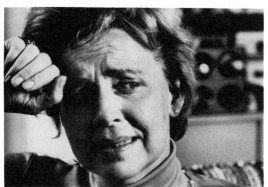

Figure 25-5.   Fatigue can be a stressor affecting the performance of family tasks.

Family Health Practices—Nutrition. A good method of assessing nutritional status is to ask the family to do a 24-hour food recall. Each person who is able to lists everything eaten in the past 24 hours and at what time. On the basis of this information, conclusions can be drawn about ade-quacy of the diet in relation to the body's daily requirements. Other questions help-ful in assessing nutrition include:

- What knowledge does the family show about food?
- Is refrigeration available?
- What cooking facilities are available?
- Who buys and prepares the food? Is the person who buys the food literate? (This affects their ability to read food labels.)
- Does the family have particular food likes and dislikes?
- Are there food allergies?
- Is anyone on a medically prescribed diet?[114]

Safety in the Home. During the home visit, the nurse can be alert to any home hazards. Providing tactful guidance to the family is a very important facet of preven-tive care. Accidents are a major killer of young children. The checklist below will guide you in determining safety in the home:

- Are drugs and poisons kept out of reach of small children?
- Do drugs have safety tops?
- Do you see peeling paint? Peeling paint may have lead in it, and ingestion by young children may lead to lead poi-soning.
- Are there guardrails at steps to protect toddlers from falls?
- Are there nonskid mats and bathtub and toilet handrails for elderly mem-bers?
- Is lighting adequate?
- Are matches kept out of reach of chil-dren?[115,116]

Provision of rest and sleep. Adequate rest and sleep contribute to feelings of mental and physical well-being. In assess-ing this aspect of family life, it is useful to note:

- How much sleep does the family get at night?
- What are the sleeping arrangements?
- What provision is made for rest and naps during the day?
- Does anyone have insomnia? How is this treated?[117]

Emotional Environment. The family provides a vehicle through which individual members develop self-images and feelings about themselves and others. The quality of personal relationships is important in overall life satisfaction.[118] Lockhard asks, "Are family members able to support one another in their daily lives?"[119] When observing the emotional climate in the family, test for the following:

- Is communication clear?
- Are feelings and words congruent?
- What are the interaction patterns like? Is anyone consistently ignored? Who speaks to whom?
- Is differentness accepted? How is it handled?
- Do family members support and encourage one another?
- How is labor divided?
- How is conflict resolved?
- How are the decisions made?
- What stresses is the family experiencing? What coping behaviors do they employ to deal with stresses?
- What functional patterns of interaction do the family use?
- What dysfunctional patterns of interaction do you observe in the family.[120]

Dysfunctional patterns of communication may occur in a family when stress is present, a family member's self-esteem is threatened, and family members don't feel free to communicate. When this happens, Satir says one of the following four com-

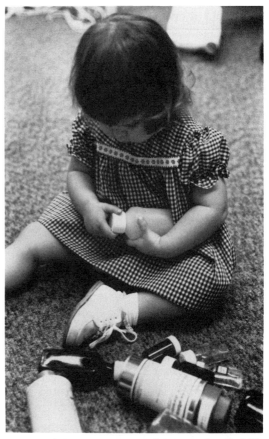

Figure 25-6.   Drugs within reach of children are an invitation to disaster. Families need to provide a safe environment for their members.

Courtesy of the Food and Drug Administration.

munication patterns emerge:

- Placating
- Blaming
- Computing
- Distracting.

The **placator** invariably tries to please the other person. He uses ingratiating behavior and apologies. He fears to disagree. The **blamer** constantly finds fault and plays the boss. If the blamer can feel superior to others, he feels better about himself. The **computer** gives a cool, calm, ultrarational appearance. This belies his feeling of vulnerability. The **distractor** uses words and does things that are not relevant to what is going on. He feels there is no place for him.[121]

Where lack of honesty is present in communication, problems exist. Dishonest communication may hide an ulterior motive and is destructive. The following list gives some examples of dysfunctional communication between couples:

- **Concerning the partner**—John consistently puts Susan in positions where she looks wrong or undesirable. This communication is dysfunctional. Its result is a "damned if you do; damned if you don't" position for Susan.

- **Tell me your problem**—In this case, Ann encourages Ted to reveal vulnerable emotion laden areas and then uses this information with family, friends, and neighbors. She uses Ted's perceived inadequacy to shore up her own feelings of inadequacy.

- **Doing something for the other**—Instead of being able to communicate her own desires or needs to William, Mary communicates that these should be obtained because he needs them.

- **Placing the burden of decisionmaking on the partner**—Although Bob is interested in the outcome of a decision, he often avoids responsibility for participating and then places the consequences of a bad decision on his wife.

- **Courtroom behavior**—Steve often verbally attacks Jean. This puts Jean in the role of defendant. She tries to justify her behavior. If a third party is present he might be called on to act as a judge. Each spouse is more interested in proving himself right than solving the conflict.[122]

- **Camouflage**—In Alice and Mark's marriage, messages are not communicated directly, but are so veiled they can barely be recognized. In this way, the person giving the message does not have to deal with rejection of his message or conflict.

Game playing runs in families and can be passed on through generations.[123] Such games represent manipulation and exploitation.

Couples that avoid discussing their conflicts display dysfunctional behavior. Tensions build in such situations. Tension also builds when couples focus on the conflict and not on the issue. Person centered attacks are common in this situation. The persons involved need to learn that it is more constructive to focus on the issue and respect the right to disagree. It is important, too, for them to learn to discuss alternatives and the pros and cons of these alternatives.[124]

Social Influences. Social influences are an integral part of a family assessment. They include culture, ethnicity, and religious practices. "Spiritual beliefs still affect the lives of most individuals. They influence such things as contraceptive practices, dietary habits, developmental transitions through rites of passage, selection of marriage partners, and reactions to health and illness."[125] Information that is helpful to gather about social influences includes the following:

- Is there a particular ethnic group with which this family identifies? What influence does this have on the family's health practices?

- Does the family practice a particular religion?

- Where does the family attend church? How frequently? What influence does religion have on the family's health attitudes, beliefs, and practices?

Recreation. "Recreation refers to activities apart from the activities of work, family, and society to which the individual and family turn at will for their relaxation, diversion, self-development, or social participation."[126] It is helpful to assess how each member of the family uses leisure time and how they each feel about it. In addition, you can note what the family

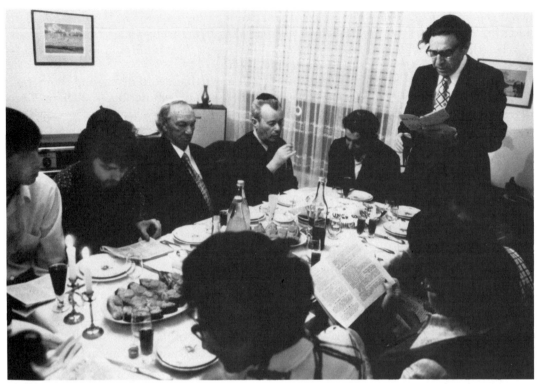

Figure 25-7.   Spiritual practices may provide a rich heritage and form cohesiveness in families.

group does for fun and whether they share activities, or each does his own thing.

Income. Lack of income can be a stressor that enhances the family's susceptibility to illness. It may mean the family is unable to provide adequate food, clothing, medical care and shelter for its members. Questions about money are sometimes difficult to ask. Ann, a student nurse, asked about income in the following way:

> "Mrs. Jones, some families have financial needs that it's helpful to share with the health department, because we may know of some community resources that can help you. Often families haven't had an opportunity to learn about these resources. I wonder if you feel your income is adequate in meeting your family's needs. Perhaps we could talk about it."

Family income may come from jobs, pensions, insurance payments, investments, or public assistance. In some situations, it is important to know the family's specific income for eligibility determinations; a number of government resources and programs require such information. Other factors to consider in determining a family's financial health are whether the family owns or rents its living quarters and what its patterns of debts and expenditures are.[127]

The family's home environment. The home in which the family lives provides clues about factors that may or may not be conducive to health. Relevant questions and observations include the following:

- How many rooms does the home have?
- What provision is made for privacy? Privacy provides space for autonomy, a place for self-exploration, and a place for protected communication.
- How is the home heated?
- Does ventilation seem adequate?
- Is there indoor plumbing?

- Are towels and soap available?
- What laundry facilities are available?[128]

Community resources. "Part of a family's successful coping is its ability to secure compliance from the environment, meaning that within the community the family is able to seek out, receive, and/or accept the appropriate resources to meet their needs for food, services, and information."[129]

- What community resources does the family use? How often?
- What are the family's feelings about the resources it uses? What are their areas of satisfaction? Dissatisfaction?
- What extended kin does the family see?

Family strengths. As data is gathered for the family assessment, it is very important to get an understanding not only of problems but also of strengths. Family strengths are those things that help the family function as a unit and feel better about itself.[130] Characteristics of strong families include the following:

- There is a facilitative process of interaction among family members.
- Families enhance individual member development.
- Relationships are structured effectively.
- Families actively attempt to cope with problems.
- There is a healthy home environment and lifestyle.
- They establish regular links with the broader community.[131]

Otto is a well-known family researcher who studied family strengths extensively. He listed the following characteristics as family strengths:

- Having enough time together

- Freedom to be alone
- Common interests
- A liking/loving/caring for each other
- Mutual commitment
- Shared faith
- Sharing of feelings
- Lots of mutual support
- Common goals, values
- Agreement on handling family finances
- Willingness to forgive
- Fostering spiritual growth in each other
- A good circle of friends
- Having a lot of fun together
- Having a sense of mission
- Good communication
- Freedom of expression
- Good sense of humor
- Respect
- Affirmation
- Shared dreams
- Sharing the work
- Self-awareness
- Good food
- Encouragement of talents
- Developing responsibility
- Capacity to reach out to the family
- Family traditions, celebrations
- Willingness to accept other lifestyles
- Freedom to grow as persons
- Sensitivity to each other's needs
- Fostering creativity in each other
- Self-worth and self-reliance building
- Structures for problem solving
- Interest in world community
- Concern.[132]

Nurses can be instrumental in helping families to recognize and use their strengths. The very act of pointing out strengths to the family can often be therapeutic and enhance coping skills and self-esteem.

Tools in family assessment. Numerous tools exist to help in conducting a family

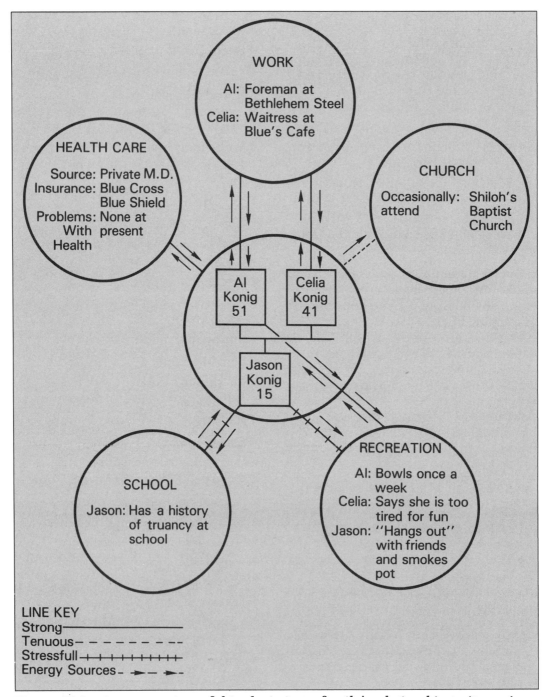

Figure 25-8. An ecomap is useful in depicting a family's relationship to its environment.

assessment. One tool is called an ecomap and is useful in depicting a family's relationship with its environment. It shows the systems with which a family relates and the strengths or weaknesses of those relationships. Developed for caseworkers by Dr. Ann Hartman, the ecomap "examines boundary maintenance aspects of family functioning. It dramatically illustrates the amount of energy used by a family to maintain its system as well as the presence or absence of situational supports and other family resources."[133]

To develop an ecomap, draw a large circle, and place the nuclear family members inside it. Squares represent males and circles represent females. Put name and age of each person in the center of the circle or square. To represent systems with which the family relates, draw circles around the family circle, just as though you were drawing planets around the sun. Examples of systems external to the family include school, work, church, the police department, and the recreation department. Depending on where the relationship exists, connect these systems to the family system or to individuals in the family. A solid line represents a strong relationship, and a line with slashes through it represents a conflict-laden relationship. Use arrows drawn along these lines to indicate direction of the flow of energy. An arrow going in only one direction indicates a unilateral energy flow. The nurse and the client can complete an ecomap together. This joint effort can foster collaboration and help the family achieve greater self-understanding. The use of the ecomap over time can show client life changes in a graphic manner.[134]

The genogram. Another useful tool in family assessment is the genogram which depicts three or more generations of a family. The genogram shows family dispersals, losses, roles, and organizational patterns. Hartman says, "Not only is each individual immersed in the complex here-and-now life space, but each individual is also part of a family saga, in an infinitely compli-

cated human system which has developed over many generations and has transmitted powerful commands, role assignments, events, patterns of living and relating down through the years."[135]

The basic structure of the genogram is described below with suggested symbolic representations. Other symbols may be used as long as a clear key defines the meaning of each symbol.

In a genogram, use circles to represent females and squares to represent males. Triangles represent unknown sex. Within these symbols write the name of the individual and the date of his birth and death. If the person lives in another place, write that underneath the symbol, along with a word or phrase that best describes the person. Draw an X through the symbol of a family member who has died. A solid line between a male and a female indicates marriage, and a dotted line represents divorce. Dates for these events should be given if they are known. Offspring of couples are shown with the older ones on the left. Households may be represented by drawing a dotted line around the particular group. Portions of families that are cut off are also shown by dotted lines. You can use colored pencils to indicate strong communication linkages as well as cutoffs.

Nursing Diagnosis. Data gathered about the individual and his family is the precursor to developing an informed opinion about the family's health status. In the process of nursing assessment, health needs and strengths the family can use to meet those needs will have been identified. Using facts from the data base and principles of client self-determination and client participation in care, the nurse and family can arrive at a list of needs and problems in the family. Because of differing backgrounds and experiences, client and nurse perceptions may not be the same. In any case, a mutually developed set of family needs is always preferable because the client will be more apt to cooperate and assist in resolving problems that he has had a

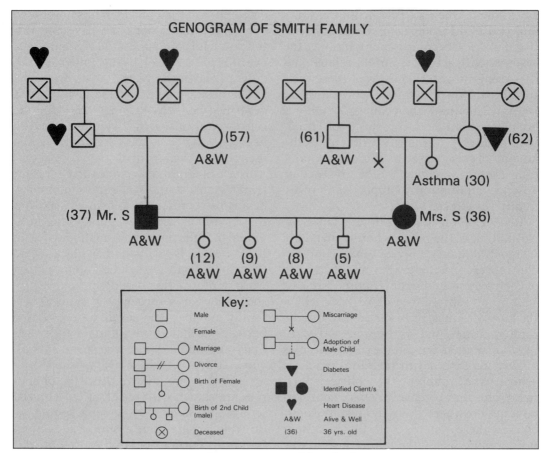

Figure 25-9.   A genogram may show patterns of family functioning across generations.

part in identifying.

It is possible that you will find no health problems. It is also possible that you will find potential stressors and problems that indicate the need for anticipatory guidance. Your nursing diagnosis may indicate the family's health status in terms of anticipated stressors, dysfunctional communication, or role conflict, for example. Problems may overlap. Gordon suggests describing problems and listing the etiological factors and their symptoms. This provides a more detailed framework for reaching goals and intervening.[136]

Efforts are underway, in several nursing practice areas, to develop specific guidelines for identifying nursing diagnoses. The following are examples of nursing diagnoses as related to the family:

- Children not receiving health care: acute, secondary to divorce and a legal custody struggle.

- Difficulty in reallocating family roles: acute, secondary to serious illness and hospitalization of an adult family member.

- Inability to accomplish stage-specific developmental tasks; chronic, secondary to dysfunctional family communication patterns.

- Economic hardship; potential, secondary to prolonged union strike.

- Acceptance of a new family members; potential, secondary to plans for adoption.

- Wife abuse; intermittent, secondary to husband's emotional illness.

- Acute medical emergencies; intermittent, secondary to family's lack of knowledge.
- System input deprivation; chronic, secondary to living in a nursing home.
- Anger; chronic, secondary to being identified as a cultural minority.
- Disruption of family transactions; acute, secondary to family reaction to discovery that a member is homosexual.[137]

As you and the family sort out the problems, rank them in order of importance to the family. This will help you to know where to begin. In multiproblem families, a long list of problems can seem overwhelming! When the client's life is at stake or community safety is jeopardized, you may not be able to begin where the client wishes.

Example
Miss Goodwin visited the Scoloni family to find out why Mrs. Scoloni hadn't brought 1-year-old Tina to the clinic for her checkup. The Scoloni's had no telephone. When Miss Goodwin arrived she found Mrs. Scoloni in tears. Mrs. Scoloni feared she was pregnant, their 3-year-old needed to be hospitalized for a hernia repair, and Mrs. Scoloni's mother had just died. Mrs. Scoloni said she needed to talk to someone about how much she missed her mother and how she feared she couldn't manage without her. Miss Goodwin wisely decided not to discuss Tina's clinic visit with Mrs. Scoloni. She listened while Mrs. Scoloni verbalized her fears. After a while Mrs. Scoloni began to relax. Miss Goodwin pointed out some of the strengths she had noticed in Mrs. Scoloni's care and warm concern for her children. She made an appointment to return in a few days to discuss Mrs. Scoloni's other concerns.

Part of problem identification is to sort out those problems you can do something about, those more effectively handled by other members of the health team, and those that can't be handled because of agency or client constraints.

Example
When Miss Goodwin was reviewing Mrs. Scoloni's case, she decided to counsel her about her feelings of loss in relation to the death of her mother. Mrs. Goodwin referred her for pregnancy testing. It turned out that Mrs. Scoloni was pregnant. Although there were abortion services in the community, abortion was not an option for Mrs. Scoloni. She was a deeply religious woman, and her religion prohibited abortion.

Planning

When problems or needs in the family have been identified, the next step is to develop a plan. "The nursing care plan serves as a blueprint for action."[138] Developing a plan with the family involves mutual goal setting and strategy formation. "A strategy is a plan, method, or series of actions designed to lead to a desired outcome. In nursing, strategies represent the general plan or methods by which nursing action may be brought to bear so as to improve the health of families."[139] Goals must be clear, acceptable to the family, specific, and measurable.

Example
Miss Goodwin was working with Mrs. Asher on improving her communication patterns. Mrs. Asher recognized that she had a tendency to make unilateral decisions in her family. She didn't give others a chance to speak. The family was going to start making vacation plans, so Mrs. Asher developed the following goals with Miss Goodwin's help: "When our family meets this Friday night to discuss vacation plans, I will not give my opinion until I have heard what others in the family think. I will let others know I have heard what they say by restating their opinions. If anyone has not spoken up, I will ask them what they think."

It is useful to set goals according to psychomotor, affective and cognitive areas. In this way goals can be set according to what the client wants to do, feel, or know. Goals should reflect whether they are client or nurse focused.[140] The former refers to goals the client is to achieve; the latter refers to goals for the nurse to achieve.

Miss Goodwin and Mrs. Asher developed the following client centered goals for Mrs. Asher:

> **Example**
> "On Miss Goodwin's next visit, I will demonstrate knowledge of good communication by listing principles of good communication (cognitive goal). I will demonstrate ability to correctly apply knowledge of congruent communication through role playing (cognitive and psychomotor goals). I will work on increasing my self-esteem by discussing at least three strengths I think I have with Miss Goodwin (affective and cognitive goals).

Miss Goodwin's goals were the following:

- In relation to Mrs. Asher's cognitive goals of learning the principles of good communication, I will review these principles with her on my next visit.
- In relation to Mrs. Asher's cognitive and psychomotor goals of being more congruent in her communication, I will review the use of "I feel" messages with her on my next visit.
- Regarding Mrs. Asher's affective goal of feeling better about herself, I will review a tape on self-affirmation with her on my visit after next.

When goals are decided, the next part of the nursing process is to list alternatives and resources for reaching them. These may include the family, the nurse, and other community resources. Pros and cons of alternatives are listed. The nurse must continually ask herself whether the alternatives will enhance the coping ability of the family and whether the family understands the various courses of action. As part of the goal setting process, the nurse and the family may develop a contract that includes the goals, the length of the contract, family and nurse responsibilities, and fees if they are charged. Not every client has the motivation, insight, or ability to participate fully in a contract setting, but many can. A contract helps clarify the purpose of the visits and encourages self-care.

Implementation.

Implementation is the third component of the nursing process and an important area for the family's involvement in its own care. Client desires, agency constraints, and cultural variables to interact to influence implementation. Components of the nursing role in implementation are:

- **Surveillance**—Your surveillance of the family's health status involves screening, monitoring through observation and interview, and physical examination.

- **Teaching**—Teaching a family about illness prevention, health maintenance, and skill development to implement a therapeutic regime are important parts of the nursing role. In teaching families, a cardinal rule is to assess learning needs first.

- **Counseling**—You may interact with the client system to help effective communication or change a behavior the client wishes to change.

- **Referring**—There are a number of health resources in the community to which you can refer the family. These resources may provide financial, educational, vocational, medical, and social services.

- **Case finding**—Determining exposure to communicable disease in family members is often the first step in preventing harmful effects of the disease.

- **Collaboration**—Working with other members of the health team is essential in providing multidisciplinary care that the family needs to achieve its optimum level of functioning.

• **Direct care**—Laying on of hands is an important part of the nurse's role.[141]

The life cycle. Part of the nursing intervention is based on the position of the family in the life cycle.

> "For about two years the average family will be childless; for the next twenty years or so, child bearing and child rearing will be central concerns, followed by about six years when children are leaving home for college, marriage or careers. For approximately 13 years the older couple will be living alone once more, and for the following 16 plus years, the family will be reduced to a widow or widower."[142]

Friedman says that health concerns vary according to stages of the family life cycle.[143] In the beginning, family sexual adjustment, role adjustment, family planning, and prenatal education are primary concerns. For a homosexual couple, sexual and role adjustment are areas of concern.

In the early childbearing stage of the family life cycle, maternity and post-partum care, family planning, well baby care, childproofing the home, obtaining knowledge about child development, and developing communication skills may be needs. Parents with preschool children have other health concerns. These include protecting children from accidents, arranging for time alone and time together, encouraging socialization of the child, integrating new family members, and caring for children who may have communicable diseases.

When the child enters school, parents need to encourage realistic school achievement for the child as well as work on maintaining a satisfactory marital relationship. As children enter their teen years, automobile, drug, and sex education are important. Parents must also tend to factors such as diet, rest, and exercise in their own lives.

When children leave home, parental health concerns may center around menopause and emerging chronic health conditions. Parents may need help adjusting to changes brought about by their roles as grandparents and also by their aging parents. They may need assistance in re-establishing communication in their own marriage.

The family in retirement may need the nurse's help in dealing with economic, housing, social, and work losses. Health problems may pose special needs. A family member's approaching death may require skilled intervention.[144]

Evaluation.

The last step in the nursing process is to evaluate the outcome of care. This means determining if objectives and goals of care have been achieved. Some goals can be measured objectively. A reduction of 20 points, systolically, in a client's blood pressure is an example. Other objectives are measured on a more subjective basis, such as when a client tells you he feels more confident about his ability to relate well to others. Questions to aid you in evaluation include the following:

• What does the family see as outcomes of care? With what areas are they satisfied and dissatisfied? Why?

• Are there any unintended results of care? What are they? (When Mrs. Sebastian went for a blood pressure checkup, the noise, crowding, and long wait in the clinic contributed to a blood pressure increase. This was an unintended outcome of care.) Unintended outcomes can be positive as well as negative.

• Could other members of the health team have intervened more effectively? What would have been the outcome in terms of cost? What benefits would have occurred in the family?

Supervisors, peers, and the nurse's own critical self-awareness are all useful components in evaluating care. This evaluation is fed back into the system and is a basis for altering care, if necessary.[145]

The nursing process is used in caring for families whether you are a community health nurse, a hospital nurse, a psychiatric nurse specializing in family therapy, or a nurse practitioner. Whenever anyone in the family is hospitalized, the patient and his family can experience it as a crisis. It is inevitable that the family will experience some disorganization. Whatever support and assistance the nurse can provide to help reestablish equilibrium and maintain family integrity will be helpful.[146] The community health nurse functions as a highly skilled generalist. Where behavioral or emotional problems are severe, she may refer the family to a colleague specializing in psychiatric nursing. Where physical problems are intractable, she may use the skills of the family nurse practitioner. All have an important role to play in helping the family to maximize its health. Most important of all is the family itself.

SUMMARY

The family system, as a concept, is very important for professional nurses to study, understand, and appreciate. All individuals have been influenced and shaped to a large degree by their family history and family relationships. Most individuals are vitally linked to some kind of family system. Patterns of health and illness frequently correlate with the strengths, emotional climate, and functional status of the family.

The structure and functions of families have evolved over the ages. Early history gives us a very sketchy view of the particulars of family life, but the concept of families being strong unifying forces within the society is evident. Historic events that have had an impact on the family include urbanization, industrialization, and science and technology. Understanding the history of and changes in family functions, values,

and attitudes gives the nurse a baseline perspective from which to better understand present day families.

Families can be studied from a variety of theoretical frameworks. Each of the six frameworks presented in this chapter provides useful ideas and approaches to family study. General systems theory and adaptation theory describe the family as an open, living, social system. The family system has distinct boundaries, functions, and patterns of communication and feedback. As an adaptive system, the family continues to change and grow within a predictable life cycle.

There are specific and fundamental functions that all families participate in. These functions can be broadly categorized into biological, economical, educational, affectual, protective, religious, and recreational. All of these functions are related and interdependent. They are carried out by various members, and by working together, family goals are achieved.

The nuclear family goes through a natural life cycle in which changes in functions and roles can be predicted. Duvall has identified an eight-stage family life cycle that begins with the young married couple and ends with retirement and death. Each of these stages has corresponding developmental tasks that are useful for family assessment and planning.

Understanding family relationships and influences on individuals is inherent in the nurse's ability to carry out the nursing process. This knowledge helps nurses to care for family units, to assess the role of the family in caring for ill members, and to be aware of the impact of illness and hospitalization on the patient's family. Family assessment is a logically planned process of gathering data about the family's physical, emotional, and social situation. It is best carried out in the home setting. The nurse focuses on family strengths as well as dysfunctions. Nursing diagnoses are statements of problems in the family or areas of need or concern. They are mutually arrived at and serve as a basis for planning and intervention.

Developing a plan for caring for the family involves mutual goal setting and strategy formation. Goals are specified both in terms of nursing and client goals. Intervention with families is carried out through health surveillance, teaching, counseling, referring, and casefinding. Evaluation is accomplished by measuring criteria to determine if objectives and goals have been achieved. Whatever the outcome of the evaluation is, it is fed back into the system as a basis for continuing or altering nursing care, as necessary.

The care of families and their individual members is practiced by nurses in every setting. The degree to which family assessment and intervention is carried out varies. Whatever the circumstance, involvement with family groups is a challenging and rewarding part of the nursing experience.

STUDY QUESTIONS

1. Give several examples of how the nurse might use her knowledge of family history in clinical situations.

2. Explain why families are often referred to as open living systems.

3. Give three examples of family subsystems.

4. Analyze the power and decisionmaking structure in a family you know. How does it compare with your own family experience?

5. Give an example of a communication problem in a family. What are some ways in which the nurse might help the family overcome the problem.

6. Draw a genogram of your family or a family you know.

7. Why is it important and therapeutic for the nurse to assess family strengths as well as problem areas?

REFERENCES

1. John Biesanz and Mavis Biesanz, **Modern Society,** (Englewood Cliffs, N.J.: Prentice-Hall, Inc., 1968) pp.209–210.
2. Dennis H. Wrong and Harry L. Gracey, **Readings in Introductory Sociology,** (New York: The Macmillan Co., 1972) p.72.
3. Evelyn Rose Benson and Joan Quinn McDevitt, **Community Health and Nursing Practice,** (Englewood Cliffs, N.J.: Prentice-Hall, Inc., 1980) p.239.
4. Cynthia J. Leitch and Richard V. Tinker, **Primary Care,** (Philadelphia: F.A. Davis Co., 1978) pp.4, 23.
5. Jean R. Miller and Ellen H. Janosik, **Family Focused Care,** (New York: McGraw-Hill Book Co., 1980) p.6.
6. Celeste R. Phillips, **Family-Centered Maternity-Newborn Care,** (St. Louis: The C.V. Mosby Co., 1980) p.207.
7. Jeanette Lancaster, **Community Mental Health Nursing,** (St. Louis: The C.V. Mosby Co., 1980) p.265.
8. Evelyn Millis Duvall, **Marriage and Family Development,** (Philadelphia: J.B. Lippincott Co., 5th ed. 1977).
9. Michael P. Farrell and Madeline H. Schmitt, "The American Family: An Historical Perspective" in **Family Health Care,** 2nd edition, Volume I, Editors: Deborah P. Hymovich and Martha U. Barnard, (New York: McGraw Hill, Inc., 1979) p.57.
10. Miller and Janosik, **Family Focused Care,** p.16.
11. Gerald R. Leslie, **The Family in Social Context,** 4th edition, (New York: Oxford University Press, 1979) pp.147, 148.
12. Ruth Murray and Judith Zentner, **Nursing**

Concepts for Health Promotion, (Englewood Cliffs, N.J.: Prentice-Hall, Inc., 1975) p.348.

13. **Ibid.**

14. Amos H. Hawley, **Urban Society,** (New York: The Ronald Press Company, 1971) pp.120–123.

15. Michael Gordon, **The Nuclear Family in Crisis,** (New York: Harper and Row Publishers, 1972) pp.6, 10.

16. William J. Goode, "Industrialization and Family Structure," in **Family,** ed. Norman W. Bell and Ezra F. Vogel (New York: The Free Press, 1968) pp.113–120.

17. Murray and Zentner, **Nursing Concepts,** pp.348, 362.

18. Irene Mortenson Burnside, **Psychosocial Nursing Care of the Aged,** (New York: McGraw-Hill Book Co., 1980) pp.2–3.

19. Robert E. Rakel, **Principles of Family Medicine,** (Philadelphia: W.B. Saunders Company, 1977) p.249.

20. Edgar W. Butler, **Urban Sociology,** (New York: Harper and Row, Publishers, 1976) p.389.

21. Elmer H. Johnson, **Social Problems of Urban Man,** (Homewood, Illinois: The Dorsey Press, 1973) p.188.

22. **Ibid,** p.97.

23. Miller and Janosik, **Family Focused Care,** p.28.

24. Goode, in Bell and Vogel, **Family,** p.113.

15. Duvall, **Marriage and Family Development,** p.47.

26. **The Washington Post,** "The Calamitous Decline of the American Family," (Washington, D.C., January 2, 1977) p.Cl.

27. Duvall, **Marriage and Family Development,** p.75.

28. **The Washington Post,** January 2, 1977, p.Cl.

29. Mary Jo Bane, **Here to Stay: American Families in the Twentieth Century** (New York: Basic Books Inc., 1976).

30. I. Nye and F. Berardo, **Emerging Conceptual Frameworks in Family Analysis,** (New York: MacMillan Co., 1966).

31. Marilyn M. Friedman, **Family Nursing, Theory and Assessment.** (New York: Appleton-Century-Crofts, 1981) p.45.

32. Arlene S. Skolnick and Jerome H. Skolnick, **Family in Transition,** (Boston: Little Brown and Co., 1971).

33. Friedman, **Family Nursing,** 44–47.

34. Catherine W. Tinkham and Eleanor F. Voorhies, **Community Health Nursing.** (New York: Appleton-Century-Crofts, 1972) pp.146, 147.

35. Friedman, **Family Nursing,** p.75.

36. Carrie Jo Braden and Nancy L. Herban, **Community Health: A Systems Approach,** (New York: Appleton-Century-Crofts, 1976) p.36.

37. Friedman, **Family Nursing,** p.8.

38. F. Ivan Nye and Felix W. Berardo, **The Family** (New York: The Macmillan Company, 1973) p.16.

39. Barbara Spradley, **Community Health Nursing—Concepts and Practices** (Boston: Little, Brown, and Co., 1981) p.239.

40. John G. Red Horse, "Family Structure and Value Orientation in American Indians," **Social Casework,** Vol. 61, No. 7 (September, 1980) pp.462–463.

41. Friedman, **Family Nursing,** p.9.

42. Spradley, **Community Health Nursing,** p.239.

43. Jay Cocks, "How Long Till Equality?" **Time,** July 12, 1982, p.24.

44. Spradley, **Community Health Nursing,** p.239.

45. Friedman, **Family Nursing,** p.8.

46. Nick Stinnett and James Walter, **Relationships in Marriage and Family** (New York: Macmillan Co., 1977) p.36.

47. Nye and Bernardo, **The Family,** p.16.

48. **Ibid.,** pp.43–46.

49. **Ibid.,** p.36.

50. **Ibid.**

51. Red Horse, "Family Structure and Value," p.462.

52. Susan L. Jones, **Family Therapy—A Comparison of Approaches** (Bowie, MD: Robert J. Brady, 1980) p.76.

53. David Kantor and William Lehr, **Inside the Family** (New York: Harper and Row, 1976), p.37.

54. **Ibid.,** p.42.

55. Robert Sommer, **Personal Space,** (Englewood Cliffs, N.J.: Prentice-Hall, Inc., 1969) p.39–57.

56. Kantor and Lehr, **Inside The Family,** p.42.

57. **Ibid.,** pp.42–44, 82–89.

58. Jones, **Family Therapy,** pp.63–64.

59. Kantor and Lehr, **Inside the Family,** pp.44–46.

60. **Ibid.,** p.91.

61. Friedman, **Family Nursing,** p.149.

62. F. Ivan Nye, **Role Structure and Analysis of the Family** (Beverly Hills: Sage Publications, 1976), p.vii.

63. Friedman, **Family Nursing,** p.149.

64. Nye and Berardo, **The Family,** p.265.

65. F. Ivan Nye and Viktor Gecas, "The Role Concept: Review and Delineation," in

Role Structure and Analysis of the Family, p.13.

66. Jay Cocks, "How Long Till Equality?", p.21.

67. Stan L. Albrecht, Howard M. Bahr, and Bruce Chadwick, "Changing Family and Sex Roles: An Assessment of Age Differences," **Journal of Marriage and the Family,** Vol 41, No. I (February, 1979) pp.41–50.

68. Audrey D. Smith, "Egalitarian Marriage Implications for Practice and Policy," **Social Casework,** Vol. 61, No. 5 (May, 1980), pp.288–295.

69. Friedman, **Family Nursing,** p.156.

70. **Ibid.**

71. **Ibid.,** p.151.

72. Nye, **Role Structure,** p.24.

73. Friedman, **Family Nursing,** p.151.

74. **Ibid.,** p.130.

75. Nye and Berardo, **The Family,** p.307.

76. Gerald W. McDonald, "Family Power: The Assessment of a Decade of Theory and Research, 1970–1979," **Journal of Marriage and The Family,** Vol. 42, No. 4 (November, 1980), 843.

77. Letha Scanzoni and John Scanzoni, "Progress in Marriage: Power, Negotiation, and Conflict" in **Family Factbook** ed. Helene Lopata, p.132.

78. Friedman, **Family Nursing,** p.131–132.

79. **Ibid.**

80. McDonald, "Family Power" p.844.

81. Friedman, **Family Nursing,** p.132.

82. **Ibid.,** p.133.

83. **Ibid.,** p.134.

84. Sara E. Archer, "Politics and Economics: How Things Really Work," in **Community Health Nursing—Patterns and Practices,** 2nd ed. by Sarah E. Archer and Ruth Fleshman (North Scituate, Massachusetts, Massachusetts: Duxbury Press, 1979) p.286.

85. Nye and Berardo, **The Family,** p.305.

86. Friedman, **Family Nursing,** p.134–135.

87. **Ibid.,** p.135–138.

88. P.H. Glasser and L.N. Glasser, **Families in Crisis,** (New York: Harper and Row, 1970) p.8.

89. Joanne E. Hall and Barbara R. Weaver **Distributive Nursing Practice,** (Philadelphia: J.B. Lippincott Co., 1977) p.110.

90. **Ibid.,** p.111.

91. Miller and Janosik, **Family-Focused Case,** p.141.

92. Virginia Satir, **Conjoint Family Therapy,** (Palo Alto, California: Science and Behavior Books, Inc., 1967).

93. Friedman, **Family Nursing,** pp.74, 78.

94. Rosemary J. McKeighen "Principles of Family Counseling" in **Family Health Care,** Vol. I by Debra Hymovich and Martha Underwood. 2nd edition (New York: McGraw-Hill Book Co., 1979) p.312.

95. Rakel, **Family Medicine,** p.264.

96. Friedman, **Family Nursing,** p.84.

97. Harold Herman and Mary Elisabeth McKay, **Community Health Services** Washington D.C.: International City Managers' Association, 1968. p.180.

98. Friedman, **Family Nursing,** p.85.

99. **Parenting: A Parent's Workbook,** (The American Red Cross, 1978) p.13.

100. Mary Jo Bane, **Here to Stay,** p.100.

101. Friedman, **Family Nursing,** p.97.

102. Evelyn Duvall, **Faith in Families,** (Chicago: Rand McNally and Company, 1970) p.32.

103. **Ibid.**

104. Daniel A. Prescott "Role of Love in Human Development" **in Marriage and Family in the Modern World,** (New York: Thomas Y. Crowell Co., 1960) p.191.

105. Rakel, **Principles of Family Medicine,** p.279.

106. Duvall, **Marriage and Family Development** p.137–148.

107. **Ibid.**

108. Friedman, **Family Nursing,** p.229.

109. Claire Tuchalski, "Identification of Needs of Goals" in **Community Health Nursing** by Ilse R. Leeser, Claire Tuchalski, and Rosine Carotenuto (Flushing, New York: Medical Examination Publishing Co., Inc., 1975) 76–83.

110. **Ibid.**

111. Helen Cohn and Joyce Tingle, **Manual for Nurses in Family and Community Health,** 2nd ed. (Boston: Little, Brown, and Co., 1974) p.10.

112. Paulette Robischon and Judith A. Smith, "Family Assessment" **in Family Centered Community Health Nursing,** Vol. I, ed. Adina M. Reinhardt and Mildred D. Quinn (St. Louis: The C.V. Mosby Co., 1977) p.45.

113. Friedman, **Family Nursing,** p.303–304.

114. **Ibid.,** p.303.

115. Tuchalski, "Identification of Needs and Goals," p.76.

116. Friedman, **Family Nursing,** p.303–304.

117. **Ibid.,** p.303.

118. **Ibid.,** p.99.

119. Carol Lockhart, "Family-Focused Community Health Nursing in the Home" in **Community Health Nursing** by Archer and Fleshman, p.165.

120. Friedman, **Family Nursing,** p.302–303.

121. Virginia Satir, **Peoplemaking** (Palo Alto, California: Science and Behavior Books, Inc., 1972), p.59–79.
122. Stinnett and Walter, **Relationships in Marriage and Family,** p.129–133.
123. **Ibid.,** p.136.
124. **Ibid.,** p.155–162.
125. Susan A. Clemem, Diane G. Eigsti, and Sandra McGuire, **Comprehensive Family and Community Health Nursing,** (New York: McGraw Hill Co., 1981), p.159.
126. Friedman, **Family Nursing,** p.97.
127. **Ibid.,** p.95–96.
128. Robischon and Smith, "Family Assessment," p.95.
129. Friedman, **Family Nursing,** p.102.
130. Spradley, **Community Health Nursing,** p.181.
131. **Ibid.,** p.182.
132. Hebert Otto, "Developing Human and Family Potential" **Building Family Strength** by Nick Stinnett, Barbara Chesser, John DeFrain (Lincoln: U. of Nebraska Press, 1979), pp.39–50.
133. Clemen, Eigsti, and McGuire, **Comprehensive Family and Community Health Nursing,** p.163.
134. Ann Hartman, "Diagrammatic Assessment of Family Relationships," **Social Casework,** Vol. 59, No. 8 (October, 1980), 465–472.
135. **Ibid.,** p.472.
136. Friedman, **Family Nursing,** p.33.
137. Lillie M. Shortridge and Juanita Lee, **Introduction to Nursing Practice** (New York: McGraw-Hill Book Co., 1980), p.496.
138. **Ibid.,** p.35.
139. Ruth B. Freeman and Janet Heinrich, **Community Health Nursing Practice,** 2nd Ed. (Philadelphia: W.B. Saunders Co., 1981) p.100.
140. Clemen, Eigsti, and McGuire, **Comprehensive Family and Community Health Nursing,** p.202.
141. Friedman, **Family Nursing,** p.37.
142. Freeman and Heinrich, **Community Health Nursing,** p.101–119.
143. **Ibid.,** p.93.
144. Friedman, **Family Nursing,** p.50–62.
145. **Ibid.,** p.38.
146. Janet Barber et al., **Adult Child Care** (St. Louis: The C.V. Mosby Co., 1977) p.162.

ANNOTATED BIBLIOGRAPHY

Duvall EM: **Marriage and Family Development,** 5th ed. Philadelphia, J.B. Lippincott, 1977. This is a classic textbook on the family and is widely known for the author's original work on the concept of the family life cycle and family developmental tasks.

Friedman MM: **Family Nursing, Theory, and Assessment.** New York, Appleton-Century-Crofts, 1981. This is an excellent nursing text on family concepts and family theory. Family health assessment is covered in detail with separate sections devoted to communication patterns in the family, power, structures, roles, family values, and numerous functions within the family. The appendix provides guidelines for family assessment including case studies and sample care plans.

Kantor D, Lehr W: **Inside the Family.** New York, Harper and Row, 1976. This book presents family dynamics with an excellent section on all types of boundaries within families. It is clearly written and gives a thorough analysis of the necessary processes that go on within a family system.

Miller JR, Janosik EH: **Family-Focused Care.** Philadelphia, F. A. Davis and Co., 1978. This general text on families and family health care uses a general systems theory framework. It provides a good overview of family theory and family development and discusses the common events with which families often need professional intervention and help. Sections on assessment, planning, and intervention processes by health care workers are delineated.

26

The Community as a System

Eliza M. Wolff

CHAPTER OUTLINE

OBJECTIVES

At the completion of this chapter the reader will be able to:

- Define the concept of community.
- Describe the epidemiological framework of the host-agent-environment.
- List rates commonly used in community health to describe the health status of a community.
- Describe the purpose of community health nursing
- Describe the role of community health nurses.
- Apply the nursing process to a community health problem.

GLOSSARY

Agent—that factor without which a disease cannot occur.

Community assessment—the determination of health needs of a community based on its health status, its ability to deal with its health problems, and ways in which it is likely to handle these problems.

Community health nursing—nursing of population groups that emphasizes prevention and health promotion, comprehensiveness and continuity of care, and application of current nursing and public health principles.

Epidemic—the outbreak of a disease above that statistically expected in terms of numbers of people affected.

Epidemiology—the study of the determinants and distribution of health, injury, and disease.

Evaluation—determination of the achievement of a goal or objective, or determination of the worth of something.

Host—a species capable of being infected by a disease.

Incidence—new cases of disease occurring in a particular time period.

Planning—the development of an interrelated series of steps to achieve a certain goal or objective.

Prevalence—cases of a disease existing at a particular point in time.

Primary prevention—the prevention of an illness before it occurs.

Secondary prevention—the early detection and treatment of an illness or condition to prevent further damage.

Tertiary prevention—maximum rehabilitation and prevention of further damage from an illness or condition.

INTRODUCTION

Understanding the basic concepts and characteristics of communities is important to nurses in any setting. A person's community often has a great deal to do with his overall health status and his ability to seek care and stay healthy. Nurses will be better able to understand, assess, plan, and evaluate nursing interventions if they can appreciate what the client's community is like. Nurses trained in community health nursing often plan broadly based nursing interventions involving the health of an entire community. For this kind of nursing, understanding community concepts is crucial, since large numbers of people are affected.

CONCEPTS IN STUDYING THE COMMUNITY

The Community as a System

A **community** is a group of people living together in a particular place. These people may share interests, values, and purposes in addition to common boundaries. Relationships as well as boundaries may bind them together. Most definitions of community emphasize people, place, and resources and the relationships that hold these elements together. Groups, organizations, towns, and countries can all be considered communities.[1]

Communities are unique systems, each

having suprasystems, subsystems, and varied inputs, throughputs, outputs, and feedback.[2] Suprasystems of a city are the state, the nation, and the world. Some subsystems of the city are its health, welfare, police, fire, and recreation departments. Suprasystems and subsystems of any community interact to give each community its unique identity.

Types of Communities

Archer and Fleshman categorize communities as **emotional, structural,** and **functional.** They stress that these categories are not mutually exclusive. **Emotional communities** are characterized by a special feeling. Such communities may be "belonging" communities, the place where a person feels at home. Another type of emotional community may be special interest groups. People committed to one another are a powerful tool in obtaining needed care for individuals and groups in that community. Family members, volunteers, churches, and philanthropic organizations may provide needed resources for patients.[3]

Structural communities, those with temporal and spatial boundaries, are divided into six categories: aggregates, face-to-face communities, communities of problem ecology, geopolitical communities, organizations, and communities of solution.

Aggregates refer to any group of people. They may simply be a group of people waiting for a bus. This concept is important when considering disease transmission. **Face-to-face communities** are close-knit, relatively small groups, such as neighborhoods and parishes. **A community of problem ecology** is a geographic area with a common problem. **Geopolitical communities** have definite legal as well as geographic boundaries. Census tracts, wards, and counties are geopolitical commu-

nities. **Organizations** are communities having purpose and structure that bind members together. A health department is an example of an organization. **Communities of solution** are those within which a problem may be defined, confronted, and resolved.

It is important to be aware of community boundaries because culture, policies, services, and reimbursement may vary according to these boundaries. Vital statistics are collected from geopolitical communities such as counties and states. Surveys of health and illness are conducted within clearly defined areas. Differences reflected in morbidity (sickness) and mortality (death) may reflect vulnerable groups needing nursing intervention.[4]

In addition to emotional and structural communities, Archer and Fleshman's third type of community is the **functional community.** The emphasis in these communities is on achievement for the common good rather than on geographic boundaries. Similarities can be seen in the concept of functional communities and the concepts of communities of special interest and problem ecology. Archer and Fleshman break functional communities into communities of identifiable need and critical mass communities. A **community of identifiable need** includes all people with a common problem but does not include boundaries. An example of such a community would be families of abused children. A **critical mass community** implies achievement. It is that combination of resources (manpower, money, equipment, and supplies) needed for the solution of a problem. The concept is an important one when considering the multiple resources that may be used in health care.[5]

The concepts of community emphasize emotion, structure, and function. Knowledge of community characteristics and their relationship and impact on patients will help the community health nurse to deliver effective patient care for individuals, families, groups, and larger populations within the community.

The Concept of Community Health

The terms community health and public health are used interchangeably. In 1920, Winslow defined public health. His definition is still applicable today. Winslow said,

Public health is the Science and Art of (1) preventing disease, (2) prolonging life, and (3) promoting health and efficiency through organized community effort for

(a) the sanitation of the environment
(b) the control of communicable infections
(c) the education of the individual in personal hygiene
(d) the organization of medical and nursing services for the early diagnosis and preventive treatment of disease, and
(e) the development of the social machinery to insure everyone a standard of living adequate for the maintenance of health,

so organizing these benefits as to enable every citizen to realize his birthright of health and longevity.[6]

Epidemiology

Epidemiology is one of the basic disciplines of community health. Epidemiology comes from several Greek words: **epi** meaning down or on, **demos** referring to people, and **logos** meaning study of knowledge. Thus, epidemiology refers to the study of what comes down on the people.[7] Epidemiology is the study of the distribution and determinants of health, injury, and illness in populations. Epidemiological studies provide evidence about the severity and impact of disease and the effectiveness of preventive and treatment measures. This information is vital for planning and evaluation purposes.[8]

In the 19th and early-20th centuries, epidemiology focused on cholera, plague, other acute infectious diseases, and nutritional deficiencies. Today it focuses on determinants of health and ills that affect mankind. Death, disease, disability, defects, social discord, and wellness come under its purview.[9] Investigations of personal and environmental factors related to an increased risk of heart attacks, cancer, and strokes; factors relating to more effective coping in activities of daily living among arthritis victims; studies of factors associated with compliance to medication regimes; studies of accident patterns; and investigations of determinants of suicide, homicide, and violence are some examples of epidemiological investigations.

Host, agent, and environment. The triad of host, agent, and environment is the framework used in epidemiological investigations. Epidemiologists study the interaction of host, agent, and environmental factors and their relationship to health outcome. Intervention may occur in any of the three areas.

Host. The host is that species capable of being affected by disease. Host factors to be discussed in this section include demographic (population) characteristics, health status, genetic susceptibility, body defenses, and health behavior. **Demographic characteristics** include age, sex, ethnicity, occupation, and marital status. Each of these factors may be related to disease. For example, the risk of stroke increases as age increases. Cancer is more common in women. Black males have the highest incidence of hypertension, and black lung disease is associated with the occupation of mining.

Another important host characteristic is **health status.** "Street people," those who have no homes and sleep on the streets, are vulnerable to poor health status. They have an increased disease risk due to lack of shelter, exposure to harsh climatic elements, and poor nutrition.

Other important host factors to consider are **genetic susceptibility** and **body defenses** such as skin, mucous membranes, and the immune system. In addition, the **health behavior** of the population is an important host factor to consider. This includes the population's dietary patterns, hygiene characteristics, health behavior, recreation, and means of handling stress.

Agent. In the host-agent-environment triad, agent refers to the presence or absence of an etiological factor or factors. Agents may be biological, physical, or chemical. Living organisms, such as bacteria, viruses, helminths, and arthropods are examples of **biological agents. Physical agents** include temperature, noise, and radiation. **Chemical agents** include gases, dusts, liquids, and vapors. An example of an **absent agent** leading to disease would be the lack of vitamin C, causing scurvy. Sometimes agents influencing health and illness are unknown.

Agents require a habitat (or reservoir), a portal of exit, means of transmission to the host, and portal of entry.[10] The reservoir may be man or animal—a rat, squirrel, or bird. The diagram in Figure 26-1 illustrates the chain of causation.

In many illnesses today, the pathway is not so straightforward. Diseases are caused by many factors that interact.

Environment. "Major components of the environment may be identified as **physical, biological, social, cultural,** and **economic.** The status of these variables within the environment may enhance or inhibit the interaction between the host and the agent."[11] **Physical** features of the environment include such factors as climate, geography, weather, and terrain. For example, the incidence of muscular dystrophy increases in cold climates.

Biological features include animal and arthropod reservoirs and food supply.[12] **Social** features may include density and crowding, for example. **Cultural** features may include knowledge, customs, language, values, and institutions transmitted from one generation to the next. **Economic** features include income level of the population, level of employment, and sources of production, distribution, and consumption.

The concept of a vulnerable host, a harmful agent or agents, and factors in the environment interacting to influence a community's health and illness patterns are important in understanding a community's health status and providing a framework for intervention.

Methods of epidemiology. The essence of epidemiological investigation is comparison. How does a group with a disease differ from one without the disease? Epidemiologists investigate the who, what, how, when, where, and why of death and disease.

Epidemiological methods encompass descriptive, analytic, and experimental studies. In **descriptive** studies, the epidemiologist describes patterns of health or illness in terms of occurrence, place of occurrence, and personal characteristics of the population affected. By studying these patterns, the scientist may develop hunches about wellness or disease causation.

In **analytic epidemiology,** the epidemiologist employs prospective (forward looking), retrospective (backward looking), or experimental studies to test hypotheses

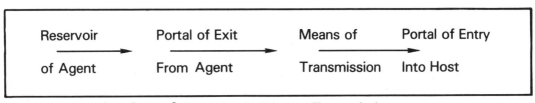

| Reservoir of Agent | → | Portal of Exit From Agent | → | Means of Transmission | → | Portal of Entry Into Host |

Figure 26-1.   The Chain of Causation in Disease Transmission.

about the determinants of health or illness. Inferences are made on the basis of comparisons.

Prospective (forward looking) studies are known as cohort studies. In these studies, the investigator studies selected characteristics of a population over time in terms of exposure to or existence of certain factors. The Framingham study is an example of a prospective study.[13] In this study, a population was studied over a number of years to determine who developed heart disease in relation to cigarette smoking, weight, levels of systolic and diastolic blood pressure, serum lipids, and other selected biochemical factors.[14] Prospective studies are a valuable means of gaining information but are time consuming and expensive to conduct.

Retrospective (backward looking) studies are referred to as case control studies. They refer to the comparison of cases with a particular health pattern or illness to those without it. Individuals without the condition are called controls. A record review to determine smoking history among patients with lung cancer and those without it is an example of a retrospective or case control study. Retrospective studies are not as expensive as prospective studies, but problems with the data may be caused by missing data and incomplete recall on the part of study subjects.

Experimental studies are conducted to determine the effectiveness of a therapeutic or preventive mode of treatment. Study subjects are assigned randomly to treatment (experimental) and control groups.[15] The experimental and control groups are similar on major variables affecting the outcome of the study, but the experimental group is given the treatment and the control group is not.

Incidence and **prevalence** are terms commonly used in epidemiological investigations. **Incidence** refers to new cases of a disease occurring within a particular period of time. Incidence is important in study-

ing the pattern of disease and in the determination of etiology. In order to determine incidence, the following formula is used:

$$\text{Incidence} = \frac{\begin{array}{c}\text{number of new cases of a}\\\text{disease in a defined popula-}\\\text{tion in a given time period}\\\times 1{,}000\end{array}}{\begin{array}{c}\text{estimated population at the}\\\text{midpoint of the time period}\end{array}}$$

Where incidence is short-lived, as in outbreaks of food poisoning, incidence rates are referred to as attack rates.[16] **Prevalence** refers to number of cases at any one point in time. Prevalence depends on the number of people having the disease and the duration of the disease. It is important to know the prevalence of illness because that helps determine resources needed for health care. The following formula is used to determine prevalence:[17]

$$\text{Prevalence} = \frac{\begin{array}{c}\text{the number of existing cases}\\\text{of a disease at one point in}\\\text{time} \times 1{,}000\end{array}}{\begin{array}{c}\text{population at that point in}\\\text{time}\end{array}}$$

Biostatistics. Facts about the health of a community may be displayed numerically with statistics. The term biostatistics refers to the use of statistics applied to biological data. Vital statistics are those events affecting the lives of population groups—births, illnesses, deaths, marriages, and divorce. Vital statistics are collected on the local level and compiled on both a state and national level.

Statistics are expressed as percentages, ratios, or rates. All of these are useful in comparing one group to another. Percentages are used to clarify relationships between numbers based on 100.[18] If 10 out of 40 children contract measles, that is 25 percent. Ratios show the proportion of one group to another and are useful in comparing data. Rates are indicators of community health. They are proportions expressed

1. **Crude birth rate** = $\dfrac{\text{number of live births in a given year} \times 1{,}000}{\text{estimated midyear population}}$

2. **Annual crude death rate** = $\dfrac{\text{number of deaths in a given year} \times 1{,}000}{\text{estimated midyear population}}$

3. **Infant mortality rate** = $\dfrac{\text{number of deaths of infants under one year of age in a given year} \times 1{,}000}{\text{number of live births during the same year}}$

4. **Neonatal mortality rate** = $\dfrac{\text{number of deaths under 28 days of age in a given year} \times 1{,}000 \text{ or } 10{,}000}{\text{number of live births during the same year}}$

5. **Fetal mortality rate** = $\dfrac{\text{number of fetal deaths of specified period of gestation in a given year} \times 1{,}000}{\text{number of live births plus number of fetal deaths of specified period of gestation during that same year}}$

6. **Perinatal mortality rate** = $\dfrac{\text{fetal deaths plus neonatal deaths in a given year} \times 1{,}000}{\text{fetal deaths plus live births in the same year}}$

7. **Maternal mortality rate** = $\dfrac{\text{number of deaths attributed to maternal conditions in a given year} \times 10{,}000 \text{ or } 100{,}000}{\text{number of live births in that same year}}$

8. **Annual age specific mortality** = $\dfrac{\text{number of deaths in a specific age group} \times 1{,}000}{\text{midyear population of the age group}}$

9. **Case specific fatality rate** = $\dfrac{\text{number of deaths in a given time period} \times 100}{\text{total number of people with the disease in the same time period}}$

10. **Annual cause specific death** = $\dfrac{\text{number of deaths from a specific cause in a given year} \times 100{,}000}{\text{estimated midyear population}}$

Table 26-1.   Specific rates commonly used in community health, expressed in terms of the population at risk.

in terms of the population at risk. Specific rates that are commonly used in community health are found in Table 26-1.

The **crude birth rate** is an important indicator in determining population increase or decrease. The estimated midyear population is used to account for population immigration and emigration through the year. The midyear usually is July 1. Crude birth rates are important as one indicator in determining need for programs, such as family planning, childbirth education, obstetrical hospital beds and manpower, schools, and recreational facilities.

Crude death rates require caution in their interpretation because they do not give information about cause of death, whether the death was preventable, and who actually died. More specific information is needed for program planning purposes and for comparing death rates of one group to another.

The **infant mortality rate** is regarded as a highly sensitive indicator of a community's health status. A high rate may reflect poor nutrition, inadequate sanitation, lack of knowledge, lack of adequate health care practices, inadequate shelter, and high infection rates. Rates vary from one location to another and from one ethnic group to another. A high infant mortality rate is a red flag signaling a need for community health intervention.[19]

The **neonatal mortality rate** reflects infants dying in the first month of life. Many infants who die in the first month of life have congenital malformation and are poorly equipped for survival. They are a highly vulnerable population.

The **fetal death rate** is derived from fetal deaths that are categorized according to period of gestation. An early fetal death refers to death prior to the 20th week of gestation. An intermediate death refers to death from the 20th to less than the 28th week of gestation. A late fetal death refers to the gestational period of 28 weeks or more. A death is described as a fetal death if there are no signs of life after expulsion by the mother. Fetal deaths are often underreported because definitions vary from state to state, and abortions are often not reported.[20]

Fetal deaths and neonatal deaths are used to derive the **perinatal mortality rate.** During the perinatal period, the risk of death is greatest until old age.[21]

The **maternal mortality rate** measures deaths associated with pregnancy, delivery, and the puerperum and extends to 90 days postpartum. You will note that in this rate, the numerator is not derived from the denominator. This rate is expressed in terms of 10,000 or 100,000 live births. Because the maternal mortality rate is so low, in order for the number to be meaningful, it must be multiplied by these larger figures.[22] Maternal mortality is an important indicator of community health status.

The **annual age-specific mortality rate** refers to the proportion of people in a particular age group who die in a given time period.

The **case-specific fatality rate** refers to the proportion of people with a particular disease who die from the disease. Note that this proportion is multiplied by 100.

The **annual case-specific death rate** refers to the proportion of the total population dying from a particular cause. Note that this proportion is multiplied by 100,000.

In addition to percentages, ratios, and rates, other statistical indices that are useful in analyzing data pertaining to groups include means, ranges, medians, and modes.

COMMUNITY HEALTH NURSING

Health care outside the hospital setting is becoming increasingly necessary due to the rising cost of hospital health care; the increase in the aging population; and the need to learn to live with chronic illness, manage stress, prevent illness, and enhance the quality of life. The 1979 Surgeon General's Report stated, ". . . of the 10 leading causes of death in the United States, at least seven could be substantially reduced if persons at risk improved just five habits: diet, smoking, lack of exercise, alcohol abuse, and use of antihypertensive medications."[23] Community health nurses can make an important contribution to their patients' health as they teach them about the importance of a healthy lifestyle and help them prevent illness and cope more effectively.

The purposes of community health nursing are to prevent illness, promote health, and provide care to individuals, families, and groups of various ages and health needs in the community. Community health nursing had its beginnings in 1859 in England when William Rathbone established visiting nurse services for the sick poor. Florence Nightingale assisted in training these nurses. In 1879, the New York Mission employed the first visiting nurses in America.[24] One hundred years later, it was estimated that there were 80,523 registered nurses working in community health in America. This was 6.5 percent of the nation's 1,235,152 employed nurses. These community health nurses worked primarily at the local level, particularly for health departments and visiting nurse associations. It was estimated that another 43,539 (3.5 percent) worked for student services, and 28,112 (2.3 percent) worked in occupational health.[25] Community health nurses, whether in a health department, school, industry, clinic, or other type of setting, have an important opportunity to emphasize the importance of preventive, continuous, and comprehensive care as they carry out the nursing process. Community health nurses work with other disciplines and play a key part in promoting the physical, social, and mental health of individuals, families, groups, and communities.

Preventing illness involves implementing and fostering three kinds of prevention. **Primary prevention** is the prevention of an illness before it occurs. **Secondary prevention** includes early detection and treatment of an illness or condition to prevent further damage. **Tertiary prevention** includes maximum rehabilitation and prevention of further damage from an existing illness or condition.

Immunizing an infant against diptheria, pertussis, tetanus, polio, and mumps is an example of primary prevention. Screening programs for hypertension, diabetes, or glaucoma, are also examples of primary prevention.

Coordinating school screening programs to detect possible vision and hearing abnormalities is an example of secondary prevention. Prompt referral and subsequent treatment of children who fail screening programs are important in the prevention of learning difficulties.

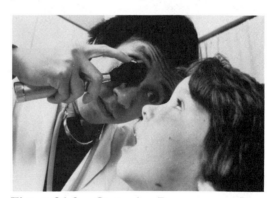

Figure 26-2. Screening Programs are Important in the Detection of Health Problems

Helping a patient revise his work schedule, minimize stress, and follow his diet after a heart attack exemplifies tertiary prevention. This type of nursing care fosters rehabilitation and lessens chances of further damage to the patient's heart.

In community health nursing, prevention of illness and the care of population groups are emphasized. Interdisciplinary care is rendered to promote the health of the whole group. Needs in the population may fall anywhere on the health-illness continuum and may be acute or chronic. Although community health care is usually given to patients outside the hospital, nurses may work in ambulatory care settings and in discharge planning within hospitals. The following example illustrates community health workers in action.

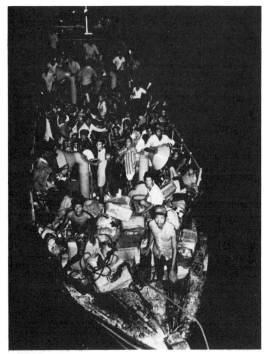

Figure 26-3.   Refugees are a Group with Special Health Needs.

Example

After the Vietnam War, a large number of Indo-Chinese refugees came to the United States. Many suffered severe economic and emotional hardships in leaving their homeland. They came with no possessions; some had lost their entire family. Many were infected with tuberculosis, malaria, and parasites. They arrived in immediate need of food, shelter, clothing, and health care. Community health nurses participated in screening and health programs for these newly arrived refugees as part of a complete health care team. Nursing and medical efforts involved primary prevention (immunizations), secondary prevention (early detection of tuberculosis), and tertiary prevention (treatment of social, emotional and physical illnesses).

Through training in public health and the physical and social sciences, community health nurses and other community health workers were sensitive to the fact that these uprooted people now faced Western values and customs totally new to them. The community health nurses prepared brochures for health care workers on Indo-Chinese customs and, for the refugees, materials on health department services. One way in which nurses assisted refugees in their cultural adaptation was by helping them find stores selling Asian foods. The nurses assisted refugees in their social adaptation by listening carefully and helping them meet other Asian families within the community. Helping refugees to adapt physically and socially was accomplished by providing care in health department clinics and by referring them for language training, schooling, and other needed services. Community health nurses provided care to meet ongoing needs that spanned the health-illness continuum.

Community and Role. This example illustrates a tenet of community health nursing—that role is shaped by health needs of the community.[26] If tuberculosis is rampant, much time may be spent in casefinding and follow-up. Where neonatal and infant mortality rates are high, the nurse may spend more time in maternal/child health programs stressing prenatal teaching and counseling, post partum follow-up, anticipatory guidance, and family planning. The community health nurse's role encompasses **all** facets of a community's health, from rodent control to enforcement of housing codes.

The American Nurses' Association describes community health nursing in the following way:

Community health nursing is a synthesis of nursing practice and public health practice applied to promoting and preserving the health of populations. The nature of this practice is general and comprehensive. It is not limited to a particular age or diagnostic group. It is continuing, not episodic. The dominant responsibility is to the population as a whole. Therefore, nursing directed to individuals, families, or groups contributes to the health of the total population. Health promotion, health maintenance, health education, coordination, and continuity of care are utilized in a holistic approach to the family, group, and community. The nurses' actions acknowledge the need for comprehensive planning, recognize the influences of social and ecological issues, give attention to populations at risk, and utilize the dynamic forces which influence change.[27]

SETTINGS FOR COMMUNITY HEALTH NURSING PRACTICE

Community health nurses practice nursing in a variety of settings. These include official and voluntary agencies, ambulatory care settings, schools, and industry.

Official Agencies

The Local Health Department. Official agencies are run by local, state, or federal government and are funded by taxes. Functions are mandated by legislation.

The official agency responsible for delivering services at the local level is the local health department. It may provide services to a city, county, or a municipality. Historically local agencies have provided programs based on the health needs of communities.[28]

Services of local health departments may include immunizations, maternal and child health care, environmental protection, vector control, family planning, school health, tuberculosis control, home care, chronic disease control, and ambulatory care.[29] The following example illustrates a typical role for a nurse employed by a local health department.

Example
Mrs. McKelvey worked as a community health nurse for a county health depart-

ment. She conducted periodic well-child clinics where children were screened for health problems and mothers were given anticipatory guidance about feeding, discipline, growth and development of their children, time management, and stress.

Mrs. McKelvey also had a caseload of families needing health supervision. Some of these families had members with chronic illness. Others were limited in their intelligence and needed community support. Mrs. McKelvey coordinated their care with members of other social agencies providing services to these families. She made referrals as necessary.

Part of Mrs. McKelvey's role was working as the nurse one day a week in the local school. She coordinated vision, hearing, and prekindergarten screening programs. She counseled teachers on signs of illness in the classroom and conducted health teaching.

Mrs. McKelvey was fortunate that her health department was well staffed. Other community health workers in the health department where she worked included physicians, sanitarians, laboratory workers, nutritionists, physical therapists, occupational therapists, speech therapists, and administrators. A multidisciplinary effort could be brought to bear on community health needs and problems. The funding for programs in which the nurses and other members of the health department worked came from local, state, and federal sources.

The State Health Department. State health departments are less involved in giving direct care to the population, but occasionally they do provide services when these services are not available at the local level. Mobile clinics may travel to local areas with needed services. Health education, environmental control, licensing, administering laws, regulating providers and insurers, financing services given by others, and supporting education and research are some of the services provided by state health departments.[30] State health departments are agencies run by health officers, ideally with training in public health. The following is an example of a nursing role at the state level.

> Miss Godfrey was a nurse who directed the Division of Child Health and Development of the state health department. She participated in policy development for child health at the state level, reviewed legislation having an impact on child health in her state, and supervised program directors in her division. She also directed budget development and deployment of resources, and supervised nursing consultants and other community health workers in her division. The nurse consultants gave inservice education programs for nurses throughout the state, often in conjunction with the assistant commissioner of health, the immunization representative, the child development specialists, and the nutritionist. The nurse consultants conducted health programs with professionals from the mental health department and the social services department. Under Miss Godfrey's direction, the nurse consultants also reviewed and commented on legislation and assisted in the development of the child health standards for the state.

The Federal Level. At the federal level, numerous departments are concerned with various aspects of the nation's health. Most health programs are under the jurisdiction of the Department of Health and Human Services (HHS), formerly the Department of Health, Education, and Welfare (HEW). This department administers the Public Health Service, which at this writing is comprised of the National Institutes of Health (NIH), the Center for Disease Control (CDC), the Health Resources and Services Administration (HRSA), the Food and Drug Administration (FDA), and the Alcohol, Drug Abuse, and Mental Health Administration (ADAMHA). Each of these agencies is concerned with setting policy, providing information and direction for the development of health legislation, giving technical and financial assistance to states, and monitoring health trends.

A number of other departments at the federal level are concerned with America's health. For example, the Department of Defense provides health care to the military, the Department of Agriculture sets daily nutritional requirements and administers feeding programs such as Women, Infants, and Children (WIC), and the Department of the Interior has programs for mine safety.

Nursing is an integral part of the health system at the federal level. Policy development, legislative direction, and monitoring trends in nursing takes place in the Division of Nursing, part of the HRSA in HHS. Specific funding for nursing education, research, and practice is provided by the Division of Nursing. The Office of the Chief Nurse of the Public Health Service also participates in the development of policy and legislation and monitors trends.

Voluntary Agencies

In addition to working for local, state, or federal government, community health nurses may work in voluntary agencies. Voluntary agencies are funded through donations from individuals, professional organizations, and philanthropic foundations. It is estimated that there are over 100,000 voluntary agencies in the United States. The most common activities of a voluntary agency are:

- To raise funds for research and educate the public about specific diseases.
- To launch vanguard programs to demonstrate the value of having the government institute certain services.
- To provide professional advisory services on a specific disease problem.
- To support official agencies.[31]

Voluntary agencies can be described according to those concerned with specific diseases, such as The American Diabetes Association; those concerned primarily with a part of the body, such as The American Heart Association; those concerned with the health of special groups, such as The American Child Health Association; and those involved with particular aspects of health, such as Planned Parenthood.[32]

One well-known community health voluntary agency is the Visiting Nurse Association which is concerned with the care of the sick at home. Community health, physical and occupational nurses, speech therapists, and social workers work as visiting nurses. Funding comes from private contributions, third party payers, and fees for service. In some localities, visiting nurse associations combine with local health departments so that care is given both to the well and the ill. Such agencies are referred to as combination agencies.

Other Settings for Practice

Other settings for community health nursing practice include ambulatory care settings, such as college clinics, industrial settings, neighborhood health centers, proprietary (for profit) home health agencies, health maintenance organizations (HMO), hospices where care to the dying and their families is provided, and prisons.

Occupational Health. Occupational health nursing involves care to individuals in the work setting. Its purpose is to prevent disease and injury and to promote health productivity and social adjustment.[33]

Occupational health nurses have a long history of participating in the protection of the American worker. In 1888, Betty Moulder was employed as a nurse by a group of coal mining companies to care for the sick and injured.[34]

There is a definite need for occupational health nursing in America today. The National Safety Council stated that in 1981, 12,300 people were killed in work accidents and 2,100,000 suffered on-the-job disabling injuries. The total cost was $32.7 billion.[35]

The occupational health nurse may work in mining centers, manufacturing plants, in construction industries, or with migrants. The work includes assessing the health status of workers, monitoring the environment, assessing and reporting hazards, caring for the sick and injured, educating the work force about preventive measures, and assisting workers in rehabilitation efforts. Giving pre-employment physicals, keeping records pertaining to accidents, and observing the workers and their environment provide important data in planning to meet employee health needs.

In large industries, members of the health team include the nurse, the physician, the industrial hygienist, and the safety officer. The industrial hygienist has special skills in environmental analysis and monitoring. The safety officer has responsibility for accident hazards. Small industries may have a one-nurse unit. Companies with less than 500 people may not have a nurse.

The nurse working in an occupational health center deals with health problems of workers that are common to the American population, such as heart disease, cancer, stroke, accidents and health needs peculiar to particular subgroups. Pregnant women are one example. Maisenbacher described an occupational health program for pregnant women in which she gave classes in growth and development of the fetus and community resources. Periodic weight and blood pressure checks were done.[36]

Other health needs requiring the skills of the occupational health nurse may result from the stress of shift work and exposure to particular hazards of the work place, whether this is coal dust in the mines, carcinogenic asbestos and beryllium, extremes of temperature, or noise. Conflict, harsh competition, and monotonous work may produce stress.[37] Other stresses may arise if workers are heads of single-parent families. The occupational health nurse has an important role to play in helping workers and their families manage stress. The nurse's role will be determined by health needs of the labor force, administrative support, professional standards, the law, and policies and resources of the company.[38]

and meeting health needs of students, and coordinates health programs for students. They also serve as a liaison between the school and community health agencies, provide necessary emergency care to children who are injured or ill at school, and work as a member of a team in meeting health needs of handicapped children.[42]

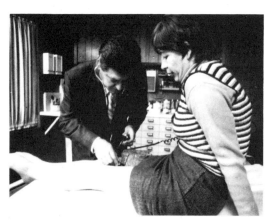

Figure 26-4. Pre-employment Physicals are an Important Part of Health Maintenance.

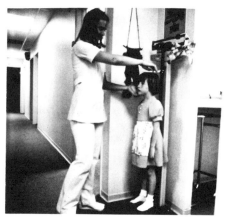

Figure 26-5. The School Nurse has a Special Role to Play.

School Health. In 1902, Lillian Wald and Lina Rogers of the Henry Street Settlement showed that decreased absenteeism in the schools occurred with nursing intervention and followup among children with communicable diseases. As a result, 12 nurses were hired for the schools.[39] Today there are almost 20,000 nurses to care for a large group of students with actual or potential health needs.[40] In 1977, over 60 million people were enrolled in educational programs through postsecondary school.[41]

School nurses may be employed by health departments, departments of education, or visiting nurse associations. An increasing number of nurse practitioners are working in the school setting. The school nurse assesses and monitors environmental hazards, appraises health status of children and refers them for needed treatment, assists teachers in recognizing

THE NURSING PROCESS

In community health nursing, the nursing process is practiced both on an individual level and a level involving families, groups, and communities. The following standards for integrating the nursing process into community health nursing were developed by Helvie and illustrate a systems approach.

- The nursing process is a systematic and continuous collection of data about the health status of the system. This data should be accessible, communicated, and recorded.

- The health-status data provides the data for nursing diagnosis.

- Nursing diagnosis forms the basis for goals and nursing care.

- Plans for nursing care include priorities and nursing measures to achieve the goals derived from nursing diagnosis.

- Nursing actions provide for a system's participation in health promotion, maintenance, and restoration.
- Nursing actions assist systems to maximize their health potential.
- The system's progress toward mutually determined goals is determined by the system and the nurse.
- Nursing actions involve ongoing reassessment, reordering of priorities, new goal setting, and revision of the nursing plan.[43]

In presenting the nursing process as applied in the community, the components of assessment and planning will be discussed primarily in terms of the community as a whole. Intervention will be looked at from the viewpoint of nurses working with individual clients. In this way, the diversity of settings in which nurses can use the nursing process in the community can be illustrated.

Assessment

The purpose of community assessment is to determine needs. These needs are based on an imbalance in the system.[44] Assessment involves collection of appropriate data, interpretation of this data, and diagnosis as a basis for nursing intervention. Community health assessment is the process of "defining a community as a system, identifying the attributes of its components and describing the pattern and organization of the community in reference to its levels of wellness."[45] Implicit in this definition of assessment is an emphasis on strengths as well as needs. There is also an emphasis on data pertaining to the population of the community as a whole. Community assessment is important in understanding influences from various systems that have an impact on individuals, families, and groups in the community. In ap-plying concepts from the epidemiological framework of host-agent-environment, this means analyzing influences from the agent and the environment on the host system. Understanding the interaction of various influences in the community gives a stronger foundation for nursing interventions. Interventions may be direct care (immunizing infants) or indirect care (testifying at a court hearing in behalf of a neglected or abused child).

In any community assessment, observations of the community are important and so are data describing the population, its health and illness patterns, health care usage patterns, health resources, and the interaction of these factors.

Observing the Community. Questions useful to ask in conducting a community assessment include the following: What does the community **look** like? Are the people pale, wan, and listless or robust? Are there a number of vacant homes? What is their condition? Are there rodents? How do people spend their time?

What does the community **sound** like? What are the major sources of noise? When is it noisiest and quietest?

What does the community **smell** like? Are the smells from lush vegetation, from industrial pollution, from sewage, or cooking pots in a small village?

Is this an urban or rural community? What is the climate like? What is the topography like?

What clues arise from the observations in terms of assets and health liabilities that exist in the community?

Using Statistics in the Assessment. In addition to observations, **statistics** are important in community assessment. They may be available from the census, the health department, or local planning groups. Other sources include the Chamber of Commerce, the police department, and the welfare department. Statistics give a numerical picture of people in a community. They show potential groups that may be at high risk.

Particular statistics the nurse will want to know are the age, sex, race, and ethnic groupings within a community. Other important population data include information about education, income, marital status, occupation, and employment rates of the population. These are important in an assessment because of their relation to health and illness. They point to groups needing certain kinds of health care services. For example, populations with large numbers of women in their childbearing years will need maternal-child health services. The elderly will need greater access to hospitals. They are likely to use three times as many hospital days as the younger population.[46]

Employment data is important, because there is increasing evidence of the relationship between exposure to harmful substances in the work environment and health.[47,48] Not only workers but families and communities are affected by hazards of the workplace. Contaminated clothing and pollution from factories may have a harmful impact on members of the community.

Health and Illness Data. Health and illness community data are important in community assessment. Although these data are useful, the nurse should know their limitations. Measuring the health status of a community is difficult because definitions of health vary. Although there are commonly accepted definitions for mortality (death) and morbidity (sickness), errors in diagnosis creep in, and this is compounded when dealing with less precise terms such as physical or social health.

Mortality and morbidity rates and health resource usage data all have been used as indicators of community health. Mortality data show the risk of dying and may be depicted by life tables or death rates. What are the causes of death in the community? How many deaths could have been prevented? How do birth and death rates compare? When considering immigration and emigration patterns as well as birth and death rates, is the community growing or shrinking?

In order to get additional data about the community's health, other questions to ask include: What is the impact of disease on this community and the community's way of dealing with the impact? How many days has the population lost from work? How has school absenteeism been affected? What can people no longer do that they were formerly able to do? How are they meeting their needs? What health resources are available to people in terms of hospitals, doctors, nurses, dentists, physical therapists, occupational therapists, social workers, clinics, nursing homes, and health departments? Are they accessible? Accredited? What is the level of care provided? Is licensing of personnel provided? Are faith healers or witch doctors used? What political, economic, and legal subsystems affect the services provided? What other subsystems contribute to health and are available, such as recreation facilities and religious institutions? What patterns of diet, exercise, rest, alcohol, and tobacco use exist in the population? Personal habits and genetics have been noted as major determinants of health outcome.[49]

Sources of data. Although data are available for the United States and for specific states and counties, data may not be available for smaller areas. There may be an opportunity for the nurse to become part of a team effort to acquire data through a survey. In such a case, the survey organizers may obtain statistical consultation to determine study subjects to be included in the sample. The team may seek advice, too, about the most appropriate tools to use for data collection.

Some data are available from local health departments, the Chamber of Commerce, law enforcement agencies, and other community agencies. Neighborhood residents may have valuable information. One source of data that may be useful to you is information from the census. The census gives a great deal of information about the population, for example, age, sex, race, and median monthly rental. Census data are collected every 10 years in the United States.

Vital statistics (births, deaths, marriages, and divorces) are collected on standardized forms developed by the National Center for Health Statistics (NCHS) of the United States Public Health Service (USPHS). They are gathered on the local level. County, state, and national data are compiled frequently to examine trends in the United States. Classifications for cause of death are based on terminology in the *International Statistical Classification of Diseases, Injuries, and Causes of Death* (ICD), which is revised every 10 years. When classifications change, it may appear that there has been a change in mortality when this is not the case.

The National Center for Health Statistics (NCHS) publishes a great deal of health information about the population that is available from the Government Printing Office (GPO). The GPO health information is based on surveys and provides a rich source of data about health patterns and practices in the United States.

Another source of data that may be useful to you is **Morbidity and Mortality Weekly Reports** (MMW). This publication provides trends on outbreaks of diseases reported to the Center for Disease Control (CDC). The World Health Organization publishes worldwide information about infectious diseases in **Weekly Epidemiological Reports** and **WHO Statistics Annual.** Volume 2 of the Annual is entitled **Infectious Diseases: Cases, Deaths, and Vaccinations.**[50]

Occasionally, a state or local area maintains a registry with information about individuals with a particular condition. This is helpful in determining incidence and prevalence of a disease although problems of definition and follow-up are common. Cancer registries exist in Connecticut, upstate New York, Utah, parts of California,

and Seattle (King County).[51] Other records that may contain useful information about various segments of the population are insurance records, school health records, and results of screening exams.

Prior to making the nursing diagnosis, the nurse should compare the community statistics to statistics of comparable communities if such data are available. This will help her determine the magnitude of a particular problem. Examining trends over time is extremely important in seeing whether a problem is on the rise or on the decline.

Problems may be categorized according to size; seriousness in relation to death, illness, and disability; economic loss to individuals and the community; potential number of people affected; effectiveness of existing and potential programs; and urgency according to public health officials and the public at large.[52] Categorization is useful because it provides a framework for looking at the magnitude of the problem. In addition to Hanlon's framework, categorizing needs according to whether they are physical, social, cognitive, or environmental provides a framework for the nursing diagnosis. Several examples of nursing diagnoses that might be found in the community setting are as follows:

- limited access to health care by home-bound residents related to discontinuing visiting nurse services.

- high incidence of venereal disease in teenagers due to a lack of health education and follow-up programs.

- inadequate social services due to a lack of information and commitment by city officials.

Any assessment involving the health of a community must look at the interplay of environmental, political, social, psychological, and biological factors within the system. Each must be weighted for its relative contribution to a problem, and judgments must be made as to which factors are amenable to change. Community assessment is a prelude to understanding forces having an impact on the population. It is a foundation for sound health planning and intervention for community health.

Planning

When a community assessment is completed, the next step is to develop a plan. In community health nursing, planning may be directed to the nursing needs of an individual or a larger group. The influences of the community on the individual or group must be kept in mind in order that the health plan be realistic. Planning involves ranking needs, developing goals and objectives, and recording the plan. Planning is important in determining needs, allocating resources, avoiding fragmentation, eliminating waste, improving organization and integrating health into other community needs.[53] "Planning is like a system in which each step is a subsystem in itself. The interdependence and interrelatedness of subsystems should prepare us to expect that any step of the process will be subject to change as a result of feedback from the activities in any other step."[54]

The first step in planning is to rank needs of the individual, group, or community. Prioritizing needs on the basis of the nursing assessment, the client's priorities, and where nursing intervention can be most effective is essential.[55] Ranking may be on the basis of numbers of people affected; seriousness of the problem in terms of death, disease, and disability; economic, social, and psychological impact of the problem; and resources available to deal with the problem. If large numbers of people are affected, this should supersede a problem that affects few, unless, for example, the nurse is dealing with the common cold versus an outbreak of polio. Diseases that kill should receive priority over those that do not, assuming there is adequate technology to deal with them. Other fac-

tors to be considered include cultural acceptability of funding, manpower, and propriety and legality of treatment.[56] Political considerations also come into play.

Goals and Objectives. After ranking the client's or community's needs, the next step is to develop goals and objectives. Goals and objectives give direction to nursing interventions. Goals are ultimate ends to be achieved. Objectives (or subgoals) are specific accomplishments or targets to achieve in realizing the goals.

An example of a specific goal for a defined population group is:

Example
In 1985 the health goal in Sawyer Elementary School is to increase immunization levels of new students by 30 percent.

Written goals are often accomplished by a needs statement or statement of justification. This is always done if the nurse is developing a formal proposal requesting additional resources in terms of nurses, money, equipment, or continuing education. An example of a needs statement follows:

Example
The literature indicates that elementary school children are particularly vulnerable to communicable diseases. In 1984, communicable disease absenteeism of 100 children at Sawyer Elementary School totaled 90 percent of all absenteeism. 400 days were lost from school. A plan is needed to reduce susceptibility to communicable disease, reduce absenteeism, and thus maximize classroom learning.

Supporting documentation from the literature and from actual experiences are both important in citing needs. When writing a formal proposal, indicate how the data was obtained. It is helpful to cite examples from the community. This lends depth and validity to the needs statement.

After writing the goals, the next step is to write objectives. Detailed material on writing objectives is given in the chapter on teaching and learning. An example of an objective for the community health nurse is shown below:

Example
The school nurse will screen 100 percent of the health records of school enterers in Sawyer Elementary School to determine which children are behind in their immunizations.

Objectives must be related to goals, because achievement of goals is measured by achievement of objectives.

Once goals and objectives are selected, then it is time to examine and decide on alternatives for reaching them. These alternatives, or strategies, should be outlined with their associated costs and benefits. The nurse may not know the actual costs and benefits of various approaches so there may be a need to consult expert nurses, health planners, or other experts. In deciding alternatives, do not forget to seek input from client groups, too. An alternative that is not acceptable to clients is not viable. When a decision is reached about the best alternative, another statement of justification is needed for writing a formal proposal.

When the alternative is selected, steps and resources necessary to ensure its completion should be drawn up. What is needed in terms of manpower, supplies, and equipment?

List dates for completion of the various tasks necessary to achieving the objective, and schedule a periodic review of accomplishments to date. It is wise to have an experienced person review the plan. Such a person will have valuable suggestions.

Implementation

The next step is implementing the plan. Implementing the plan is putting it into action. It involves carrying out strategies to meet goals and objectives and may require action on both the nurse's and the client's part.

Direct intervention requires a basis of trust between nurse and client. It is important to keep the client's goals in mind and try to see things through his eyes. Careful attention to communication skills and relationship building is essential.

Three types of nursing intervention that are particularly applicable in the community have been described. These are called: **supplemental, facilitative,** and **developmental.**[57] **Supplemental** intervention means doing things for your clients that they cannot do for themselves. Remember that intervention may be not only at the individual level but also at the larger level of family, group, or community.

Example
Mr. George Stevens, the nurse, made weekly home visits to Mr. Smith, a 65-year-old diabetic. Mr. Smith had poor vision and was not able to draw up his insulin. Mr. Stevens drew up the insulin for Mr. Smith, who stored the filled syringes in his refrigerator. Mr. Stevens provided supplemental intervention for Mr. Smith by filling his syringes, an activity he was not able to do for himself.

Facilitative intervention means removing barriers to care, whether they are physical, emotional, cultural, cognitive, or economic.

Example
Mrs. Cary made a home visit to Mr. and Mrs. Jones. Mrs. Jones had recently given birth to a premature infant, Wanda. When Mrs. Cary finished her family assessment, she was concerned about Mr. and Mrs. Jones' lack of nutritional knowledge. Mrs. Cary knew the family was eligible for a supplemental feeding program in the community. She explained the program to Mr. and Mrs. Jones and told them how the foods would be beneficial to the health of their family. Mrs. Cary completed a referral to the supplemental feeding program for the Jones' family. Mr. and Mrs. Jones were able to obtain milk, juice, cereal, and eggs for their family at reduced cost. By removing cognitive and economic barriers, Mrs. Cary intervened so that the family could meet its nutritional needs more effectively.

Developmental intervention is directed to helping the client act more positively in his own behalf.

Example

Mrs. Schroeder was concerned about the obesity among a group of high school girls in one of her schools. The girls were continually downgrading themselves. Their self-esteem was low. They wanted to lose weight and increase their confidence. Through a program of weight control and counseling, Mrs. Schroeder helped the girls lose weight, focus on their strengths, and increase their self-esteem. Mrs. Schroeder provided developmental intervention in helping the girls act more positively in their own behalf.

In supplemental, facilitative, and developmental interventions, the nurse's role may require **referring** clients to other resources for needed care. These resources may include health, counseling, welfare, and educational resources. When making a referral, it is important for the nurse to introduce the client, either on the phone or through a referral form, summarize the client's needs, and state the expectation of the referral.

The nurse's role also may require **coordination** with other health care workers in providing care to clients. This prevents fragmentation and duplication of services. Care may need to be **delegated** to other members of the health care team such as a home health aide. Other jobs of the nurse may be **screening, casefinding, follow-up** and **research.** In screening programs, the nurse tests clients for the presence or absence of disease. In casefinding, the nurse looks for contacts of persons with a particular disease, such as TB or hepatitis, in order to screen them for disease and refer them for needed treatment. Follow-up of such clients involves seeing that they obtained treatment. Research might involve investigating those factors that influenced the client's seeking care and complying with treatment.

Evaluation

The next step in the nursing process is evaluation, "the process of determining value or the amount of success in achieving a predetermined objective."[58] It is important in determining which interventions are most effective with particular groups. Determining how well objectives have been met with client groups necessitates the development of criteria and tools to measure attainment of objectives. It means determining the success level of nursing care and client achievements.

When evaluating nursing care, questions useful to ask include: Was the care effective? Was it efficient? What was the quality of nursing performance?

Effectiveness means looking at what was accomplished in terms of the objectives. What fostered positive results? What contributed to negative results? Did the patient learn what was taught?

Efficiency is accomplishing nursing care in the least costly manner. Nurses are accountable to the organization where they work, the nursing profession, and themselves. It is important not to squander resources. This means not wasting time, energy, supplies, or being careless with equipment.

Quality includes looking at the care provided in terms of whether it was appropriate and whether it conformed to professional standards. Freeman and Heinrich indicated that quality is an elusive goal but that care should be examined in terms of comprehensiveness, sensitivity, responsible stewardship, and continued updating of skills. Quality implies a well-defined sense of priorities since resources are limited.[59]

Quality can be evaluated in terms of **structure, process,** and **outcome.**[60] This evaluation framework can be applied to any health setting. Donabedian stressed that quality of care is not a unitary concept. It involves multiple dimensions. **Structure** refers to the environment in which care is given. Dimensions of structure include "referring to and formulating criteria for adequate physical facilities, good administrative processes, well-qualified staff, good communications, and staff development processes."[61] The assumption is that these are necessary to the provision of good care.

Process refers to what the nurse, as caregiver, does for the patient. This includes both technical and interpersonal skills. Dimensions of process evaluation include interactions between the nurse and clients and decisions made in relation to clients. It also includes the interaction between the client and other health care providers. Categories for rating within the process category include information related to knowledge, organizational skills, skills in human relations, observational ability, and technical skills. Process may refer to activities the patient must perform to achieve a certain level of wellness. Other authors prefer to put patient behavior under outcomes.

Outcome in the structure-process-outcome model refers primarily to alterations on the health-illness continuum for the client. Changes may occur in the areas of attitude, learning, physiological parameters, developmental milestones, prevention, maintenance, and rehabilitation. Other common outcome measures include death, disease, disability, discomfort, and dissatisfaction. It is important to know the weaknesses of these measures. For example, in using patient records to evaluate quality of care, mortality statistics may be available, but the records may be incomplete. In using disease as a measure, it is important to consider the accuracy of the diagnosis. Disease categories don't identify level of discomfort. Disability denotes the inability to perform one's normal activities. Such data may be obtained by self-report and may be subject to bias. Measures of discomfort and dissatisfaction are both obtained by self-report and may be subject to bias.[62]

It is often difficult to know if outcome is related to process or other extraneous factors. Although writers in the field have stressed the importance of linking structure, process, and outcome criteria, results to date have been less than conclusive.[63,64]

Part of the evaluation of care entails not only what to measure, but how to measure it. Sources of data include the patient's record, incident reports, reports from third party payers, staff interviews and observations, morbidity reports, and patient surveys. Tests, interviews, reports, observations, and samples of a product can also be included as data sources.[65]

Data may be obtained while the patient is still being served, concurrently, or after he has been discharged from care, retrospectively. Concurrent data may be obtained from the patient's chart, from patient interview and inspection, and from staff conferences, interviews, or observation. Retrospective data may be obtained from the patient's chart, patient interview or questionnaire, and staff conferences.

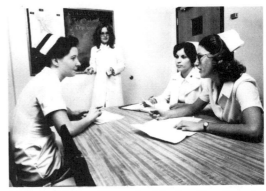

Figure 26-6.   Chart Audits Are One Way to Strive for Excellence.

The nursing process provides a framework for a rational, systematic approach to patient care. In community health nursing, this approach is applied to individuals as well as families, groups, and whole communities. Careful, accurate, population based assessment, planning, implementation, and evaluation are necessary in striving for optimal community health.

SUMMARY

This chapter has introduced concepts of community tools used in community health, the purpose of community health nursing, roles and settings of community health nurses, and the nursing process in community health. The concept of community was defined and highlighted as a system with its own inputs, throughputs, outputs, and feedback. Community systems were described according to emotional, structural, and functional communities. Community health was defined. Epidemiology and biostatistics were described in terms of knowledge they provide in analyzing community health, aiding the community health nurse in looking at the community as a whole and highlighting groups needing particular interventions. The purpose of community health nursing was discussed as was the setting for practice. Roles of community health nurses working in local and state health departments, occupational health, and school health settings were depicted. The nursing process as it applies to community health nursing was described.

Community health nursing demands all that the nurse can bring to it in terms of commitment, intellectual integrity, skill, and caring. The health problems affecting not only the nation's, but also the world's population are great and reflect a need for skilled nurses who can promote maximum physical, social, and emotional health.

STUDY QUESTIONS

1. Traffic accidents are a major killer in the United States today. Describe primary, secondary, and tertiary prevention efforts that might be effective in reducing mortality from this cause.

2. Using your nursing school as an example of a community, describe suprasystem and subsystem influences that affect its health status. In what ways would you describe your school as an emotional community? A structural community? A functional community?

3. A number of individuals in your case load have hypertension. Using the nursing process and the concept of host-agent-environment, describe the application of these concepts to the nursing care of this particular population group.

4. In a community for which you are developing a health plan, TB and diabetes are the chief causes of morbidity and mortality. If you only had limited resources, what principles of health planning would you use to attack these problems? What rates would you use in assessing the scope of the problem?

5. In conducting a childbirth education class for pregnant women, how would you go about evaluating the effectiveness of your nursing care? What health status indicators would you use? Why?

REFERENCES

1. Evelyn Benson and Joan McDevitt, **Community Health and Nursing Practice** (Englewood Cliffs, New Jersey: Prentice-Hall, 1980), p.256.
2. Effie Hanchett, **Community Health Assessment: A Conceptual Tool Kit** (New York: John Wiley and Sons, 1979), p.10.
3. Sarah Archer, "Selected Concepts for Community Health Nurses," **Community Health Nursing-Patterns and Practices,** 2nd ed. rev. by Sarah Archer and Ruth Fleshman (Massachusetts: Duxbury Press, 1979), pp.23–24.
4. **Ibid.,** pp.24–27.
5. **Ibid.,** pp.27–29.
6. John Hanlon and George Pickett, **Public Health—Administration and Practice,** 7th ed. rev. (St. Louis: C.V. Mosby Co., 1979), p.4.
7. Ilse R. Leeser, "The Community as a Patient," in **Community Health Nursing** by Ilse R. Leeser, Claire Tuchalski, and Rosine Carotenuto (New York: Medical Examination Publishing Co., Inc., 1975), p.89.
8. Sarah E. Archer and Ruth P. Fleshman, "Epidemiology and Some Applications to

Primary Prevention," in **Community Health Nurse** ed. Sarah E. Archer and Ruth P. Fleshman, p.219.

9. Benson and McDevitt, **Community Health,** p.62.

10. Barbara Spradley, **Community Health Nursing, Concepts and Practices** (Boston: Little Brown and Company, 1981), p.207.

11. Lesser, "The Community as a Patient," p.90.

12. Benson and McDevitt, **Community Health,** p.69.

13. Ruth B. Freeman and Janet Heinrich, **Community Health Nursing Practice,** 2nd ed. rev. (Philadelphia: W.B. Saunders Co., 1981), p.145.

14. Phillip E. Sartwell and John M. Last, "Epidemiology," in **Public Health and Preventive Medicine,** 11th ed. rev., ed. John M. Last (New York: Appleton-Century-Crofts, 1980), p.47.

15. Grace Wyshak, "Epidemiology," in **Community Health Care and the Nursing Process** by Margot J. Fromer (St. Louis: C.V. Mosby, 1979), pp.215–221.

16. **Ibid.,** p.224.

17. Archer and Fleshman, **Community Health Nursing,** p.224.

18. Benson and McDevitt, **Community Health,** p.81.

19. Sartwell and Last, "Epidemiology," p.21.

20. Benson and McDevitt, **Community Health,** p.83–84.

21. **Ibid.,** p.84.

22. **Ibid.**

23. U.S. Department of Health, Education and Welfare, **Healthy People—The Surgeon General's Report on Health Promotion and Disease Prevention.** DHEW Publication No. 79–55071 (Washington: U.S. Government Printing Office, 1979), p.14.

24. Spradley, **Community Health Nursing—Concepts and Practices,** p.30.

25. "Nurses Today—A Statistical Portrait," **American Journal of Nursing,** 82, 3 (March, 1982), 448–451.

26. Freeman and Heinrich, **Community Health Nursing Practice,** p.1.

27. The Executive Committee and the Standards Committee of the American Nurses' Association Division on Community Health Nursing Practice, **Standards of Community Health Nursing Practice,** (Kansas City, Missouri: ANA, 1974), p.10.

28. **Ibid.,** p.15.

29. Steven Jones, "Provisions of Public Health Services," **Public Health and Preventive Medicine,** ed. John M. Last, p.16.

30. Leahy, Cobb, and Jones, **Community Health Nursing,** p.17.

31. Jonas, "Provisions of Public Health Services," p.1626.

32. John Hanlon, **Public Health Administration and Practice,** 6th ed. rev. (St. Louis: C.V. Mosby, 1974), p.243.

33. Marjorie J. Keller, "Health Needs and Nursing Care of the Labor Force," in **Community Health Care** by Margot J. Fromer, p.413.

34. Carol A. Silberstein, "Nursing Role in Occupational Health," **Community Health Nursing: Keeping the Public Healthy,** ed. Linda Jarvis (Philadelphia: F.A. Davis Co., 1981), p.127.

35. **Accident Facts—1982 Preliminary Condensed Edition.** National Safety Council (Chicago, Illinois: March, 1982).

36. Kim Maisenbacher. "Prenatal Preparation: An Industrial Application," **Occupational Health Nursing,** 29, 2 (February 1981), 19–20.

37. Freeman and Heinrich, **Community Health Nursing,** p.514.

38. Anna Mae Tichy, "Wellness, the Workers, and the Nurse," **Occupational Health Nursing,** 29, 2 (February, 1981), 22.

39. Freeman and Heinrich, **Community Health Nursing,** p.489.

40. Dorothy S. Oda, "A Viewpoint of School Nursing," **American Journal of Nursing,** 81, 9 (September, 1981), 1677.

41. Freeman and Heinrich, **Community Health Nursing,** p.490.

42. Marilyn Stember. "Nursing Role in School Health," **Community Health Nursing,** ed. Linda Jarvis, p.143.

43. Carl D. Helvie, **Community Health Nursing,** Philadelphia: Harper and Row, 1981, p.136.

44. **Ibid.**

45. Hanchett, **Community Health Assessment,** p.35.

46. William Shonick, "Health Planning," in **Public Health and Preventive Medicine,** ed. John M. Last, p.1604.

47. Barry I. Castleman and Manuel J. Vera Vera, "Impending Proliferation of Asbestos," **International Journal of Health Services,** 10, 3 (1980), 389–403.

48. Russell W. Peterson, "Health and Ecological Effects of Energy Systems: An Overview," **Environmental Health** Perspectives. 32 (1979), 235–239.

49. Victor Fuchs, "Economics, Health and Post Industrial Society," **Milbank Memorial Fund Quarterly,** 52, 2, (Spring 1979), 153–182.

50. Last, ed., **Public Health,** p.27.

51. **Ibid.,** p.29.
52. Hanlon, **Public Health Administration and Practice,** pp.280–291.
53. **Ibid.,** p.280.
54. Sarah Archer. "Selected Community Health Processes," **Community Health Nursing-Patterns and Practices,** by Archer and Fleshman, p.73.
55. **Ibid.,** p.79.
56. Hanlon, **Public Health Administration,** p.285.
57. Freeman and Heinrich, **Community Health Nursing,** p.72.
58. George James, "Evaluation in Public Practice," in **Program Evaluation in the Health Fields,** ed. Herbert C. Schulberg, Alan Sheldon, and Frank Baker (New York: Behavioral Publications, 1969), p.29.
59. Freeman and Heinrich, **Community Health Nursing,** p.83.
60. Avedis Donabedian, "Evaluating the Quality of Medical Care," **Program Evaluation in the Health Fields,** ed. Schulberg, Sheldon, and Baker, pp.186–189.
61. Marlene A. Mayers, Ronald B. Norby, and Anita Watson, **Quality Assurance for Patient Care** (New York: Appleton-Century-Cforts, 1977), p.6.
62. Allen D. Spiegel and Herbert Hyman, **Basic Health Planning Methods,** (Germantown, Maryland: Aspen Systems Corporation, 1978), pp.340–341.
63. William E. McAuliffe, "Measuring the Quality of Medical Care: Process Versus Outcome," **Millbank Memorial Fund Quarterly,** 57, 1 (Winter, 1979), 118–152.
64. Robert Brook, Kathleen Williams, and Allyson Avery, "Quality Assurance Today and Tomorrow: Forecast for the Future," **Annals of Internal Medicine,** 85, 6, (1976), 809–817.
65. Spiegel and Hyman, **Basic Health Planning,** p.392.

ANNOTATED BIBLIOGRAPHY

Freeman RB, Heinrich J: **Community Health Nursing Practice.** Philadelphia, W.B. Saunders Co., 1981. This is a classic textbook on community health nursing that provides a systematic approach to community assessment and risk assessment of families. It provides methodologies for data collection including a tool for identifying nursing needs of families.

Fromer MJ: **Community Health Care and The Nursing Process.** St. Louis, The C.V. Mosby Co., 1979. This text presents an introduction to community nursing with emphasis on the holistic approach to health and health care.

Hanlon JJ, Pickett G: **Public Health Administration and Practice,** 7th ed. St. Louis, The C.V. Mosby Co., 1979. This classic textbook is a very comprehensive resource on the field of public health. The many dimensions of health in the community setting are explored in depth. Selected topics include historic roots, international health issues, public health analysis and planning, ecology and health, epidemiology, and health care delivery services.

Jarvis LL: **Community Health Nursing: Keeping the Public Healthy.** Philadelphia, F.A. Davis Co., 1981. This text presents a comprehensive view of the community, community health nursing, and many specific social and environmental issues that impact upon public health and nursing. Selected nursing roles in the community are defined and discussed with examples.

Warren RL: **Studying Your Community.** New York, The Free Press, 1965. This book presents practical descriptions of community concepts. Selected sections include the economic structure of communities, community planning, housing, recreation, and communication in communities. It is comprehensive in its coverage of recommended topics to consider in community assessment.

27

Environmental Aspects

Phyllis B. Heffron
Janet-Beth Flynn

CHAPTER OUTLINE

OBJECTIVES

At the completion of this chapter, the reader will be able to:

- Define the ecological model.
- Discuss the relationship between air pollution and human health.
- Discuss the effects of water pollution on health and safety.
- List the health effects of at least six toxic substances in the environment.
- List three sources of ionizing radiation in the environment.
- State at least four ways nurses can assist clients in controlling noise pollution.
- Describe the role of the occupational health nurse in reducing environmentally induced health effects.
- Describe a safe hospital environment.
- List factors needed to make a comfortable hospital environment.
- Describe nursing actions that can be carried out to protect patients from environmental injury.

GLOSSARY

Acute toxicity—Any poisonous effect produced by a single short-term exposure that results in severe biological harm or death.

Agricultural pollution—The liquid and solid wastes of farming, including runoff from pesticides, fertilizers, and feedlots; erosion and dust from plowing; animal manure and carcasses, crop residues and debris.

Air pollution—The presence of contaminant substances in the air that do not disperse properly and interfere with human health.

Bioaccumulation—The concentration of certain substances as they move up the food chain. An important mechanism in concentrating pesticides and heavy metals in organisms such as fish.

Biodegradable—Any substance that decomposes quickly through the action of microorganisms.

Carcinogenic—Cancer producing.

Decibel—A unit of relative sound measurement.

Decomposition—The breakdown of matter by bacteria; change in the chemical makeup and physical appearance of materials.

Ecology—The study of the relationships of living things to one another and to their environment.

Ecosystem—The interacting system of a biological community and its nonliving surroundings.

Electrical threshold—The minimum amount of current to which the human body responds.

Environment—In ecological terms, the sum of all external conditions affecting the life, development, and survival of an organism.

Hazardous waste—Waste materials that, by their nature, are inherently dangerous to handle or dispose of, such as old explosives, radioactive materials, some chemicals, and some biological wastes; usually produced in industrial operations.

Herbicide—A chemical that controls or destroys undesirable plants.

Humidity—The amount of moisture in the air.

Infection—A disease process caused by an infectious agent such as a bacteria, virus, or other microorganism.

Mutagenic—Causing a change in the genetic structure of an organism in subsequent generations.

Noise—Any undesired sound.

Nosocomial infection—An infection originating in a medical facility such as a hospital; includes infection with symptoms that may not show up until after the patient's discharge, and infections occur among staff members.

Oncogenic—Tumor causing, whether benign or malignant.

Pesticide—Any substance used to control pests ranging from rats, weeds, and insects, to algae and fungi.

Pollutant—Any introduced substance that adversely effects the usefulness of a resource.

GLOSSARY Continued

Pollution—The presence of matter or energy whose nature, location, or quality produces undesired environmental effects.

Potable water—Appetizing water that is safe for drinking or use in cooking.

Radiation—The emission of particles or rays by the nucleus of an atom.

Radioactive—Substances that emit rays either naturally or as a result of scientific manipulation.

Radioisotopes—Radioactive forms of chemical compounds, such as cobalt-60, used in the treatment of diseases.

Recycling—Converting solid waste into new products by using the resources contained in discarded materials.

REM—Acronym for roentgen equivalent man, a measure of radiation by biological effect on human tissue.

Smog—Air pollution associated with oxidants.

Solid waste disposal—The final placement of refuse that cannot be salvaged or recycled.

Thermal pollution—Discharge of heated water from industrial processes that can affect the life processes of aquatic plants and animals.

Teratogenic—Substances that are suspected of causing malformations or serious deviations from the normal type that cannot be inherited, in or on animal embryos or fetuses.

Toxic substance—A chemical or mixture that may produce an unreasonable risk of injury to health or the environment.

Water pollution—The addition of enough harmful or objectionable material to damage or contaminate water quality.

INTRODUCTION

The term environment is one of those elusive words that can be defined in a multitude of ways. Its definitions and usages vary in complexity and context. In its broadest and most simple definition, environment is around or outside of something. In relation to man, the environment most commonly refers to the physical surroundings—air, water, sunlight, noise, and organic and inorganic objects. In a systems framework, the external environment is whatever exists outside the identified system boundary and includes other systems and subsystems. The internal environment exists inside the system's boundary. The immediate environment may be a community, a neighborhood, a house, room, or other enclosure. Environment may refer to social or psychological atmosphere. In actuality, man's environment includes everything that affects him.

Throughout the ages, man has been adapting to his natural environment and has made many attempts to control and shape it.[1] These attempts have resulted in a wide base of knowledge about the complex relationships that exist among living systems. One of the major characteristics of the man/environment relationship is reciprocity. Man acts on the environment and receives from the environment.[2] In recent years, the effects of man's acts on the environment, e.g., industrialization, biomedical, and engineering technology, have become increasingly evident and widely studied in terms of ecology, environmental hazards, and human health.

The immediate environment of man in terms of community and city planning, institutional design and safety, and environmentally induced psychosocial stressors has received increasing attention as related to the quality of life and individual health status.[3,4]

The nursing profession has been concerned with aspects of man's environment since the days of Florence Nightingale.[5] Basic nursing texts always have emphasized the importance of safety, cleanliness, air quality, and temperature control as integral aspects of total patient care and nursing responsibility. Community health nurses extend environmental concerns to areas of preventive health care and maintenance of general public health. Ecological issues impact individuals, families, and communities.[6] Nurses need to be sensitive to and have a basic understanding of these issues as they affect health and the environment. It is natural for clients to seek out the nurse to provide facts, answers, and opinions on a variety of these issues.[7]

The focus of this chapter is man's relationship to his environment and how it relates to nursing and health. An emphasis on man's external physical environment requires two major areas of discussion: ecology and man's general quality of life, and the immediate environments of man as related to health care settings and the home.

The Ecological Model

The condition of the environment in which we live, the air, water, buildings, and grounds, determine to a large extent how we live, what we eat, which diseases we are likely to contract, our state of health, and ability to adapt. The science of ecology is

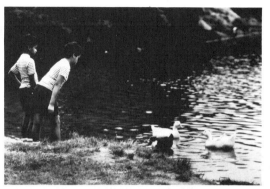

Figure 27-1.   The quality of the environment affects individuals, families, and communities.

primarily a biological science that studies the environment and environmental factors affecting man. Of primary concern to ecologists are the dynamic relationships between living things and their surroundings.[8]

This ecological model gives us a broad and suitable framework from which to view environmental issues as they affect clients and the practice of nursing. Ecology encompasses a holistic, systems theory approach that can provide insights into environmental hazards and stresses that affect health adaptation.[9]

Human ecology is concerned very specifically with the man/environment relationship. In addition to the biological and physical interrelationship that come immediately to mind, cultural, technological, social, and behavioral aspects of man's adaptive responses are also included.[10] An important concept of basic ecology is the ecosystem. An **ecosystem** is a total collection of adapted organic and inorganic parts that support a chain of life within a selected area.[11] More simply, an ecosystem is the home or habitat where groups of plants and animals live together in harmonious balance. Our earth is well endowed with ecosystems of a wide variety of sizes, shapes, and content. The entire earth is actually one giant ecosystem, as are ponds, rivers, deserts, forests, and

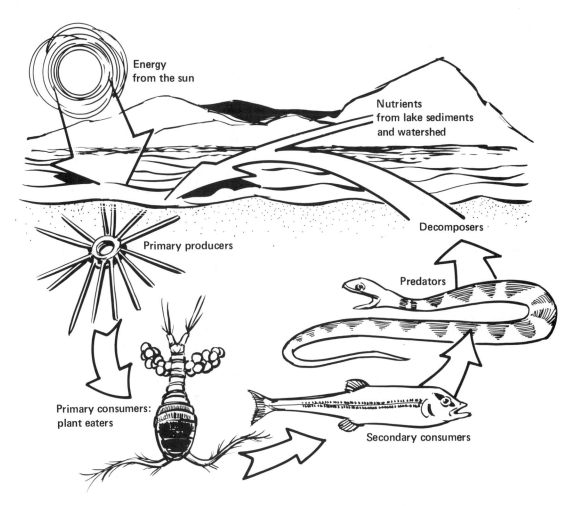

Figure 27-2.   The components of an ecosystem are in dynamic equilibrium with their environment.

caves. These ecosystems are all physically and biologically different, but they function in the same general way: predictably and in a chain-like fashion.

Radiant energy from the sun sets the chain in motion as the process of photosynthesis allows solar energy to become fixed and stored in green plants. The energy stored by plants is passed along through the ecosystem in a series of steps that involve eating and being eaten, decomposing, and recycling back into green plants.[12] In ecology, the living parts of an ecosystem work together in what is called a food chain and are divided into producers (the green plants), consumers (plant eaters and meat eaters), and decomposers (primarily bacteria). Plant and animal growth within these food chains are dependent on the nonliving materials in the ecosystem, such as water, carbon dioxide, oxygen, and minerals dissolved in the water. These nonliving materials have their own cycles that also occur predictably and interdependently. The water cycle, for example, involves evaporation and condensation. Water vapor in the earth's atmosphere is distributed and moves via air currents, then cools and forms clouds. Rain falls on the earth, soaks into the soil, and fills the springs, rivers, and oceans. Surface water from these open bodies of water evaporates when the sun shines and returns water vapor to the atmosphere. Other cycles that are highly interrelated within the ecosystem are the carbon and oxygen cycle and the nitrogen cycle. These minerals and other nonliving materials are constantly recycled through the ecosystem from soil, atmosphere, and water to plants, animals, decomposers, and back again.[13]

Ecosystem functioning is important to understand when studying human health and the environment. Man-made interferences, such as chemical substances introduced into the environment, can profoundly disturb ecosystems and their equilibrium. "It is because of this biogeochemical cycling that DDT sprayed in an Indian hut to kill the *Anopheles* mosquitoes, or laid down on a California farm to kill cotton pests, appears in penguins in Antarctica and in human mother's milk in New York City."[14] Another example that illustrates a direct "cause and effect" disruption to ecosystems involves the disposal of water used to cool nuclear reactors. When this waste water is discharged into streams or lakes in its heated state, it causes irreversible damage to fish and plant life.[15]

When considering man's total environment, ecological issues are germaine to the interest of professional nurses. The list is virtually endless when one considers all the possible hazards, adverse effects, and stresses with which man comes in contact. Several of these health related issues—environmental pollution, toxic substances, radiation, noise, and various psychosocial topics—have been selected for further discussion.

Environmental Pollution

Pollution is described in the dictionary as a state or act of uncleanliness, defilement, or impurity. Environmental pollution refers primarily to the pollution of man's physical environment, the atmosphere, the waterways, and the land. The menace of such pollution—smog, garbage heaps of plastic containers, bottles, and pop-top cans, and stagnant pools of foul water—has been growing over the past years, particularly following the postwar period of abundance and high technology achievement.[16]

Air Pollution. Air pollution began to receive a great deal of attention when urban smog surfaced as a major public health problem in the early 1960s. Smog, an innovative term meaning the chemical pollution that occurs when automobile exhaust emissions react with sunlight, was particularly evident in cities with high concentrations of cars and aircraft, such as Chicago and Los Angeles.[17] Large industrial cities like Pittsburg, Pennsylvania, and Newark, New Jersey, were characterized by a pall of sooty, murky air that tended to build up during periods of low wind velocity and certain other atmospheric conditions. People breathing this contaminated air were subject to a variety of respiratory ailments and, in some cases, the smog was directly related to morbidity and mortality.[18]

As general concern for the environment escalated, special interest groups formed to study, support, and lobby to clear up the air. It became evident that air pollution affected humans indirectly as well as directly by damaging plants, materials, and other animals.[19] Crops were destroyed by smog and fluoride in the air, wild and domestic animals died from airborne dioxin, and stone on buildings crumbled from the presence of acid in the air.[20]

The leading cause of air pollution is from industrial manufacturing, and the second major cause is automobile exhaust.[21] The smoky by-products of combustion, particularly the burning of coal to generate electricity, disperse large amounts of solid and liquid particles, such as dust, ash, soot, and various metals and chemicals.[22] Poisonous gases, such as sulfur dioxide from industrial processes and hydrocarbons and nitrogen oxide from motor vehicle exhaust, account for numerous adverse health effects that include irritation of the eyes, nose, and throat, respiratory irritation, impairment of cardiac function, and possible mutagenic and carcinogenic effects.[23]

In 1970, Congress passed the Clean Air Act of 1970 (amended from the Clean Air Act of 1963), which governs all types of air pollution. This act, administered by the Environmental Protection Agency (EPA), required automobile and industrial manufacturers to reduce poisonous emissions from car exhausts and industrial smokestacks over a 10-year period.[24] Amended again in 1977, the Clean Air Act gave even broader power to the EPA to set standards for any category of industry whose air pollution causes or contributes to the endangerment of public health.[25] Although fraught with political pressures and red tape within and outside the government, this legislation has proved worthwhile, and there is evidence that our air quality has improved. It is recognized increasingly, however, that governmental regulations that impose restrictions, controls, and fines are only one way to attack the problem of air pollution.[26] Knowledge about atmospheric chemistry, air transport, and control are also imperative in understanding and solving the problem.[27]

Water Pollution. Over the ages, various forms of water pollution have plagued man and the environment. In this country, early laws regarding water pollution were aimed at the prevention of waterborne diseases, such as typhoid fever, cholera, and others. In 1914, the first drinking water standards were enacted, and in 1948 Congress passed the Water Pollution Act.[28] Since that time and increasingly in the past decade, water pollution has come to mean contamination from a number of sources other than infection causing organisms. With the onset of the industrial revolution in America, the

industrial and manufacturing needs shifted from power to the need for water as an agent for cooling and processing. It was this shift that resulted in the release of highly toxic pollutants into our streams and rivers. The quantity of pollutants exceeded the capacity of the water to be naturally cleansed through recycling, and water pollution occurred on a massive scale. In addition, the rapid population growth in the United States also had an effect on water pollution. Many local water treatment plants have been unable to purify water fast enough, and there is greater risk of contamination. Along with more people, there is more new construction, more high technology farming, and more disruption of natural resources, for example, through mining. Water runoff from mines, farms, construction sites, and city streets have resulted in an increase of both toxic and nontoxic pollutants entering the nation's waterways.[29]

Water pollution can be categorized according to its source. The major sources of water pollution are common organic sewage, bacteria, organic and chemical plant nutrients, earth sediments from soil erosion, radioactive materials, and thermal pollution (waste heat from nuclear power plants).[30] Water pollution also can be expanded to include the presence of unsightly garbage and litter thrown into our rivers and lakes.[31]

The effects of water pollution on human health can range from minor skin irritation to death, and can affect us directly or indirectly. We can become sick or injured from drinking or coming into skin contact with contaminated water. We are also affected directly by shortages of drinking water or by diminished food shortages. Indirectly, we can become ill from eating foods or green plants that have come into contact with polluted water. Water pollution can affect psychological health as well, when water looks bad, smells bad, or tastes bad, regardless of its safety. Water pollution can affect people economically, such as fisherman who have lost their livelihood due to fish contaminated with mercury.[32] Thermal pollution, which results when heated water is discharged into rivers or streams, can significantly upset ecological relationships. Clams, snails, crabs, and worms have totally disappeared from much of Florida's Biscayne Bay because of thermal pollution from two power plants.[33]

The responsibility for reducing pollution of our waterways rests with local, state, and federal agencies as well as with the public at large. On the federal level, the EPA administers a number of water pollution control programs under the auspices of the Clean Water Act of 1972 (amended in 1981), and the Safe Drinking Water Act of 1974 (amended in 1977). The Clean Water Act provides funds for modification of municipal sewage treatment systems, provides regional planning assistance for waste water treatment facilities, sets limits for effluents (liquid industrial discharges into waterways), and sets water quality standards.[34] The effects of water pollution on health must be looked at in terms of the total "quality of life" of individuals, and their physical, mental, and social well-being.[35]

Toxic Substances. Human beings and the environment are being exposed each year to a large number of chemical substances. In addition to the air we breathe, almost everything we touch, eat, or drink contains them. Among the chemical substances and mixtures being developed and produced, there are some whose manufacture, use, or method of disposal presents unreasonable risks of injury to health or the environment.[36] The term "toxic substances" commonly refers to those chemicals or mixtures of chemicals that produce adverse health effects to humans or animals, either directly or indirectly.

Toxic substances include a number of manufactured chemicals, as well as naturally occurring substances, such as mercury or lead, that are mined and released into the environment. It is estimated that nearly 60,000 chemicals are in use in the United States today, and approximately 800 new chemical substances are proposed each year for manufacture.[37]

In 1976, the Toxic Substances Control Act (TSCA) was enacted by Congress. This Act, administered by the EPA, is mandated to protect public health and the environment from chemical risks. The EPA gathers information on chemical substances, requires testing on those that are potentially toxic, and identifies those that are harmful. Testing requirements to determine specific health effects include studies for carcinogenicity, mutagenicity, teratogenicity, and behavioral toxicity. Regulations are passed by the EPA for those chemicals posing a threat to health. The regulations may range from a complete ban of the substance to a minor relabeling modification.[38]

The EPA also has responsibility for controlling another group of chemical substances that act as pesticides. Authority for this action was enacted most recently in 1980 under amendments to the 1947 law: The Federal Insecticide, Fungicide, and Rodenticide Act (FIFRA). Pesticides are chemical or biological substances used to control pests, such as rats, weeds, insects, and fungi. They are used on farms, in homes, hospitals, and commercial and government establishments.[39] Misuse of pesticides can contaminate the environment and result in their accumulation in ecological food chains.

Additional toxic substances, such as drugs, food, food additives, and cosmetics, are regulated within various other government agencies, like the Food and Drug Administration and the Department of Agriculture.

Health effects from all of these toxic substances vary tremendously, and persons can be exposed to them in many ways, including air and water pollution. The EPA gives priority to chemical substances that may produce chronic health effects or those with irreversible and debilitating effects, e.g., oncogenic, mutagenic, teratogenic, and neurotoxic chemicals. Other known health effects are cardiovascular, respiratory, immunological, dermatological, and reproductive. Figure 27-3 summarizes some of the most significant toxic substances in the environment, their principal characteristics, uses, and health effects.

Toxic Substance	Characteristics & Use	Principal Health Effects
ARSENIC	• highly toxic poison • occurs naturally in coal and oil • past uses in pesticides and herbicides • currently has very limited agricultural uses and as a weed killer • used in paint, glass, and ceramic industries • large quantities produced from smelting of lead and other metals, from cotton gins and coal burning • compounds of arsenic are the most toxic	• severity of toxic reaction depends on concentration and type of compounds • acute systemic poisoning with gastrointestinal inflammation, nausea, vomiting, diarrhea, cardiac toxicity, and death • acute occupational exposure can lead to nasal cancer and teratogenic effects • chronic exposure can lead to muscle weakness, anorexia, gastrointestinal symptoms and mucous membrane irritation • a carcinogen in the workplace
ASBESTOS	• a widely naturally occurring fiber • used in road building construction, insulation, cement, floor tiles, pipes, filters, and numerous other sources • can be a source of pollution in drinking water • acid rain component	• occupational exposure to airborne asbestos can cause asbestosis (lung fibrosis), lung cancer, pleural & peritoneal mesothelioma, and gastrointestinal cancer • waterborne asbestos, poorly understood but some connection with generalized mesothelioma in the public
BERYLLIUM	• a highly toxic nonradioactive metal • used in copper alloys and machine manufacture • significant past use in fluorescent light industry discontinued in 1949 because of high incidence occupational disease: berylliosis • used today primarily in industrial settings that refine it or use it in alloying, e.g., machine shops, ceramic and propellant plants, and foundries	• route of entry through lungs • acute poisoning symptoms include multiple respiratory system problems, weakness, weight loss, anemia • chronic exposure leads to degeneration and death • beryllium poisoning can affect people living near beryllium factories
CADMIUM	• soft, heavy metal similar to zinc and mercury • a harmful toxin in the form of sulfides of carbonate in zinc, copper, and lead ores	• route of entry through inhalation, ingestion, and absorption • occupational exposure produces general malaise, nervousness, dry mouth, impaired

Toxic Substance	Characteristics & Use	Principal Health Effects
CADMIUM (cont.)	• 50 percent of all the cadmium in United States is used by electroplating industries • used to manufacture batteries, plastics, paints, metal alloys, photographic supplies, glass and rubber products • present as a fine mist during burning of products containing cadmium • food contamination an important source of exposure	sense of smell, shortness of breath, sore throat, chest cramps, back pain, and anorexia • long term exposure may produce emphysema, liver and kidney symptoms, central nervous system impairment and adverse cardiovascular effects • suspected correlation with hypertension • carcinogenic implications
CHLORINE	• dense green-yellow gas • strong oxidizing agent • used in the preparation, processing and liquification of chlorine • also used in chemical, pulp, and paper processes	• pulmonary edema • pneumonitis • bronchitis
CHROMIUM	• a hard metal • contaminates the environment as an aerosol or dust • used in electroplating, manufacturing stainless steel, tanning and photographic supplies, combustion of coal and refuse	• carcinogenic • direct contact causes dermatitis, skin ulcers
FLUORIDE	• a highly reactive gas as hydrogen fluoride • a corrosive, poisonous, and gaseous chemical element as a compound of fluorine • used to produce phosphate fertilizers, aluminum brick, tile, steel, and glass • by-product of coal combustion • ocean dumping of waste fluoride can cause air pollution	• accumulates more readily in children • in areas subjected to fluoride pollution from industry, the following symptoms have been reported: polycythemia, fluoride in teeth, nails, urine, and hair of children • chronic exposure of high doses can lead to depression of collagen formation and bone resorption
MERCURY	• a heavy metal • occurs naturally from erosion and weathering • pollution results from mining, refining of mercury, combustion of fuels and refuse, use of pesticides containing mercury use as a fungicide, use in paper and pulp industry, and numerous other sources • can cause water pollution from industrial waste and agricultural runoff	• greatest risk to general population is from consumption of contaminated fish • route of entry often inhalation in occupational sites • health effects are mostly neurotoxic with progression to deafness, blindness, paralysis, kidney failure, and death

Toxic Substance	Characteristics & Use	Principal Health Effects
NICKEL	• a hard metal • occurs most commonly in oil and coal deposits • used in manufacture of stainless steel and other metal processes • found in nickel-aluminum compounds associated with many industrial uses • used as fuel additives • found in asbestos, coal, and crude oil • air pollution comes from burning of coal and petroleum products	• contact dermatitis • atmospheric nickel can be inhaled or absorbed through the skin; foods contaminated in processing can be ingested • gaseous nickel carbonyl, very toxic and can produce lung cancer; acute poisoning produces chest pain, vertigo, and vomiting • disease from chronic occupational exposure may take up 20 years to develop
CHLORINATED HYDROCARBONS (Pesticides)	• man-made chemical compounds including DDT, benzene hexachloride, heptachlor, and others • used as pesticides • do not break down into nontoxic substances in the environment • nearly all uses of DDT, other similarly highly toxic compounds have been banned in the United States	• DDT widely studied in terms of its health effects • early symptoms of poisoning include headache, dizziness, and anorexia; some evidence of changes in liver function • major documented effects of DDT poisoning are neurotoxic and include hyperactivity and muscle tremors • carcinogenicity and genetic changes documented in animals • enzyme changes, e.g., can cause a drop in certain hormone levels, such as estrogen
ORGANOPHOS- PHATES (Pesticides)	• a group of synthetic pesticides that largely have replaced chlorinated hydrocarbon pesticides, such as DDT • some common compounds in this group include atrazine, simazine, parathion, malathion, and others • can be highly toxic, but do not persist in the environment as long as chlorinated hydrocarbons • very poisonous to both harmful and beneficial insects	• heavy occupational exposure can cause headache, nausea and vomiting, stomach cramps • several deaths reported each year from acute occupational exposure • parathion most toxic to man • chronic exposure to agricultural workers often misdiagnosed as food poisoning, heat stroke, or gastroenteritis • long-term health effects not known
HERBICIDES	• defoliant compounds used to destroy noxious weeds and shrubs along highways and for lawn and garden use • includes chlorophenoxy acids, urea derivatives, fenuron and diuron, triazines, acylanilides	• generally of low toxicity when exposure occurs; may cause some irritation and discomfort • indirect health effects more important; may destroy food supplies for animals, disrupts plant and waste ecosystems by

Toxic Substance	Characteristics & Use	Principal Health Effects
HERBICIDES (cont.)		• using of O_2 in water and affecting fish life • teratogenic and carcinogenic effects in lab animals
FUNGICIDES	• two widely used fungicides are captan and folpet (phthalimides)	• have been shown to be carcinogenic, teratogenic, and mutagenic to experimental animals
NITROSAMINES	• include any of a series of organic compounds derived from amines (derivative of ammonia) and containing the divalent = N.NO radical • occur throughout the environment in food, drugs, tobacco, drinking water, and air • principal sources: direct discharges from industrial processes; formed when natural amines in food (amino acids) combine with polluted air containing nitrogen compounds; formed in human stomach when nitrates (found in some meat and poultry products) are ingested	• laboratory tests have shown these substances to be carcinogenic and mutagenic
POLYCHLORINATED BIPHENYLS (PCBs)	• widely used industrial compound, chemically similar to DDT • very prevalent in the environment; a partial listing of uses include electrical equipment, lumber, metal, concrete, paint, printing ink, solvents, varnishes, and floor tile • released in industrial wastes • does not break down readily and is passed along through the food chain, e.g., found in fish and wild animals	• correlated to lethal effects in game birds and reduced reproductive capacity in fish eating mammals, minks, and seals • etiological agent in "Yusho Disease" (first reported in Japan following accidental ingestion of high concentration of PCBs) characterized by severe skin disorders, eye discharge, loss of hair, numbness of extremities, headaches, gastrointestinal symptoms, deformed nails, joints, and bones • aftereffects of disease can include permanent central nervous system damage • carcinogenic in rodents • occupationally exposed persons have experienced nausea, vertigo, eye and nasal irritation, asthmatic bronchitis, dermatitis, fungus, and acne
	• a plasticizer used in the production of polyvinyl chloride (PCV), the most commonly	• affects calcium metabolism and shows an increase in abortion and fetal abnormalities

Toxic Substance	Characteristics & Use	Principal Health Effects
VINYL CHLORIDE (VC)	used clear plastic • escapes in air and water as a pollutant • occupational exposure occurs in polyvinyl chloride plants • general public is exposed via aerosol containers, plastic wraps on foods, and drinking water; also used widely in industry, home and medical science, in wall coverings, upholstery, appliances, cosmetic, and perfumes • polyvinyl chloride releases hydrochloric acid when burned	when given to lab animals at relatively low doses • associated with liver cancer and other carcinomas • studies have also suggested increased rates of birth defects in communities where PVC manufacturing plants are located
POLYBROMINATED BIPHENYLS (PBBs)	• highly toxic flame retardant • it is persistent in the environment and bioaccumulates • added to fibers and plasticized materials, such as typewriter and calculator casings, shavers, and hand tools • released to environment during manufacturing process	• long-term toxicity unknown • short-term toxicity studies show impaired reproductive and liver function, nervous disorders, and teratogenic effects
KEPONE	• highly poisonous chlorinated organic compound • long life in the environment, and bioaccumulates • used as fire retardants, plasticizers, and pesticides • released in waste water and atmosphere during manufacture • seafood contamination another threat to humans	• has produced serious illness among workers in Kepone manufacturing plants; symptoms include neurological disorders, skin changes, muscle spasms, sterility, liver lesions, cancer, and others • has produced adverse reproductive effects in rats

Figure 27-3.   Selected Toxic Substances in the Environment.

Adapted from: William J. Baumol, Wallace E. Oates, **Economics, Environmental Policy, and the Quality of Life,** ©1979, pp.48–57. By permission of Prentice-Hall, Inc., Englewood Cliffs, NJ.[40]

Solid Waste Disposal. One of the most indisputable environmental problems, which is intertwined with most other forms of pollution, is the accumulation of garbage, litter, and other unwanted materials known as solid wastes. Solid waste, refers to garbage (waste resulting from growing, preparing, cooking, and preserving foods), dead animals, demolition waste (bricks, masonry, piping, and lumber), sewage treatment residue, industrial wastes, and other refuse.[41]

Solid waste disposal in communities always has been a problem. In recent times, the United States has experienced a tremendous increase in the problem. Residential and commercial sources generate solid waste at the rate of 132 million metric tons per year.[42] Industrial waste is more than double that amount, totaling 350 million metric tons a year, of which approximately 41 million metric tons are hazardous wastes.[43] Economic and population growth and the production of plastic, glass, aluminum, and other disposables all contribute to the problem. In 1970, nearly 73,000 cars were abandoned in New York City.[44]

The problems of solid waste disposal, particularly of toxic, hazardous wastes, constitute a number of public health and environmental dangers. The health effects of toxic chemical wastes are summarized in Figure 27-3, and sewage disposal problems were discussed earlier in this chapter. The control and eradication of solid waste problems has been mandated to the EPA under the auspices of The Resource Conservation and Recovery Act of 1976 (RCRA), which regulates current and future waste practices, and the Comprehensive Environmental Response, Compensation, and Liability Act (CERCLA), known as Superfund, which is responsible for cleaning up old and abandoned toxic waste sites.[45] In addition, many voluntary programs throughout the country have contributed to consciousness raising and the elimination of some solid waste through recycling efforts.

It is beyond the scope of this chapter to discuss the specifics of solid waste disposal and to compare methods. For many years "the old attitude towards solid waste disposal has been to dump it, burn it, or bury it."[46] This attitude still prevails among many people who are not concerned with environmental issues or who are not aware of all the complexities and hazards. With the help of government agencies on all levels and various private interest groups, there are continuing, concerted efforts to deal with solid waste management problems, its treatment, storage, transportation, and disposal.

Radiation. Radiation is yet another form of pollution in our environment. It occurs naturally in the atmosphere as well as from manmade sources, such as nuclear reactions and x-rays.

Radiation was first described by Henri Becquerel, a French scientist who accidentally discovered that one element can spontaneously change into another.[47] An element or material is said to be **radioactive** when energy or particles are emitted from the nucleus of its atoms. The actual particles or "rays" that are emitted are called **radiation.**[48]

There are three types of radiation: alpha, beta, and gamma. Each is associated with the type of energy ray or particle emitted from the nucleus. Alpha particles are actually changed nuclei, such as a helium nucleus being emitted from a uranium isotope. Beta particles are electrons emitted from the nucleus, and gamma rays are emissions of high-energy light.

Ionizing radiation refers to the ability of radiation to make molecular changes. Ionization is a process that removes electrons from atoms and creates charged atoms and molecules. Ionizing radiation is of most concern to human health, as it can disrupt molecules within the body cells and cause destruction leading to cell death or other abnormal deviations.

Of the three types of radiation, gamma radiation is the most damaging to the human body.[49] It has a relatively low ionization capability but is high in its ability to penetrate body tissues. Gamma radiation also has a cumulative effect in the body, and small doses over a long period of time can be devastating. Alpha particles are high ionizers but low penetrators. Emitters of alpha radiation, such as uranium and plutonium, are dangerous to human health, because they can be ingested through food and water or inhaled into the lungs. Once in the body, these heavy metals have a tendency to concentrate in the bones; subsequent damage to bone marrow and blood forming cells can occur and lead to leukemia.[50]

Beta radiation has a moderate ability to ionize and are low in penetration. Health effects from this type of exposure are primarily skin and surface abnormalities, such as eye cataracts.

Everyone is subject to a certain amount of radiation from natural sources in the environment. These natural sources include cosmic radiation from the sun, radiation in the soil and rocks, and small amounts of radiation that are emitted within the body.[51] Other sources are from manmade sources, such as fallout from nuclear bomb tests, exposure and leakage from nuclear power plants and from x-rays in medicine and dentistry.

The use of radiation in medical and dental practice is well-established. There are applications in both diagnosis and therapy, and various measures exist to safeguard the health of patients and health workers alike. A complete discussion of radiation in health care settings follows in the next section.

The use of nuclear power plants and the degree to which they are hazardous to health has been a running public and political debate for some time. There are currently over 60 operating nuclear plants in the United States.[52] These nuclear plants, or reactors, use radioactive isotopes like uranium or plutonium as their fuel source. By a process of fission (splitting of the atom, which produces heat and radiation), steam is produced from water, and electricity is generated.[53] The process is technical and complex, but the major concerns for health and safety center around leakage of radiation from these reactors, exposure to workers, and contamination from toxic wastes.

Radioactive pollutants from these reactors can be in the form of liquids, solids, and gases.[54] Waste disposal, particularly of highly radioactive used fuel elements and fission products, is a critical problem. Presently these wastes are buried in cement drums or million-gallon stainless steel tanks under the sea or 14 feet underground.[55]

The concern regarding adverse effects of manmade nuclear energy has prompted a number of national and international efforts to control environmental and population contamination. In the United States, the Atomic Energy Commission (AEC) was created in 1946 to regulate nuclear power. In 1975, the AEC was abolished and replaced by the Nuclear Regulatory Commission (NRC) and the Energy Research and Development Administration (ERDA).

At present, a number of federal agencies are responsible for protecting the public from unnecessary radiation exposure. The EPA, working in conjunction with a number of these agencies, has responsibility for setting standards and carrying out environmental monitoring. EPA standards exist to limit radioactive releases from nuclear power plants and from the processing of uranium. The EPA is developing standards for disposal of radioactive wastes and working on guidelines for nuclear accident prevention.[56]

Noise. Unwanted sound, loud or soft, make us nervous, irritable, angry, listless, or unable to sleep. The amount and intensity of environmental noise is a growing problem in the United States. Noise is considered a pollutant because of its ability to permanently damage the ear and contribute to a variety of other physical and mental ills.

Sources of excessive noise are frequently associated with urban areas and include general industrial activity, building construction, motor vehicles, and jet airplanes.[57] Building construction, in particular, is a major environmental problem. More and more people who work in the construction business or live around areas of continual construction experience gradual but permanent hearing loss. Portable compressors, for example, produce some of the most objectionable noise, as do jack hammers, power saws, pneumatic wrenches, concrete mixers, and dump trucks. In the home, electrical appliances are a major contributor of noise pollution:

radios, TVs, stereos, typewriters, vacuum cleaners, dishwashers, blenders, exhaust fans, hair dryers, and power tools.

The major health effects of excessive noise are summarized below:

- permanent inner ear damage ranging from slight impairment to total deafness
- temporary, leading to chronic hearing losses
- masking of warning signals (e.g., vehicular horns) that can lead to industrial and domestic accidents
- disturbance of sleep, rest, and relaxation
- interference with speech communication
- a source of annoyance, frayed nerves, and other psychological disturbances
- reduction of the opportunity for privacy
- constriction of blood flow throughout the body.[58,59]

The ear is very vulnerable to harm from noise, because it cannot close itself like an eyelid; it is designed by nature always to be alert.[60] The decibel is the most commonly used measure of sound. Environmental readings can be taken on a standard noise meter in units of decibels. A reading of zero represents the threshhold of audible sound for normal human hearing.[61] The higher the decibel level, the louder the noise. Scientists believe that continuous eight-hour exposure to levels of 85 decibels can result in permanent hearing loss.[62] Some common environmental sources of noise and their associated decibel levels appear in Figure 27-4.

Noise control is one of the most difficult environmental problems because it involves virtually everyone in all the activities of daily living. There are a number of ways to reduce and control noise. Quieter airplanes, cars, trucks, and motorcycles can be built. Flight plans of aircraft can be restricted, and noise barriers can be placed along highways and in industrial plants. The EPA and other organizations, such as the American Speech-Learning-Hearing Association, are working toward preventing noise-induced hearing impairment and reducing environmental noise. In addition, local governments and community organizations are developing noise standards and educating the public about the health hazards of noise pollution and its prevention.

The EPA's Office of Noise Abatement and Control recommends the following actions for noise reduction in the home:

- Install exhaust fans on rubber mounts.
- Caulk windows and install storm windows to cut down outside noise and conserve energy.

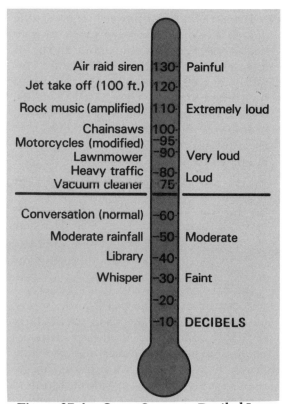

Figure 27-4.   Some Common Decibel Levels in Everyday Life

- Use vinyl flooring or thick linoleum in kitchens and bathrooms.
- Use wall-to-wall and stair carpeting with felt or rubber padding to dampen noise.
- Use drapes to help absorb noise.
- Keep radios, televisions, and stereos at a lower volume.
- Use vibration mounts under large electrical appliances such as washers, dryers, and dishwashers.
- Place foam pads or towels under electric typewriters, blenders, and other small appliances.
- Replace metal garbage cans with plastic ones.[63]

ECOLOGICAL ISSUES AND THE NURSING PROCESS

Nurses traditionally have been concerned about various environmental issues that affect man's immediate surroundings. Safety and comfort measures within the home and hospital, for example, have been well-documented as major health determinants and important components of nursing care. Occupational health nurses, particularly in industrial manufacturing settings, have taken an active role in promoting the importance of job safety and the prevention of illness associated with the workplace environment.

As nurses continue to look at health and illness in a holistic fashion, concerns about health and the environment are accentuated in importance and broadened in scope. The ecological perspective of the man-environment relationship provides nurses with additional knowledge about acute and chronic health effects, methods of illness prevention, and influences on the general quality of life.

The quality and success of the nursing process is dependent to a large extent on the nurse's ability to gather significant data, apply knowledge, and analyze facts. These actions set the stage for making nursing diagnoses and developing care plans. The ways in which nurses can apply their understanding of environmental issues to this process include research, client and community assessment, health teaching, and other methods of therapeutic intervention that promote client adaptation.

Certain aspects of a client's environment need to be considered when taking a nursing history or conducting a general assessment. These include type and location of housing, specifics of employment, e.g., where employed, known occupational hazards, and length of employment, leisure activities, and personal habits. Chapters 7, 25, and 26 elaborate on some of these assessment areas and give more specific direction regarding how to elicit environmental information.

Community health nurses and nurses who work in schools, industries, and other settings have more opportunities to assess the environment directly, whereas hospital based nurses have to rely on subjective data gathered from the patient interview or from previous health records.

Occupational health nurses have a primary responsibility in assessment of environmental hazards and conditions that influence health status. Under the Occupational Health and Safety Act of 1970 (OSHA) health professionals who work in occupational health settings are mandated to seek information and facilitate detection of relationships between the physical and mental ill health of workers and their job environment.[64] OSHA requires that all employers must provide workplaces that will not endanger the safety or health of employees. Catherine Tinkham, a community health nurse leader and author, has developed a data collection tool for use by nurses in setting up industrial nursing services. Some of the assessment questions contained in this tool follow:

- Types of industry?
  —Centralized or decentralized?
  —How many buildings?
  —Are the buildings close together or far apart?
- What product is produced?
- What operations and activities are carried out?
- What occupational hazards are present that could affect health, e.g., gases, radiation, weather, noise?
- What kinds of illnesses and injuries are reported among the employees?
- Number of workers who have chronic illnesses?
- Number of workers with physical handicaps including visual and learning conditions?[65]

Another part of the environmental assessment process is direct observation. Community health nurses must be alert for health hazards in the home and look for potential environmental pollution problems that might exist in the geographic area. Occupational health nurses need to make visual inspections of the worksite and watch workers as they carry out tasks. Periodic screening of persons at high risk for environmentally induced illnesses is another assessment method that nurses can use. Blood tests to determine levels of lead and chemical substances and routine chest x-rays for miners are examples.

It is also important for nurses to identify aspects of the environment that influence health positively and to encourage adaptive behaviors that help people cope with the environment.[66] Citizen participation in community efforts to reduce pollution and conserve our natural resources is one way people attempt to adapt. Car-pooling and recycling of solid waste are also examples.

Nursing interventions associated with environmental problems vary according to the knowledge and position of the nurse

and the nature of the problem. Direct nursing care for acute illnesses caused by environmental problems is carried out by occupational health nurses, emergency room nurses, and hospital nurses. In these settings, familiarity with causative agents, e.g., toxic substances, and their treatments is crucial.

In the long run, efforts directed toward primary prevention of environmentally induced health problems is the most effective nursing intervention. Educating the public about the effects and prevention of noise, pollution, cancer causing agents, radiation exposure, and lead poisoning can be done through various mass media techniques and one-to-one communication. Health education is not a panacea for eliminating environmental health effects or guaranteeing major changes in peoples' health behaviors, but it can serve to provide clients with enough information for them ultimately to make rational decisions on their own.

These decisions may range from electing to use ear protectors in a noisy work environment to major life changes, such as moving to another state or starting a new job. The more factual information the nurse has about the total health effects involved and of the preventive measures available, the more help she can give the client. Although community based nurses are often thought to be associated with this kind of health intervention, hospital based nurses also have opportunities to effect changes. A popular theory in health education, the Health Belief Model, holds that clients are more apt to change their health behaviors if they truly believe that the behavior in question will continue to cause ill effects. In the hospital, a client experiencing acute ill effects is more vulnerable to understanding and accepting such information.

Environmental health effects concern all of us. Awareness of what the problems are, which populations are most likely to be affected, and what kind of prevention is most effective is of vital concern to professional nurses everywhere. The challenges involve supporting community and global efforts to preserve our resources, motivating clients to change their behavior, and working to maintain a healthy environment in the best interest of the community.

ENVIRONMENTAL CONTROL IN THE HOSPITAL SETTING

Healthy individuals are capable of adapting or adjusting their environment and can manipulate it to suit themselves by controlling heating, lighting, ventilation, coloring, and many other things. Individuals can create a pleasant environment in which they feel comfortable. When individuals become ill and enter the hospital, they can no longer control or manipulate their surroundings as they wish.

Loss of control over the environment can affect how individuals adapt to hospitalization. Because of this, nurses must serve as patient advocates and assist patients to adapt to the environment, as well as adapt it for them so that it is safe and comfortable.

A safe environment is one in which there is freedom from injury from electrical hazards, thermal hazards, radiation, fire, drug chemical hazards, pollution, microorganisms, and psychological trauma. A comfortable environment is one in which unpleasant stimuli, such as extremes of temperature, color, odors, and noise, are controlled. A comfortable patient environment is also one in which there is adequate space for patients and staff, and one in which privacy is assured. Besides nursing, other hospital departments are involved in protecting patients from hazards and unpleasant surroundings. One example is the maintenance department, which frequently checks all electrical equipment for safety and repairs any damaged or broken

parts. This department also repairs any broken items in patients' rooms, such as windows, light bulbs, and plumbing. The housekeeping department or environmental control department (as it is known in some agencies) is responsible for keeping patients' rooms clean and odor free. Many agencies now employ nurse epidemiologists (see Chapter 3) who assess the potential for spread of infection and keep it to a minimum. Many agencies also have frequent visits from the community's fire marshall, who assesses the environment for fire hazards. Other agencies monitor radiation and building safety. Everyone on the health care team works together to provide a safe and comfortable hospital environment for patients.

All patients are at risk for injury, and nurses should assess carefully all patient areas with safety in mind. There are patients, however, who tend to be more susceptible to environmental hazards. These include the elderly, the very young, the handicapped, the emotionally disturbed, the patient with a lower resistance to disease, and the patient experiencing sensory alterations or deficits.

The Hospital Environment and the Nurse

The hospital environment is controlled in order to meet patient needs, but it reaches beyond each individual patient's unit into every corner of the agency. It even reaches beyond the agency in some instances, such as in agencies with home care departments. Nurses need to be aware of the impact of the hospital environment on the patients they assist.

In assessing the environment, nurses can begin with the patient's immediate unit. Since proper and adequate respiration is a primary need for all patients, an assessment of air quality is a good place to begin.

Air Quality. Air quality refers to the adequacy and cleanliness of air available. Mechanisms should be available to circulate the air in the room. Air conditioners with air circulation devices are useful, and most agencies today have them. If not, large circulating fans are often available from the housekeeping department. If an air conditioning unit alone is used to provide circulation, it may be necessary to use a room humidifier to replace some of the humidity in the air.

Humidity. Humidity is the amount of moisture present in the air. Geographic location, weather, and time of the year can contribute to the amount of humidity.

Air that is too dry, or too low in humidity, can cause excessive drying of the skin, which can cause skin to crack and break down. The mucous membranes dry as well, and this may cause irritation to the nose and throat, inability to cough up secretions, and excessive drying of the mouth and tongue. Conversely, environments that have high humidity can cause joint pain and other feelings of discomfort. This discomfort may be caused because the body regulates its temperature partly by perspiring. High humidity air affects the rate at which perspiration evaporates and makes individuals uncomfortable.

Temperature. Room temperature contributes to patients' feelings of comfort. Room temperature is a personal preference, however, and varies from individual to individual, and culture to culture. A room temperature of 68–72°F (20–22°C) is considered comfortable by most people, although babies and older people may prefer a warmer room temperature.

Odors. Many smells in the hospital environment are unpleasant and need to be assessed and controlled. Odors may come from trash cans, body wastes, strong chemicals, cigarette smoke, body odors, and many other things. Even strong perfumes on hospital personnel or visitors can be overwhelming for patients who are ill, and should be eliminated if possible. All units should be kept free of body waste, trash, dirty linens, and other objects that have strong or disturbing odors.

Allergens and Pollutants. Other factors related to an adequate environment for respiration include assessment of any allergens present in it. Several things contribute to "interior pollution." Air pollutants include plants, flowers, dust, perfumes, and cigarette smoke. These all can be controlled by eliminating them from the patient unit, particularly if patients are allergic to them.

Many agencies now have policies against smoking in patient units. Smoking is only permitted in designated smoking areas, and patients and visitors must use these areas if they wish to smoke.

Lighting. The amount and quality of lighting contributes to the patients' comfort and safety. When lighting is not adequate, eyestrain, headaches, irritability, and altered visual perceptions may occur. Conversely, when light is too bright and turned on for 24 hours a day, it is difficult for patients to get high-quality rest and sleep. (See Chapter 19 on Sensory Alterations). Nurses should regulate light so that it is not too bright, not too dull, and it duplicates nature's day/night cycle by turning lights on during the waking hours and turning down or off during the sleeping hours. Lighting during the daylight hours should support outdoor lighting, not replace it. Ideally, patients should have access to windows to help keep their spirits up and to keep them oriented to the day/night cycle (see Figure 27-5).

Children and older people may find night lights comforting, but this is a personal preference and should be assessed individually. Night lights serve to orient patients to strange surroundings at night and adds a safety feature if patients use the bathroom at night.

Noise. Noise, as an environmental hazard, recently has been classified by some authorities as a pollutant. Surprisingly, hospitals very often are guilty of noise pollution. One would like to think of hospitals

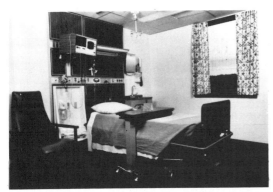

Figure 27-5. A. Daylight should be used to enhance room lighting.

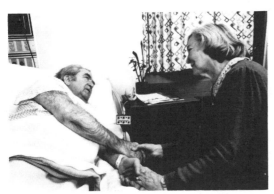

B. Lighting should be adequate in the evening.

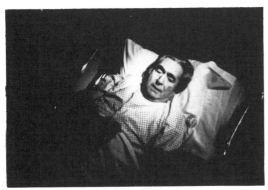

C. Lighting should reflect the day/night cycle.

as quiet places where the sick go to get well. While it is true that the sick go to hospitals to get well, it is not true that they are quiet places. Hospitals are large action oriented agencies that employ hundreds of people to care for their patients. Whenever hundreds of human beings are engaged in action oriented tasks, a great deal of noise is created.

Loud noises can be irritating and fatiguing to well individuals and even more so to individuals who are ill or in pain. Persons who are ill and hospitalized may be disturbed by noises that would not normally bother them. Loud talking or a television, for example, may disturb their rest and even produce complaints or outbursts of anger.

Some noises tend to be more irritating than others. Sudden loud noises, such as a metal item being dropped, cause a fright response. Squeaking wheels and doors are another. Telephones disturb patients, as do loud talking and laughing. Some of these things can be expected and tolerated during the day, but at night they can be particularly troublesome to patients.

If nurses realize the extent to which loud noises are disturbing, they can begin to be more aware and assess noise levels on their units. It then becomes possible to eliminate, control, or correct the noise level.

Decor and Other Factors.

Environmental decor can be manipulated to provide a pleasant atmosphere for patients. Hospitals are getting away from the white on white decor favored in the past. Research has demonstrated that use of colors can contribute to the way people feel.

Color. Soft colors tend to contribute favorably to patients' feelings. Blues, greens, pale yellows, and soft pinks are restful, and can be used in and around patient units. Bright colors, such as red and canary yellow, are stimulating colors and are best used in lounges and corridors located away from patient units. Grays, blacks, and browns are depressing somber colors and, unless used on floors and baseboards, are not good choices.

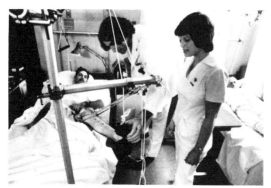

Figure 27-6.   Hospitals are noisy, action-oriented agencies.

Many agencies are now using more color in room divider curtains, draperies, bedspreads and blankets, on walls, ceilings, and floors. Well-selected colors brighten the environment and make it more cheerful.

Furnishings. Rooms in hospital units are traditionally equipped with high-low hospital beds, over-the-bed tables, bedside cabinets, comfortable chairs, lamps, and occasionally desks and desk chairs. In addition to these, there are usually wall communication units and call bell cords for patients to call for assistance when in need. Most patient units contain a lavatory with a sink and toilet. Some lavatories contain a shower stall or a bathtub as well. Usually there is additional equipment such as sphygmomanometers, oxygen and suction sources, and in intensive care units, there may be more high-technology equipment.

Since most hospital furnishings are quite different from home furnishings, their purpose and use should be explained to patients on admission. Special care should be given to explaining how the call bell and communication unit works. Patients also should be oriented to their room, the rest of the floor, and shown where the toilet and bath facilities are located. Finally, newly admitted patients should be introduced to their roommate and the staff who will be caring for them.

Privacy. Individuals who are hospi-

talized have, to some extent, lost control over their privacy, and it is important to remember that they still need privacy. Nurses need to be aware of this and assess this need. Closed doors, drawn curtains, and appropriate draping are several means for meeting this need.

Nurses also need to be aware of the legal aspects of invasion of privacy (See Chapter 8). Avoid this problem by knocking before entering a patient's room, asking permission to go into the closet or bedside cabinet, and so forth.

Neatness. Clutter is always unappealing, and this is true in the hospital as well as other settings. Nothing makes a unit more unattractive than yesterday's newspaper, remnants of breakfast, and medical supplies and equipment littering the top of every available surface. The patient's permission, however, should be obtained before disposing of personal items. Dead or dying flowers should be removed, again after receiving the patient's permission.

Space. Although nurses do not have much control over the amount of space available, they usually are able to provide patients with some space that is defined as their own. The concept of space, like privacy, requires that nurses assess the need for personal space and respect it. Many of the same actions used to ensure privacy are employed to provide patients with the feeling of their own territory. Boundaries should be assessed and respected and permission asked before entering a patient's space. Some hospitals, for example, have rules about staff members sitting on the edge of patients' beds. This may or may not be appropriate, but it is a good example of what it means to invade a patient's space.

Safety at the Bedside. The need for safety at the bedside is another component of the general environmental assessment. The most common injuries that bedfast patients sustain are related to burns and falls.

Fire dangers are the most frightening.

Burns from fire generally result from smoking in bed. Patients drop off to sleep or drop lighted cigarettes onto their beds, pajamas, or into wastebaskets. If patients are permitted to smoke in their rooms, ashtrays should be provided, and smoking should be monitored to prevent this hazard. Prevention is the best defense against burns. Should a fire start, prompt, safe, and efficient actions must be taken by hospital staff. The first step in the procedure is to remove patients from immediate danger. The second step is to attempt to contain the fire by using fire extinguishers and closing windows and fire doors. All accredited hospitals are required to have detailed fire plans and hold regularly scheduled drills and educational sessions.

Burns can be caused by scalding liquids, chemicals, radiation, light bulbs used for heat treatments, hot water bottles, heating pads, electric blankets, and lamps. Careful testing of bath water and other solutions with thermometers will help prevent injury from scalding liquids. Safe storage of caustic chemicals and radioactive materials will decrease that type of burn. Monitor patients undergoing heat lamp treatment and position lamps carefully to reduce the chance of injuring them. Wrapping a hot water bottle in several layers of towels and placing it in a securely fastened pillow case will reduce this type of burn. Eliminating the use of electric heating pads and electric blankets is the most effective way of controlling this type of injury.

Falls are the next most common injury sustained by hospital patients. Although they occur often with older patients, patients of all ages are at risk for suffering injuries due to falls. Most falls occur when patients get up too fast and faint; stay up too long and become weakened; or attempt to function independently before they are strong enough. Some of the reasons these falls occur are because health care providers do not respond quickly enough to

call lights, patients do not understand how to call the nurse, they overestimate the amount of strength they have, and they are confused or disoriented. Nurses need to assess their patients' abilities and strengths, and the various hazards to patient safety.

Specific actions can be taken by nurses to provide a more secure environment. These include:

- keeping the bed in the low position
- raising all side rails when patients are in bed
- raising the furthest side rail when patients are out of bed
- encouraging patients to wear slippers with firm nonskid surfaces or shoes when out of bed
- keeping floors free of trash, electric cords, and water
- assuring that walking devices, such as canes and crutches, have intact rubber tips
- assuring that all beds, wheelchairs, and stretchers have locked wheels before transferring patients
- providing adequate personnel to move patients
- keeping all medications locked in medicine room
- placing safety caps on lotions and powders
- assessing patients for suicide potential and taking appropriate actions
- using restraints such as posey jackets and wrist restraints as needed.

By assuring the above safety measures, patient safety is enhanced. In the event that a patient does fall, a careful assessment needs to be done and charted. Check to see if all of the items above were used appropriately. The patient's condition must be assessed and noted. If injury is sustained, can the patient be moved safely? If the decision is made to move him, he should be returned to bed and examined by a physician. If not, the patient must be examined wherever he is and the best method for movement determined.

Sanitation in the Hospital. Microorganisms are always present in the environment, and this is particularly true in the hospital. These organisms tend to congregate in hospitals, because patients may be harboring contagious bacteria, viruses, or other disease producing agents. Also, illness and debilitation increase the susceptibility of persons to a secondary infection.

Illnesses produced by microorganisms or viruses are called infections. No body system or component is immune to the risk of becoming infected. For infections to begin, a series of six factors must be present:

- Infectious Agent (example: streptococcus)
- Reservoirs (example: throat)
- Exit from Reservoir (example: nose)
- Mode of Transmission (example: air droplet)
- Portal of Entry (example: mouth)
- Susceptible Person (example: the patient)

If any of the above factors are absent, infections cannot be transmitted. See Figure 26-1, page 637, for further reference.

Infections that are acquired by hospitalized patients are called **nosocomial infections.** Unfortunately the incidence of this type of infection is not as low as health care providers would like it to be. It appears to be related to the overuse of antibiotics, resistant strains of microorganisms, and faulty handwashing techniques or disinfecting procedures of the health care providers.

All patients and health care providers are at risk for developing nosocomial infections, but certain groups can be identified as high risk. These include infants and young children, the elderly, the chronically ill, the debilitated, the poorly nourished, the burned, the postoperative, the immunosuppressed, the patient with a low white blood count, and the extremely anxious. Staff members who work continually with infected patients or contaminated equipment are also at high risk for nosocomial infections.

Means of spread of infection must be assessed by nurses and nursing actions employed to decrease the chance of nosocomial infections. These methods are quite diverse and depend on the means of transmission. The most important of these is employing careful handwashing techniques after having any contact with patients or their supplies and equipment. All patients with identified contagious infections should be placed in isolation rooms, and correct isolation procedures in caring for them should be observed. All health care providers or visitors who have infections should be kept away from patients, especially those designated as high risk. If this is not possible or practical, they should wash their hands carefully and put on a mask and, if appropriate, a gown. Dirty laundry never should be placed on the floor. It should be placed in a hamper, and the hamper should be emptied when it reaches about four to six inches from the top. Dirty laundry in hampers should be disposed of often and not allowed to sit on the unit all day. Laundry can serve as a media for bacteria growth. Trash also should be discarded frequently, as it provides good media for the growth of microorganisms.

Careful techniques of food storage in hospital kitchens and on hospital units can reduce this type of infection. It is not pleasant to suffer from food poisoning when well, and it can be very harmful for debilitated patients. Food never should be stored on hospital units for longer than 24 hours. All foodstuffs placed in the refrigerator should have a time and a date on it. Any foods or liquids that do not smell or look appropriate should be discarded. Foodstuffs should be kept in pest-resistant containers to keep down vermin. Pests such as mice, flies, and other insects must be exterminated. If all of these factors are assessed and controlled, the number of nosocomial infections can be reduced.

Electrical Hazards. All health care providers in direct contact with patients should be aware of the safe use of electricity, electrical equipment, and the hazards of using electricity. Understanding how to use electrical equipment safely is particularly important in instances where more than one piece of electrical equipment is being used for one patient.[67] It is additionally important when it is used for patients who are especially vulnerable to electrical injury, such as those with indwelling catheters or wet dressings.[68]

According to Ohm's law (of electricity), anyone in contact with an electrical appliance can become a part of the electrical circuit.[69] This can occur because of a mechanical defect in the electrical equipment or because of normal leakage of current from equipment. The insulating material must be sufficient to reduce the level of electrical leakage, so that it is kept below threshold. The threshold level of electricity is the minimum amount of current to which the human body responds. Threshold levels vary depending on whether the skin is intact or wet.

Protecting patients from electrical hazards is one of the nurse's roles. She must assess many factors in determining electrical safety and hazards (see Figure 27-7). Once the needs are assessed, patient units and other spaces should be kept free of electrical hazards.

Mechanical pacemakers that stimulate the heart are frequent in hospitalized individuals. Many of these pacemakers are known as demand pacemakers and function only on the absence of an electrical impulse from the heart. If electrical impulses,—stimuli in wavelength to the pacemaker— are present in the environment, the pacemaker will not perceive the ab-

---

ELECTRICAL HAZARDS

- Overloaded circuits
- Defective wiring
- Inadequate or overloaded fuses
- Excessive current
- Inadequate grounding
- Damaged plugs
- Frayed cords
- Insecure sockets
- Handling electrical equipment with hands
- Excessive use of extension cords

Figure 27-7. Nurses must assess the environment for electrical hazards.

---

sence of the electrical impulse from the heart, and ventricular contractions will not occur. It is, therefore, vitally important for nurses to assess the potential threat to patient safety.

Radiation. Although radiation does not fall directly within the practice of nursing, it is used extensively in the health care system as a means of diagnosis and treatment. Because of the use of radioactive materials, in the form of x-rays, scans, and radioactive implants, nurses need to assess their hazards and take steps to assure safety for patients, staff, visitors, and for themselves.

Radioactive materials are supplied in sealed sources (radioactive chemicals sealed in a coating), unsealed sources (radioactive chemicals not sealed in a coating) and x-rays.[70] Patients who are treated with x-rays or other radioactive materials receive treatment in specially designed rooms, and there should be no radioactivity outside of these treatment rooms. The United States government has designed regulations to guide the installation of x-ray equipment.

Health care agencies have specially trained personnel who work in the x-ray and radiotherapy departments. These personnel control their exposure to radioactive material by:

- reducing the time spent in contact with radiation
- increasing distance from the source of radiation
- wearing lead aprons, gloves, or drapes
- standing behind lead barriers
- wearing metered tags that are sent periodically for exposure analysis.

Nurses can use the above methods in practice as well as when assisting patients who are being treated with radiation or who are receiving radioactive materials as a part of the diagnostic process. Even if the duration of the exposure to the radioactive material is brief, nurses should keep in mind that brief exposures to radiation over long periods of time may be equal to one long dose of radiation and may be hazardous to their health. Women who are pregnant should not be exposed to radiation, if possible.

Patients who have received temporary radioactive material as implants act as another source of radiation in the environment. Limits should be set on the amount of time nurses spend with these patients, and nurses should wear lead aprons and gloves when in contact with them. Patients should have their own bathrooms when in this type of isolation, and all radioactive body discharges (feces, urine, vomitus, etc.) must be dealt with safely. In most instances, nurses should wear rubber gloves and sometimes may need to dispose of certain discharges in special containers. If any of these contaminated wastes get on the nurse's gloved hands, they should be carefully washed under running water with soap and then carefully removed, so that the hands do not come into direct contact with radioactive wastes.

Obviously, patients experiencing treatment with radioactive material and subsequent isolation are going to experience anxiety, fear, and stress. Nurses need to be supportive to both patients and their families during the duration of the treatment.

Toxic Substances in the Hospital. Due to their nature, hospitals have numerous toxic substances and chemicals in the form of drugs, medications, and strong disinfectants. Nurses always should assure that these substances are labeled properly, stored in secure areas designated for the purpose, and are in safe containers with childproof tops. The latter is especially true in areas of the hospital where children and confused or disoriented patients are diagnosed and treated.

A potential danger from drugs or chemicals arises from the use of outdated or deteriorated substances. Any drug or chemical that has changed in its appearance, texture, or odor, or has passed its expiration date should be discarded or returned to the pharmacy, since it may no longer be safe to use. Should any altered drug or chemical be administered accidently, a physician should be notified immediately and the hospital procedure for such instances followed.

Building Safety. Buildings that are used for any type of patient care always should be kept in the safest possible condition. This entails keeping everything in good repair and well lighted. Fire exits should be clearly marked and have easy access. In addition, stairwells should be well-marked, unlocked, and well-lighted.

Discovery of loose tiles, faulty equipment, burned out lights, etc., should be reported to the appropriate department (housekeeping, environment control, maintenance, buildings and grounds, etc.) immediately.

A SAFE ENVIRONMENT FOR NURSING PRACTICE

Nurses, like the patients they care for, are also exposed to environmental hazards. Part of the nursing responsibility, which benefits nurses as well as their patients, is to follow good health practices and maintain a high level of wellness. In order to accomplish this, a number of health practices should be observed.

Maintaining good nutrition is one of the most basic areas that nurses can set an example for, as well as keeping themselves alert and healthy. Nurses are busy people, and those who work in acute care settings often have long hours of duty, irregular shift assignments, and overloaded patient care responsibilities. These very problems, which often make it difficult to observe good nutritional habits, are some of the reasons why adequate nutrition is so necessary. Nurses need to plan menus around the basic food groups and avoid such practices as meal skipping and junk food snacking. Professional consultation should be sought for weight problems or other eating disorders.

Another basic area of good health practice is obtaining adequate rest, relaxation, and sleep. An adequate number of hours of sleep should be obtained every 24 hours and relaxing activities planned for off hours. Activities such as jogging, yoga, or exercise, may be very helpful in reducing stress as will pursuing hobbies or other special interests.

Dental and health checkups should be at least yearly and immunizations kept up-to-date. Another important and frequently overlooked health behavior is staying home when ill. Illness needs to be treated with rest, and nurses, when ill, should remain home. Going to work when ill not only reduces one's ability to get well, but also exposes patients to illness.

In maintaining a high level of wellness, nurses are able to function at their best and serve as a role model for patients and the general public.

Protection Against Injury and Disease in the Environment. Nurses can observe specific behaviors based on scientific principles in order to prevent disease or injury to themselves. These include the use of proper body mechanics, good personal hygiene and handwashing, proper body treatment of contaminated materials, correct use of equipment, and careful manipulation of toxic substances.

Body Mechanics. There are basic principles underlying the practice of good body mechanics. These principles include:

- the use of major muscle groups
- the use of a broad base of support
- the center of gravity in the middle
- the preparation of the muscles before moving
- the use of the nurse's own weight to push or pull
- the avoidance of working against gravity
- the use of as little effort as possible
- the reduction of friction
- the prevention of muscle fatigue
- the use of lifting aides or the use of other staff members
- the use of good assessment and judgment.

If nurses use these basic principles consistently, they will avoid most serious injuries to themselves and their patients.

Personal Hygiene. Good personal hygiene habits and good handwashing techniques reduces the chance of cross contamination. Nurses always should wash their hands after touching patients, bed linens, bedpans, secretions, and toxic substances. Soap, friction, and running water should be used, and the fingernails, knuckles, and wrists should be washed as well. Nurses should use their assessment skills to assess their own skin condition for drying, cracking, hangnails, cuts, or abrasions. Hangnails should be clipped, nails trimmed (and free of snags), cuts and abrasions treated, and a moisture lotion used.

Toxic Substances. Nurses frequently are called upon to prepare medications or manipulate substances that are harmful to body surfaces. Studies have shown links between the use of anti-cancer drugs and subsequent precancerous lesions or new primary growth.[71] The risk for nurses handling such drugs has not yet been identified, but it has been shown that nurses working with drugs to treat cancer have mutagens in their urine.[72]

Extensive research to validate these hypotheses has not been conducted, so there is little to support the banning of these drugs. It is vital for nurses to know about the dangers of handling such drugs.

Other more common drugs can produce allergic dermatitis. Some of these drugs include aminophylline, benzocaine, cytoxics, mycin drugs, penicillin, and phenothiazides, and streptomycin. Nurses should take special care when manipulating the above drugs.

Nurses handle a variety of chemicals as well as drugs. The chemicals encountered include antiseptics, detergents, alcohol, dyes, bacteriostatic agents, and other chemicals, such as anaesthetic liquids and gases. In addition to being harmful to skin and mucous membrances, many chemicals and gases are highly flammable and increase the chances for fire.

For protection from drugs and chemicals, nurses should know:

- the chemical name of the substance
- the trade name
- the hazards
- poisoning antidotes
- the precautions for storage
- the precautions for use.

By observing simple safety precautions, nurses can avoid side effects from manipulating strong or harmful substances in the work environment.

SUMMARY

The environment of man includes everything that affects him, his physical environment, his social and psychological environment, and his internal environment. Man's relationship with his environment is interdependent and reciprocal. This give and take relationship is central to the adaptation process of which all living things are a part. The characteristics and consequences of the man/environment relationship have a direct affect on human health, survival, and the quality of life. The nursing profession is interested in what these relationships are, how their characteristics are manifested, and what the consequences of selected man/environment actions are.

Ecology is the science that studies the dynamic relationships of living things to one another and to their environment. The ecological model encompasses a holistic approach that can provide insights into environmental hazards and stresses that can affect human health and the ability to adapt. An important concept within ecology is the ecosystem. The ecosystem is very simply a collection of adapted living organisms within a particular environment. Knowledge about environmental conditions and hazards comes from studying these ecosystems and how they relate with natural cycles such as the water cycle, nitrogen cycle, atmospheric movements, and so forth.

There are many conditions within man's environment that affect health status and the general quality of life. Some of the major ecological issues that have been identified include air pollution, water pollution, toxic substances, solid waste accumulation, ionizing radiation, and noise. Each of these issues has some unique health effects, and many have related and overlapping consequences. Radiation, for example, can pollute air and water as well as result in a hazardous waste disposal problem.

Nurses can use their knowledge about ecology and environmental hazards as they carry out the nursing process. Knowledge about environmentally induced acute illnesses, e.g., chemical poisoning and water borne diseases, can assist them in the assessment process and in choosing appropriate interventions, including health education and other methods of prevention.

Community health nurses and occupational health nurses have assessment responsibilities in the home and work setting. Occupational health nurses have an opportunity to reach large number of people within educational programs that emphasize hazard identification and prevention of industrial accidents and work-related illnesses. Nurses in the community are engaged in other forms of primary prevention, too, such as mass screening programs.

Nurses are also concerned about effects of the immediate environment on the hospitalized patient. Hospitalized patients, to some extent, lose control over their environment. This can affect how they feel, behave, and adapt. Nurses are in a good position to serve as patient advocates in this area and assist patients by providing a safe and comfortable environment.

A safe environment is free from electrical hazards, physical barriers that contribute to falls, thermal hazards, radiation, fire, drug and chemical hazards, pests, pollution, harmful microorganisms, and psychological trauma. A comfortable environment is free from unpleasant stimuli, such as extremes of temperature, color, unpleasant or strong odors, and excessive noise. In addition, a comfortable environment attends to space and privacy needs.

Nurses who work in institutional settings are exposed to many of the same environmental hazards as patients. Repeated radiation exposure and frequent contact with toxic substances and microorganisms are several occupational hazards that nurses need to be aware of. The responsibility to identify these hazards and take action to eliminate them rests with each individual and the institution. Nurses and other health professionals have an additional responsibility to maintain their own personal health status and serve as role models in the promotion of good nutrition and other beneficial health practices.

STUDY QUESTIONS

1. List the various causes of air pollution in your community. What evidence, if any, do you see that indicates that people are concerned about it and its health effects?

2. Identify a major river or other body of water in your area. What are some actual or potential sources of water pollution affecting it?

3. Contact your city or county health department to learn what environmental health services are offered. How do these services affect such things as solid waste disposal and noise pollution? Are radiation levels in the area monitored?

4. Visit the office of an occupational health nurse and describe the nurse's role. List areas where primary prevention might lessen or eliminate health effects of environmental hazards.

5. Interview a hospitalized patient and list the things he likes and dislikes about his immediate environment. Identify any

nursing measures that could improve or enhance the quality of this particular environment.

6. Describe the role of a nurse epidemiologist in the hospital setting. What kinds of input can this person provide for the prevention of nosocomial infections?

7. List at least four occupational hazards that can affect the health of nursing personnel. How can the ill effects of these hazards be prevented?

REFERENCES

1. James M. Fitch, **American Building: The Environmental Forces that Shape It.** (New York: Schocken Books, 1975) p.4.
2. **Ibid.**
3. **Ibid,** pp.4–14.
4. Jack Smolensky, **Principles of Community Health,** 4th edition, (Philadelphia: W.B. Saunders Co., 1977) p.1.
5. Lillian DeYoung, **Dynamics of Nursing,** (St. Louis: The C.V. Mosby Co., 1981) pp.12–13.
6. Linda Jarvis, **Community Health Nursing: Keeping the Public Healthy,** (Philadelphia: F.A. Davis Co., 1982) p.621.
7. Ruth Murray and Judith Zentner, **Nursing Concepts for Health Promotion,** (Englewood Cliffs, N.J.: Prentice-Hall, Inc., 1975) p.250.
8. Smolensky, **Principles of Community Health,** p.25.
9. Jeanette Lancaster, **Community Mental Health Nursing,** (St. Louis: The C.V. Mosby Co., 1980) p.22.
10. **Ibid.,** p.10.
11. Smolensky, **Principles of Community Health,** p.26.
12. Robert Leo Smith, **The Ecology of Man: An Ecosystem Approach,** (New York: Harper & Row Publishers, 1972), pp.3, 5.
13. **Ibid.,** pp.14, 15.
14. Osborn Segerberg, Jr., **Where Have All the Flowers, Fishes, Birds, Trees, Water and Air Gone?** (New York: David McKay Company, Inc. 1971) p.54.
15. Evelyn Rose Benson and Joan Quinn McDevitt, **Community Health and Nursing Practice,** 2nd ed. (Englewood Cliffs, N.J.: Prentice-Hall, Inc., 1980) p.58.
16. **Ibid.,** p.53.
17. William J. Baumol and Wallace E. Oates, **Economics, Environmental Policy, and the Quality of Life,** (Englewood Cliffs, N.J.: Prentice-Hall, Inc., 1979) p.46.
18. Barbara Ward and René Dubos, **Only One Earth,** (New York: W.W. Norton & Co., Inc., 1972) p.57.
19. Parker C. Reist "Air Pollution," in **Community Health Nursing,** by Linda Jarvis, (Philadelphia: F.A. Davis Co., 1981) p.642.
20. **Ibid.,** p.644.
21. **Ibid.,** p.434.
22. Baumol & Oats, **Economics, Environmental Policy,** p.47.
23. **Ibid.,** pp.45–47.
24. William O. Douglas, **The Three Hundred Year War,** (New York: Random House, 1972).
25. Reist, "Air Pollution," **Community Health Nursing,** p.645.
26. **Ibid.**
27. **Ibid.**
28. Murray and Zentner, **Nursing Concepts,** p.251.
29. U.S. Environmental Protection Agency, **Your Guide to the U.S. Environmental Protection Agency,** (Wash., D.C.: Office of Public Affairs A-107, 1982) p.7.
30. Edgar W. Butler, **Urban Sociology,** (New York: Harper & Row, Publishers, 1976) p.448.
31. Melvin A. Bernarde, **Our Precious Habitat,** (New York: W.W. Norton & Co., Inc., 1973) p.149.
32. David P. Spath "Water Pollution," in **Community Health Nursing,** by Linda Jarvis (Philadelphia: F.A. Davis Co., 1981) p.660.
33. **As We Live and Breathe: The Challenge of Our Environment,** (Wash., D.C.: The National Geographic Society, 1971) p.96.
34. U.S. Environmental Protection Agency, **Your Guide,** pp.8, 9.
35. Spath "Water Pollution," **Community Health Nursing,** p.660.
36. U.S. Environmental Protection Agency, **Your Guide,** p.17.
37. "Toxic Substances Control Act," Public Laws 94–669, October 11, 1976, p.90 Stat. 2003.
38. **Ibid.**
39. "The Federal Insecticide, Fungicide, and Rodenticide Act," Public Law 92–516, pp.86 STAT 973–999.
40. James W. Berry, David W. Osgood, and Phil-

ip A. St. John, Chemical Villians, A Biology of Pollution (St. Louis: C.V. Mosby Company, 1974); George L. Waldbott, M.D., Health Effects of Environmental Pollutants (St. Louis: C.V. Mosby Company, 1973); World Health Organization, Health Hazards of the Human Environment (Geneva: World Health Organization, 1972); M.A.Q. Khan and John P. Berderka, Jr., eds., Survival in Toxic Environments (New York: Academic Press, Inc., 1974); Henry A. Schroeder, M.D., The Poisons Around Us: Toxic Metals in Food, Air, and Water (Bloomington, Ind.: Indiana University Press, 1974); Environmental Quality, The Sixth Annual Report of the Council on Environmental Quality (Washington, D.C.: U.S. Government Printing Office, 1975); T.H. Maugh, "Polychlorinated Biphenyls: Still Prevalent but Less of a Problem" Science 173 (1972):338; M.G. Mustafa, P.A. Peterson, R.J. Munn, C.E. Cross, "Effects of Cadmium Ion on Metabolism of Lung Cells" in Proceedings of the Second International Clean Air Congress, ed. H.M. Englund and W.T. Beery (New York: Academic Press, Inc., 1971); P. Kotin and H.L. Falk, "The Role and Action of Environmental Agents in the Pathogenesis of Lung Cancer: Part I, Air Pollutants" Cancer 12 (1959):147; Environmental Protection Agency [FRL 454-1] [40 CFR Part 61] National Emission Standards for Hazardous Air Pollutants, Proposed Standard for Vinyl Chloride; Summary Characterization of Selected Chemicals of Near-Term Interest, Office of Toxic Substances (U.S. Environmental Protection Agency, Washington, D.C., April 1976); Environmental Quality, The Seventh Annual Report of the Council on Environmental Quality (Washington, D.C.: U.S. Government Printing Office, 1976); John M. Wood, "A Progress Report on Mecury," Environment 14, No. 1 (January–February, 1972), pp.33–39.

41. Bernarde, **Our Precious Habitat**, p.179.
42. U.S. Environmental Protection Agency Statistics, Office of Public Affairs, Wash., D.C., 1982.
43. **Ibid.**
44. Bernarde, **Our Precious Habitat**, p.178.
45. U.S. Environmental Protection Agency Reports, Office of Public Affairs, Wash., D.C., 1982.
46. Bernarde, **Our Precious Habitat**, p.183.
47. Leo J. Malone, **Basic Concepts of Chemistry** (New York: John Wiley and Sons, 1981) pp.54–59.

48. **Ibid.**
49. **Ibid.**
50. **Ibid.**
51. Carol A. Silberstein, "Ionizing Radiation and Community Health," in **Community Health Nursing** by Linda Jarvis (Philadelphia: F.A. Davis Co., 1981) p.682.
52. Ralph Nader and John Abbott, **The Menace of Atomic Energy,** (New York: W.W. Norton and Company, Inc., 1979) p.10.
53. **Ibid.,** p.38.
54. Richard W. Wagner, **Environment and Man,** (New York: W.W. Norton and Co., Inc., 1971) p.213.
55. **Ibid.,** p.214.
56. U.S. Environmental Protection Agency, **Your Guide,** p.19.
57. Joseph J. Seneca and Michael K. Taussig, **Environmental Economics,** 2nd ed., (Englewood Cliffs, N.J.: Prentice-Hall, Inc., 1979) p.191.
58. **Ibid.,** p.194.
59. James D. Miller, **Efforts of Noise on People** (Wash., D.C.: The U.S. Environmental Protection Agency, 1971).
60. Henry Still, **In Quest of Quiet,** (Harrisburg, PA: Stackpole Books, 1970) p.13.
61. Seneca & Taussig, **Environmental Economics,** p.191.
62. **Noise From Heavy Construction** (Wash., D.C.: The U.S. Environmental Protection Agency, 1972).
63. U.S. Environmental Protection Agency, Office of Noise Abatement and Control, Wash., D.C. 1978.
64. Mary Louise Brown "The Quality of the Work Environment," **American Journal of Nursing,** Vol. 75, No. 10, October 1975, pp.1756–57.
65. Catherine W. Tinkham "The Plant as the Patient of the Occupational Health Nurse," Nursing Clinics of North America, Vol. 7, #1, March 1972, pp.100–102.
66. Evelyn R. Benson and Joan Q. McDevitt, **Community Health Nursing Practice,** (Englewood Cliffs, N.J.: Prentice-Hall, Inc., 1980) p.59.
67. I.M. Meth, "Electrical Safety in the Hospital," **American Journal of Nursing, 80** (1980) pp.1344–48.
68. **Ibid.,** p.1344.
69. Nurse Action Group, "Protection is Better than Curie," **Nursing Mirror,** 152 (1981), pp.26–30.
70. Nurses Action Group "Beware of the Drug," **Nursing Mirror** 152 (1981) 34–38.
71. **Ibid.**
72. **Ibid.**

ANNOTATED BIBLIOGRAPHY

Clark CC: **Enhancing Wellness: A Guide for Self-Care.** New York, Springer Publishing Co., 1981. Included in this text are self-assessment tools for personal living, work, and play environments. Discusses high-risk groups related to harmful substances and protective measures.

Dickey LD: **Clinical Ecology.** Springfield, Thomas Publishing Co., 1976. This is a basic textbook on the clinical study of the effects of chemicals, food, allergenic substances, and other environmental agents on the individual.

Friedman FB: **Restraints: When all Else Fails, There Still are Alternatives.** RN 46:1:79–88; January 1983. Uses of restraints and alternatives to them are discussed in this useful article.

Kirkis J. **Tactics to Hold Microbes at Bay.** RN 45:6:81; June 1982. This brief article summarizes how infection spreads and how to reduce it.

Lee PS, Pash BJ: **Preventing Patient Falls.** Nurs 83 13:2:118–120; February 1983. This article gives several reasons why patients fall and suggests a nursing checklist to prevent falls.

Maddocks G: **A Childproof Environment.** Nurs Mirror 152:21:i–vii; May 1981. This discusses safety features that can be used to protect infants and young children from injury.

Maddocks G: **Careful—Don't Touch.** Nurs Mirror 152:21:ii–iv; May 1981. This article discusses how children are injured and the types of injuries most frequently encountered.

Maddocks G: **Growing to Independence.** Nurs Mirror 152:21:viii–xiv; May 1981. This article discusses safety in children of school age through adolescence.

Mattia MA: **Hazards in the Hospital Environment.** Am J Nurs 83:1:73–77; January 1983. This article discusses the health risks associated with working with selected gases and suggests ways of minimizing these risks.

Mattia MA: **Hazards in the Hospital. The Sterilants: Ethylene Oxide and Formaldehyde.** Am J Nurs 83:240–243; February 1983. This article discusses the hazards of selected toxic chemicals and suggests ways of reducing these hazards.

Meth IM: **Electrical Safety in the Hospital.** Am J Nurs 80:7:1344–1348; July 1980. This excellent article discusses the concept of electricity and applies it to environmental safety.

Nurse Action Group: **Protection is Better than Curie.** Nurs Mirror 152:8:26–30; February 1981. This article from a British journal discusses radiation, treatment, and relevant nursing action.

Nurse Action Group: **Beware of the Drug.** Nurs Mirror 152:6; February 1981. This article discusses chemical and drug hazards present in the work environment and steps to take to avoid injury.

Odum EP: **Fundamentals of Ecology,** 3rd ed. Philadelphia, W.B. Saunders, 1971. A basic ecology textbook that stresses ecosystem dynamics.

Witte NS: **Why the Elderly Fall.** Am J Nurs 79:11:1950–1952; November 1979. Falls are the second leading cause of death in the United States, and the elderly were susceptible to falling for a variety of reasons. This article explains the reasons, gives examples, and suggests actions to prevent falls.

Index